SMALL ANIMAL
MEDICAL
THERAPEUTICS

SMALL ANIMAL MEDICAL THERAPEUTICS

Michael D. Lorenz, B.S., D.V.M.

Diplomate, American College of Veterinary Internal Medicine—
Internal Medicine
Dean of College of Veterinary Medicine
College of Veterinary Medicine
Kansas State University
Manhattan, Kansas

Larry M. Cornelius, D.V.M., Ph.D.

Diplomate, American College of Veterinary Internal Medicine—
Internal Medicine
Professor of Small Animal Medicine
College of Veterinary Medicine
The University of Georgia
Athens, Georgia

Duncan C. Ferguson, V.M.D., Ph.D.

Diplomate, American College of Veterinary Internal Medicine—
Internal Medicine
Associate Professor of Physiology and Pharmacology
College of Veterinary Medicine
The University of Georgia
Athens, Georgia

With 12 Contributors

J.B. Lippincott Company   Philadelphia

New York   London   Hagerstown

Acquisitions Editor: Mary K. Smith
Sponsoring Editor: Anne Geyer
Cover Design: Anita R. Curry
Production Supervisor:
  Robert D. Bartleson

Production Service: Nan Nagy
Compositor: Publication Services, Inc.
Printer/Binder: R.R. Donnelley &
  Sons Company

1   3   5   6   4   2

Library of Congress Cataloging in Publication Data

Small animal medical therapeutics / edited by Michael D. Lorenz, Larry
    M. Cornelius, Duncan C. Ferguson.
        p. cm.
    Includes bibliographical references and index.
    ISBN 0-397-50994-4
    1. Dogs—Diseases—Treatment. 2. Cats—Diseases—Treatment.
I. Lorenz, Michael D. II. Cornelius, Larry M. III. Ferguson,
Duncan C.
SF991.S593 1991
636.089—dc20   91-27802
                                                                         CIP

The authors and publisher have exerted every effort to ensure that drug selection and dosage set forth in this text are in accord with current recommendations and practice at the time of publication. However, in view of ongoing research, changes in government regulations, and the constant flow of information relating to drug therapy and drug reactions, the reader is urged to check the package insert for each drug for any change in indications and dosage and for added warnings and precautions. This is particularly important when the recommended agent is a new or infrequently employed drug.

CONTRIBUTORS

Scott A. Brown, V.M.D., Ph.D. Diplomate, American College of Veterinary Internal Medicine—Internal Medicine; Assistant Professor of Physiology and Pharmacology, College of Veterinary Medicine, The University of Georgia, Athens, Georgia

Steven C. Budsberg, D.V.M., M.S. Diplomate, American College of Veterinary Surgeons; Assistant Professor of Small Animal Medicine, Department of Small Animal Medicine, College of Veterinary Medicine, The University of Georgia, Athens, Georgia

Clay A. Calvert, D.V.M. Diplomate, American College of Veterinary Internal Medicine—Internal Medicine; Associate Professor of Small Animal Medicine, Department of Small Animal Medicine, College of Veterinary Medicine, The University of Georgia, Athens, Georgia

Margarethe Hoenig, Dr. Med. Vet., Ph.D. Associate Professor of Physiology and Pharmacology and Small Animal Medicine, College of Veterinary Medicine, The University of Georgia, Athens, Georgia

Gilbert J. Jacobs, D.V.M. Diplomate, American College of Veterinary Internal Medicine—Cardiology; Associate Professor of Small Animal Medicine, College of Veterinary Medicine, The University of Georgia, Athens, Georgia

Michael R. Lappin, D.V.M., Ph.D. Diplomate, American College of Veterinary Internal Medicine—Internal Medicine; Assistant Professor of Small Animal Medicine, College of Veterinary Medicine and Biomedical Sciences, Colorado State University, Fort Collins, Colorado

Linda Medleau, D.V.M., M.S. Diplomate, American College of Veterinary Dermatology; Associate Professor of Dermatology, Department of Small Animal Medicine, College of Veterinary Medicine, The University of Georgia, Athens, Georgia

John E. Oliver, D.V.M., M.S., Ph.D. Diplomate, American College of Veterinary Internal Medicine—Neurology; Professor of Small Animal Medicine, Department of Small Animal Medicine, College of Veterinary Medicine, The University of Georgia, Athens, Georgia

Cynthia M. Otto, D.V.M. Georgia Heart Association, Research Fellow, Department of Small Animal Medicine, College of Veterinary Medicine, The University of Georgia, Athens, Georgia

Victoria W. Pentlarge, D.V.M. Diplomate, American College of Veterinary Internal Medicine—Internal Medicine; Animal Eye Care Clinic, Athens, Georgia

Pauline M. Rakich, D.V.M., Ph.D. Assistant Professor of Pathology, Athens Diagnostic Laboratory, College of Veterinary Medicine, The University of Georgia, Athens, Georgia

Laura Smallwood, D.V.M. Small Animal Medicine Resident, College of Veterinary Medicine, The University of Georgia, Athens, Georgia

PREFACE

In 1987, the textbook *Small Animal Medical Diagnosis* was published by the editors. This book emphasized a problem-oriented diagnostic approach to case management and proved to be a unique and valuable resource for veterinary students and small animal practitioners. Although symptomatic therapy of various problems was briefly described, in-depth treatment was omitted. *Small Animal Medical Therapeutics* attempts to provide readers a concise review of the treatment procedures utilized for the most common medical conditions of dogs and cats. By focusing entirely on therapy, the authors are able to provide details of management protocols often omitted from standard textbooks and still offer reasonable brevity for busy readers. Therapies are discussed in three levels: standard therapy, alternative therapy, and investigational therapy. Drug regimens, potential side effects, supportive care, and patient monitoring are described. Extensive use is made of summary tables in individual chapters to facilitate finding specific information regarding drug usage. A drug dosage appendix is included at the end of the book that lists all drugs discussed in the chapters as well as their most common uses and dosages.

Small Animal Medical Therapeutics is written by experienced clinicians. It is an ideal companion text to *Small Animal Medical Diagnosis*. We hope that the concise presentation of up-to-date treatment methods for common canine and feline medical problems will be useful to busy students and practitioners.

Michael D. Lorenz, B.S., D.V.M.
Larry M. Cornelius, D.V.M., Ph.D.
Duncan C. Ferguson, V.M.D., Ph.D.

ACKNOWLEDGMENTS

The editors are indebted to many people for their assistance in the completion of this book. First and foremost, we sincerely appreciate the hard work and cooperation of each author. We know from first-hand experience how much of a challenge it is for already overcommitted clinicians to find the time to write. Their willingness to take on and complete this task for little more than the satisfaction of a job well done is testimony to their enthusiasm and dedication for veterinary education and practice.

Many others were an essential part of this production. Two people deserve special mention. Nancy Mullins was consistently helpful and always patient. Her attention to detail and her no-nonsense approach kept us on track and moving toward a sometimes elusive-appearing goal of completion on time. Anne Geyer, editorial assistant at J.B. Lippincott, always dealt with us in a friendly, thorough, and professional manner, and we are most appreciative.

We thank our secretaries, Sharon Humbert, Diane Embrick, Randi Gilbert, and Mamie Watson, for their efforts and good cheer despite the seemingly never-ending requests for "just a few more changes."

Special mention and recognition must be conveyed to our colleagues (faculty) and colleagues in training (students, interns, residents) at our respective institutions of higher learning (Kansas State University and the University of Georgia). Their dedication to excellence in patient care and their zeal for learning are two major reasons we were motivated to complete this book.

We thank our families for their support and sacrifice, without which the task would have been much more difficult or not possible.

Finally, we are indebted to the J.B. Lippincott Company for their confidence in us in publishing this textbook.

Michael D. Lorenz, B.S., D.V.M.
Larry M. Cornelius, D.V.M., Ph.D.
Duncan C. Ferguson, V.M.D., Ph.D.

TABLE OF CONTENTS

CHAPTER ONE

Fluid, Electrolyte, and Acid-Base Therapy

Larry M. Cornelius

Recognition and treatment of fluid and electrolyte disorders are common to daily small animal practice. A number of abnormalities, medical and surgical, can disrupt normal homeostasis and result in potentially life-threatening fluid, electrolyte, and acid-base imbalances. The primary purpose of this chapter is to present information about fluid therapy that is helpful to practicing veterinarians.

The major objectives of fluid, electrolyte, and acid-base therapy are to: 1) treat shock (see Chapter 17); 2) replace water and correct electrolyte imbalances; 3) provide daily maintenance needs of water and electrolytes; 4) correct acid-base disorders; and 5) avoid causing new problems as a result of treatment.

DEHYDRATION

Dehydration is defined as a deficit of body water and is often accompanied by losses of body electrolytes and changes in acid-base balance. Signs of dehydration include loss of skin elasticity (turgor), dry mucous membranes, and prolonged capillary refilling time. Severe dehydration may cause weakness, depression, and cardiovascular collapse (shock). Common laboratory abnormalities that often present are increased packed cell volume (PCV), plasma protein, and urine specific gravity (usually higher than 1.035). Despite the complexities of biochemical alterations often associated with dehydration, effective fluid volume replacement is of primary concern. Mild to moderate electrolyte and acid-base abnormalities may be corrected by body compensatory mechanisms once the patient is rehydrated.

Standard Therapy

The clinician should routinely take the time to plan fluid volume therapy rather than haphazardly guess about the appropriate treatment. This approach prevents such common errors as overtreating small patients and markedly undertreating large dogs.

Fluid Volume Requirements. The plan for fluid volume therapy should consider *existing deficit* requirements, *maintenance needs*, and abnormal *continuing losses*. The existing deficit is the quantity of water lost prior to examination and is estimated by considering the history, physical examination, and laboratory data (Table 1-1). Maintenance fluid needs should be supplied when the patient cannot or will not ingest sufficient water to replace normal insensible losses from urine, feces, respiratory tract, and skin (about 40–60 ml/kg/day). The volume of abnormal continuing losses of fluid should be estimated and included in replacement therapy. Shown in Table 1-2 are sample calculations illustrating the method used to determine fluid volume requirements of a dehydrated animal. It is well to remember when using these or other guidelines in this chapter that there is a patient at the end of the needle. Highest priorities are to treat and monitor the patient, not to blindly follow calculated (estimated) fluid, electrolyte, and acid-base requirements.

Solutions for Fluid Therapy. Table 1-3 outlines commercially available electrolyte solutions often used for fluid and electrolyte therapy in dogs and cats. Many other special-purpose fluids are available but are not often necessary. It is best to stock a limited number of solutions appropriate for treatment of common fluid and electrolyte problems and become proficient at using them.

The choice of fluid should be based on the abnormalities that need correction (Table 1-4). Generally polyionic, isotonic fluids, e.g., lactated Ringer's solution, are the most versatile because their composition is similar to that of extracellular fluid (ECF). Lactated Ringer's solution is an alkalinizing fluid because it contains lactate, which is a bicarbonate precursor. Ringer's solution contains increased amounts of chloride instead of lactate and is an acidifying fluid. Lactated Ringer's and Ringer's solutions contain only a small quantity of potassium. Addition of potassium chloride to these fluids may be necessary for patients with conditions associated with increased loss of body potassium (see Hypokalemia, below).

Isotonic sodium chloride solution (0.9%), or saline, is often (incorrectly) called physiologic or normal saline. Isotonic saline contains 154 mEq of sodium and 154 mEq of chloride. The sodium concentration is similar to that in ECF, but the chloride concentration is higher. The increased chloride content can cause acidification of ECF (hyperchloremic metabolic acidosis). Also, saline does not contain other electrolytes found in ECF. For these reasons, use of 0.9% saline should be limited to conditions associated with significant sodium loss, e.g., adrenocortical insufficiency, also known as Addison's disease (see Hyponatremia, below). Half-strength saline (0.45%) is occasionally used for conditions characterized by hypernatremic dehydration (see Hypernatremia, below).

A 5% glucose solution is approximately isotonic. Its primary use is to supply water to alleviate the dehydration characterized by loss of nearly pure water

TABLE 1-1. Estimating Fluid Volume Deficit from the History, Physical
Examination, and Laboratory Data

Severity of Dehydration	Percent of Dehydration	Typical History	Usual Physical Findings	Laboratory Data
Mild	<5	Short-term anorexia, vomiting	Normal	Slightly increased PCV, plasma protein, BUN, and urine specific gravity
Moderate	6–8	More prolonged anorexia, vomiting, diarrhea	Decreased skin turgor, dry mucous membranes, prolonged capillary refilling time	More marked increases in above values
Severe	10–12	Prolonged anorexia, profuse vomiting, chronic, polyuric renal failure	More severe signs as noted above	More marked increases in above values
Shock	12–15	Profuse vomiting, heat stroke, severe diarrhea	More severe signs as noted above plus depression, tachycardia, weak pulse	More marked increases in above values

(hypernatremic dehydration), such as occurs with intense panting due to
hyperthermia. Pure water cannot be administered parenterally because it is
markedly hypotonic and would cause erythrocytes to swell and hemolyze.
Because 5% dextrose contains no electrolytes, it should not be used in patients
with disorders characterized by significant electrolyte losses. Glucose solutions
at 10%, 20%, and even 50% concentration can be given intravenously if
administered slowly to allow adequate mixing and dilution. They are used
primarily to supply calories and to cause osmotic diuresis in animals with renal
insufficiency. Glucose solutions should be administered only intravenously.

As mentioned above, supplementation of the above solutions may be
required to correct specific problems such as potassium depletion and metabolic acidosis or alkalosis. Concentrated potassium chloride solution is available to add to Ringer's and lactated Ringer's solutions. For severe metabolic
acidosis, hypertonic sodium bicarbonate can be added to 5% dextrose or 0.45%
saline. Sodium bicarbonate should not be added to calcium-containing fluids,

TABLE 1-2.   Example Calculations for Estimation of Fluid Volume Requirements

Existing deficit (ml) = body wt (kg) × %dehydration × 1000
Maintenance requirements = body wt (kg) × 40–60 ml/kg/day
Continuing losses = estimation of fluid volume loss (ml/day)

Example: A 20-kg dog is dehydrated because of anorexia and profuse watery diarrhea of 3 days' duration. The patient has decreased skin elasticity, dry mucous membranes, and slightly prolonged capillary refilling time. PCV is 57%, plasma protein 8.6 g/dl, BUN 38 mg/dl, and urine specific gravity 1.060. Dehydration is estimated to be 8%.

Question: What volume of fluid does this patient need?

Answer: Existing deficit (ml) = 20 kg × 0.08 (8%) × 1000   = 1600
Maintenance requirements (ml) = 20 kg × 50 ml/kg/day = 1000
Continuing losses—estimated (ml)   = 400
Total (ml)   3000

---

e.g., lactated Ringer's, because it causes calcium precipitation. Supplementation of 0.9% saline with sodium bicarbonate is not advisable since the resultant solution contains a high sodium concentration.

Routes of Administration.   Both medical and practical considerations may affect the choice of route for fluid therapy in the dog and cat. Of the routes available for fluid administration, the oral, intravenous, and subcutaneous routes are the most useful. The intraosseus route is occasionally used for blood or fluid administration to puppies and kittens or to adult patients who do not have an accessible vein.

If the patient will drink and vomiting is not present, the oral route is an excellent choice for treatment of mild dehydration. Within limits, fluids that differ significantly from ECF may be administered orally. Entrolyte (Smith-Kline Beecham) is marketed for oral rehydration therapy for dogs and cats, and most animals drink it voluntarily. Several commercial electrolyte products are manufactured for oral administration to humans, including Pedialyte (Ross Laboratories) and Gatorade (USV Laboratories). Many dogs will drink these fluids; but if they will not, forced administration with a large syringe can be tried. The oral route is the most practical and economic means of nutritional supplementation, assuming that vomiting or severe gastrointestinal tract disorders are not present.

If the patient will not eat, force-feeding or preferably placement of a feeding tube (nasoesophageal, pharyngostomy, gastrostomy, jejunostomy) may be necessary. A thin gruel can be made by mixing canned dog or cat food with water in an electric blender. Commercial liquid products for enteral tube feeding of dogs and cats are available (Canine CliniCare, Feline CliniCare, Pet Ag Co.). Enteral tube feeding is an excellent method of meeting fluid, electrolyte, and nutrient requirements in sick dogs and cats (unless vomiting or

TABLE 1-3. Selected Solutions and Additives Used for Basic Fluid and Electrolyte Therapy in Dogs and Cats

Fluid or Additive	Na	K	Cl	HCO$_3$	Ca	Mg	kcal/L	Tonicity	Usual Use
Water and electrolyte solutions (mEq/L)									
Lactated Ringer's	130	4	109	28[a]	3	0	9	Isotonic	Polyionic fluid replacement, alkalizer
Ringer's	147	4	156	0	5	0	0	Isotonic	Polyionic fluid replacement, acidifier
Saline									
0.45%	77	0	77	0	0	0	0	Hypotonic	Correction of hypernatremic dehydration
0.9%	154	0	154	0	0	0	0	Isotonic	Correction of hyponatremic dehydration
Dextrose									
2.5%	0	0	0	0	0	0	85	Hypotonic	Correction of hypernatremic dehydration
5%	0	0	0	0	0	0	170	Isotonic	Correction of hypernatremic dehydration
10%	0	0	0	0	0	0	340	Hypertonic	Osmotic diuresis, correction of hypoglycemia
20%	0	0	0	0	0	0	510	Hypertonic	Osmotic diuresis, correction of hypoglycemia
Additives for parenteral use (mEq/ml)									
7.5% Sodium bicarbonate	1	0	0	1	0	0	0	Hypertonic	Correction of severe metabolic acidosis
14.9% Potassium chloride	0	2	2	0	0	0	0	Hypertonic	Correction of potassium deficiency
10% Calcium gluconate	0	0	0	0	0.465	0	0	Hypertonic	Correction of hypocalcemia

(continued)

TABLE 1-3.   *(continued)*

Fluid or Additive	Na	K	Cl	HCO3	Ca	Mg	kcal/L	Tonicity	Usual Use
Additives for oral use									
Potassium gluconate elixir[b] (mEq/ml)	0	1.33	0	0	0	0	0	Hypertonic	Correction of potassium deficiency
Potassium gluconate powder[c] (mEq/tsp)	0	8	0	0	0	0	0		Correction of potassium deficiency
Sodium bicarbonate tablets (mEq/tablet)									
5 grain	3.9	0	0	3.9	0	0	0		Correction of metabolic acidosis
10 grain	7.8	0	0	7.8	0	0	0		Correction of metabolic acidosis
Special fluids									
Whole blood			Variable			0		Isotonic	Anemia, shock
Plasma			Variable			0		Isotonic	Hypoalbuminemia, maintenance of microcirculation

[a]Lactate is metabolized to HCO3 by the liver.
[b]Kaon, Adria Laboratories.
[c]Tumil-K, Daniel's Pharmaceuticals.

serious gastrointestinal disease is present). Discussion of nutritional therapy is beyond the scope of this chapter (see Suggested Readings, below for articles on this topic).

Rapid restoration of the ECF volume and dispersion within the body is usually best accomplished by intravenous fluid administration. In general, the intravenous route is preferred when dehydration is moderate to severe or when fluid loss has occurred rapidly. Usually, the more acute the fluid loss, the more imperative it is to replace existing deficits rapidly. For example, an animal in hemorrhagic shock caused by a gunshot wound may require fluid replacement at as rapid a rate as possible; here the fluid is administered by gravity flow

TABLE 1-4. Common Fluid, Electrolyte, and Acid-Base Disturbances in Selected Clinical Disorders and Suggested Treatment

Condition	Dehydration[a] Iso	Hyper	Hypo	Potassium[b] Status Norm	Hyper	Hypo	Sodium[c] Status Norm	Hyper	Hypo	Acid-Base[d] Status Normal	Met. Acid.	Met. Alk.	Resp. Alk.	Initial Fluid Therapy[e] LR Soln.	R Soln.	0.9% NaCl Soln.	5% Glu.	Additive KCl Soln.	HCO₃ Soln.
Adrenocortical insufficiency			×		×				×		×			±		×			
Anorexia, chronic	×	±		×			×			×				×				×	
Congestive heart failure	×			×			±			×	±			±			×		
Diabetes mellitus	×		±	±	±	×	×		±		×			×				×	
Diarrhea, severe	×			×			×	±			×			×					
Heat stroke		×		×			±	×			×			×			± ×		
Hepatic failure	×		±			×	×				±	×		±			×	×	
Pancreatitis, acute	×		±			×	×	±	±			×		±	×	×		×	
Renal failure, oliguric	×				×		×				×			×	×				
Renal failure, polyuric	×		±	±		×	×		±		×				×				
Shock, endotoxic	×			×			×				×			×					
Shock, hemorrhagic[f]	×			×			×				×			×					
Urethral obstruction	×	±			×		×	±			×			×					±
Vomiting, profuse			×			×			×			×			×	×		×	

± Condition occasionally present or treatment sometimes indicated.

[a] Iso = isotonic; Hyper, Hypo = hyper-, hyponatremic.
[b] Norm, Hyper, Hypo = normo-, hyper-, hypokalemia.
[c] Norm, Hyper, Hypo = normo-, hyper-, hyponatremia.
[d] Met = metabolic; Acid = acidosis; alk = alkalosis; resp = respiratory.
[e] LR = lactated Ringer's; R = Ringer's; glu = glucose.
[f] Blood transfusion usually indicated.

through one or more large-bore needles. Conversely, whenever losses have occurred over a period of days or weeks, body homeostatic mechanisms have had time to adjust, and slow fluid replacement is generally more appropriate. As was mentioned in regard to the oral route, within limits, solutions that differ in composition from ECF may be administered intravenously.

Disadvantages of the intravenous route include 1) a greater chance of side effects (phlebitis, bacteremia/septicemia, overhydration); 2) the time-consuming nature of the procedure; and 3) the need for assistance to restrain the patient. The latter dilemmas can be partially overcome by using indwelling venous catheters.

Advantages of indwelling venous catheters are that they: 1) provide immediate access to the circulation in an emergency; 2) allow continuous intravenous infusion or multiple intravenous administrations or blood samplings without vein destruction; 3) facilitate administration of irritating solutions with less risk of perivascular leakage; and 4) allow measurement of central venous pressure (jugular catheter). Commercial venous catheters are usually of two types: long, flexible polyethylene catheters (Delmed I-Cath, Delmed, Inc.), and short, more rigid polyethylene catheters (Sovereign Indwelling Catheter, Sherwood Medical). Breakaway cannula catheters (L-CATH, Luther Medical Products), which allow the needle to break away after insertion, are now available for instillation into the jugular vein. Flexible catheters are generally best 1) whenever the unit is to be left in place for longer than 24 hours and 2) for placement into a jugular or saphenous vein (see next paragraph). Aseptic technique and meticulous maintenance should be adhered to whenever placing and using an intravenous catheter. With practice, it is generally possible to complete the entire placement procedure in less than 15 minutes.

Usual sites for placing an indwelling venous catheter are the jugular, cephalic, and medial saphenous veins. Large-bore catheters can be placed in the jugular vein, which allows rapid fluid administration and makes it easy to obtain blood samples. Use of cephalic catheters is usually limited to short-term (24–48 hours) events, e.g., during anesthesia and surgery and for immediate postoperative care. It is generally difficult to obtain blood samples from cephalic catheters, and they are difficult to keep clean, dry, and in place. Use of longer, flexible polyethylene catheters (12–18 inches) in the medial saphenous vein is frequently a good alternative to jugular catheter placement in small patients such as cats (especially obese cats with small jugular veins). If the animal is uncooperative, induction of general anesthesia with isoflurane (Forane, Anaquest) and use of an induction chamber is generally safe and convenient. If the catheter is properly secured by bandaging and good catheter care is applied, medial saphenous catheters are stable and can be kept patent over several days for fluid infusion. As was the case for cephalic catheters, blood sampling from medial saphenous catheters is difficult.

Use of indwelling intraosseus catheters is usually restricted to patients in which it is not feasible to use an indwelling venous catheter (puppies and kittens or adult patients that do not have an accessible vein, e.g., an animal in shock with collapsed veins or one that has had its veins damaged by repeated venipuncture or previous catheter use). The rate of fluid delivery is usually limited to about 11 ml/minute with gravity flow, but can be increased to 24 ml/minute by using a pressure infusion cuff and applying 300 mm Hg pressure.

One milliliter of heparinized saline solution (10 units of heparin/ml of saline) should be instilled into the catheter immediately following placement, following each blood sampling, and at least three or four times daily in order to decrease the chances of catheter occlusion. When sampling blood from a catheter, the first 1 ml of blood should be either discarded or saved in the syringe for reinfusion after a second blood sample is drawn for needed laboratory testing. This technique lessens the chances of contaminating the sample with the heparinized saline in the catheter lumen.

Affordable automated infusion pumps are becoming available for use in small animal patients. These pumps markedly enhance patient care by providing an accurate method of regulating the rate and quantity of fluids administered (e.g., electrolytes, drugs, nutrients). Infusion pumps do not eliminate the need for careful patient monitoring.

Serious complications sometimes associated with the use of indwelling venous catheters include thrombophlebitis, thromboembolism, septicemia, and bacterial endocarditis. The following recommendations should help reduce the incidence and seriousness of catheter-related side effects.

1. Use an indwelling venous catheter only when it is definitely needed.
2. Use aseptic technique when placing the catheter.
3. Place a gauze sponge covered with povidone-iodine ointment (Betadine) over the site of entry and carefully secure the catheter by bandaging.
4. Check the catheter site regularly for redness and swelling and watch for signs of fever, leukocytosis, or arrhythmia. If any of these signs are observed, remove the catheter and submit the tip for bacterial culture and antimicrobial sensitivity testing if possible. Administration of an antibiotic, e.g., cephradine (Velosef, Squibb), at a dosage of 20 mg/kg every 8 hours IV or PO may be indicated while awaiting results of sensitivity testing.
5. Remove the catheter when it is no longer required, or replace it with another catheter in a different vein every 4–5 days if continued catheter use is imperative.

The subcutaneous route is practical in dogs and cats, especially for short-term maintenance fluid therapy. Fluids may be administered as rapidly as feasible by gravity flow through an 18- to 20-gauge needle; however, absorption and dispersion within the body are significantly slower than when the intravenous route is utilized. Absorption may be markedly prolonged in hypotensive animals, and it is recommended that the intravenous route be used first to rehydrate the patient and improve circulation to the subcutaneous tissues. Only isotonic and nonirritating solutions should be administered subcutaneously. Although 5% dextrose solution is isotonic, it should not be given subcutaneously to severely dehydrated animals because ECF electrolytes diffuse into the electrolyte-free subcutaneous pool of 5% dextrose solution followed by extracellular water. The ECF volume may then be temporarily decreased until equilibration between the 5% dextrose solution and ECF has occurred. When using the subcutaneous route for fluid therapy, one should carefully observe the patient prior to each treatment to be certain that fluid previously administered subcutaneously has been adequately absorbed. If it has not, further subcutaneous fluid administration may cause circulatory compromise and severe tissue slough.

By using a combined approach of initial deficit replacement intravenously, followed by administration of maintenance requirements subcutaneously, the practicing veterinarian can rapidly expand the ECF volume, improve renal blood flow, and avoid the labor-intensive task of prolonged slow intravenous drip protocols in some dehydrated patients.

Rates of Fluid Administration. Some of the factors that affect the rate at which fluids are administered to a patient are 1) the route being utilized; 2) the primary disease present; 3) the clinical condition of the patient; 4) the purpose of therapy; 5) the composition of fluid being administered; and 6) the degree of restraint required.

Knowledge of normal daily fluid maintenance requirements can serve as a basis for estimating intravenous fluid infusion rates for dehydrated animals. Normal fluid maintenance requirements are 40–60 ml/kg/day or 1.7–2.5 ml/kg/hr (roughly 1 ml/lb/hr). A common method of rehydrating mild to moderately dehydrated patients is to replace fairly rapidly at least one-half of the estimated fluid deficit requirements during the first 4–8 hours (assuming that cardiopulmonary function and urine production are adequate). It is done by infusing a polyionic fluid, e.g., lactated Ringer's solution at a rate of approximately two or three times the normal hourly maintenance rate (3.4–7.5 ml/kg/hr or roughly 1.5–3.0 ml/kg/hr) until about one-half of the estimated deficit has been replaced. Remaining fluid needs (about one-half of the estimated deficit, maintenance, and continuing losses) are administered more slowly over the subsequent 16–20 hours by contin-uous intravenous infusion at a rate of 1.5–2.0 times the hourly maintenance requirements (2.5–5.0 ml/kg/hr or roughly 1.0–2.5 ml/lb/hr). Once deficit needs have been replaced and abnormal continuing losses are no longer occurring, the rate of fluid administration can be reduced to maintenance amounts (1.7–2.5 ml/kg/hr or roughly 1 ml/lb/hr). As previously mentioned, consideration should be given to changing to the subcutaneous route for administration of maintenance fluid needs.

In everyday practice situations, deviations from the ideal slow rate of fluid administration (or continuous intravenous infusion) may be necessary. Rapid intravenous administration of fluids is also indicated for patients in shock. For fluids that are isotonic and similar in composition to plasma (e.g., lactated Ringer's solution, Ringer's solution), the following formula may be used as a guideline to estimate the maximal safe rate of intravenous fluid infusion (except for patients with serious cardiovascular disease or oliguric renal failure).

$$\text{Body weight (kg)} \times 90 = \text{ml fluid/hour}$$

Using body size as a basis for estimating the rate of fluid administration is an aid in selecting an appropriate rate of fluid administration for the individual animal. It is imperative to closely observe the patient for signs of overhydration; if such signs appear, the rate of administration is slowed or stopped, as necessary. Signs of excessive rate of fluid administration (overhydration) include restlessness, shivering, tachycardia, serous nasal discharge, tachypnea, moist rales, coughing, protrusion of the eye from the orbit, vomiting, and diarrhea.

Patient Monitoring

With careful periodic monitoring, the occurrence of the above complications is relatively uncommon. It is helpful to record fluid input on a regular basis (e.g., every 4 hours) and record totals every 24 hours including the estimated urine output. Parameters to be checked and the frequency of monitoring depend on the individual case. It is important to record all values on a flow sheet in order to observe trends in the data. For most patients receiving fluid therapy, PCV (microhematocrit tube), plasma total protein (refractometer), and accurate body weight should be checked at least daily. Depending on the rate of decline of the PCV, a value of 12–15% or less may be an indication for whole blood administration. Colloid osmotic pressure of plasma is more closely related to plasma albumin than to total plasma protein. However, a decrease in plasma total protein to less than 3.0–3.5 g/dl may be justification for slowing or decreasing fluid administration and considering plasma or whole blood transfusion (see Chapter 17).

Other important biochemical parameters to monitor include blood urea nitrogen (BUN) and serum electrolytes, especially potassium. An increasing BUN may indicate decreased renal blood flow (prerenal) and signify that the volume of fluid being administered is inadequate. On the other hand, a decreasing BUN is often a favorable prognostic sign associated with a good response to fluid therapy. Hypokalemia occurs frequently during parenteral fluid therapy of several days' duration, especially when using solutions with a composition similar to that of plasma, e.g., lactated Ringer's solution. Checking the serum potassium regularly every 2–3 days may be warranted (see Hypokalemia, below).

Urine production can be estimated in most patients by palpating the bladder and observing urination. If urine production is uncertain, it may be important to measure urine output more accurately. This is usually done by using a metabolic cage or a grate and pan with a conventional cage, or by placing and securing an indwelling urinary catheter. A significant disadvantage of using indwelling urinary catheters is the high risk of inducing a urinary tract infection. The consensus is that while an indwelling urinary catheter is in place, the patient should not be on an antibiotic because of the hazard of a resistant bacterial infection developing. Meticulous attention to the volume of fluid input and careful patient monitoring are critical in the oliguric patient to prevent overhydration and subsequent pulmonary edema.

Whenever the risk of fluid volume overload is greater than usual (presence of cardiovascular compromise, oliguria, or anuria; poor response to initial volume loading in shock; pulmonary contusions; severe acute pancreatitis with pulmonary damage), central venous pressure (CVP) monitoring during intravenous fluid administration can help prevent pulmonary edema. CVP is measured through an indwelling jugular catheter whose tip is located well in the intrathoracic jugular vein, preferably near the right atrium. Commercial disposable kits consisting of a water manometer, tubing, and three-way valves are available, although similar devices may be constructed less expensively. The manometer and tubing are interposed between the bottle of fluid being administered and the jugular catheter, making it possible to periodically interrupt fluid administration, fill the manometer, and measure CVP.

Central venous pressure is an indication of the capacity of the heart to effectively pump a given blood volume. Its primary usefulness during intravenous fluid therapy is to warn of impending left heart failure and potentially fatal pulmonary edema. CVP more closely reflects right atrial pressure than left atrial pressure. Therefore, it is possible for pulmonary edema to occur despite a normal CVP. Changes in CVP during fluid administration are probably of more significance than is the absolute CVP value. Normal CVP is approximately 0–5 cm of water, and at these pressures fluid administration can probably safely continue. CVP values between 5 and 10 cm of water are slightly increased; and if additional fluids are required, they should be administered cautiously. When CVP exceeds 10 cm of water, fluid administration should be discontinued in order to avoid impending pulmonary edema.

ELECTROLYTE IMBALANCES

Electrolytes of most common concern during fluid therapy in everyday small animal practice are sodium and potassium. Although total body stores of these electrolytes do not always correlate with their plasma concentrations, it is far more practical to evaluate the latter.

Sodium Abnormalities

Sodium salts are primarily responsible for the osmolality of ECF and are the major determinants of ECF volume and distribution of water between extracellular and intracellular fluids. Plasma sodium concentration is closely regulated and maintained within narrow limits despite large variations in dietary sodium intake.

Hyponatremia. Hyponatremia can be due to decreased sodium intake, increased sodium excretion, overhydration, or combinations of these causes. Hyponatremia may occur with decreased, increased, or normal body fluid volume. Causes of hyponatremia with decreased body fluid volume (hyponatremic dehydration) including vomiting, diarrhea, adrenocortical insufficiency, renal disease, postobstructive diuresis, removal of large quantities of ascitic fluid by paracentesis, and diuretic therapy. Causes of hyponatremia with increased body water are uncommon and include the syndrome of inappropriate antidiuretic hormone (ADH) secretion and excessive 5% dextrose infusion, especially to patients with oliguric renal failure. Hyponatremia with normal body fluid volume can occur with unusual syndromes characterized by primary polydipsia (e.g., psychogenic polydipsia) and with resetting of the thirst center osmostats in the hypothalamus.

Pseudohyponatremia sometimes results from hyperlipidemia, hyperproteinemia, and increased plasma osmolality due to marked hyperglycemia or mannitol administration. Treatment of the primary cause generally corrects the decreased plasma sodium concentration.

Clinical signs of hyponatremia are nonspecific and usually reflect the status of ECF volume. Hyponatremic dehydration may cause severe decrease of ECF volume and signs of shock. Hyponatremia associated with overhydration may cause signs of water intoxication, such as weakness and central nervous system abnormalities (restlessness, tremors, seizures, delirium).

Standard Therapy. Treatment of hyponatremia includes reducing the plasma sodium concentration and correcting the underlying cause. Before initiating treatment for hyponatremia, one should determine whether the patient is dehydrated, overhydrated, or euhydrated because the appropriate therapy for these conditions is significantly different. In general, sodium-containing fluids should be administered to dehydrated, hyponatremic patients; and water restriction, diuretics, or both should be used for overhydrated or normally hydrated patients. It is usually safer to normalize serum sodium gradually, over a period of 24–48 hours, because rapid normalization of chronic hyponatremia can cause dangerous brain shrinkage, as neurons may not be able to synthesize idiogenic osmoles this rapidly. For most patients with hyponatremic dehydration, either 0.9% sodium chloride or Ringer's solution is preferred. Fluid volume requirements are estimated as previously described (see the discussion on fluid volume requirements, above). Serum sodium should be measured every day or two and hydration status evaluated frequently to assess the adequacy of therapy for hyponatremic dehydration.

If the serum sodium concentration is low (< 110 mEq/L), rapidly increasing the serum sodium level by administering hypertonic saline solution (3% saline) may be necessary to prevent irreversible neurologic damage. The serum sodium concentration should be monitored frequently in these critically ill patients (preferably twice daily) until it stabilizes.

Treatment of hyponatremia associated with overhydration depends on the cause. Water restriction (to a quantity less than the urine output) is warranted for patients in this category. The syndrome of inappropriate secretion of ADH has been observed in dogs with heartworm disease and is characterized by water overload and increased renal sodium excretion. Water restriction and heartworm treatment are indicated for these patients. If administration of excessive 5% dextrose solution is the cause of hyponatremia and overhydration, cessation of its administration usually corrects the hyponatremia.

Hypernatremia. Hypernatremia can occur as a result of excessive water loss, decreased water intake, excessive sodium retention, increased sodium intake, or combinations of these factors. Dehydration may or may not be present. Basic causes of hypernatremic dehydration include inadequate water intake and excessive water loss. Inadequate water intake may occur when too little water is provided for injured and debilitated animals, and in patients with central nervous system disease with diminished thirst perception. Excessive water loss, usually with inadequate water intake, occurs with intense panting to dissipate heat, renal water loss (nephrogenic diabetes insipidus, central diabetes insipidus, administration of osmotic diuretics), gastrointestinal losses in certain cases of vomiting or diarrhea, and water loss into cells (seizures, rhabdomyolysis). Basic causes of hypernatremia with minimal or no dehydration are excessive sodium intake and increased sodium retention. Specific etiologies include parenteral administration of fluids with excessive sodium concentration, e.g., hypertonic saline solution, and excessive sodium bicarbonate added to other fluids.

Signs of hypernatremia are the result of ECF hypertonicity. Plasma osmolality can be estimated from the following formula.

$$P_{osm}(mOsm/L) = 2(Na + K) + glucose/18 + BUN/2.8*$$

Dogs and cats apparently are more resistant to the CNS effects of hypernatremia than are people, but clinical signs are often observed when plasma osmolality exceeds 375 mOsm/L. With severe ECF hyperosmolality (plasma osmolality >400 mOsm/L), weakness and depression may progress to stupor, coma, and death within a few hours unless the hypernatremia is reversed. Dangerous hypernatremia is more likely to occur when the serum sodium level exceeds 180 mEq/L, but careful monitoring for trends is warranted when the serum sodium exceeds 170 mEq/L.

Standard Therapy. Appropriate treatment of hypernatremia depends on the presence or absence of dehydration. For hypernatremic dehydration, the particular treatment regimen depends on the severity of hypernatremia and

---

*Some investigators omit the BUN from this formula because urea is freely diffusible across cell membranes and does not contribute to effective plasma osmolality.

the underlying disorder. If too little water has been offered or the patient has been too debilitated to drink and is mildly dehydrated, simply making sure the animal drinks water may be adequate. In the rare case of a defective central nervous system thirst center, adding water to the patient's food is necessary. If dehydration associated with hypernatremia is moderate to severe, parenteral fluid therapy is indicated. When the serum sodium level is less than 170 mEq/L and the plasma osmolality is less than 375 mOsm/L in such patients, correction of hypernatremia can be accomplished with either 5% dextrose or 0.45% saline solution infused intravenously over a 6- to 12-hour period with the fluid volume required estimated by the methods previously discussed (see the discussion on fluid volume requirements, above).

For the management of severe hypernatremia (serum sodium > 180 mEq/L, plasma osmolality > 400 mOsm/kg), *the rate of reduction of plasma osmolality is critically important.* Lowering the serum sodium concentration too slowly may allow irreversible brain damage due to neuronal dehydration, whereas a too-rapid reduction can cause "rebound" cerebral edema and death. The serum sodium concentration should decline by about 1.0 mEq/L/hr. These animals are critical care patients and require close supervision and monitoring until the serum sodium normalizes. Experience with severe hypernatremia in dogs and cats suggests that serum sodium is usually difficult to decrease and that aggressive treatment is generally necessary.

Either 5% dextrose or 0.45% saline solution given by slow intravenous drip should be tried first. Plasma osmolality should be corrected steadily over a 24-hour period. It is imperative that the animal's neurologic status be closely observed and that the serum sodium concentration be frequently determined (at least every 6–8 hours). If significant reduction of serum sodium does not occur within 6 hours, or worsening of the neurologic status is observed, more aggressive efforts to decrease serum sodium should be made immediately. Intravenous furosemide (Lasix), 1–2 mg/kg every 6–8 hours, and 2.5% dextrose by slow (5–10 ml/kg/hr) intravenous drip should be started. Careful monitoring of serum sodium and neurologic status must be continued until serum sodium normalizes.

The prognosis depends on how early severe hyperosmolality is recognized and reversed. Once plasma osmolality exceeds 400 mOsm/kg, progression to death often occurs within a matter of a few hours.

If hypernatremia resulted from excessive sodium administration or ingestion (little or no dehydration), cessation of sodium administration or ingestion and supplying water for drinking in increasing quantities over a 4- to 6-hour period are indicated.

Potassium Abnormalities

Almost 98% of body potassium is located intracellularly at a concentration of about 150 mEq/L. The remaining 2%, in the ECF, is closely maintained at a normal concentration of about 3.7–5.6 mEq/L. The distribution of potassium between the extracellular and intracellular fluids is critical for many physiologic processes and is affected by several factors, including the pH of the ECF. Alkalosis causes "shifting" of potassium from the extracellular space to the intracellular space, whereas acidosis promotes transfer of potassium into the ECF. Normal total body potassium content is determined by the balance between intake and excretion. Daily potassium ingestion equals or exceeds the amount of potassium in ECF. Therefore, appropriate renal excretion of excessive potassium is vital to avoid fatal hyperkalemia. Serum potassium may not be correlated with total body potassium stores.

Hypokalemia. Hypokalemia is a common and important disorder in canine and feline patients and may be present in association with decreased, normal, or increased body potassium content. Chronic anorexia, especially when associated with administration of fluids low in potassium, can cause hypokalemia and body potassium depletion. Disorders associated with alkalosis (e.g., profuse vomiting) or administration of alkalinizing compounds such as lactate or bicarbonate are particularly likely to cause hypokalemia and body potassium depletion because of the alkalosis-induced "shifting" of potassium from the extracellular to the intracellular space and the enhancement of renal potassium excretion. Also, excessive parenteral administration of fluids low in potassium, especially alkalinizing fluids such as lactated Ringer's solution, often cause hypokalemia and body potassium loss. Polyuric renal failure, particularly in cats, may be associated with excessive potassium losses in the urine, eventually resulting in serious hypokalemia and body potassium deficit. Postobstructive diuresis, often observed for a few days after relief of urethral obstruction, may result in hypokalemia. Furosemide, mineralocorticoid, and amphotericin B administration cause renal potassium loss. Insulin causes cellular uptake of glucose and potassium and can result in hypokalemia.

Clinical signs of potassium deficit and hypokalemia (anorexia, weakness, ileus, poor renal concentrating ability) often go unrecognized because they are nonspecific and may be attributed to the primary disease itself. Correction of potassium deficiency usually alleviates these signs.

Standard Therapy. Treatment of hypokalemia usually requires administration of potassium, although correction of alkalosis (see Acid-Base Imbalances, below) normalizes serum potassium in some patients. Precise amounts of potassium for the treatment of hypokalemia cannot be accurately quantitated because there is no predictable method of measuring cellular potassium deficit and uptake of the administered potassium. Therefore, when treating potassium deficiency, it is important to measure serum potassium periodically to assess the efficacy of therapy and adjust the dosage accordingly. Estimates of required quantities of potassium are usually derived from the history, physical examination, and laboratory data, especially the serum potassium level and total carbon dioxide level (TCO_2). In general, hypokalemia associated with

TABLE 1-5. Parenteral Potassium Supplementation[a]

Severity of Potassium Depletion	Serum Potassium (mEq/L)	Potassium Dosage (mEq/kg/day)	KCl (mEq) Added to 250 ml Fluid
Mild	3.0–3.7	1–3	7
Moderate	2.5–3.0	4–6	10
Severe	<2.5	7–9	15–20

[a]Be certain urine output is adequate prior to potassium administration. If the intravenous route is used, do not exceed 0.5 mEq KCl/kg/hr. It is preferable to administer potassium-containing fluids orally unless vomiting is present. The subcutaneous route can also be used, and concentrations of potassium of up to 40 mEq/L can be so administered.

acidosis indicates more serious potassium deficit than does hypokalemia accompanied by normal blood pH or alkalosis.

Guidelines for potassium supplementation are shown in Table 1-5. These figures are *approximations* derived from knowledge of normal daily potassium requirements and clinical experience with various diseases. *Before administering potassium, one should be certain that urine production is adequate.* Otherwise, potentially fatal hyperkalemia may result.

The route and rate of potassium supplementation depend on the severity of the clinical signs and the cause of potassium loss. Because life-threatening hypokalemia that requires intravenous potassium infusion is uncommon and fatal cardiotoxicity from hyperkalemia is more likely during intravenous potassium administration, either the oral (in the absence of vomiting) or the subcutaneous route of administration is preferred. Most commercial dog and cat foods contain sufficient potassium to correct mild potassium deficiencies. For moderate and severe deficits, potassium gluconate supplements, in both liquid (Kaon) and powder (Tumil-K) formulations, and potassium chloride tablets for oral use are available. Enteric coated potassium chloride tablets are poorly absorbed and should not be used.

Whenever the oral route is impractical and renal function is good, subcutaneous administration of polyionic, isotonic fluids, e.g., lactated Ringer's or Ringer's solutions fortified with 30–40 mEq of potassium chloride per liter, is a safe, effective method of potassium replacement.

If potassium is administered intravenously, it is generally safer to rehydrate the patient first with fluids low in potassium (lactated Ringer's, Ringer's, 0.9% saline solutions) prior to administering potassium-enriched fluid. An exception is treatment of the severely hypokalemic cat (see below). The rate of intravenous infusion of potassium should not exceed 0.5 mEq potassium/kg/hr without careful patient monitoring. The use of an automated constant-infusion pump and careful monitoring by personnel qualified to recognize early signs of cardiotoxicity—including electrocardiographic (ECG) monitoring—are suggested.

Recommended treatment protocols for cats showing signs of muscle weakness due to hypokalemia depend on the severity of hypokalemia and clinical signs. Oral treatment alone is recommended for all but the most severely affected cats. Parenteral administration of fluids, even those enriched with potassium, should be avoided if possible because of their tendency to further lower serum potassium and cause potentially fatal hypokalemia. Kaon is suggested at an oral dosage of 2.5–4.0 mEq of potassium every 12 hours. Serum potassium should be checked daily until it is in the normal range. Most cats show evidence of increased strength and improved appetite and attitude within 2–3 days, but complete return of muscle strength may take several weeks. Administration of supplemental potassium (Kaon or Tumil-K) should be continued at home on a long-term basis. The dosage is generally about 2–4 mEq potassium/day PO, although there is considerable variation among cats. The serum potassium level should be monitored weekly and the supplemental potassium dosage increased or decreased accordingly.

Intravenous potassium administration is occasionally necessary for a cat with profound hypokalemia and signs of severe weakness and impending respiratory paralysis. These critically affected cats require intensive care and monitoring. Intravenous administration of concentrated potassium solution can cause cardiotoxicity, and therefore use of an automated infusion pump and continuous ECG monitoring are advised. A maximal rate of an intravenous potassium infusion of 0.4 mEq/kg/hr is recommended. The following example illustrates the calculations necessary for treating a severely hypokalemic cat.

A 7-year-old domestic shorthair cat is presented with signs of marked weakness due to hypokalemic polymyopathy. Dehydration is estimated at 6%. Serum potassium is 2.2 mEq/L. The cat weighs 3 kg.

Question: What is an appropriate treatment protocol?
Answer: Priority should be given to rapid correction of the profound hypokalemia followed by correction of dehydration. The intravenous route is advised because of the severe signs and potential death of the patient unless serum potassium is increased rapidly.

0.4 mEq/kg/hr × 3 kg
= 1.2 mEq potassium/hour or 0.02 mEq potassium/minute

Add 56 mEq KCl to 1 L of lactated Ringer's solution that already contains 4 mEq potassium/L for a final potassium concentration of 60 mEq/L or 0.06 mEq potassium/ml of enriched solution.

Use a pediatric minidrip infusion set at 60 drops/ml and an automated constant-infusion pump.

Question: How many drops per minute must be infused to deliver 1.2 mEq potassium/hour or 0.02 mEq potassium/minute to this patient?
Answer: 0.06 mEq potassium/1 ml of enriched solution *and*
              60 drops/ml for pediatric minidrip infusion set

Therefore 0.06 mEq of potassium/60 drops *or*
0.001 mEq of potassium/1 drop
To deliver 0.02 mEq of potassium/minute:

$$\frac{0.02 \text{ mEq potassium/minute}}{0.001 \text{ mEq of potassium/drop}}$$

= 20 drops/minute, or 1 drop every 3 seconds

When infusing potassium intravenously, the serum potassium level should be determined every 4–6 hours and the potassium infusion slowed by about one-half once the serum potassium level increases to 3.5 mEq/L. When serum potassium is in the normal range, the potassium infusion should be stopped. Intravenous infusion of dopamine (Elkins-Sinn) at a dosage of 0.5 μg/kg/min via a constant-infusion pump reportedly can be lifesaving in some severely hypokalemic cats because it causes transient redistribution of potassium from the intracellular fluid to the ECF. Administration of potassium gluconate orally should be initiated immediately in these patients.

Hypokalemia due to redistribution of potassium may be corrected by appropriate treatment of the primary cause (i.e., correction of alkalosis, reduction of insulin dosage).

Hyperkalemia. In most cases of hyperkalemia, total body potassium stores are normal. Cardiotoxicity caused by hyperkalemia is potentially life-threatening.

Basic causes of hyperkalemia include increased potassium intake, decreased renal potassium excretion (most common), and "shifting" of potassium from cells into ECF. Hyperkalemia due to increased potassium intake is rare with the exceptions being excessive intravenous potassium chloride or potassium penicillin administration, especially in small patients. Decreased urinary excretion of potassium occurs with conditions such as urethral obstruction, ruptured urinary tract and uroabdomen, oliguric renal failure, hypoadrenocorticism (Addison's disease), administration of aldosterone-inhibiting diuretics, and acidemia. Causes of potassium redistribution into the ECF include massive crush injuries, acidosis, and hyperkalemic periodic paralysis (rare).

Signs of hyperkalemia include bradycardia, cardiac arrhythmia (most common), weakness, shock, and death. The onset and severity of signs are not always predictable from the serum potassium concentration; however, onset of signs can be anticipated when the serum potassium concentration reaches 6.5–7.0 mEq/L. Whenever the serum potassium concentration exceeds 8 mEq/L, immediate treatment of hyperkalemia should take precedence over diagnostic procedures.

Standard Therapy. Treatment of hyperkalemia can be accomplished by administering low-potassium, alkalinizing fluids to cause urinary potassium excretion, enhancing the redistribution of potassium into cells by using alkalinizing fluids or an insulin-glucose mixture, or antagonizing the cardiac effects of potassium by infusing a calcium-containing solution. The use of exchange resins in the colon or peritoneal dialysis to decrease serum potassium is not usually practical in dogs and cats.

The particular treatment used depends on the cause and severity of the hyperkalemia. Most cases of mild to moderate hyperkalemia (serum potassium 6.5–8.0 mEq/L) can be effectively managed by intravenous administration of a low-potassium, isotonic, alkalinizing fluid (lactated Ringer's solution) in sufficient quantities to rehydrate the patient and cause mild diuresis. Increased delivery of sodium, bicarbonate, and water to the distal nephron increases renal potassium excretion. Alkalinization of ECF causes redistribution of potassium into cells.

For moderately severe hyperkalemia (serum potassium >8.0–8.5 mEq/L with ECG abnormalities), either sodium bicarbonate *or* glucose-insulin solution (not both) may be infused intravenously to cause cellular uptake of potassium. Cellular uptake of potassium caused by insulin temporarily decreases the serum potassium concentration while the underlying problem is corrected. Sodium bicarbonate is recommended whenever the hyperkalemic patient has serious metabolic acidosis (plasma TCO_2 or HCO_3 < 10 mEq/L). Recommended dosage is 2–3 mEq $NaHCO_3$/kg body weight administered intravenously over 30 minutes. Because rapid administration of sodium bicarbonate can cause serious side effects (see discussion on treatment of metabolic acidosis, below), use of this compound is not advised unless laboratory measurement of plasma TCO_2 or HCO_3 has confirmed metabolic acidosis. Intravenous administration of regular insulin and 20% glucose solution (10 units of regular insulin per deciliter of 20% glucose solution) is occasionally necessary. For dogs, the rate of administration of this insulin-glucose mixture should be based on an insulin dosage of 5 units/kg/hr (50 ml/kg/hr). In the cat, regular insulin may be administered as an intravenous injection of 0.5 units/kg followed immediately by an intravenous bolus of 2 g of dextrose per unit of insulin given (10 ml of 20% dextrose). For example, a 4-kg cat would receive 2 units of regular insulin intravenously followed by an intravenous bolus of 4 g of dextrose (20 ml of 20% dextrose). Continuous ECG monitoring is advised. Blood glucose should be checked hourly (Chemstrip bG, AccuCheck II, Boehringer Mannheim), and serum potassium measurement should be repeated in 2–3 hours. Based on these values, appropriate adjustments can be made in the administration of the sodium bicarbonate or glucose-insulin solution. Once serum potassium declines to less than 7.5–8.0 mEq/L, it is preferable to stop the sodium bicarbonate or glucose-insulin infusion and begin intravenous administration of lactated Ringer's solution as described above for treating mild to moderate hyperkalemia.

If cardiac arrhythmias associated with extreme hyperkalemia (serum potassium >9.5–10.0 mEq/L) are severe and death is believed to be imminent, calcium should be used to directly counteract the cardiotoxic effects of the high serum potassium concentration. A 10% calcium gluconate solution should be administered by slow intravenous infusion (over a period of 10–15 minutes) at a dosage of 0.5 ml/kg. Because the effective dosage of calcium gluconate is variable, the heart rate or ECG should be carefully monitored during the infusion. The infusion should be stopped when the heart rate increases or the ECG begins to normalize.

Appropriate treatment of the underlying cause of hyperkalemia must be initiated without delay.

ACID-BASE IMBALANCES

Acidosis and alkalosis refer to pathologic processes that cause accumulation of acids and alkali within body fluids, and if not halted cause a change in blood pH. When the serum bicarbonate concentration is altered, the patient is said to have metabolic acidosis or alkalosis; whereas changes in the blood partial pressure of carbon dioxide (PCO_2) are termed respiratory acidosis or alkalosis.

The patient's history may be helpful for assessing the type of acid-base disturbance present. By considering the severity and duration of signs of the primary disorder, it may be possible to predict if an acid-base disorder is likely and whether it is mild or severe. A physical examination is unreliable for predicting either the type or the severity of acid-base disturbances. From knowledge of the usual imbalances caused by various clinical disorders it is often possible to predict the type of acid-base disturbance in a patient (Table 1-4). However, there is no substitute for adequate laboratory data for an accurate assessment of the acid-base balance. Ideally, arterial blood is collected for measurement of pH, PCO_2, PO_2, and calculated bicarbonate. The TCO_2, which comprises about 97% bicarbonate, is a practical way to evaluate the metabolic component of acid-base disorders. Evaluation of the anion gap (AG)

$$AG = [Na + K] - [Cl + HCO_3]$$

is also helpful in the interpretation of acid-base balance.

Metabolic acidosis (decreased serum bicarbonate) is the most common acid-base abnormality in dogs and cats. Common causes of metabolic acidosis include azotemia (prerenal, renal, postrenal), diabetic ketoacidosis, lactic acidosis (poor tissue perfusion, especially in shock), toxins such as ethylene glycol, drugs such as ammonium chloride, and profuse diarrhea. *Metabolic alkalosis* (increased serum bicarbonate) may be caused by profuse vomiting, especially when associated with loss of mostly gastric juice, excessive administration of bicarbonate, lactate, citrate, or acetate, and prolonged use of diuretics such as furosemide.

Respiratory acidosis (increased arterial PCO_2) indicates decreased or ineffective ventilation and may occur with central nervous system depression associated with anesthesia, sedation, or damage to the respiratory centers. Additional causes are airway obstruction; severe, diffuse parenchymal lung diseases such as pneumonia; restrictive airway diseases such as pleural effusion; and injuries that limit expansion of the thoracic cage such as flail chest. Neuromuscular disorders that compromise the ability to ventilate effectively (phrenic nerve paralysis, botulism, coonhound paralysis) may also cause respiratory acidosis. Causes of *respiratory alkalosis* (decreased PCO_2) include mild or moderate parenchymal lung diseases such as pneumonia or pulmonary edema, mild or moderate restrictive airway diseases such as pleural effusion, pronounced panting, excessive mechanical ventilation, and stimulation of the central nervous system respiratory centers (fever, endotoxemia, hyperammonemia).

Standard Therapy

Appropriate therapy of acid-base disorders depends on the type of disturbance and the cause and severity of the primary disease.

Metabolic Acidosis. Mild metabolic acidosis may not require specific treatment if the primary disease is quickly resolved. Bicarbonate may be given by the oral route if vomiting is not present and if need is not immediate. Sodium bicarbonate tablets are available in 5 grain (325 mg) and 10 grain (650 mg) sizes. Five grains of sodium bicarbonate has almost 4 mEq of sodium and bicarbonate, respectively. Sodium bicarbonate powder (baking soda) is also suitable but is not often used in dogs and cats.

For mild to moderate metabolic acidosis (serum TCO_2 10–16 mEq/L) associated with dehydration, parenteral treatment with lactated Ringer's solution is recommended. Fluids containing acetate instead of lactate are also available and are acceptable in most instances. Lactate and acetate are metabolized by the liver to bicarbonate (1 mEq of lactate or acetate equals 1 mEq of bicarbonate). For severe metabolic acidosis (serum TCO_2 < 10 mEq/L), use of sodium bicarbonate solution, usually as an additive to either 0.45% saline or 5% glucose solution, may be warranted.

The approximate amount of lactate, acetate, or bicarbonate required to correct metabolic acidosis can be estimated from the following formula.

$$\text{Body wt. (kg)} \times 0.5 \times HCO_3 \text{ deficit}$$
$$(\text{where } HCO_3 \text{ deficit} = \text{normal serum } HCO_3 - \text{patient's serum } HCO_3)$$

Experimental studies in dogs have shown that the bicarbonate space of distribution varies depending on the severity of metabolic acidosis, and therefore formulas used to calculate bicarbonate requirements provide only rough estimates.

In general, metabolic acidosis should be corrected over a 24- to 48-hour period. For most cases, a conservative approach to treating metabolic acidosis using lactate or acetate instead of bicarbonate is preferred. For life-threatening metabolic acidemia, intravenous administration of one-half of the estimated bicarbonate requirements during the first 4–6 hours is warranted. Reported serious side effects of excessively rapid intravenous sodium bicarbonate administration are paradoxical cerebrospinal fluid acidosis (whenever sodium bicarbonate is infused too rapidly), decreased ionized serum calcium, hypokalemia, left shifting of the oxyhemoglobin dissociation curve resulting in reduced oxygenation of tissues, and plasma hyperosmolality due to hypernatremia. Serum TCO_2 and anion gap should be monitored frequently to assess results of therapy.

Metabolic Alkalosis. Metabolic alkalosis caused by excessive treatment with alkali generally responds to stopping administration of the alkali; further treatment is generally not required. Metabolic alkalosis due to vomiting is associated with dehydration, chloride depletion, and often significant potassium deficit. In most cases, expansion of the extracellular space by the administration of solutions high in chloride and supplemental potassium are effective. Ringer's solution enriched with potassium chloride is preferred (see discussion on treatment of hypokalemia, above).

Respiratory Acidosis. Treatment of respiratory acidosis involves restoring effective ventilation and correcting the primary cause whenever possible. Ventilatory assistance may be needed. Oxygen administration without assisted ventilation may worsen respiratory acidosis because animals with chronic respiratory acidosis maintain ventilation by hypoxic drive.

Respiratory Alkalosis. Symptomatic therapy of respiratory alkalosis is not usually necessary. Treatment requires alleviation of hyperventilation and correction of the primary cause whenever possible.

SUGGESTED READINGS

Bell FW, Osborne CA: Treatment of hypokalemia. In: Kirk RW, ed. Current Veterinary Therapy IX. Philadelphia: WB Saunders, 1986;101.

Bell FW, Osborne CA: Maintenance fluid therapy. In: Kirk RW, ed. Current Veterinary Therapy X. Philadelphia: WB Saunders, 1989;37.

Dow SW, LeCouteur RA: Hypokalemic polymyopathy of cats. In: Kirk RW, ed. Current Veterinary Therapy X. Philadelphia: WB Saunders, 1989;812.

Lippert AC, Armstrong PJ: Parenteral nutritional support. In: Kirk RW, ed. Current Veterinary Therapy X. Philadelphia: WB Saunders, 1989;25.

Otto CM, McCall Kaufmann G, Crowe DT: Intraosseous infusion of fluids and therapeutics. Compend Contin Ed Pract Vet 1989;11:421.

Polzin DJ: Disorders of potassium balance. In: Proceedings of the 8th ACVIM Forum, Washington, DC, 1990;305.

Polzin DJ: Disorders of sodium balance. In: Proceedings of the 8th ACVIM Forum, Washington, DC, 1990;301.

Senior DF: Fluid therapy, electrolyte, and acid-base control. In: Ettinger SJ, ed. Textbook of Veterinary Internal Medicine. Philadelphia: WB Saunders, 1989;429.

Wheeler SL, McGuire BH: Enteral nutritional support. In: Kirk RW, ed. Current Veterinary Therapy X. Philadelphia: WB Saunders, 1989;30.

Willard MD: Treatment of hyperkalemia. In: Kirk RW, ed. Current Veterinary Therapy IX. Philadelphia: WB Saunders, 1986;94.

Zenger E, Willard MD: Oral rehydration therapy in companion animals. Compan Anim Pract 1989;19:6.

CHAPTER TWO

General (Polysystemic) Problems: Pyrexia, Anorexia, Weight Loss, and Obesity

Michael D. Lorenz

PYREXIA

Pyrexia (fever) is an elevation of body temperature caused by disease. Pyrexia is produced by substances that are capable of resetting the brain's thermoregulatory center at a higher than normal body temperature. Called endogenous pyrogens, these substances are released from neutrophils, monocytes, and eosinophils in response to several exogenous stimuli such as bacterial endotoxins, bacteria, viruses, and allergens. Fever is a problem encountered frequently in dogs and cats.

Hyperthermia is a marked elevation in body temperature caused by high environmental temperature and the reduced ability of dogs and cats to efficiently dissipate body heat. Pyrogen activation and release are not involved in the pathogenesis of hyperthermia (heat stroke), although rare, high fever may lead to heat stroke if the ambient temperature is above 80°–85°F. The treatment for hyperthermia is discussed in Chapter 17.

Standard Therapy

The symptomatic suppression of fever is not usually necessary unless the rectal temperature exceeds 105°F (40.6°C) or when prolonged anorexia and depression occur secondary to fever. Several drugs have antipyretic effects, and they do not lower body temperature unless fever is present. Aspirin and other salicylate-like antipyretics do not affect the production of endogenous pyrogens. They probably decrease the effect that pyrogens exert in resetting the thermostat in the hypothalamus to a higher temperature. Aspirin and dipyrone are the drugs most commonly used in small animals. Aspirin is the initial drug of choice at a dosage of 10 mg/kg q12h PO in dogs and 10 mg/kg PO q48h in cats. Aspirin may cause gastric mucosal irritation and decreased platelet aggregation.

Acetaminophen can be used in dogs to suppress fever. A dosage of 10 mg/kg q12h PO is recommended. Rarely, hepatic necrosis has been associated with acetaminophen therapy in dogs. Because of its toxicity, acetaminophen is not recommended in cats.

Dipyrone (Novin, Haver) is a nonsteroidal anti-inflammatory agent that has antipyretic properties in dogs and cats. It is available as a solution for subcutaneous, intramuscular, or intravenous administration at a dosage of 25 mg/kg. Dipyrone causes leukopenia, agranulocytosis, gastritis, and decreased coagulation in dogs and cats. Its administration is therefore limited to the immediate suppression of fever.

Animals with fever should be well hydrated and maintained on sufficient calories to prevent weight loss. Constipation may be a complication of fever and should be corrected with enemas or bulk laxatives (or both). The ideal ambient temperature is controlled at 72°–75°F (22.2°–23.9°C), and the room is well ventilated.

Animals with fevers above 106°F (41°C) should be cooled with ice packs, alcohol rubdowns, or cool water enemas. Treatment is repeated as necessary to keep the body temperature below 105°F (40.6°C).

Alternative Therapy

Glucocorticoids have potent antipyretic effects, as they reduce the amount of endogenous pyrogen released from leukocytes in response to endotoxin and sepsis. Glucocorticoids suppress leukocyte migration, local inflammatory responses, and immunologically mediated processes that stimulate endogenous pyrogen release. Glucocorticoids may also inhibit prostaglandin release, an effect that inhibits fever production centrally. However, glucocorticoids may potentiate the harmful effects of infectious diseases and are contraindicated for these diseases. Glucocorticoids are most useful as antipyretic agents for neoplastic or immune-mediated diseases.

Phenothiazine tranquilizers may lower body temperature by causing profound peripheral vasodilatation. Sedation, ataxia, and profound hypotension are serious side effects that usually preclude the use of phenothiazines as antipyretic agents.

ANOREXIA

Anorexia is the lack of or disinterest in the ingestion of food. Total anorexia is the pathologic absence of hunger. Anorexia occurs with many disease processes that directly inhibit or suppress activity of the hunger center in the brain stem. Anorexia may be partial or complete, pathologic, physiologic, or psychological. Because anorexia is frequently associated with many disease processes, the major task is to determine and correct its underlying cause.

Standard Therapy

There are several medical therapies that help stimulate eating in anorectic dogs and cats regardless of etiology. The treatment for weight loss (caloric malnutrition), a serious sequela to anorexia, is described in subsequent sections of this chapter.

The most effective means for maintaining nutrition is the voluntary consumption of food. Therefore every effort should be made to entice anorectic dogs and cats to eat voluntarily before attempts are made to chemically stimulate the appetite or to provide enteral nutritional support. Diet composition, feeding intervals, and environmental factors contribute significantly to the eating habits of dogs and cats. These parameters are disturbed frequently in the hospital, and every effort should be made to duplicate the home environment.

Diet. Cats are typically more selective about their food than are dogs. Cats should be offered the same diet as they receive at home, but the diet should be energy-dense. Most cats prefer moist, warm food, although some cats are addicted to dry or semimoist cat food. Their preference should be established in the medical history. Because cats rely heavily on their sense of smell, diets with a strong meat, fish, or cheese odor may stimulate eating. The food should be warmed to body temperature to volatilize odors (a microwave oven is recommended) and presented to the cat in small amounts several times a day. Most cats prefer to eat in isolation, and efforts must be made to avoid noise or other distractions. Sometimes placing a towel over the cage door entices a cat to eat, and stroking or petting may stimulate eating. Placing a small amount of food on the front paws may stimulate licking, which sometimes carries over into eating. Most cats prefer to eat from large, shallow dishes or directly from the floor.

Dogs like more variation in their diet and eat a larger selection of foods. Dogs may be attracted to sweet foods, but most prefer diets high in protein and fat. Foods with strong odors, such as canned cat food or dog food warmed to body temperature, are recommended. The addition of small quantities of garlic salt or meat tenderizer may increase the appeal of meat diets. Some dogs can be encouraged to eat by petting, whereas others prefer to eat alone. As with cats, feeding small amounts frequently is usually more successful than leaving food in the cage.

Chemical Stimulation. Several drugs are known to stimulate appetite in dogs and cats. The benzodiazepine derivatives and cyproheptadine have short-term appetite-stimulating activity. Diazepam (Valium, Roche) is most effective when administered intravenously at a dose of 0.2 mg/kg not to exceed a maximum total dose of 5 mg. Feeding usually begins within 5 minutes and may last 20 minutes. Diazepam should be given two times a day. Appetite stimulation in anorectic animals tends to decrease with multiple injections of diazepam. Oxazepam (Serax, Wyeth) has been used in cats for appetite stimulation at a dose of 2.5 mg/cat PO. Sedation and ataxia are side effects of diazepam and oxazepam therapy.

Cyproheptadine (Periactin, Merck) stimulates the appetite of cats but not that of dogs. A dose of 2–4 mg/kg/day PO is recommended. Excitability and aggressive behavior are side effects in some cats.

Glucocorticoids nonspecifically stimulate appetite in dogs and cats. Unless contraindicated by underlying diseases, prednisolone at a dosage of 0.25 mg/kg/day PO may be effective. Therapy is usually maintained for 5–7 days. Anabolic steroids such as stanozolol (Winstrol, Winthrop-Breon) stimulate appetite in some animals. A dose of 1–2 mg PO twice a day or 25–50 mg IM once a week is recommended.

Despite little evidence of clinical efficiency, B vitamins have been used clinically to stimulate appetite in cats. Because cats have a high requirement for B vitamins in their diets, it is important to supplement anorectic cats with parenteral B vitamins.

WEIGHT LOSS

Weight loss results from a negative caloric balance, such as when metabolic utilization exceeds the supply. Although weight loss may result from the loss of body fluids, as with dehydration, in this section only weight loss due to undernutrition (calorie deficiency, protein deficiency, or both) is discussed.

Standard Therapy

In general, there is but a single cause of weight loss: insufficient calories to meet metabolic needs. Caloric deficiency may be divided into three major categories: 1) inadequate food intake (anorexia, deficient diet); 2) malassimilation; and 3) excessive caloric expenditure. Definitive therapy of pathologic weight loss is dependent on diagnosis and correction of the underlying disease. The symptomatic therapy for anorexia has been described in previous sections. The therapy of malassimilation is described in Chapter 8.

Enteral alimentation is the most effective method to correct caloric and protein malnutrition in anorectic animals with normal gastric and small intestinal function. Gruels made from energy-dense foods are given through oral, pharyngostomy, or gastrostomy tubes. Caloric and protein requirements are calculated based on estimates of normal body weight. Requirements are increased 25–30% for conditions that increase the metabolic demands of the body (i.e., fever, cancer, increased thyroid secretion). The diet should be divided into three or four equal meals and given slowly through the feeding tube at appropriate times. Appropriate vitamin and mineral therapy should also be given. Repeated oral tube feeding in cats is stressful. Pharyngostomy or gastrostomy tubes allow enteral administration of well-balanced cat food gruels without the need for extreme restraint. Cats tolerate gastrostomy tubes better than pharyngostomy tubes.

The use of special diets for the management of various diseases is described in appropriate sections throughout this book. The reader should consult these sections for specific dietary recommendations for the enteral alimentation of animals with specific diseases.

OBESITY

Obesity (body weight in excess of 15% of normal weight) is a common nutritional disorder caused by excessive body fat. The probable cause of the increasing incidence of obesity in dogs and cats is that highly palatable energy-dense foods are widely available and pets undergo inadequate exercise relative to caloric intake. Common or simple obesity refers to adipose tissue in a normal body distribution pattern. Hyperplastic obesity is caused by an excessive number of adipocytes, which may be genetically controlled but is certainly associated with overeating early in life. Hypertrophic obesity, caused by increased size of adipocytes, is the major form of common obesity encountered in veterinary practice.

Standard Therapy

Obesity results when prolonged caloric intake exceeds metabolic needs. It is usually associated with overeating and insufficient physical activity. The mainstays of weight reduction are calorie restriction and increased physical activity.

The most important component of a weight reduction program is owner cooperation. Owners who accept the diagnosis of obesity and the many potential health problems it causes are generally successful with managed weight reduction programs. The program must be described in writing and evaluated weekly. Owners should record dietary consumption, exercise frequency and duration, and body weight on a daily basis, and such records should be reviewed once a week by the veterinarian. Prior to instituting the program, each pet should be evaluated thoroughly for any underlying medical problems. Laboratory tests, such as a complete blood count, biochemical profile, and urinalysis, should be completed.

Reduced Caloric Intake. The basic diet may be available commercially (r/d Canine and Feline, Hill's Pet Products; Cycle 3, Gaines Foods, Inc.; Fit'n'Trim, Purina) or homemade. Caloric requirements are based on providing 60% of the maintenance requirements of the estimated normal weight. This reduced diet is divided and given three or four times a day if possible. *No* snacks are allowed. Some clients demand the need to give snacks, in which case high fiber wafers are recommended. Generally, 8–12 weeks are required to achieve the ideal weight. Weight reduction should occur at a rate of 0.5–2.0 pounds per week. When weight loss does not occur and the owner is in compliance with the diet, calories should be reduced by an additional 25%.

More rapid loss can be achieved by total caloric restriction. The animal is hospitalized, and care is exercised to supply a balanced vitamin–mineral supplement and to closely monitor the animal's clinical condition. Desired weight reduction can be achieved in approximately 6 weeks. This treatment is *not* recommended for cats, as it may cause hepatic lipidosis and liver failure.

Increased Physical Activity. A physical exercise program can be instituted for dogs but is not practical for cats. Dogs can be exercised through walks on a leash and intensive play. Specific goals should be outlined, but most dogs need to walk at least 1 mile each day. Some owners have trained their dogs to walk on a motorized home treadmill.

Appetite Suppressants. Most of the drugs used for appetite suppression in humans are not effective in dogs and cats. Experimentally, threochlorocitric acid has induced satiety by slowing the gastric emptying time; and sucrose polyester, an indigestible food additive with the taste of fat, has increased palatability. Both compounds may be available in the future, as they have demonstrated effectiveness in experimental dogs.

SUGGESTED READINGS

Brown SA: Obesity. In: Lorenz MD, Cornelius LM, eds. Small Animal Medical Diagnosis. Philadelphia: JB Lippincott, 1987;98.

Lorenz MD: Disturbances of food intake: anorexia and polyphagia. In: Lorenz MD, Cornelius LM, eds. Small Animal Medical Diagnosis. Philadelphia: JB Lippincott, 1987;23.

Lorenz MD: Pyrexia (fever). In: Lorenz MD, Cornelius LM, eds. Small Animal Medical Diagnosis. Philadelphia: JB Lippincott, 1987;15.

Lorenz MD: Weight loss. In: Lorenz MD, Cornelius LM, eds. Small Animal Medical Diagnosis. Philadelphia: JB Lippincott, 1987;90.

Macy DW, Ralston SL: Cause and control of decreased appetite. In: Kirk RW, ed. Current Veterinary Therapy X. Philadelphia: WB Saunders, 1989;18.

CHAPTER THREE

Dermatologic Diseases

Linda Medleau and Pauline M. Rakich

ALLERGIC SKIN DISORDERS

Allergic skin disorders in dogs and cats include urticaria, angioedema, atopy, allergic contact dermatitis, food allergy, drug eruption, and parasitic hypersensitivities. Frequently, the allergic animal is hypersensitive to more than one thing, i.e., fleas, pollens, and food.

Urticaria and angioedema are cutaneous forms of anaphylaxis. Urticaria is characterized by areas of superficial dermal edema (wheals, hives), whereas the edema of angioedema occurs in the deeper dermis and subcutaneous tissue and is more diffuse. Urticaria and angioedema are caused by exposure to something that has induced an immediate hypersensitivity reaction (e.g., drugs, food, vaccines, bacterins, stinging or biting insects, allergenic extracts, plants, excess heat or cold).

Atopy (inhalant allergic dermatitis) is common in dogs and occurs also in cats. Atopy is characterized by a pruritic skin problem that may be seasonal or nonseasonal. Clinical signs in dogs include face rubbing, feet licking or chewing, armpit or inguinal pruritus, and otitis externa. In severe or chronic cases, there may be generalized skin involvement. Secondary conjunctivitis may be seen with face rubbing, and secondary pyoderma and seborrhea are common. In cats, the clinical signs of atopy include miliary dermatitis, eosinophilic granuloma complex lesions, head and neck pruritus, and symmetric (psychogenic) alopecia.

Food allergy is characterized by a nonseasonal, pruritic dermatitis. The clinical signs are variable. In dogs, the clinical signs include atopic-like or flea allergic-like skin disease, generalized pruritic folliculitis, seborrheic skin disease, otitis externa, and urticaria–angioedema. Food allergic cats may present with miliary dermatitis, head and neck pruritus, generalized pruritus, eosinophilic granuloma complex lesions, or symmetric (psychogenic) alopecia. Concurrent gastrointestinal signs, such as vomiting, diarrhea, and excessive flatulence, are rarely seen in food allergic dogs and cats.

There are two types of contact dermatitis. One is caused by contact with a primary, irritant substance such as a caustic chemical. The other type, allergic contact dermatitis, is seen in animals only when they have a delayed hypersensitivity reaction to substances such as cleaning agents, wool, grass, topical medications, collars, and vinyl toys or food bowls. The lesions of contact dermatitis include erythema, papules, alopecia, ulcers, necrosis, and pruritus or pain. Chronic lesions are often thickened, lichenified, and hyperpigmented. Typically, thin-haired areas that come in contact with the ground such as the ventral interdigital aspects of the paws, ventral aspects of the abdomen, tail, thorax, and neck, scrotum, chin, and inner ear pinnae are affected. The neck is involved in animals allergic to flea collars. If the allergen is a topical insecticide or shampoo, the haired areas of the skin are also affected. In dogs that develop allergic contact dermatitis from exposure to dishes or chew toys, the nose and lips are involved.

Drug eruptions are the rarest of the hypersensitivity disorders. Any drug, systemic or topical, can cause a reaction. Pruritus may not be present. The clinical signs are variable and include papules, pustules, exfoliation, vesicles, bullae, purpura, erythema, urticaria, angioedema, alopecia, toxic epidermal necrolysis, erythema multiforme, ulcerations, and otitis externa.

The clinical signs and treatment of parasitic hypersensitivities are discussed in the section on parasitic skin diseases.

Treatment of Allergic Dermatitis

Treatment of allergic skin disorders generally involves symptomatically treating the skin condition while the underlying cause is eliminated. In cases where the underlying cause of the allergy cannot be determined, the skin condition is controlled with long-term symptomatic medical management. The objectives are to make the animal more comfortable by 1) reducing inflammation and pruritus, 2) treating secondary pyoderma or seborrhea, and 3) eliminating the underlying cause from the animal's environment if possible.

Specific Therapies. *Urticaria and Angioedema.* Mild reactions may require no treatment. With more severe reactions, the use of prednisolone, 2 mg/kg PO, IM, or IV is indicated. Antihistamine therapy may help prevent new lesions from developing. With angioedema, cold packs may help quicken the regression of the edema. For anaphylactic reactions, epinephrine is also administered. The underlying cause(s) of the urticaria or angioedema should be identified and avoided.

Atopy. Three options are available for the management of atopy. Preferably, the offending antigen is removed from the animal's environment. For instance, wool or feather-containing material should be removed if the animal is wool or feather allergic. Likewise, dogs that are allergic to cat or horse dander should not contact these species. Dust control measures should be employed if the animal is allergic to housedust. Because mattresses are sources of dust and molds, they should be encased in vinyl zippered protectors. Carpeting and furniture should be vacuumed regularly. Canister type vacuum cleaners are better than upright vacuum cleaners because with upright vacuum cleaners dust can return to the air as it passes through the bag. Periodically cleaning the ducts of home heating and cooling systems and using electrostatic and activated charcoal filters are recommended. To prevent house dust mites from proliferating, humidifiers or dehumidifiers (or both) should be used to keep the relative humidity between 30 and 50%.

If avoidance of the offending allergen is not possible (e.g., pollens), symptomatic therapy with corticosteroids and antihistamines or immunotherapy with antigenic extracts can be used. Immunotherapy is usually indicated in animals that do not tolerate corticosteroid therapy, do not improve with antihistamine therapy, or have clinical signs of atopy for more than 4 months a year. The use of corticosteroids and antihistamines is discussed in this section on adjunctive therapies. With immunotherapy, the animal is given serial subcutaneous injections of progressively larger amounts of the offending allergens. Pharmaceutical companies that manufacture allergenic extracts include Center Laboratories (Port Washington, NY), Greer Laboratories (Lenoir, NC), and Hollister-Stier (Rexdale, Ontario). The regimen we use for dogs and cats is outlined in Table 3-1. Although some animals show improvement immediately, others take up to 1 year before improvement is noted. Symptomatic therapy with antihistamines, fatty acid supplements, or anti-inflammatory doses of glucocorticosteroids does not interfere with immunotherapy and can be used concurrently if needed. Good to excellent results with immunotherapy are seen in 50–65% of the cases. To maintain its effectiveness, immunotherapy must be continued for life. The most common reasons for immunotherapy failure include stopping the injections, parasitic infestations, bacterial skin infections, other undiagnosed allergies (e.g., food), and newly acquired inhalant allergies.

Adverse reactions to immunotherapy are rare in dogs and cats but may include temporary intensification of pruritus, localized edema, pain or pruritus at the injection site, and anaphylaxis. If intensification of pruritus is seen, the dosage of the extract should be lowered or anti-inflammatory doses of prednisone should be administered orally on the day of injection. If anaphylaxis occurs, the animal is treated with prednisolone, antihistamines, and epinephrine as described for urticaria–angioedema.

Food Allergy. The diagnosis and treatment of food allergic dermatitis begins by feeding the animal a hypoallergenic diet. The diet should be fed for at least 10 weeks to dogs and cats. The hypoallergenic diet should contain a single protein and single carbohydrate source that has never been part of the regular diet. Suggested diets in dogs include home cooked lamb, chicken, rabbit, venison, or fish with rice or potatoes, or canned or dry Prescription Diet Canine d/d (Hill's Pet Products). Please note that approximately 20% of food allergic dogs do not improve when fed canned Prescription Diet Canine d/d. This lack of response may reflect an allergy to metal, which leaches from the can into the food. During the trial diet no table scraps, dog treats, rawhide chews, flavored nylon chewbones, flavored heartworm preventative, flavored vitamin supplements, or flavored antibiotic suspensions should be given to the dog. Hypoallergenic diet

TABLE 3-1. Hyposensitization Schedule for Subcutaneous Injections of Allergenic Extracts to Dogs and Cats

	Dose (cc)		
Day	VIAL 1 (100–200 PNU/ml)	VIAL 2 (1000–2000 PNU/ml)	VIAL 3 (10,000–20,000 PNU/ml)
1	0.2		
3	0.4		
5	0.6		
7	0.8		
9	1.0		
11		0.2	
13		0.4	
15		0.6	
17		0.8	
19		1.0	
21			0.2
23			0.4
25			0.5

Continue with 0.5 cc from vial 3 every 7 days.

suggestions for cats include home cooked lamb or pork, lamb baby food (Gerber's), or canned Prescription Diet Canine d/d. Similar to dogs, some food allergic cats do not improve when fed canned d/d. For cats that will not eat a hypoallergenic diet, an alternative is to feed a commercial cat food that contains a different protein source than that usually fed. For finicky eaters on semimoist diets, feed a commercial canned or dry cat food because some cats are allergic to the additives in semimoist diets. During the diet trial, cats should not be given table scraps, any milk products, flavored vitamin supplements, or flavored antibiotic suspensions.

If the animal is food allergic, the pruritus should decrease markedly within 10 weeks of the change in diet. Partial response to a hypoallergenic diet suggests that other types of allergy may also be present.

A definitive diagnosis of food allergy is made when the animal becomes pruritic upon provocative exposure to its previous diet. Pruritus may occur within several hours or its occurrence may be delayed for 3–5 days. Single ingredients from the previous diet should be added to the hypoallergenic diet for 7-day periods each to determine the allergenic components.

Food-allergic animals must be fed diets that do not contain the offending allergens, as these animals may not benefit from symptomatic corticosteroid therapy. If commercial diets fail to control clinical signs, the test diet must be

TABLE 3-2.   Hypoallergenic Diet for Dogs

Cooked lamb ¼ lb (115 g)
Cooked rice 1 cup (175 g)
Vegetable oil 1 t (5 g)
Dicalcium phosphate 1½ t (7 g)
Potassium chloride ⅛ t (0.6 g)

Combine all ingredients and mix well. Yield: ⅔ lb (300 g) (795 kcal/lb).

From Lewis LD, Morris ML, Hand MS. *Small Animal Clinical Nutrition.* Topeka: Mark Morris Associates, 1989. t = teaspoon

used for maintenance. Home cooked diets must include adequate levels of vitamins and minerals and, for cats, taurine. For cats on home cooked diets, the meat should be baked or roasted. Boiling usually reduces the taurine content of meat by approximately 50% of baked values unless the cooking fluid remains with the food. The minimum daily taurine requirement for cats is unknown; the current recommendation is 100–250 mg/day. A sample home cooked hypoallergenic diet that is balanced and fulfills the canine minimum daily requirements for all vitamins and minerals is shown in Table 3-2. For diets in which taurine supplementation is desired, pure taurine (500 mg capsules) is available at human health food stores. Although clams are high in taurine (1017 mg/kg), clam juice should not be used as a source of taurine because its taurine content is negligible. Canned Prescription Diet Canine d/d has enough protein and taurine to be used as a maintenance diet for cats.

Contact Dermatitis. The definitive treatment for contact dermatitis is removal of the offending substance. Erythematous, inflamed lesions can be treated symptomatically with topical corticosteroids. Ulcerated or necrotic lesions are clipped and cleaned and then treated topically with Domeboro's solution (Miles) two or three times daily for 5–15 minutes. To make up the solution, two packets of powder or two tablets are added to 0.5 L (1 pt) of water. Domeboro's solution can be used for 1 week, after which it should be discarded and a fresh solution made up. For animals that have widespread lesions or intense pruritus, oral corticosteroid therapy is administered as discussed under the adjunctive therapies in this section. Systemic antibiotic therapy may also be necessary if the lesions are secondarily infected (see section on pyodermas).

Mechanical barriers such as T-shirts and socks may be useful to prevent contact with irritants or allergens that cannot be removed from the animal's environment. Long-term therapy with systemic corticosteroids is often only partially successful because most cases become refractory with time.

Drug Eruptions. Stop administration of the offending drug. Symptomatic therapy with topical wet dressings or soaks may be indicated if lesions are exudative. Localized lesions should be treated topically with Domeboro's solution (Miles) two or three times daily for 15–30 minutes. Two packets of powder or two tablets should be added to 0.5 L (1 pt) of water. Once made up, the solution can be used for 1 week, after which it should be discarded and a fresh solution made up. For generalized crusting or exudative eruptions, whirlpool baths to which an antiseptic such as chlorhexidine (Nolvasan Solution, Fort Dodge), 5 ml/L water, has been added should be used for 30-minute periods once or twice daily to cleanse the lesions gently. Response to systemic corticosteroid therapy (as described below) is unpredictable. Systemic antibiotic therapy as described in the section on pyodermas is indicated if eruptions are generalized to help prevent secondary bacterial skin infections from developing. Provocative challenge with the suspect drug is not advised, and future use of the drug or any chemically related compounds must be avoided.

Adjunctive Therapies. Adjunctive therapies in the management of allergic skin disorders include the use of glucocorticoids, antihistamines, essential fatty acids, progesterones, antibiotics for secondary pyoderma, flea control, and antiseborrheic therapy.

Glucocorticoids. Systemic glucocorticoids may provide pruritus control while the underlying cause is managed. Glucocorticoids are most effective in animals that are pruritic for less than 5 months of the year. Animals that scratch for most of the year tend to develop glucocorticoid refractoriness. In dogs, side effects of glucocorticoids are more easily prevented if short-acting oral preparations (prednisolone, prednisone, methylprednisolone) are used. To break the itch–scratch cycle, short-acting glucocorticoids are administered every day. Pruritus is usually controlled within 5–7 days; and if maintenance therapy is needed, every-other-day short-acting glucocorticoid administration is highly recommended. The drug dosages for induction and maintenance control of pruritus are listed in Table 3-3. For long-term therapy, the lowest possible dose of glucocorticoids necessary to keep the dog comfortable should be used. The author has treated some dogs that failed to respond to relatively high doses of steroids given every other day yet were well controlled on low doses given every day. Also, the concurrent use of antihistamines or essential fatty acid supplements may allow further reduction in the dose of glucocorticoids necessary to control pruritus. Dogs that develop polyuria and polydipsia on prednisone or prednisolone may have fewer side effects with methylprednisolone (Medrol, Upjohn). However, methylprednisolone is more expensive than prednisolone or prednisone.

Cats require higher doses of oral prednisolone for pruritus control than do dogs. Because cats are fairly resistant to developing iatrogenic hyperadrenocorticism, oral or injectable glucocorticoids can be used for induction (Table 3-3). For maintenance therapy, every-other-day administration of oral prednisone or prednisolone is preferred. For long-term therapy, the lowest possible dose of glucocorticoids necessary to keep the cat comfortable should be used.

Side effects of glucocorticoids include polyuria, polydipsia, polyphagia, weight gain, and other signs of Cushing's disease. Long-term therapy with

TABLE 3-3. Glucocorticoid Therapy for Allergic Dermatitis in Dogs and Cats

Steroid	Induction Dosage	Maintenance Dosage
Prednisone or prednisolone	0.2–0.5 mg/kg q12h PO (dog) 1–2 mg/kg q12h PO (cat)	0.2–0.6 mg/kg q48h PO (dog) 1–2 mg/kg q48h PO (cat)
Methylprednisolone (Medrol)	0.16–0.4 mg/kg q12h PO (dog)	0.16–0.5 mg/kg q48h PO (dog)
Methylprednisolone acetate (Depo-Medrol)	4 mg/kg SC or IM (cat)	

steroids may also result in immunosuppression with increased susceptibility to pyoderma, demodectic mange, urinary tract infections, and upper respiratory tract infections. Sudden withdrawal of glucocorticoids may cause signs of adrenal insufficiency because chronic glucocorticoid therapy produces varying degrees of adrenocortical suppression. Animals on continual steroid therapy should have routine veterinary checkups every 6 months. At each checkup, a urinalysis should be performed because asymptomatic urinary tract infections are common occurrences in dogs undergoing long-term therapy with glucocorticoids.

Antihistamines. Antihistamines control pruritus in approximately 40% of atopic dogs. An antihistamine that works in one dog may not be effective in another. Thus a different antihistamine should be tried for 1-week periods until a satisfactory response is produced (Table 3-4). Antihistamines are usually only partially effective, but their concurrent use with glucocorticoids may allow a marked reduction in glucocorticoid dosage. In cats, chlorpheniramine 2–4 mg twice daily may be effective in controlling pruritus.

The most common side effect of antihistamines is sedation. Less commonly, hyperexcitability may occur. Antihistamines, especially hydroxyzine (Atarax), are potentially teratogenic and should not be used in pregnant animals.

Essential Fatty Acid Supplements. These products may be effective in reducing pruritus by blocking the metabolism of arachidonic acid, thereby decreasing the release of inflammatory mediators. Oral preparations containing these fatty acids include Derm Caps (DVM) and EfaVet (Vet-Kem). Response to this treatment can take up to 2 months, so other antipruritic drugs may be needed initially. Even if the fatty acid supplement is not completely effective by itself, its concurrent use with glucocorticoids may allow a marked reduction in glucocorticoid dosage.

Progestational Compounds. Although progestational compounds are often used to relieve pruritus in cats, we do not recommend them because of their potential serious side effects (see below). Glucocorticoids are as effective and safer in most cases. Also, progestational compounds are not approved for use in cats. The recommended dosage of megestrol acetate (Ovaban, Schering;

TABLE 3-4. Antihistamines for Atopy in Dogs

Generic Name	Trade Name	Oral Dosage	Supplied As	
Over the counter				
Chlorpheniramine	Chlor-Trimeton (Schering)	2–12 mg q8–12h	Tablets: Capsules: Syrup:	4, 8, 12 mg 8, 12 mg 2 mg/5 ml
Diphenhydramine HCl	Benadryl (Parke-Davis)	2–4 mg/kg q8h	Tablets: Capsules: Elixir: Syrup:	25, 50 mg 25, 50 mg 12.5 mg/5 ml 12.5 mg/5 ml
Prescription				
Trimeprazine	Temaril (Herbert)	1–2 mg/kg q8h	Tablets:	2.5 mg
Cyproheptadine	Periactin (Merck Sharp & Dohme)	0.3–2.0 mg/kg q12h	Tablets: Syrup:	4 mg 2 mg/5 ml
Hydroxyzine HCl	Atarax (Roerig)	2 mg/kg q8h	Tablets: Syrup:	10, 25, 50, 100 mg 10 mg/5 ml
Terfenadine	Seldane (Merrell Dow)	4–10 mg/kg q12h	Tablets:	60 mg

Megace, Mead-Johnson) is 2.5–5.0 mg PO q48h to effect and then 2.5–5.0 mg q1–2weeks for maintenance. The dosage of medroxyprogesterone (Depo-Provera, Upjohn) is 10 mg/kg IM or SC once and then only as needed.

Side effects are common, especially with injectable progesterones. Side effects in cats include polyphagia, weight gain, personality changes, pyometra, decreased spermatogenesis and infertility in males, diabetes mellitus that may be transient or permanent, mammary gland hyperplasia, mammary adeno-carcinoma (in males and females), and adrenal suppression.

Antibiotic Therapy. Because dogs with allergic skin diseases are predisposed to secondary pyoderma, antibiotic therapy is indicated whenever bacterial skin infection develops. The dosage and regimen for antibiotic therapy are discussed in the section on pyoderma.

Topical Therapy. Topical therapy is used to reduce the scaling, greasiness, inflammation, pruritus, and odor in dogs with secondary seborrhea. For localized pruritic lesions, topical steroid preparations can be applied to the lesions two to three times daily. Powdered Aveeno Colloidal Oatmeal, mixed with cool water and applied as a rinse, may reduce pruritus for 1–3 days. The use of shampoos and rinses is discussed in the section on seborrhea.

PYODERMA

Pyoderma is a pyogenic bacterial infection of the skin. For purposes of therapy, pyodermas are classified according to depth of infection, i.e., surface, superficial, or deep.

Surface pyodermas involve the epidermis primarily and include acute moist dermatitis ("hot spots," pyotraumatic dermatitis, or moist eczema) and skin fold pyoderma. Acute moist dermatitis results from trauma to the skin, which allows overgrowth of resident bacteria. It is a self-induced lesion the dog creates when it licks, chews, or scratches an area of irritation initiated by fleas, other ectoparasites, allergic skin disease, anal sac disease, otitis externa, folliculitis, trauma and wounds, foreign body, dirty matted wet haircoat, or psychosis. The lesions are rapidly progressive and characteristically erythematous, moist, exudative, and usually painful. Skin fold dermatitis (skin fold pyoderma) results from constant friction of the skin, poor air circulation, and accumulation of moisture due to an anatomic defect involving the face (facial fold dermatitis), lip (lip fold dermatitis), body (body fold dermatitis), vulva (vulvar fold dermatitis), or tail (tail fold dermatitis).

Superficial pyodermas involve the epidermis and hair follicles. They are usually caused by *Staphylococcus* spp. and present as either superficial pustular dermatitis (impetigo) or folliculitis. Impetigo is seen most commonly in young dogs prior to puberty and may be associated with parasitism, viral infections, poor nutrition, or a dirty environment. Lesions of superficial pyoderma may include papules, pustules, crusts, epidermal collarettes (circular erythematous lesions rimmed by scale and frequently with hyperpigmented centers), and alopecia. Pruritus varies from absent to intense. Most commonly the lesions are mistaken for demodicosis or dermatophytosis, which can be ruled out by skin scrapes and fungal culture, respectively. When infection is recurrent despite appropriate antibacterial therapy, an underlying predisposing condition should be sought, e.g., ectoparasites, allergy, seborrhea, hypothyroidism, or hyperadrenocorticism.

Deep pyodermas involve tissues deeper than hair follicles. Infection is usually secondary to an underlying cause such as foreign body, trauma, ectoparasitism, hypothyroidism, hyperadrenocorticism, or neoplasia. Middle-aged German shepherd dogs appear to be predisposed to recurrent deep pyodermas that may be refractory to therapy. In contrast to superficial pyodermas, many organisms may be isolated from deep pyodermas, including *Staphylococcus* spp., various gram-negative bacteria, *Actinomyces* or *Nocardia* spp., *Mycobacterium* spp., and *Mycoplasma* spp. and related organisms. Lesions of deep pyoderma typically consist of alopecia, hyperpigmentation, ulcers, crusts, draining fistulas, subcutaneous nodules, and cellulitis. Because of the serious nature of the infection and the possibility of multiple infections, bacterial and fungal culture and sensitivity tests are always indicated. Skin scrapes should be performed to rule out demodicosis. Mycobacterial, actinomycotic, nocardial, and *Mycoplasma* and related infections should be considered in dogs and cats with chronic nonhealing ulcers, abscesses, and draining subcutaneous nodules that respond poorly to antibiotics and routine therapy. Diagnosis of such infections is based on characteristic histologic changes in biopsy specimens from lesions, demonstration of organisms with special stains, and cultural identification.

Treatment of Pyoderma

Standard Therapy. Therapy of pyoderma is usually based on systemic antibiotics. Although treatment is fairly straightforward in most cases, failures are common, the reasons for which include choosing an inappropriate antibiotic, using an appropriate antibiotic at an inappropriate dose, administering an antibiotic for an inadequate duration, and using corticosteroids concurrently with antibiotics.

Most pyodermas in dogs and cats are caused by coagulase-positive *Staphylococcus* spp., many of which produce the enzyme penicillinase. Consequently, an antibacterial drug known to be active against staphylococci and resistant to penicillinase should be chosen. Penicillin, ampicillin, amoxicillin, hetacillin, and carbenicillin are inactivated by penicillinase and thus are not appropriate empiric choices for treating pyodermas. Resistance to tetracycline is also frequent. Narrow-spectrum antibiotics that are effective against coagulase-positive staphylococci include erythromycin (17.6–22.0 mg/kg three times daily), lincomycin (15.4–22.0 mg/kg three times daily), and oxacillin, cloxacillin, or dicloxacillin (22.0 mg/kg three times daily). Erythromycin and lincomycin are usually good drugs for treating pyodermas, but they should not be used empirically to treat infections that have been treated with antibiotics previously. The reason is that bacterial resistance to erythromycin and lincomycin develops frequently with previous antibiotic treatment. In addition, erythromycin and lincomycin exhibit cross resistance; and if one is ineffective for treating a pyoderma, the other is similarly ineffective.

Broad-spectrum antibacterial drugs effective against staphylococci include chloramphenicol (44.0–55.0 mg/kg three times daily; 50 mg twice daily may be a more appropriate dose for cats), trimethoprim-sulfonamide (15.4–22.0 mg/kg twice daily), and cephalosporins such as cefadroxil, cephalexin, and cephradine (15.4–22.0 mg/kg three times daily). Chloramphenicol and trimethoprim-sulfonamide combinations may not be clinically effective regardless of the results of in vitro sensitivity testing. This situation appears to be true especially for deep pyodermas, so neither drug is a good choice for treatment of deep pyoderma. A combination drug (Clavamox, SmithKline Beecham Animal Health Laboratories) incorporates amoxicillin with clavulanic acid, which binds to bacterial penicillinase and inactivates it. Therapeutic failures are frequent at the manufacturer's recommended dose of 13.75 mg/kg twice daily; but when given at a dosage of 13.75–22.0 mg/kg three times daily, Clavamox is effective in treating pyodermas. Aminoglycosides such as gentamicin have good in vitro activity against staphylococci but are impractical because of the potential for nephrotoxicity and because they must be administered parenterally. Gentamicin is usually reserved for severe infections with organisms resistant to other less toxic antibiotics. Enrofloxacin is a broad-spectrum bactericidal fluoroquinolone drug that has become available for veterinary use (Baytril, Mobay Animal Health). The manufacturer's recommended dose is 2.5 mg/kg PO twice daily for a maximum of 10 days; but we have found, from a limited number of cases, that a dose of 5.0 mg/kg PO twice daily and a treatment interval of longer than 10 days may be more appropriate for pyodermas.

The temptation to use decreased doses of antibiotics in order to reduce the cost for a client should be resisted because using too low a dose promotes development of resistant organisms, which ultimately necessitates using even more expensive antibiotics. Concurrent use of corticosteroids is contraindicated for most bacterial skin infections. Although corticosteroids induce apparent clinical improvement by inhibiting inflammation, they impair the host's ability to eliminate pathogenic organisms.

Side Effects. The most common side effects of antibacterial therapy are gastrointestinal disturbances such as vomiting and diarrhea. Vomiting is especially common with erythromycin and can be minimized by administering the first three doses with a small amount of food. Although a major problem in humans, bone marrow dyscrasias are reported rarely in animals treated with chloramphenicol. Chloramphenicol appears to be more toxic to cats than to dogs. Healthy cats given doses ranging from 25 to 120 mg/kg/day for 14–21 days developed dose-dependent central nervous system (CNS) depression, dehydration, anorexia, weight loss, vomiting, diarrhea, and reversible bone marrow suppression. Because of the duration and dose required to treat pyodermas, chloramphenicol may not be an appropriate antibiotic for cats. The aminoglycosides are potentially nephrotoxic, and frequent monitoring of renal function [via urinalysis and blood urea nitrogen (BUN)] is necessary when using them. Enrofloxacin can cause erosion of cartilage of the weight-bearing joints in growing dogs and for this reason should be avoided in immature animals. In rare instances, antibacterial agents induce idiopathic reactions manifested as oral, cutaneous, and mucocutaneous eruptions or as vasculitis with polyarthritis, lymphadenopathy, and fever. Many drugs have been reported to cause drug eruptions or reactions in dogs and cats, but most commonly these reactions are reported to occur with sulfadiazine and sulfamethoxazole-trimethoprim. The reaction usually resolves after drug administration is discontinued.

Treatment of Acute Moist Dermatitis

Standard Therapy. Therapy of acute moist dermatitis involves symptomatic treatment as well as correcting the underlying initiating cause. The affected area should be clipped and cleaned (Betadine, Purdue Frederick Co.; Nolvasan,

Fort Dodge Laboratories). Sedation may be necessary when treating dogs with painful lesions. Wet soaks with an astringent such as aluminum acetate solution (Domeboro, Miles Laboratories) 5–10 minutes two to four times daily helps dry up the lesions. Treatment with any type of ointment is contraindicated because ointments are occlusive and prevent drying. A topical steroid cream, however, may be applied two to three times daily to decrease pruritus and inflammation. If pruritus is severe, oral prednisolone may be administered for 7–10 days at a dose of 0.55–1.10 mg/kg/day.

Alternative Therapy. In some instances, especially in golden retriever and St. Bernard dogs, response to standard therapy may be poor. It has been suggested that failure to respond to therapy is due to extension of inflammation to hair follicles and deep dermal structures. In such cases, systemic antibiotics are necessary to resolve the lesion.

Treatment of Skin Fold Dermatitis

In most cases of skin fold dermatitis, the only permanent treatment is surgical correction of the skin fold or tail amputation. Because the standards for some breeds require a facial fold, however, surgical ablation would produce a serious fault in a show dog. In the case of obese dogs, weight reduction eliminates or minimizes the problem. Medical therapy is palliative and usually long term. Inflammation can be minimized by routine (daily to once or twice weekly) cleansing with 2.5–5.0% benzoyl peroxide (OxyDex Gel, DVM), rinsing, and application of an astringent (Domeboro solution). Body fold dermatitis may involve larger areas of skin, necessitating more generalized therapy such as frequent antibacterial and antiseborrheic shampoos (OxyDex, DVM; Sebbafon, Winthrop Laboratories).

Treatment of Superficial Pyoderma

If the infection is mild and localized, no therapy may be necessary other than eliminating the underlying cause(s). In most instances, daily antibacterial shampoos (OxyDex) speed recovery. When lesions are extensive, systemic antibiotic therapy is indicated. The infection is almost always due to staphylococcal organisms, so for an initial episode of superficial pyoderma an appropriate antibiotic is chosen empirically without aid of culture and sensitivity testing. Systemic antibacterial therapy should be continued at the standard therapeutic dose until lesions are completely resolved plus an additional week (minimum 3 weeks). Failure to clear lesions completely prior to stopping antibacterial therapy is a frequent cause of recurrent infection. Any predisposing causes should be corrected. If none can be found and the pyoderma recurs repeatedly, adjunctive therapy may be used (see alternative therapy for recurrent pyoderma).

Treatment of Deep Pyoderma

Hair around lesions or on the entire body, if lesions are generalized, should be clipped. Daily antibacterial shampoos (OxyDex) or whirlpool baths (Betadine) help flush out draining tracts and dry up lesions. The antibacterial therapy is chosen based on bacterial culture and sensitivity testing, keeping in mind that chloramphenicol and trimethoprim-sulfonamide frequently are minimally effective despite good in vitro activity. Because staphylococcal organisms are common pathogens in pyodermas, if no staphylococci are isolated reculturing may be warranted. In instances in which two or more organisms are cultured (most commonly *Staphylococcus* spp. plus a gram-negative organism), an antibiotic effective against both or all organisms is chosen. If it is not possible, an antibiotic effective against the staphylococcal organism should be used because the other organisms are often secondary invaders that are eliminated with resolution of the staphylococcal infection. Antibacterial therapy should be continued at full therapeutic dosage until lesions completely resolve, plus an additional 2 weeks: usually a minimum of 6–8 weeks of therapy is required. Any underlying causes should be corrected. If pyoderma recurs despite appropriate antibacterial therapy and no underlying contributing cause can be found, adjunctive therapy may be considered (see alternative therapy for recurrent pyoderma).

Mycobacterial Infections. Treatment of cutaneous tuberculosis is discouraged because of the public health hazard. Surgical excision is the treatment of choice for feline leprosy. Wide surgical excision is also recommended for treatment of atypical mycobacterial infections. However, postoperative wound dehiscence and recurrence, frequently many months after apparent healing, occur commonly. Long-term antibiotic therapy based on sensitivity testing is helpful in some instances but is generally unrewarding. Rarely remission occurs without therapy.

Actinomycosis and Nocardiosis. Treatment for actinomycosis and nocardiosis is similar except for the choice of antibiotics. Both conditions are treated with a combination of local and systemic therapy (see Chapter 16). Lesions are surgically débrided, exudate drained, and the area extensively lavaged. Long-term antibacterial therapy is necessary. High doses of penicillin (80,000–100,000 units/kg/day) are most commonly recommended for treatment of actinomycosis. Erythromycin, cephaloridine, and minocycline have in vitro activity against *Actinomyces* spp. Cephalothin, ampicillin, lincomycin, clindamycin, tetracycline, doxycycline, and chloramphenicol are less active but may still be effective, whereas oxacillin, dicloxacillin, cephalexin, and aminoglycosides are ineffective and should not be used for treating actinomycosis. Nocardiosis is most commonly treated with sulfonamides, especially sulfadiazine (220 mg/kg initial dose, then 110 mg/kg twice daily). Triple sulfa (20 mg/kg three times daily), sulfadimethoxine (25 mg/kg/day), and trimethoprim-sulfonamide (15.4–22.0 mg/

kg twice daily) have also been used. Erythromycin and ampicillin combinations have been shown to be synergistic and have been used successfully to treat nocardiosis in people. Antibacterial therapy should be continued 4 weeks beyond resolution of lesions.

Mycoplasma **and Related Bacteria.** Subcutaneous infections with *Mycoplasma* and related bacteria are unresponsive to all broad-spectrum antibiotics but resolve with tetracycline therapy (22.0 mg/kg three times daily). Wound flushing with tetracycline solution and dressing with tetracycline ointment have been used as adjuncts to systemic tetracycline.

Alternative Therapy of Recurrent Pyoderma. In cases of recurrent pyoderma in which unusual etiologic agents and neoplasia have been ruled out and no underlying cause can be found, immune modulation or long-term once-daily antibiotic therapy may be useful for preventing further recurrences.

A variety of bacterial products have been found to be immunostimulatory. Staphage Lysate (Delmont Labs, Swarthmore, PA) is a sterile staphylococcal bacterin that is used as a nonspecific T-lymphocyte stimulator for antibiotic-responsive recurrent staphylococcal pyodermas. When active pyoderma is present, antibiotics are given concurrently with the bacterin until lesions resolve; then bacterin is used alone. Several protocols can be used.

	Dose (ml SC)	
Week	Superficial Pyoderma	Deep Pyoderma
1	0.1 ml	0.25 ml
2	0.2	0.50
3	0.3	0.75
4	0.4	1.00
5	Then 0.5 weekly	Then 1.0–2.0 weekly

An abbreviated protocol consists of 1.0 ml SC per week for a minimum of 12 weeks. After pyoderma is cleared with antibiotics, bacterin is used as the sole form of therapy and is given every 10–30 days as needed to prevent recurrence. Side effects of Staphage Lysate, which are rare, include reaction at the site of injection, malaise, fever, vomiting, and quivering; one case of polyarthritis has been reported. In a study evaluating the usefulness of Staphage Lysate for treating dogs with idiopathic recurrent superficial pyoderma, dogs receiving antibiotics and 0.5 ml bacterin SC twice weekly had better clinical resolution of lesions than those receiving antibiotics and placebo.

Immunoregulin (ImmunoVet, Inc., Tampa, FL), a suspension of nonviable *Propionibacterium acnes*, is given intravenously to stimulate the reticuloendothelial system. In one study, dogs with chronic recurrent pyoderma were treated with *P. acnes* and antibiotics or with antibiotics alone. Eighty percent (12 of 15) of the dogs treated with antibiotics and *P. acnes* compared to 38% (5 of 13) of the dogs treated with antibiotics alone responded with significant improvement or complete remission of lesions at the end of the 12-week study. Other investigators have found this product to be less efficacious. The current treatment schedule for Immunoregulin consists of two injections per week for the first 2 weeks and one injection per week for weeks 3 through 12. Immunoregulin is administered according to the following dosage: less than 7 kg (15 lb), 0.25 ml; 7 to 20 kg (15–45 lb), 0.50 ml; 21–34 kg (46–75 lb), 1.00 ml; more than 34 kg (75 lb), 2.00 ml. Side effects of Immunoregulin therapy include mild anaphylactoid reactions, including vomiting, anorexia, malaise, and fever. Extravasation of the material can result in local inflammation and swelling.

Levamisole (Levasole, Pitman-Moore) is an anthelmintic drug with nonspecific T-cell stimulating activity when given at a dose of 2.2 mg/kg PO every other day. Accurate dosing is important because a higher or lower dose is immunosuppressive. Antibiotics are administered concurrently until infection is under control. If effective, levamisole is continued for life. Side effects are rare but can include gastrointestinal disturbances, lethargy, neurotoxicity, leukopenia, and drug eruptions.

Cimetidine (Tagamet, SmithKline) is an H_2 histamine receptor blocker that is thought to act as an immune stimulator by reversing T-suppressor cell-mediated immunosuppression in patients with chronic infections. The recommended dose for dogs is 3.0–4.0 mg/kg PO twice daily used in conjunction with antibiotics until the pyoderma resolves. It is then continued alone for a minimum of 12 weeks. If effective, cimetidine is continued for life.

In some instances recurrent pyoderma may be maintained in remission with a single daily dose of antibiotics. Standard therapeutic doses are administered initially during active infection. Once the pyoderma is cleared completely, a single dose of the antibiotic is given once daily. If the pyoderma fails to recur, once-daily antibiotic administration is continued indefinitely.

DERMATOPHYTOSIS

Dermatophytosis is a fungal infection of the skin, hair, or nails that is caused by a dermatophyte. The three major dermatophytes causing disease in dogs and cats are *Microsporum canis*, *Microsporum gypseum*, and *Trichophyton mentagrophytes*.

The lesions of dermatophytosis vary considerably in dogs. Clinical signs may include folliculitis, alopecia, scales, and crusts. The lesions may range from barely visible scaly patches of partial alopecia with little evidence of inflammation to raised, erythematous nodules called kerions. The distribution of the lesions may be focal (especially involving the head and legs), multifocal, or diffuse.

TABLE 3-5. Topical Antifungals for Localized Dermatophytosis

Generic Name	Trade Name
Chlorhexidine ointment	Nolvasan (Fort Dodge)
Povidone-iodine ointment	Betadine (Purdue Frederick)
Thiabendazole	Tresaderm (MSD Agvet)
Miconazole cream or solution	Micatin (Advanced Care) Conofite (Pitman-Moore) Monistat (Ortho)
Haloprogin cream or solution	Halotex (Westwood)
Econazole cream	Spectrazole (Ortho)
Clotrimazole	Lotrimin (Schering) Mycelex (Miles)

In cats, circumscribed patches of alopecia that may be crusty are typical. Other signs may include areas of broken-off hairs, miliary dermatitis, and dermal or subcutaneous nodules. Lesions are often localized, especially on the head and ears, but may also be multifocal or generalized. Many cats are asymptomatic carriers of *M. canis,* and infection may not be noticed until dermatophytosis develops in a human or animal contact.

Because fungi are not a common cause of skin disease in dogs and cats, a definitive diagnosis of dermatophytosis should be made prior to initiating treatment. Diagnostic aids commonly used include ultraviolet Wood's light examination, direct microscopic examination of scales and hairs, histopathologic examination of skin biopsies, and fungal culture. Of these measures, fungal culture is the most reliable method for confirming dermatophyte infection.

Treatment of Localized Dermatophytosis

Standard Therapy. Localized dermatophytosis can be a self-limiting disease, with spontaneous resolution possible. Nevertheless, localized dermatophytosis can also generalize and is potentially contagious to other animals and people. Therapy is indicated. The affected area(s) should be clipped and the lesion(s) treated twice daily with a topical antifungal product. The antifungal product is also applied to the skin and hairs surrounding the lesion to prevent the fungal infection from spreading outward. Treatment is continued 1 week beyond apparent clinical cure. Antifungal products that may be used for treating localized lesions are listed in Table 3-5.

Tresaderm (MSD Agvet) contains neomycin, which occasionally induces contact sensitivity. Povidone-iodine ointment is messy to use, may be irritating to the skin (especially in cats), and may stain the haircoat, carpeting, and furniture.

Alternative Therapy. There are several topical products that are effective against human dermatophytosis but have not been investigated in dogs or cats. Such products include ketoconazole cream (Nizoral, Janssen Pharmaceutica), sulconazole nitrate cream and solution (Exelderm, Westwood Pharmaceuticals); oxiconazole nitrate cream (Oxistat, Glaxo), and naftifine hydrochloride cream (Naftin, Herbert Laboratories). Animals refractory to localized topical treatment should be treated with the regimen used to treat generalized dermatophytosis.

Investigational Therapy. Several imidazole antifungal drugs are undergoing clinical tests but are not yet available for topical use. Such drugs include tioconazole, bifonazole, isoconazole, and enilconazole. Tioconazole has fungicidal activity and may lead to more rapid clearing of infection than the other imidazoles. Terconazole, a triazole antifungal agent, is also in an investigational phase and is not yet available in the United States. It may be more active against dermatophytes than are the imidazoles.

Treatment of Generalized Dermatophytosis

Standard Therapy. Therapy for generalized dermatophytosis involves long-term treatment with both topical and systemic antifungal products. The general objectives of treatment are to: 1) resolve the dermatophytosis; 2) eliminate environmental sources of reinfection; and 3) prevent in-contact animals and people from becoming infected.

Topical Treatment. Affected animals with medium- to long-haired coats should be clipped with a No. 10 cutting blade in order to remove infected hairs. The animal's entire body should be treated with an antifungal solution (dipped) once or twice a week until fungal cultures are negative or 2 weeks past clinical cure (minimum is 4 weeks of treatment). Antifungal products for topical treatment of generalized fungal lesions include lime sulfur solution (Lymdip, DVM), chlorhexidine solution (Nolvasan, Fort Dodge), povidone-iodine solution (Betadine, Purdue Frederick), Captan (Orthocide Garden Fungicide), and sodium hypochlorite (Clorox). Their dilutions for use are listed in Table 3-6. Jewelry should be removed and protective clothing and rubber gloves worn by the individual doing the treatment. The solution is applied to the animal's body with a sponge until the haircoat and skin are completely saturated. The entire body is treated including the face, but contact with the eyes should be avoided. The solution is not rinsed off but is allowed to air-dry on the animal. Povidone-iodine may be irritating to the skin, especially in cats. Captan is a potential contact sensitizer in people; rubber gloves must be worn when it is handled. Sodium hypochlorite may cause yellow discoloration of white haircoats.

Enilconazole solution (Imaverol, Janssen), 20 ml/L of water, is effective for the topical treatment of dermatophytosis in dogs. This product is available in Europe and Canada but is not yet licensed for use in the United States.

TABLE 3-6. Topical Antifungals for Treating Generalized Dermatophytosis

Generic Name	Trade Name	Dilution
Lime sulfur solution	Lymdip (DVM)	25 ml/L water
Chlorhexidine solution	Nolvasan (Fort Dodge)	25 ml/L water
Povidone-iodine solution	Betadine (Purdue Frederick)	42 ml/L water
Captan 50% powder	Orthocide Garden Fungicide	1.5 teaspoons/L water
Sodium hypochlorite	Clorox	100 ml/L water

Systemic Antifungal Therapy. *Griseofulvin* is the systemic drug of choice but should be used in conjunction with topical antifungal therapy. Griseofulvin, which *must* be administered every day, is poorly absorbed unless given with a high fat meal. The particle size of griseofulvin affects absorption, and microsize or ultramicrosize forms should be used. The dosage of microsize griseofulvin (Fulvicin-U/F, Schering) is 50 mg/kg PO once daily or divided into two daily doses. The dose of ultramicrosize griseofulvin (Gris-PEG, Herbert Laboratories) is 30 mg/kg/day. If no response is seen after 2 weeks of treatment, the dosage should be doubled. Treatment is continued until fungal cultures are negative or 2 weeks past clinical cure (minimum 4 weeks).

Griseofulvin is teratogenic and is contraindicated in pregnant animals. Gastrointestinal side effects (nausea, vomiting, diarrhea) may be alleviated by administering the drug with food and dividing the total daily dose into two or three doses. Idiosyncratic reactions in cats have also been reported and include anemia, leukopenia, depression, ataxia, and pruritus. During treatment in cats, CBCs should be monitored every 2 weeks. If idiosyncratic side effects develop, griseofulvin should be discontinued.

Ketoconazole (Nizoral, Janssen Pharmaceutica) is also effective for the treatment of dermatophyte infections but is not licensed for animal use. The administration of ketoconazole, 10–20 mg/kg given once daily or divided into two daily doses, is usually effective. Giving it with food may enhance its absorption. Treatment with ketoconazole must continue until fungal cultures are negative or for 2 weeks beyond clinical cure. Ketoconazole alone (with no coat clipping or topical treatment) has been used successfully to treat generalized dermatophytosis in dogs and cats. The average duration of treatment was 6 weeks.

Anorexia, diarrhea, vomiting, elevated serum liver enzyme levels (alanine aminotransferase, ALT), and icterus have been associated with ketoconazole administration in dogs and cats. If anorexia develops, ketoconazole therapy should be halted and the animal's liver enzyme levels (especially ALT) measured. Therapy is reinstituted at a lower dosage, given on an alternate-day basis, or both after the serum ALT level returns to normal and the animal regains its normal appetite. Giving ketoconazole with food and dividing the total daily dosage into two or three doses may help alleviate signs of anorexia and vomiting. Reversible change in coat color (lightening or graying) during ketoconazole therapy has been observed occasionally in dogs. Ketoconazole is teratogenic in laboratory animals and should not be administered to pregnant animals.

Investigational Therapy. Itraconazole and fluconazole are triazole antifungal agents being developed for oral use. These drugs appear to be at least as effective, with fewer side effects, than ketoconazole.

Environmental Treatment. Because infected hairs that are shed may remain infective for more than a year, animal hairs must be removed from the environment to prevent reinfection. Carpeted areas should be vacuumed at least once weekly. Likewise, hard surfaces (floors, countertops, cages) with which the animal comes in contact must be disinfected at least once a week with sodium hypochlorite (Clorox) diluted 1:10 in water.

Other Precautions. Because dermatophytosis is a zoonotic disease, strict hygiene is important. Infected animals should be kept isolated from noninfected animals and people (especially young children and the elderly) to prevent spread of the disease. When handling infected animals, rubber gloves should be worn and the hands washed afterward. All in-contact animals should be examined, so mildly affected animals and asymptomatic carriers can be identified and treated. Exposed, noninfected animals can be treated prophylactically with griseofulvin, 50 mg/kg daily, for 10–14 days. Cats that are asymptomatic carriers should be treated with the same regimen used to treat animals with generalized dermatophytosis.

ECTOPARASITISM

Ectoparasites are common causes of skin disease in dogs and cats. The effects of ectoparasites vary from minor irritation to severe generalized skin disease. In addition, secondary systemic diseases can be transmitted by ectoparasites to the animal host and associated humans. The diagnosis of ectoparasitism is based on the history, appearance, and distribution of lesions and finding parasites on physical examination, skin scrapings, or skin biopsy. In all cases, the goal of therapy is to eliminate the ectoparasite from the animal and its environment while minimizing exposure of the animal, owner, and environment to potentially toxic chemicals. Although hundreds of parasites can affect dogs and cats, only a small number are common problems and are discussed here: cheyletiellosis, demodicosis, fleas, notoedric mange, otodectic mange, pediculosis, sarcoptic mange, and trombiculidiasis.

Cheyletiellosis ("Walking Dandruff")

Standard Therapy. *Cheyletiella* sp. mites are usually easily killed by most parasiticides, including those routinely used for fleas (Table 3-7). Dips, shampoos, or powders containing lime sulfur, pyrethroids, carbamates, or organophosphates can be used for treating dogs. Cats and rabbits should be treated with lime sulfur, pyrethrins, or carbaryl. The affected animal and all in-contact animals should be treated once weekly for 4–8 weeks. An antiseborrheic shampoo prior to treatment may be useful if hair and skin are excessively oily (see section on seborrhea). Environmental control is important to prevent reinfestation. The premises should be cleaned and an insecticide applied (Table 3-8).

Alternative Therapy. Cheyletiellosis in dogs has also been treated successfully with ivermectin. A dose of 0.2 mg/kg SC repeated in 3 weeks was effective, and no adverse reactions were seen. Ivermectin is not licensed for this use in dogs. Because *Cheyletiella* sp. mites are usually susceptible to most common insecticides, ivermectin is not recommended except in kennel situations where many dogs are involved or in unusual cases that are resistant to standard forms of therapy.

Canine Localized Demodicosis

Localized demodicosis is a mild disease, with 90% of cases resolving spontaneously. There is little evidence to indicate that treatment prevents development of generalized demodicosis in the small number of cases of localized demodicosis that ultimately become generalized. However, if therapy is considered necessary, 1% rotenone ointment (Goodwinol ointment, Goodwinol Products), benzoyl peroxide gel (OxyDex Gel, DVM; Pyoben Gel, Allerderm), or benzyl benzoate lotion can be rubbed into the lesion(s) once daily. Treatment usually produces an initial irritation of lesions that should not be interpreted as worsening of the disease.

Because immunosuppression is involved in the development of demodicosis, corticosteroids must be avoided. Stress should be minimized by providing a good diet, preventing infectious disease with immunizations, and eliminating internal parasites. The dog should be reevaluated in 4–8 weeks. If skin lesions have increased in number or size or increased numbers or immature forms of *Demodex* are seen in skin scrapings, the disease should be treated as a case of generalized demodicosis.

Generalized Canine Demodicosis

Generalized demodicosis is a severe disease that is difficult and expensive to treat. However, the long-term prognosis has improved, and therapy has become less complicated and toxic with the advent of the mitacide amitraz

TABLE 3-7. Examples of Insecticides for Dogs and Cats

Active Ingredient (Class)	Trade Name	Manufacturer	Dogs	Cats
			Approved For	
Dips				
Pyrethrin (B)	Hartz 2 in 1 Flea & Tick Dip	Hartz Mountain	X	X
Rotenone-pyrethrin (B)	DuraKyl Pet Dip*	DVM	X	
d-Limonene (B)	Flea Stop	Pet Chemicals	X†	X‡
	Hill's VIP Organic Dips*	Hill's Pet Products	X†	X‡
Permethrin (SP)	Expar 3.2% EC*	Coopers Animal Health	X	
Malathion (OP)	Sergeant's Flea & Tick Dip	A. H. Robins	X	
	Adams Flea Off Dip*	Adams Veterinary Research Labs	X	X
Phosmet (OP)	Paramite*	Vet-Kem	X	X
Chlorpyrifos (OP)	Duratrol*	Animal Care Products/3M	X	
Powders				
Synergized pyrethrin-carbamate	Adams Flea Off Dust*	Adams Veterinary Research Labs	X	X
	Diryl Flea Powder for Dogs and Cats	Pitman-Moore	X	X
Carbamate	Wellcome Flea Powder for Cats	Coopers Animal Health		X
	Sevin	Carson Chemicals/ Union Carbide	X†	X†
Supona (OP)	Dermaton Dust*	Coopers Animal Health	X	
Sprays				
Synergized pyrethrin (B)	Hartz 2 in 1 Flea & Tick Killer	Hartz Mountain	X	X
Synergized pyrethrin Alcohol base (B)	Adams Flea Off Mist*	Adams Veterinary Research Labs	X	X
Water base (B)	Mycodex Aqua-Spray*	Beecham Labs	X	X
Synergized, microencapsulated pyrethrin (B)	Sectrol Two Way Pet Spray*	Animal Care Products/3M	X	X

(*continued*)

TABLE 3-7. *(continued)*

Active Ingredient (Class)	Trade Name	Manufacturer	Approved For	
			Dogs	Cats
Synthetic pyrethroid	Rid A Flea	Kenco	X	X
Synthetic pyrethroid-carbamate	Sergeant's Pump Flea & Tick Spray	A. H. Robins	X	X
Carbamate	Sergeant's Pump Cat Flea & Tick Spray	A. H. Robins		X
Dichlorvos (OP)	Hartz 2 in 1 Flea & Tick Spray with deodorant	Hartz Mountain	X	X
Synergized pyrethrin-carbamate	Sulfodene Scratchex Dog and Cat Spray	Combe Inc.	X	X
Pyrethrin-methoprene	Ovitrol Plus*	Vet-Kem	X	X
Foams				
Synergized, microencapsulated pyrethrin	Sectrol foam*	Animal Care Products/3M	X	X

B = botanical; OP = organophosphate.
*Available only from licensed veterinarians or pest control operators.
†Also safe for puppies.
‡Also safe for kittens.

(Mitaban, Upjohn). Even dogs that cannot be completely cured may be kept asymptomatic by intermittent dips continued indefinitely.

A hereditary predisposition to juvenile-onset generalized demodicosis is suspected based on the fact that certain breeds and lines of dogs have an increased tendency to develop the disease. For this reason, the American Academy of Veterinary Dermatology recommends that any dog developing generalized demodicosis be neutered. In addition, estrus or pregnancy may trigger relapses that can be prevented by neutering recovered females. In older dogs, underlying immunosuppressive factors are frequently associated with generalized demodicosis. Such conditions as endogenous or exogenous hyperglucocorticism, neoplasia, diabetes mellitus, or liver disease must also be controlled in order to treat the demodicosis successfully. *Systemic corticosteroids must always be avoided in dogs with demodicosis.*

Standard Therapy. Currently, the only use of amitraz approved by the U.S. Food and Drug Administration is at a concentration of 0.025% applied every 2 weeks. This concentration is prepared by diluting one vial (10.6 ml) in 2 gallons of warm water or one-half vial (5.3 ml) in 1 gallon of water immediately before each use.

TABLE 3-8. Examples of Insecticides for Environmental Flea Control

Active Ingredient	Class	Trade Name	Manufacturer
Pyrethrin	B	Various	—
Microencapsulated synergized pyrethrin	B	Sectrol*	Animal Care Products/3M
Resmethrin	SP	Rid A Flea	Kenco
Fenvalerate	SP	VIP Concentrated Yard Spray	Hill's Pet Chemicals
Carbaryl	C	Sevin	Union Carbide
Bendiocarb	C	Ficam*	W. Fisons Inc.
Propoxur	C	Baygon*	Mobay Chemical Corp.
Malathion	OP	Various	—
Chlorpyrifos	OP	Rid A Bug	Kenco
		Vet-Kem Yard & Kennel Spray*	Vet-Kem
		Dursban	Dow Pharmaceuticals
Microencapsulated chlorpyrifos	OP	Duratrol Yard and Kennel Flea Spray Concentrate*	Animal Care Products/3M
Diazinon	OP	Spectracide	Ciba-Geigy
Microencapsulated diazinon	OP	Knox Out 2FM*	Pennwalt
Propetamphos	OP	Safrotin*	Sandoz Inc.
Dichlorvos	OP	Various	—
Methoprene	IGR	Precor,* Siphotrol*	Vet-Kem
Fenoxycarb	IGR	Torus 2E	Maag
Synergized pyrethrin-methoprene	B, IGR	Siphotrol Premise Spray*	Vet-Kem
Permethrin-methoprene	SP, IGR	Siphotrol Plus Fogger*	Vet-Kem
Chlorpyrifos-methoprene	OP, IGR	Duratrol Household Flea Spray*	Animal Care Products/3M
Synergized pyrethrin-chlorpyrifos-methoprene	B, OP, IGR	Siphotrol Plus II House Treatment*	Vet-Kem

B = botanical; SP = synthetic pyrethroid; C = carbamate; OP = organophosphate; IGR = insect growth regulator.
*Available only from licensed veterinarians or pest control operators.

Prior to the first dip, the haircoat should be clipped on medium- and long-haired dogs. The dog should be shampooed to remove scales and crusts using a shampoo containing benzoyl peroxide (OxyDex, DVM; Pyoben, Allerderm). Benzoyl peroxide is recommended because it is antibacterial and has follicular flushing activity, which improves penetration of the mitacide. The dog is towel- or blow-dried, and then freshly prepared dip is sponged onto the entire body. The dog is allowed to air-dry. Response to therapy is monitored by skin scrapings prior to each dip. Therapy should be continued for 4 weeks after skin scrapings from multiple sites become negative.

The ears of all dogs with generalized demodicosis should be swabbed for mites because concurrent demodectic otitis externa occurs commonly. Demodectic otitis can be treated with rotenone (Canex, Pitman-Moore) in mineral oil (1:3) daily until no mites are found on subsequent swabs and then continued once weekly for the duration of the amitraz dips.

Antibacterial therapy is indicated in all cases with secondary bacterial infection. The choice of antibacterial agent should be based on sensitivity testing, and therapy should be continued for a minimum of 4 weeks.

The most common side effect with amitraz therapy is transient sedation, which may last up to 72 hours. It occurs most often in toy breeds, and using half the recommended concentration for the first two treatments has been suggested to minimize adverse reactions. Anorexia, polyuria, polydipsia, transient pruritus, hypothermia, increased glucose concentration, seizures, ataxia, and rare deaths also may occur.

Alternative Therapy. Although approved for use only every 14 days, amitraz has been found to be much more effective when applied weekly. Consequently, some veterinary dermatologists prefer to treat all dogs with generalized demodicosis with the approved concentration of 0.025% amitraz but at weekly intervals. If skin scrapings contain increased numbers of mites after four to six treatments, the concentration of amitraz can be doubled.

Demodectic otitis can be treated with amitraz in mineral oil (1:9) instilled into the ear canals once or twice weekly. Mitaban diluted in mineral oil may be stable for up to 1 week but is not approved for this use.

Demodectic pododermatitis is especially difficult to treat and may not resolve with approved therapy. Mitaban can be applied to the feet once or twice during the interval between whole body dips. Each treatment should consist of soaking the feet in dip for 10 minutes. Another means of treating demodectic pododermatitis consists of applying a solution of 0.2 ml amitraz per 30 ml mineral oil every 3 days to the feet. Neither of these uses of amitraz is approved.

In some dogs, amitraz treatment results in resolution of skin lesions but does not completely eliminate the mites. In such dogs, lesions can be kept in remission by applying amitraz at 2- to 8-week intervals indefinitely.

Ivermectin has not been found to be effective for treatment of demodicosis.

Feline Demodicosis

Feline demodicosis is a rare disease that is frequently associated with underlying immunosuppressive factors such as diabetes mellitus, feline leukemia virus, systemic lupus erythematosus, toxoplasmosis, and feline immunodeficiency virus.

Standard Therapy. Localized demodicosis can be treated with once-daily application of rotenone ointment (Goodwinol ointment, Goodwinol Products). Generalized demodicosis in cats has been treated successfully with phosmet (Paramite, Vet-Kem), malathion, and lime sulfur dips applied at weekly intervals until skin scrapes are negative.

Alternative Therapy. Amitraz is not licensed for use in cats in the United States, but it has been used successfully to treat feline demodicosis. Application of 0.025% amitraz to affected areas twice weekly and whole body treatment with 0.0125% amitraz at weekly intervals was effective in one cat with localized demodicosis and one cat with generalized demodicosis, respectively. Side effects from the first whole body dip included mild sedation, salivation, and hiding for approximately 12 hours.

Fleas

Effective flea control requires a coordinated effort involving treatment of all animals as well as their indoor and outdoor environment. Hundreds of flea control products are available that can lead to confusion regarding which products are best. However, with a basic understanding of the major classes of insecticides, it is relatively simple to design an effective and safe flea control program. No single standardized program is appropriate for every animal.

The general goals of a flea control program are to keep the animal as free of fleas as possible, to minimize environmental contamination and human and animal exposure to toxic insecticides, and to prevent development of resistance.

Classes of Insecticides. The most commonly used insecticide is *pyrethrin*, which is a natural extract of chrysanthemums. Pyrethrin kills fleas quickly but has little residual activity because it is rapidly degraded by ultraviolet light. It has low potential for mammalian toxicity and is approved for use on both dogs and cats. Pyrethrin is found in many formulations, including shampoos, sprays, dusts, dips, foggers, and premise spray. It is frequently combined with other insecticides to increase the residual activity of the product. Newer pyrethrins have been synergized and microencapsulated to improve residual activity. Development of resistance to pyrethrin is thought to be rare.

Pyrethroids are synthetic compounds that resemble pyrethrin structurally but are more stable on exposure to sunlight and therefore have longer residual activity. Pyrethroids are similar to pyrethrins in action and toxicity. Examples include permethrin, resmethrin, fenvalerate, and allethrin. Pyrethroids are used in premise and animal products. Some pyrethroid products are approved for use on dogs and cats, whereas others are safe only for dogs. The label of a pyrethroid-containing product should be read carefully prior to use.

d-*Limonene*, another botanical insecticide, is derived from citrus peel. It is toxic to all stages of the flea, including the egg. *d*-Limonene has been incorporated into shampoos, dips, and sprays approved for use on both dogs and cats. The residual activity of *d*-limonene is less than that of synergized microencapsulated pyrethrins. Adverse effects in cats include mild hypersalivation and muscle tremors. At 5–15 times the recommended concentration, hypersalivation, ataxia, muscle tremors, and hypothermia become increasingly more severe but resolve by 6 hours after treatment. No adverse effects have been reported in dogs.

Two groups of potent insecticides, carbamates and organophosphates, are *cholinesterase inhibitors* that have the potential for serious adverse reactions. Carbamates are found in shampoos, powders, dips, and sprays for use on dogs and cats as well as in preparations for indoor and outdoor use. Carbaryl (Sevin, Union Carbide) is the most frequently used carbamate and is most commonly used as a dust. Bendiocarb (Ficam) is commonly used by professional exterminators for premise control of fleas. It is safe, odorless, and nonstaining; and it has good residual activity even after vacuuming a treated carpet.

Organophosphates, the second group of cholinesterase inhibitors, are unstable and do not persist in the environment. They are primarily adulticidal and are among the most toxic insecticides. They should not be used on puppies and kittens, and most should not be used on cats. The two exceptions are malathion and phosmet (Paramite, Vet-Kem), which are relatively safe for use on adult cats. Chlorfenvinphos (Supona) is formulated into dips and powders for dogs and premise products. Chlorpyrifos (Dursban) is an exception to strictly adulticidal activity because it is also larvicidal. It is incorporated into sprays and dips for dogs and premise products, and a microencapsulated form with long residual activity is available for treatment of the indoors and outdoors. Diazinon, an organophosphate with long residual activity and little tendency to induce resistance, is used in various formulations for indoor and outdoor premise use. Two organophosphate compounds, fenthion and cythioate, are used for their systemic insecticidal effects.

Signs of acute carbamate and organophosphate intoxication are similar: salivation, defecation, urination, emesis, weakness, muscle tremors, myosis, ataxia, and convulsions. Respiratory paralysis is the ultimate cause of death.

The *insect growth regulators* methoprene and fenoxycarb are synthetic compounds that mimic a juvenile hormone and thereby prevent maturation of larval fleas to adults. They are ovicidal and larvicidal but do not kill adults. For this reason, they are frequently combined with an adulticide for immediate flea kill. Both compounds are safe and essentially nontoxic to mammals. They are stable in an indoor environment and have long residual activity (60–90 days in combination products). Methoprene is degraded by ultraviolet light and is therefore useful only for indoor premise treatment, whereas fenoxycarb is relatively photostable and can be used outdoors. Methoprene is used in foggers and premise sprays alone or in combination with synergized pyrethrin, permethrin, or chlorpyriphos. A methoprene-pyrethrin spray has been approved for use on dogs and cats (Ovitrol Plus, Vet-Kem). Fenoxycarb was available originally only to professional exterminators, but it has now been marketed in combination with adulticides in foggers and premise sprays for sale through veterinarians and over the counter (EctoGard House & Carpet Spray and Fogger, Fermenta Animal Health; PT 400 Ultraban, Enviromed).

Treatment of Environment. Because most of the flea's life cycle is spent off the host, the key to successful flea control is effective treatment of the environment, both indoors and outdoors. Unless the environment is treated simultaneously with the animal, the yard and house serve as constant sources of reinfestation that no amount of insecticide applied to the animal can stem. Mechanical cleaning and insecticide application (see Table 3-8) are equally important aspects of environmental treatment.

In the house, all hard floors should be mopped and any blankets or rugs on which the animal sleeps should be washed weekly at the hottest setting. Vacuuming carpets regularly removes larvae and eggs as well as organic material that can serve as food for flea larvae. Because the vacuum cleaner bag provides an ideal environment for flea development, it should be discarded immediately after use to prevent reinfestation. Putting insecticide powder or portions of flea collars into the bag can prevent flea development, but this practice can also release additional and unwanted quantities of insecticide into the environment when the vacuum cleaner is used again later. Steam-cleaning carpets is the most reliable means of killing flea eggs. Difficult to reach areas of the house, such as floor cracks, floorboards, under furniture, and closets, should be sprayed or dusted. The major portion of the house can be treated with carpet shampoos, aerosol sprays, hand-held pump sprays, spray tanks, or foggers. A combination product consisting of larvicidal and adulticidal ingredients is best. In households with crawling infants, the safest insecticides are pyrethrin and growth regulators. Insecticide application should be repeated twice more at 14- to 21-day intervals. The second and third treatments need contain only an adulticide. After this initial treatment, the house should be treated periodically as needed, e.g., every 6–8 weeks in the southeastern United States. In regions where the temperature is conducive for flea breeding all year long, insecticide use is virtually continual and can result in development of resistance. To prevent resistance, insecticides should be rotated routinely.

In the yard or kennel, all areas in which the animal rests should be cleaned. Areas protected from sunlight and where the soil is moist provide optimum conditions for flea development. Such areas should be mowed or raked to remove organic debris. Animals should be prevented access to areas under a house, porch, or trailer, which are optimal flea breeding grounds. Shady areas of the yard or kennel should be treated with insecticide sprays, dusts, or granules. The reapplication rate depends on the weather and levels of reinfestation. During periods of rainy weather it may be necessary to treat every 1–2 weeks, whereas in dry weather the residual activity may last for more than a month.

Standard Treatment of the Animal. For best results, flea control on the animal must be done in concert with environmental treatment. All animals in a household must be treated to eliminate all sources of reinfestation. The specific class and formulation of insecticide depends on the particular animal, degree of infestation, and owner's personality (Table 3-7). To prevent overexposure to a single class of insecticide, which could lead to toxicity, a different class of insecticide should be used for treatment of animals and the environment.

When environmental control is thorough, nonresidual treatments, such as a pyrethrin-based shampoo, may be sufficient. Shampoos kill fleas only during the time they are on the animal. Once rinsed off, the shampoos have no residual activity. In addition, the lather must remain in contact with the skin for an adequate period to be effectively insecticidal. Contact time varies with each product and can be determined from the label. A pyrethrin-based shampoo can be used on severely infested puppies and kittens.

Sprays and foams containing pyrethrins, microencapsulated pyrethrins, synthetic pyrethroids, or *d*-limonene have short residual activity. Water-based and alcohol-based sprays are available. Water-based flea sprays are less expensive, are less irritating to skin, take longer to dry, and kill fleas slowly. Alcohol-based flea sprays are more expensive, have more odor, are flammable, and are drying and irritating to damaged skin; but they have rapid flea killing action. Foams may be better tolerated by nervous dogs and cats than sprays. Sprays and foams should not be used on puppies and kittens less than 2 months old.

Powders or dusts have slightly more residual activity than sprays and foam; but to be effective, the powder must be worked thoroughly through the haircoat down to the skin. An old sock filled with the insecticidal powder rubbed back and forth through the hair works well. Dusting must be repeated two or three times per week. It is messy, drying to the skin, and irritating to mucous membranes. Pyrethrin and carbamates are the most common insecticides in dusts. Carbaryl (Sevin) is the most frequently used carbamate. Our suggested usage is as follows: 10% concentration for adult dogs, 5% concentration for adult cats, and 2.5% concentration (diluted with cornstarch) for puppies and kittens. Carbaryl should not be used on kittens younger than 4 weeks, nursing puppies, or pregnant or lactating animals.

When environmental control is poor or the animals roam freely, products with more residual activity are necessary. Products with the longest residual activity are dips. Dips are insecticidal solutions that are sponged onto the entire body and allowed to dry on the hair and skin without rinsing. Dips penetrate all haircoats and have the most effective immediate action. If the hair is matted, dirty, or greasy or the skin is infected, the animal should be washed first with an appropriate shampoo. Most dips must be repeated every 7–10 days, but the product label must be consulted for the recommended rate of application. Not all dips are safe for use on cats, and the label should be read before any dip is used on these animals. Dips are also not safe for puppies and kittens younger than 4 months. When used for extended periods, dips are drying to the skin and hair. This drying action can be counteracted by adding bath oil to the dip. Skin-So-Soft® bath oil (Avon Products) is a good choice because it not only lubricates the skin but also repels fleas. Although inadequate as the sole method of flea control, it has significant flea repellent activity and is a useful adjunct to insecticide treatment. Addition of 1.5 ounce of Skin-So-Soft® per gallon of dip provides an optimum compromise between flea repellency and oiliness.

Two systemic organophosphates are available for flea control. Both are approved for use in dogs only. Fenthion is a topically applied organophosphate that is systemically absorbed and kills the flea after it takes a blood meal. It is an oily liquid with a strong, unpleasant odor. The product approved for use on the dog (Pro-Spot, Haver-Mobay) is used at a dose of 4.0–8.0 mg/kg every 2 weeks, which appears to be safe but not very effective. The second systemic organophosphate approved for flea control on dogs is cythioate (Proban, Haver-Mobay). The dose is 3.0 mg/kg PO twice weekly. It is not approved for use in cats. Effective blood levels are maintained for only 6–12 hours after administration, and the flea must bite the dog to be killed. Neither of these products has been effective in our experience.

Mechanical removal of fleas with a flea comb (32 teeth per inch) is useful for young puppies and kittens or for animals whose owners want to minimize or eliminate chemical use. Flea combs are appropriate only for short haired dogs and cats. The animal must be combed daily or every other day and any fleas combed out killed by immersing in alcohol.

Flea collars, ultrasonic flea collars, brewer's yeast, B complex vitamins, elemental sulfur, garlic, and hyposensitization are of questionable efficacy. Flea collars are ineffective and cause systemic toxicosis and contact irritation in some individuals. A broad spectrum of ultrasound has not been found to repel fleas, affect their jumping rates, or interfere with flea reproduction or development; and there are no published data to indicate that ultrasonic collars work. Controlled studies using brewer's yeast, B vitamins, and elemental sulfur have shown them to be ineffective as flea repellents. Similarly, hyposensitization has been found to be ineffective for treatment of flea-bite hypersensitivity.

Adjunctive therapy for flea infestation includes antiseborrheic shampoos for seborrhea (see section on seborrhea), antibacterial shampoos and systemic antibiotics (see section on pyoderma), and antihistamines and corticosteroids for severe pruritus and flea-bite allergy (see section on allergy).

Alternative Treatment of the Animal. Spotton (Bayvet), which is a 20% (weight/volume) solution of fenthion for control of *Hypoderma* and lice on cattle, has been found to be an effective means of flea control for dogs when used at a dose of 20.0 mg/kg applied directly to the skin of the back every 2–3 weeks. A dose of 10.0 mg/kg Spotton has been used on cats. This product has a high potential for toxicity and is not approved for use in either dogs or cats. Reported adverse effects include animal deaths, weight loss, anorexia, depression, and muscle tremors of the head and neck. Muscle tremors are especially common in small dogs weighing less than 7 kg. Signs usually resolve within 6–8 weeks of discontinuing fenthion use but recur if fenthion treatment is resumed. Peripheral neuropathies have been reported in people exposed to Spotton. At the suggested dose of 20.0 mg/kg, fenthion is microfilaricidal, and heartworm status should be evaluated prior to instituting treatment. Because of the potential for serious side effects in both animals and humans, we use this product only in exceptional cases.

Notoedric Mange (Feline Scabies)

The hair should be clipped from affected areas and the cat bathed to remove scales and crusts if scabies is present. The least toxic parasiticidal agent is 2–3% lime sulfur dip. It is the treatment of choice for young kittens or pregnant or debilitated cats. The only drawback to lime sulfur is a residual odor of rotten eggs left on the hair. Malathion and phosmet (Paramite, Vet-Kem) dips are also effective and relatively safe in adult cats. The dip is applied once weekly until lesions resolve and then is continued for an additional 1–2 weeks. All in-contact animals, including dogs and pet rabbits, should also be treated. The environment should be cleaned to prevent reinfestation; and in instances of multiple cat involvement, such as in a cattery, the premises should be treated with an insecticide (Table 3-8). If pruritus is intense, systemic corticosteroids can be administered (e.g., 20 mg methylprednisolone acetate per cat SC or IM). Systemic antibiotics should be given to cats with secondary bacterial infection (see section on pyoderma).

Treatments that have been reported to be effective but are not approved for use in cats are 0.025% amitraz solution (Mitaban, Upjohn) applied once or twice at a one-week interval and ivermectin used at a dosage of 0.2 mg/kg PO or SC twice at 2-week intervals.

Otodectic Mange (Ear Mites, Otoacariasis)

See the section on otitis externa in this chapter for a detailed description of therapy for ear mites. The affected animal as well as all in-contact animals should be treated. Ears should be cleaned with a ceruminolytic agent prior to instilling a parasiticide. Effective treatments include rotenone (Canex, Pitman-Moore) (must be diluted 1:3 with mineral oil for use in cats), pyrethrins

(OtiCare-M, ARC Laboratories; Cerumite, Evsco Pharmaceutical), thiabenda-zole (Tresaderm, Merck Sharpe & Dohme), and carbaryl (Mitox, Norden Laboratories). Because this mite can survive on other parts of the body, a topical flea preparation should be applied once weekly for 4 weeks (Table 3-7).

An alternative method of treatment is ivermectin at a dose of 0.2 or 0.4 mg/kg SC given one time. Ivermectin is not approved for use in dogs or cats at this dose.

Pediculosis (Lice)

Lice are easily killed with most insecticides, including lime sulfur, pyrethrins, or carbamates. The infected animal and all in-contact animals should be treated once weekly for 4 weeks with an insecticidal shampoo, dip, or powder. The premises, animal's bedding, combs, brushes, and collars should be cleaned. Appropriate supportive care may be necessary for severely debilitated animals.

Sarcoptic Mange (Canine Scabies)

Standard Therapy. The animal affected by canine scabies should be clipped and bathed with an antiseborrheic shampoo (see section on seborrhea). An acaricidal preparation should be applied to the entire body, including the face. Various dips are effective, and each should be applied once weekly until lesions resolve; treatment continues for an additional 2 weeks (minimum 5 weeks). The least toxic product is 2–4% lime sulfur. It is safe for use on young, sick, or debilitated dogs. Additional properties of lime sulfur useful for treatment of sarcoptic mange are its antipruritic and antibacterial actions. Lindane should not be used on puppies or cats. Phosmet (Paramite, Vet-Kem) and malathion can also be used. Lindane dips (ParaDip, Haver-Lockhart; GammaRx, Carson Chemicals) are effective when used at a concentration 25% over the recom-mended level.

If pruritus is severe, systemic corticosteroids (e.g., prednisolone 0.55–1.10 mg/kg/day) may be given for 2 or 3 days. Systemic antibiotics should be admin-istered if secondary pyoderma is present (see section on pyoderma). In long-standing cases, the dog may become debilitated and require supportive care.

All in-contact animals should also be treated. Although cats are rarely infected with canine scabies, they can harbor the mite for short periods and should be treated with a safe acaricide (e.g., 2–3% lime sulfur). *Sarcoptes scabiei* is highly contagious, and the environment, including cages, crates, collars, and grooming equipment, must be cleaned thoroughly and treated with an insec-ticide (e.g., malathion).

Alternative Therapy. Amitraz (Mitaban, Upjohn) is effective against sar-coptic mange when applied at a concentration of 0.025% (5.3 ml/gallon of water) and repeated 2 weeks later. Mitaban is not licensed for treatment of sarcoptic mange in dogs. Ivermectin at a dose of 0.2 mg/kg SC or PO and repeated in 2 weeks also eliminates *Sarcoptes* mites but is not licensed for this use in dogs. Ivermectin at this dose is frequently toxic to collie dogs and should not be used in this breed. Signs of ivermectin-induced toxicosis in sensitized or overdosed dogs are salivation, vomiting, ataxia, tremors, depression, disorientation, recumbency, coma, and death. Because ivermectin is microfilaricidal, heartworm status must be evaluated prior to administering the drug.

Trombiculidiasis (Chiggers, Harvest Mites)

Chiggers are easily eliminated with one or two applications of an insecticidal shampoo, dip, or powder. Lime sulfur and pyrethrins are safe and effective. If the ears are involved, thiabendazole drops (Tresaderm) should be instilled into the ears. Tresaderm also contains dexamethasone, which is helpful in controlling pruritus. If pruritus is severe and generalized, systemic corticosteroids can be given for 2 or 3 days (prednisolone 0.55–1.10 mg/kg/day). Contaminated areas must be avoided to prevent reinfestation of the animal.

SEBORRHEA

Seborrhea is characterized by increased scaling of the skin with or without increased sebum production. Seborrheic skin disease is much more common in dogs than in cats. Seborrhea in the dog may be characterized by dry skin with excessive scaling (seborrhea sicca), greasy and malodorous skin (seborrhea oleosa), or a combination of the two. Inflammation and erythema (seborrheic dermatitis) may also be present. In dogs, seborrheic skin disease is almost always secondary to some other problem, so a thorough search for an underlying cause should always be made. Seborrhea may be associated with endocrine disorders (especially hypothyroidism and sex hormone imbalances), dietary deficiencies, malabsorption-maldigestion disorders, intestinal parasitism, ectoparasitism, dermatophytosis, allergic dermatoses, environmental causes (low humidity, excessive bathing), autoimmune skin diseases, cutaneous lymphosarcoma, and pyoderma. Other disorders that may be associated with seborrhea in dogs include vitamin A-responsive dermatosis (reported in cocker spaniels, schnauzers, and Labrador retrievers), zinc-responsive dermatosis, and granulomatous sebaceous adenitis.

Vitamin A-responsive dermatosis is characterized by generalized scaling with focal, thick, inflamed, crusty lesions and frond-like keratinous plugs.

Zinc deficiency may occur in any breed dog, but Siberian huskies, malamutes, Doberman pinschers, and Great Danes are predisposed. It is most common in dogs less than 1 year of age, although older animals may also be affected. Affected dogs develop a crusting dermatosis that typically involves skin around the eyes and mouth, ears, and pressure points. Hyperkeratotic footpads, secondary pyoderma, pyrexia, lymphadenopathy, anorexia, and pitting edema of the limbs may also be present.

Secondary skin infection with the yeast *Malassezia pachydermatis* may contribute to or cause seborrhea. Although a normal inhabitant of skin, *Malassezia* may overgrow in dogs that have been on chronic antibiotic therapy for recurrent pyodermas associated with allergic or seborrheic skin disease. A tentative diagnosis is made cytologically by finding budding peanut- or footprint-shaped yeasts of *Malassezia* in direct smears or skin scrapings taken from affected skin. A definitive diagnosis is made histologically by finding numerous yeast organisms in crusts, stratum corneum, or hair follicles.

Treatment

Standard Therapy. Therapy of secondary seborrhea involves symptomatically treating the skin condition while correcting the underlying cause. In cases where no underlying cause can be found (primary idiopathic seborrhea), the skin condition is controlled with long-term symptomatic management.

The general objectives are to 1) reduce scales, crusts, and grease; 2) reduce body odor; 3) control secondary pyoderma; and 4) reduce pruritus. These objectives may be met by identifying and eliminating any underlying cause, weight reduction if the animal is obese, dietary changes including dietary fat supplementation, topical antiseborrheic therapy, antibiotic therapy, and corticosteroid therapy.

Specific Therapies. The treatment of such underlying causes as endocrine disorders, malabsorption-maldigestion, endoparasites, ectoparasites, dermatophytosis, allergic diseases, autoimmune skin diseases, and pyoderma are discussed elsewhere in this textbook.

Vitamin A-Responsive Dermatosis. The treatment is vitamin A supplementation, 10,000 units PO once daily for small- to medium-sized dogs such as cocker spaniels and 50,000 units PO once daily for large dogs such as Labrador retrievers. Improvement is usually seen within 1–2 months, although treatment is continued for life. To date, vitamin A toxicosis has not been reported in dogs receiving long-term vitamin A therapy for this disorder.

Zinc-Responsive Dermatosis. Treatment of zinc-responsive dermatosis includes correcting any dietary imbalance. Diets high in calcium or cereal are contraindicated because they inhibit zinc absorption. Oversupplementation with minerals and vitamins may also prevent normal zinc absorption. Zinc supplementation should be instituted with zinc sulfate in large breed dogs, 100–200 mg PO twice daily, or zinc methionine (Zinpro, Norden) in any sized dog, 1.7 mg/kg PO once daily. Zinc supplementation can be discontinued at maturity in some dogs; in others, relapse occurs if zinc supplementation is stopped.

Oversupplementation with zinc may result in vomiting or diarrhea. Because hemolytic anemia from zinc toxicosis has been reported in puppies that ingested new pennies, care should be taken to make sure that dogs are not oversupplemented with zinc.

Granulomatous Sebaceous Adenitis. The prognosis for cure of granulomatous sebaceous adenitis is guarded to poor. In some dogs, treatment with prednisone or prednisolone, 2.2 mg/kg PO once daily, controls the skin problem. If improvement is seen, the corticosteroid dosage is then tapered to the lowest possible needed. Isotretinoin (Accutane, Roche Dermatologics), 1 mg/kg PO once daily, has been reported to be effective in some dogs.

Malassezia *Skin Infection.* Topical treatment with 1% selenium disulfide shampoo (Vet-Kem) once or twice weekly and ketoconazole (Nizoral, Janssen Pharmaceutica), 10 mg/kg PO daily, should result in dramatic improvement of *Malassezia* skin infection within 2 weeks. If only partial improvement is seen and no yeasts are found on follow-up skin scrapings, an underlying or concurrent skin problem (e.g., pyoderma, allergic dermatitis) is present that needs to be managed.

One of us (L.M.) treated a West Highland white terrier puppy with itraconazole, 10 mg/kg PO daily, for *Malassezia* skin infection secondary to idiopathic seborrhea. The *Malassezia* skin infection was resolved after 2 weeks of therapy. No topical therapy was used.

Adjunctive Therapies. *Weight Reduction.* In obese dogs moisture and surface lipids accumulate in skin folds and frictional areas (e.g., axillae) and may aggravate seborrheic skin disease. Thus weight reduction is indicated in overweight seborrheic dogs.

Dietary Changes. The diet should be changed in dogs that are fed generic dog foods (non-American Association of Feed Control Officials approved dog foods such as some store brands), semimoist dog foods, dry dog foods, or table food. Generic dog food may not be balanced; and it may contain substances that inhibit absorption of nutrients or food substances that are not easily digested. Dogs should not be fed semimoist dog foods because, for unknown reasons, they often aggravate seborrheic skin conditions. Dry dog foods are often low in fat; when they are used, dietary fat supplementation should be instituted (see below). Home cooked diets are not recommended unless balanced for vitamins, protein, fat, and minerals.

Interestingly, dogs that are deficient in dietary fat may have either dry or greasy haircoats. Thus dietary fat supplementation should be considered in any seborrheic dog. Unsaturated fats (vegetable oil) should be used. Adding 1 teaspoon of oil per 8-ounce measuring cup of dry food should supply sufficient linoleic acid to improve the haircoat. Improvement in the haircoat, which is usually gradual, should be noted within 2 months. Oversupplementation of fat may result in obesity, soft stools, frank diarrhea, or pancreatitis.

Alternative Therapy. There are several commercial fat supplements that can be used instead of vegetable oil. These products, which include Efa-Z Plus

(Allerderm), Derm Caps (DVM, Inc.), EfaVet (Vet-Kem), Diet-Derm (Vet-A-Mix), and Nutri-Sol (Norden), have the advantages of being less messy and easier to use but are more expensive.

Topical Therapy. Topical therapy is used to reduce scaling, greasiness, inflammation, pruritus, and odor. The duration of treatment is variable. In dogs with correctable underlying causes of seborrhea, topical therapy can be discontinued eventually. In dogs with idiopathic seborrhea, topical therapy is usually continued indefinitely. The type and frequency of treatment must be individualized for each dog. Some dogs require daily or alternate-day shampoos, whereas others need baths only twice a month to control seborrhea. Topical therapy includes the use of shampoos and rinses.

Shampoos. There are several shampoos available commercially. The type of shampoo chosen depends on whether the animal has dry, oily, or "combination" skin. Antiseborrheic shampoos remove dandruff by being keratolytic or keratoplastic. Keratolytic agents soften excessively keratinized tissue so it can be removed mechanically. Keratoplastic agents exert a "normalizing" effect on the keratinization process by an unknown mechanism. Antiseborrheic shampoos usually contain salicylic acid, sulfur, tar, selenium sulfide, or benzoyl peroxide in various strengths and combinations. Salicylic acid is mildly antipruritic, bacteriostatic, and keratolytic. Sulfur is mildly antibacterial, antipruritic, keratolytic, and keratoplastic, but it is not a good degreaser. When salicylic acid is combined with sulfur, a synergistic effect may occur. Tar preparations are antipruritic, keratolytic, and keratoplastic. Selenium sulfide shampoos are keratolytic and degreasing. Benzoyl peroxide shampoos are antibacterial, antipruritic, keratolytic, and degreasing.

Dry Skin Conditions. Hypoallergenic shampoos are good for dry to normal skin. Also effective for dry, flaky skin are shampoos that contain sulfur and sodium salicylate in an emollient base (Table 3-9).

Combination or Oily Skin Conditions. Tar shampoos are good for oily or "combination" skin (Table 3-10) but should not be used on dogs with normal or dry skin conditions. They can be irritating, and too frequent use may result in dry, flaky skin. In cats, tar shampoos are potentially toxic and should not be used.

Oily Skin Conditions. Shampoos containing 0.9–1.0% selenium sulfide or selenium disulfide may be used to treat oily skin (Table 3-4). These products may stain the haircoats and can be irritating, especially in cats. Shampoos containing benzoyl peroxide are excellent for treating oily skin (Table 3-11). However, they can be irritating, especially if used on dry skin.

Rinses and Sprays. Rinses and sprays are used as adjuncts to shampoos to add luster to dry skin (Table 3-12). They are either sprayed on and then combed into the haircoat or are applied as a conditioning rinse following the bath. The human product Alpha Keri bath oil (Westwood) can also be used as a final rinse by adding 1 capful to 1–2 quarts of water. Overuse of topical rinses or sprays may result in a greasy haircoat.

TABLE 3-9.   Shampoos for Dry Skin

Trade Name	Comments
Allergroom (Allerderm)	Hypoallergenic
HyLyt (DVM)	Hypoallergenic
Soothing Hypo-Allergenic Shampoo (Vet-Kem)	Hypoallergenic
Sebaffon (Winthrop)	Contains 0.5% sulfur/0.5% sodium salicylate
Sebolux (Allerderm)	Contains 2% sulfur/2.3% sodium salicylate
Sebalyt (DVM)	Contains 2% sulfur/2% salicylic acid/0.5% triclosan
Micro Pearls Skin and Coat Moisturizing Shampoo (Evsco)	Soap-free
Medicated Shampoo (Vet-Kem)	Contains 0.5% salicylic acid/aloe vera

TABLE 3-10.   Tar Shampoos for Oily or "Combination" Skin*

Trade Name	Contents
Lytar (DVM)	3% Refined tar, 2% sulfur, 2% salicylic acid
Mycodex Tar and Sulfur Shampoo (Beecham)	0.5% Coal tar, 5% sulfur, 1% salicylic acid
Pragmatar (Norden)	0.5% Cetyl alcohol coal tar distillate
Allerseb T (Allerderm)	3% Coal tar, 2% sulfur, 2% salicylic acid
Medicated Tar and Sulfur Shampoo (Vet-Kem)	0.5% USP crude coal tar, 5% colloidal sulfur, 1% salicylic acid
MicroPearls Coal Tar Shampoo (Evsco)	5% USP coal tar

*Do not use on dogs with normal or dry skin or on cats.

Antibiotic Therapy. Because dogs with seborrhea are predisposed to secondary pyoderma, antibiotic therapy is indicated whenever bacterial skin infection develops. The dosages and regimens for antibiotic therapy are discussed in the section on pyoderma.

Corticosteroid Therapy. The judicious use of low doses of oral corticosteroids is often useful for alleviating pruritus. Prednisone or prednisolone is given at a dosage of 0.2–0.5 mg/kg q12h PO. Pruritus is usually controlled within 10 days. If maintenance therapy is needed, prednisone or prednisolone, 0.2–0.6 mg/kg PO, is continued on an alternate-day basis. Long-term corticosteroid therapy is not recommended because iatrogenic hyperadrenocorticism, pyoderma, and urinary tract infections may result. Also, corticosteroid therapy can

TABLE 3-11. Shampoos for Oily Skin

Selenium sulfide/disulfide shampoos*
Seleen (Ceva)
Selenium Disulfide Shampoo (Vet-Kem)
Selsun Blue

Benzoyl peroxide shampoos
Pyoben (Allerderm)
Oxydex (DVM)
Sulfoxydex (DVM)
Micro Pearls Benzoyl Peroxide Shampoo (Evsco)

*Do not use on cats.

TABLE 3-12. Rinses and Sprays for the Treatment of Seborrheic Skin Disorders

Hy-Lyt EFA (DVM)
Humilac (Allerderm)
Hypo-Allergenic Dermal Spray (Vet-Kem)
Hypo-Allergenic Skin Cream and Coat Conditioner (Vet-Kem)
Micro Pearls Humectant Spray (Evsco)
Micro Pearls Cream Rinse (Evsco)

eventually aggravate seborrhea by causing the skin to become dry and flaky and the haircoat to become dry and brittle. The dosage and regimen for short-term corticosteroid therapy is discussed in the section on allergic skin disorders.

OTITIS EXTERNA

Low numbers of bacteria and yeast are normally found in the external ear canals of dogs and cats. Disturbances of the normal flora allow bacteria and yeast organisms to overgrow the ear canal. A thorough search for an underlying cause should always be made.

The most common cause of otitis externa in cats is infection with *Otodectes cynotis*. Dogs also are commonly affected. Typically, there is black ear debris of "coffee-ground" consistency, although in some animals otic discharge may be minimal to absent.

Other ectoparasitic diseases that may cause or contribute to otitis externa include sarcoptic mange in dogs, notoedric mange in cats, chiggers, spinous ear ticks (*Otobius megnini*), and demodicosis. Demodicosis may cause ceruminous otitis in dogs and cats. A diagnosis of demodectic otitis is made by microscopic identification of *Demodex* in ear exudate.

Dogs may be anatomically predisposed to recurring ear infections if they have heavy, pendulous ears or excess hair in their ear canals. The accumulation of cerumen and moisture from poor air circulation predisposes these dogs to secondary ear infections. Yeast otitis may occur in dogs that swim or get water in their ears during baths. Dogs with allergic disease such as atopy and food allergy are prone to develop recurring ear infections. Typically, the inner surface of the ear pinnae becomes erythematous, and the dog may scratch or shake its ears. In chronic cases, the ear canals become inflamed, and secondary yeast otitis may develop.

Other causes of otitis externa include dermatophytosis, foreign bodies, and neoplasia. A foreign body should always be ruled out, especially when only one ear is involved. Neoplasia may cause otitis or, in the case of small polyps, serve as a nidus for secondary infection. Lastly, otitis externa frequently occurs in dogs with primary idiopathic seborrhea.

Diagnostic evaluation routinely includes an otoscopic examination, microscopic examination of ear debris, and Gram stain of ear exudate. A bacterial-fungal culture is indicated if the ear problem is chronic, severe, or recurring, or if the tympanic membrane is ruptured and signs of otitis media are present.

Infections may worsen during treatment if the owner applies the medication inadequately or is rough when treating or cleaning the ear, if the wrong medication has been prescribed, or if a contact allergy develops to the otic preparation.

Animals that relapse shortly after otic therapy is discontinued do so because the underlying problem has not been eliminated or because the treatment has not been continued long enough. Weekly otoscopic examinations are necessary to assess progress and to determine when the otitis has resolved completely.

Treatment

Standard Therapy. Treatment of otitis externa generally involves symptomatically treating the ear infection while the underlying cause is corrected. The objectives of therapy are to 1) reduce inflammation, pain, and pruritus; 2) treat secondary bacterial or yeast infections; and 3) correct the underlying cause.

Specific Therapies. Treatment of the underlying causes—sarcoptic mange, notedric mange, chiggers, atopy, food allergy, flea allergic dermatitis, seborrhea, hypothyroidism, and autoimmune skin disease—is discussed elsewhere in this textbook.

Otodectes cynotis. There are several factors to consider when treating *Otodectes* otitis externa. Excessive ear debris must be removed. Because in-contact animals can be asymptomatic carriers, all household dogs and cats must be treated. Some dogs and cats treated for *Otodectes* otitis with otic preparations develop pruritic skin problems due to mites on the body. Skin scrapings may be positive for otodectic mites even though there are no mites or inflammation in these animals' ear canals. Topical insecticidal products and miticidal otic preparations should be used concurrently. The affected animal and all other household dogs and cats should be topically treated with flea sprays or flea powders twice weekly or with flea dips once weekly for 4 weeks. Otic preparations effective against ear mites include those that contain thiabendazole (Tresaderm, Merck & Co.), rotenone (Canex, Pitman-Moore) in mineral oil (1:3), pyrethrin (Mitecide Otic Solution, Eli Lilly; Cerumite, Evsco Pharmaceutical; Oticare, ARC), and carbaryl (Mitox, Norden). Tresaderm should be applied in the ears one or two times daily for 2 weeks; the other products must be used every 1–3 days for 1 month. Localized allergic or irritant reactions characterized by pain, inflammation, or pinnal hair loss may occur with topical preparations.

Although not approved for this use in dogs and cats, ivermectin (Ivomec, Merck), when given as a single subcutaneous injection of 0.2 mg/kg, is effective against otodectic mites. No topical or otic treatment is needed with ivermectin unless secondary bacterial or yeast infection is present.

Adverse reactions to ivermectin may occur, especially if the animal is accidentally overdosed with the large-animal formulations. The use of ivermectin is contraindicated in collies and collie crosses because these dogs are sensitive to the toxic effects of this drug. Adverse side effects have not been reported in cats. Adverse effects associated with ivermectin in dogs include drooling, vomiting, ataxia, tremors, weakness, recumbency, stupor, and coma. Good supportive care usually results in complete recovery, although convalescence may take several weeks, and severely affected animals may die. Symptomatic care includes fluid therapy and nutritional support. If the dog is recumbent it needs appropriate bedding and frequent turning to prevent the development of decubital ulcers. If the dog is bradycardic, glycopyrrolate (Robinul-V, Robins), 0.01 mg/kg IV, IM, or SC, is given as needed to maintain a heart rate over 80 beats per minute.

Demodectic Otitis. Rotenone (Canex, Pitman-Moore) in mineral oil (1:3) or amitraz (Mitaban, Upjohn) in mineral oil (1:9) is applied in the ears every other day until two follow-up ear swabs taken 1–2 weeks apart fail to reveal mites. If the animal is being treated for generalized demodectic mange, the ear canals should be treated prophylactically with the rotenone-mineral oil or amitraz-mineral oil solution once a week for the duration of therapy.

Adjunctive Therapies. *Ear Cleaning.* Topical medication on top of ear debris is not effective. If the ears are severely inflamed and painful, treatment is given for 3–5 days. The ear canals are then reexamined and thoroughly cleaned. A few drops of topical anesthetic with 2–4% lidocaine (Lidocaine HCl Injection, Elkins-Sinn) or 0.5% proparacaine hydrochloride ophthalmic solution (Ophthaine Solution, ER Squibb & Sons) applied in the ears every 5 minutes may be helpful when cleaning ears that are mildly painful. Sedation or anesthesia may be needed if there is a lot of debris or if the animal's ears are severely painful. A ceruminolytic agent is instilled in the ear canal if there is waxy or thick debris in order to soften the debris and make it easier to remove. There are many veterinary ceruminolytic and cleaning preparations available (Table

TABLE 3-13. Veterinary Ceruminolytic and Otic Cleaning Preparations

Name	Contents
Clear X Ear Cleaning Solution (DVM)	dioctyl sodium sulfosuccinate, urea, peroxide, lidocaine hydrochloride
Panoprep (Solvay)	carbamide, peroxide, glycerin
Adams Pan-Otic (Norden)	dioctyl sodium sulfosuccinate, aloe vera, alcohol, propylene glycol
Epi-Otic Cleanser (Allerderm)	lactic acid, salicylic acid, propylene glycol
Nolvasan Otic Cleaning Solution (Fort Dodge)	chlorhexidine
Oti Clens (SmithKline Beecham)	malic acid, benzoic acid, salicylic acid, alcohol, propylene glycol

3-13). To remove the debris, the canal is irrigated with a flushing solution that is instilled under gentle pressure alternating with suction from a bulb syringe placed loosely, deep in the ear canal. Chlorhexidine solution (Nolvasan solution, Fort Dodge) 4 ml/L water or povidone-iodine solution (Betadine, Purdue Frederick) 10 ml/L of water can be used as a flushing solution. However, neither chlorhexidine nor povidone-iodine solution should be used in animals with ruptured tympanic membranes. To aspirate residual fluid, the bulb syringe or small catheter attached to a 12-ml syringe can be used. The irrigation and aspiration are continued until all debris has been removed and the tympanic membrane can be visualized. If debris cannot be removed with aspiration, it may be removed mechanically with a 7-inch alligator forceps, curette, or ear loop passed through the otoscopic cone.

The owner should be instructed on how periodically to clean the animal's ear canals. Cotton-tipped applicators should not be used because they tend to push ear debris from the vertical canal into the horizontal canal. A ceruminolytic agent or cleaning solution (Table 3-13) is instilled in the ear canals, and the ear canals are gently massaged. The animal is allowed to shake its head, after which excess fluid and debris are gently wiped from the orifice of the ear canals with cotton balls or gauze pads. The ear canals should be treated as frequently as needed to remove wax buildup. Overzealous or too frequent cleaning may cause a contact irritant otitis to occur.

Animals with painful or pruritic otitis externa should receive short-term treatment with systemic corticosteroids. Oral prednisone or prednisolone is administered at the dosage of 0.5–1.0 mg/kg/day for 5–14 days. Topical otic preparations that contain corticosteroids should be used concurrently. *The use of corticosteroids in dogs and cats with demodicosis is contraindicated.*

Dogs that suffer from allergic otitis or idiopathic ceruminous otitis may benefit from the topical use of an otic corticosteroid-DMSO solution (Synotic, Syntex). Two to five drops of Synotic are placed in the ear canals one or two times daily until inflammation is controlled and then as frequently as needed to control the problem.

The corticosteroids in otic preparations may be absorbed systemically, and long-term therapy could result in iatrogenic hyperadrenocorticism and immunosuppression. Corticosteroids may also predispose to secondary bacterial infections and yeast overgrowth.

Fungal/Yeast Otitis. The most common cause of mycotic otitis is super-infection with the yeast *Malassezia pachydermatis*. Less commonly, otitis externa is associated with *Candida albicans* or dermatophyte infection. Topical products containing thiabendazole (Tresaderm, Merck) are effective against *Malassezia, Candida*, and the dermatophytes. Topical preparations containing nystatin (Panalog, Solvay) are effective only against *Candida*. Polyhydroxydine (Xenodyne, Solvay) is reported to be effective against fungi and yeast, but we have had more success using it as a preventive agent (e.g., prophylactically after swimming) than as a therapeutic agent for preexisting infection. Acetic acid solutions such as Otic Domeboro (Miles Pharmaceuticals), or white vinegar diluted 1:2 with water may also help prevent otitis from occurring in dogs worked in water. The acetic acid solution Hydro-B 1020 (Butler) also contains hydrocortisone and is useful when mild inflammation is present.

Bacterial Otitis. Moist, exudative, ceruminous bacterial otitides should be treated with topical antibacterial solutions, whereas dry, scaly otitides should be treated with oil- or ointment-based medications. Antibacterial otic preparations include those that contain chloramphenicol (Chloromycetin Otic, Parke-Davis; Liquichlor, Evsco), neomycin (Tresaderm, Merck; Panalog, Solvay), polymyxin B and neomycin (Cortisporin Otic Solution, Burroughs Wellcome; Forte-Topical, Upjohn), and gentamicin (Gentocin Otic, Schering). Gram-positive organisms are frequently susceptible to all of the aforementioned antibiotics, whereas gram-negative organisms may be resistant to chloramphenicol. *Pseudomonas* sp. are especially resistant to most antibiotics. Otic preparations that may be effective against *Pseudomonas* sp. infection include Domeboro solution (organisms cannot survive in an acidic environment), povidone-iodine or polyhydroxydine solution (Xenodyne, Solvay), and Tris EDTA solution. Tris EDTA solution is made by mixing 1.2 g of EDTA Disodium and 6.05 g of Tris buffer in a container. Distilled or deionized water is added to bring the volume of solution to 1 L. The pH of the solution is adjusted to 8.0 by adding sodium hydroxide or hydrochloric acid. The solution should then be sterilized with a bacterial filter or autoclaved. If desired, either gentamicin 3 mg/ml or amikacin 9 mg/ml can be added to the solution to enhance its effectiveness against *Pseudomonas*. For treatment, 3–5 drops are instilled in the ears every 12 hours.

Aminoglycosides (neomycin, gentamicin, amikacin) and iodine (povidone-iodine, polyhydroxydine) are potentially ototoxic if the tympanic membrane is not intact. Neomycin may cause allergic contact sensitization.

AUTOIMMUNE DISEASES

Autoimmune skin diseases are a diverse group of conditions that result from an inappropriate immune response to various body components. They vary from mild and limited to severe and generalized with systemic signs. In comparison to all other skin diseases, autoimmune diseases are rare and constitute only about 1% of all skin conditions in dogs and cats. Other, more common diseases, such as infectious, parasitic, metabolic, and neoplastic conditions, that can be mistaken for autoimmune disease must be ruled out. An accurate diagnosis is essential because of the serious nature of many of these diseases and the frequent need for lifelong therapy. Except in rare instances, immunosuppressive therapy should be withheld until the diagnosis of autoimmune disease is made with certainty. Diagnosis of these conditions is based on a combination of history and clinical appearance, typical histologic lesions, and characteristic antibody or complement deposition as demonstrated by immunofluorescence or immunoperoxidase testing.

Standard Therapy

Most animals with autoimmune skin disease require immunosuppressive therapy for their entire lives. Because most of the agents used to treat autoimmune diseases have serious and possibly fatal side effects, the potential benefits to be gained from their use must be balanced against the potential adverse effects. The best results are obtained by individualizing therapy for each patient rather than attempting to apply a rigid therapeutic regimen to each case. In addition, frequent examinations are essential to monitor therapy closely and readjust medications as needed. Despite careful monitoring relapses are common, and some cases may not respond to any therapy. In rare instances, an apparent "cure" is achieved.

The general objectives are to 1) achieve maximum skin healing while 2) minimizing side effects of the therapeutic agents.

Corticosteroids. Systemic corticosteroids, usually prednisone or prednisolone, are the drugs of choice for the initial treatment of most autoimmune skin diseases. However, these drugs have the potential for serious side effects, which ultimately may be worse than the disease. Consequently, the benefits of corticosteroid usage must be weighed against the possible adverse effects. In animals with mild manifestations of autoimmune skin disease, other forms of therapy with less potential for adverse effects would be more appropriate. To minimize the side effects, corticosteroids should be used at the lowest dose possible and administered as infrequently as possible.

Corticosteroids are initially used at immunosuppressive doses (induction therapy) until lesions completely resolve, and then they are slowly tapered to the lowest dose that maintains the disease in remission (maintenance therapy). Typical induction doses of prednisolone range from 2.2 to 6.6 mg/kg/day, divided into two equal doses given morning and evening. In a long-term retrospective study of a large number of dogs with various autoimmune skin diseases 2.2 mg/kg/day was usually ineffective, and a 6.6 mg/kg/day dose was frequently accompanied by severe and unacceptable side effects; a dose of 4.4 mg/kg/day was found to be an optimum induction dose for dogs. In general, cats require approximately twice the dose used in dogs for induction and maintenance therapy; and a successful induction dose for cats was 6.6 mg/kg/day. The immunosuppressive dose is administered until lesions completely resolve, approximately 10–21 days. Maintenance therapy is then begun by administering the total daily dose used for induction therapy as a single massive dose every other morning (dogs) or evening (cats). This alternate-day dose is reduced by 50% each week until the lowest maintenance dose is achieved. Relapses commonly occur because the corticosteroid dose is decreased too rapidly or before disease activity is completely suppressed.

In some instances, a better clinical response is seen and fewer side effects develop when equipotent doses of dexamethasone are used for maintenance therapy. Doses ranging from 0.03 to 0.10 mg/kg PO every other day have been used successfully to maintain remission in dogs. Cats with pemphigus foliaceus have been maintained successfully with combination therapy including dexamethasone 0.5 mg/kg once weekly. Injectable steroids are used only rarely for therapy of autoimmune skin diseases. Occasionally, they are the only means of treating fractious cats. Injectable methylprednisolone acetate (Depo-Medrol, Upjohn) administered at 8- to 10-week intervals has been used successfully to maintain remission in a cat with systemic lupus erythematosus.

Topical corticosteroids are indicated when the skin condition is limited in distribution such as may occur with pemphigus erythematosus or discoid lupus erythematosus. However, topical therapy appears to be less efficacious in animals with pemphigus erythematosus than in people with this condition. Hydrocortisone is the least potent topical corticosteroid and is useful for maintenance therapy. More potent fluorinated corticosteroids are usually necessary to achieve resolution of lesions initially. The biologic activity of ointments is usually greater than that of creams and lotions. The preparation should be applied three or four times daily until lesions resolve, and then administration is decreased to the lowest possible dose (ideally, once daily or every other day application of hydrocortisone). Therapy can alternate between the two types of corticosteroid depending on disease activity. To prevent unintentional medication of the individual treating the animal, the corticosteroid preparation should not be applied with bare fingers.

Side Effects. Adverse side effects of systemic corticosteroids are common in dogs treated for autoimmune skin diseases. They include severe polyuria and polydipsia, polyphagia, muscle wasting and weakness, hepatopathy, secondary respiratory and urinary tract infections, pancreatitis, diarrhea, and depression.

Side effects are rare in cats but are similar to those seen in dogs. Side effects produced by topical corticosteroid therapy are usually less severe and include local cutaneous atrophy, focal alopecia, focal pigmentary disturbances, and contact dermatitis. Iatrogenic hyperglucocorticism is possible when large areas are treated for prolonged periods. Side effects are less severe with topical hydrocortisone therapy than with more potent fluorinated corticosteroids.

Combination Immunosuppressive Therapy. Treatment of most autoimmune skin diseases with corticosteroids alone is frequently unsuccessful, either because of unacceptable side effects or lack of response. These drawbacks can be overcome or minimized by combination therapy consisting of lower doses of corticosteroids in conjunction with another immunosuppressive agent. Combination therapy is recommended when substantial improvement is not seen within 10 days of initiating induction therapy or when the maintenance dose of corticosteroids (< 1.0 mg/kg every other day) cannot be achieved within 3–4 weeks. Alternatively, combination therapy can be used immediately during initial treatment. In such cases, lower induction doses of corticosteroids may be used (e.g., prednisolone 2.2 mg/kg/day). Typically, combination therapy consists of a corticosteroid plus gold salts, a cytotoxic immunosuppressive drug, or vitamin E. Both drugs are continued until lesions completely resolve. When the disease is in remission, the corticosteroid is tapered to every other day administration. The cytotoxic drug is then discontinued, and the disease is maintained in remission with alternate-day steroids. If relapse occurs remission is again achieved with combination therapy and is maintained with the lowest possible dose of corticosteroid and cytotoxic drug. In contrast, when a gold salt or vitamin E is used, the corticosteroid dosage is progressively decreased and discontinued, if possible, and remission is maintained with gold salts or vitamin E alone or in combination with the lowest possible alternate-day corticosteroid dose.

Chrysotherapy. The use of gold salts is termed chrysotherapy. Indications for gold therapy are pemphigus diseases and bullous pemphigoid in dogs and cats. Chrysotherapy for treatment of cutaneous lupus is currently in disfavor because no benefit of oral gold was seen in human patients with systemic lupus erythematosus. However, a dog with systemic lupus erythematosus was treated successfully with a combination of aurothioglucose and alternate-day dexamethasone. Gold can be used in combination with a corticosteroid or can be used alone as the sole means of therapy for mild cases. There is a 4- to 12-week lag phase before clinical response is seen with chrysotherapy. In some instances, gold therapy can be stopped and the disease stays in remission, especially pemphigus foliaceus in both dogs and cats.

Injectable and oral forms of gold are presently available. The two forms have different properties of circulation, tissue distribution, and excretion, which account for differences in toxicity. Parenteral gold has been the standard form of chrysotherapy for autoimmune skin diseases in animals. Aurothioglucose

(Solganol, Schering) is a water-soluble gold salt suspended in sterile sesame oil. The drug is administered according to the following schedule.

	Test Dose (mg IM)	
	Cats, Small Dogs	Dogs > 10 kg
Week 1	1	5
Week 2	2	10

If no adverse reactions are seen, the dose is 1 mg/kg/week IM until remission (6–12 weeks); then 1 mg/kg IM every 2 weeks for 1–2 months; then 1 mg/kg IM every 4–8 weeks. If no clinical response is seen in 16 weeks, the dose can be increased to 1.5 mg/kg/week.

An alternative method of chrysotherapy is by oral administration. Experience with the oral form of gold, auranofin (Ridaura, SmithKline & French), in veterinary medicine is limited. The dosage used in dogs has been 0.05–0.20 mg/kg twice daily. The maximum dose is 9.0 mg/day because the clinical effectiveness may not be better at higher doses, and side effects increase with increasing doses. Oral gold can be administered concurrently with corticosteroids or nonsteroidal antiinflammatory agents.

Side Effects. Side effects of parenteral chrysotherapy are not common and usually occur early in therapy. Most of the adverse effects are benign and resolve when therapy is discontinued. The most common adverse effect is a pruritic exfoliative dermatitis. Renal toxicity is less common, and blood dyscrasias such as thrombocytopenia are rare. Chrysotherapy can be resumed with lower doses after signs of toxicosis subside. Adverse effects in dogs receiving oral gold salts include thrombocytopenia with hemolytic anemia and spherocytosis and diarrhea. The incidence of dermatologic side effects is much lower for auranofin than for aurothioglucose in people; none have been reported in dogs.

Monitoring of parenteral chrysotherapy includes physical examination, hemogram with platelet count, BUN, and urinalysis prior to each injection during the first 2 months of therapy. During maintenance, monthly to quarterly evaluation is sufficient. Treatment should be discontinued at the first sign of any adverse reaction. During oral chrysotherapy, the dog should be monitored with a hemogram with platelet count and creatinine prior to therapy, every 2 weeks for the first month, monthly for the second and third months, and then every 3–4 months. A biochemical profile should be evaluated before therapy and every 6 months thereafter.

Contraindications to parenteral chrysotherapy are renal disease, hepatic dysfunction, blood dyscrasias, pregnancy, systemic lupus erythematosus with renal involvement, uncontrolled diabetes mellitus, and concomitant use of an antimalarial, immunosuppressants other than corticosteroids, phenylbutazone, and oxyphenbutazone (because of the potential for these drugs to cause blood dyscrasias).

Cyclophosphamide. Cyclophosphamide (Cytoxan, Mead Johnson), a cytotoxic drug with immunosuppressive activity, is used to lower the dose or completely eliminate corticosteroids in therapy of pemphigus vulgaris, pemphigus foliaceus, pemphigus vegetans, bullous pemphigoid, and systemic lupus erythematosus in dogs and cats. The drug is given orally, and various dosing schedules can be used: 50 mg/m^2 every other day, 1.5 mg/kg/day for 4 days then off for 3 days, or 1.5–2.5 mg/kg every other day.

The most common toxic effects with cyclophosphamide use are myelosuppression, hemorrhagic cystitis (in dogs), and gastroenteritis. The risk of cystitis may be minimized by encouraging water consumption and frequent urination. Other adverse effects include urinary bladder fibrosis and neoplasia, infertility, teratogenicity, carcinogenesis, alopecia, and altered wound healing. During the initial phase of therapy, a hemogram with platelet count and urinalysis should be performed weekly. Therapy should be discontinued if the white blood cell count drops below 4000/μl or the platelet count is less than 120,000/μl. When cell numbers return to normal, therapy can be resumed with 75% of the original dose. Therapy should be discontinued immediately if hematuria develops. If the hematuria does not resolve despite drug withdrawal, additional diagnostic tests are indicated to determine the cause. Clinical signs of vomiting, diarrhea, fever, or depression warrant laboratory evaluation. Because of the propensity for cystitis to develop, cyclophosphamide is not an appropriate drug for long-term maintenance therapy in dogs.

Azathioprine. Azathioprine (Imuran, Burroughs Wellcome) is another cytotoxic drug used in dogs for treatment of pemphigus diseases, bullous pemphigoid, systemic lupus erythematosus, cold agglutinin disease, and uveodermatologic (Vogt-Koyanagi-Harada-like) syndrome. It is usually used in combination with corticosteroids. Various oral doses have been used: 1.1–2.2 mg/kg once daily or every other day, 2.2 mg/kg every other day, and 1.5 mg/kg/day. Once lesions are in remission, the dose is decreased to the lowest effective level. A 3- to 6-week lag phase occurs before clinical response is seen.

Adverse effects of azathioprine include bone marrow suppression, hepatotoxicosis, increased susceptibility to infection, teratogenicity, and skin eruptions. Pancreatitis has been reported in dogs treated with azathioprine and prednisolone for immune-mediated conditions. Laboratory monitoring consists of a hemogram with platelet count and determination of liver enzyme values every 1–2 weeks during initial therapy and then every 1–2 months once maintenance is achieved. If leukopenia, thrombocytopenia, or anemia develops or liver enzymes become elevated, azathioprine should be discontinued. When values return to normal, therapy can be resumed at 50–75% of the original dose. Azathioprine can be myelosuppressive in cats, and so its use in cats is discouraged.

Chlorambucil. Chlorambucil (Leukeran, Burroughs Wellcome) is the least toxic of the alkylating agents used to treat immune-mediated dermatoses in dogs. It is usually used in conjunction with prednisone. The dose is 0.1–0.2 mg/kg/day or every other day. A lag phase of 4–8 weeks is usual prior to clinical response. Toxic effects are rare and consist of myelosuppression and gastrointestinal effects.

Vitamin E. Vitamin E (*dl*-α-tocopherol), an oil-soluble vitamin, is used for treatment of discoid lupus erythematosus and pemphigus erythematosus in dogs. Vitamin E is usually used in conjunction with a corticosteroid to decrease the steroid dose, but disease in some dogs can be controlled with vitamin E alone. A dose of 400 IU is given twice daily, and the acetate or succinate form of the vitamin is recommended. It should be given 2 hours before or after a meal to maximize efficacy. Vitamin E appears to have a 30- to 60-day lag phase before a clinical response is seen. If a more immediate clinical response is desired, topical or systemic corticosteroids can be used during this lag time. No side effects have been reported in dogs treated with vitamin E. Because of its apparent lack of adverse effects, vitamin E is the treatment of choice for dogs with mild or limited disease.

Dapsone. Dapsone (Avlosulfon, Ayerst) is a sulfone used in dogs to treat sterile neutrophilic and eosinophilic diseases, including pemphigus erythematosus and linear immunoglobulin A (IgA) dermatosis. It has been used with limited success for the treatment of pemphigus foliaceus. The dose is 1.0 mg/kg two or three times daily for induction. A response should be seen within 4–6 weeks, after which the number of doses is reduced as much as possible. Side effects of dapsone are potentially serious and include anemia, neutropenia, thrombocytopenia, hepatotoxicity, gastrointestinal signs, and skin reactions. Laboratory monitoring of dapsone therapy should consist of a hemogram with platelet count and biochemical profile every 2 weeks during the first 6 weeks of therapy and then less frequently as the number of doses is decreased.

Alternative Therapy

An alternative method for induction therapy consists of *corticosteroid pulse therapy*, which is the parenteral administration of suprapharmacologic doses of methylprednisolone sodium succinate for short periods. The use of pulse therapy has been reported in one dog with pemphigus vulgaris, three dogs with pemphigus foliaceus, and one dog with systemic lupus erythematosus. The following protocol was used: Dogs were hospitalized for 4 days; methylprednisolone sodium succinate (Elkins-Sinn) was administered at a dose of 11.0 mg/kg IV in 250 ml of 5% dextrose in water over 1 hour for three consecutive days; cimetidine was given at a dose of 4.0 mg/kg q8h PO during the 3 days; dogs were discharged 24 hours after the last treatment. This form of therapy was rapidly active, and no side effects were seen; however, skin disease recurred in all five dogs within 4 weeks of completion of pulse therapy. Combination immunosuppressive therapy, consisting of 1.1 mg prednisolone/

kg every 24 hours plus azathioprine or gold, was required to keep skin disease in remission. Therapy was monitored with a hemogram and biochemical profile at the time of admission, after each treatment, and 24 hours after the last treatment. Serum lipase was measured at admission and 24 hours after the last treatment. The dogs were reexamined 1, 2, 4, and 6 weeks after therapy.

Cyclosporine is an immunosuppressive drug used most commonly in humans for prevention of organ rejection. Currently it is used in people for treatment of various immune-mediated conditions. It has been used with limited success in only a small number of dogs and cats for treatment of pemphigus foliaceus, pemphigus erythematosus, and cutaneous lupus erythematosus. The usual dose for dogs and cats is 20.0 mg/kg/day PO, but a range of 10.0–30.0 mg/kg/day has been used. The drug should be divided into two equal doses and given on an empty stomach. The major adverse effects in people are nephrotoxicity and hepatotoxicity. Dogs and cats appear to be more refractory to cyclosporine-induced renal and hepatic impairment. Side effects reported in dogs have usually been transient but occasionally are severe enough to necessitate cessation of therapy. Toxic signs include periodic vomiting or diarrhea, anorexia, gingival hyperplasia, pyoderma, bacteriuria, and a proliferative papillomatous dermatosis. Side effects in cats appear to be minor. Monitoring for toxic effects consists of a complete blood count, biochemical profile, and urinalysis weekly for the first month, every other week for 1–2 months, and then monthly.

Heparin therapy was reported useful for the management of pemphigus vulgaris in one dog. Heparin has been used since the 1950s for treatment of pemphigus vulgaris in people when clinical trials indicated a good response with heparin alone or heparin in conjunction with moderate doses of corticosteroids. The mechanism of action is unknown, but heparin is thought to alter lymphocyte activity and have an antiprotease effect. The dose of heparin used in the dog was 100 IU/kg SC twice daily. Injections were given until lesions resolved. Monitoring during heparin therapy consisted of coagulation studies every 15 days. No abnormalities were detected.

Adjunctive Therapy

Sun avoidance, topical sunscreens, and application of indelible ink are recommended to minimize exposure to ultraviolet light, which is reported to induce exacerbations in animals with pemphigus erythematosus, discoid lupus erythematosus, and bullous pemphigoid. When skin disease is severe, daily whirlpool baths during initial therapy are soothing and helpful for removing crusts and exudate. Systemic antibiotics should be administered to animals with ulcerative lesions during treatment with high levels of immunosuppressive agents, which could render them susceptible to secondary bacterial infection.

MISCELLANEOUS SKIN CONDITIONS

The treatments for eosinophilic granuloma complex in dogs and cats, canine acral lick dermatitis, sterile pyogranulomas in dogs, and psychogenic alopecia in cats are discussed in this section.

Canine Eosinophilic Granuloma

Eosinophilic granulomas in dogs are characterized by nodular to plaque-like lesions in the oral cavity, on the skin, or in the external ear canal. Histologically, there are foci of collagen degeneration surrounded by eosinophilic and histiocytic infiltrates. Treatment with prednisone or prednisolone 0.5–2.2 mg/kg PO daily for 10–20 days is usually effective. The treatment can be discontinued once the lesions have completely regressed.

Feline Eosinophilic Granuloma Complex

Eosinophilic granuloma lesions in cats include indolent ulcers, eosinophilic plaques, and linear granulomas. These lesions may be associated with an underlying allergic disorder (flea allergic dermatitis, atopy, food hypersensitivity), or they may be idiopathic. The prognosis is better for lesions in which a correctable underlying cause can be found than for lesions that are idiopathic.

Standard Therapy. Treatment includes removing or treating the underlying cause (e.g., immunotherapy for atopy) and medically managing the lesions. Therapy with systemic glucocorticoids is usually effective. The cat is given prednisone or prednisolone 2.2 mg/kg PO twice daily until the lesions have completely resolved. If the glucocorticoids are discontinued before the lesion has completely healed, it will recur. A good alternative to oral glucocorticoid therapy is methylprednisolone acetate (Depo-Medrol, Upjohn), 4 mg/kg or 20 mg/cat SC. The methylprednisolone acetate is administered every 2 weeks for up to three treatments. If after the third treatment the lesion is still not completely healed, oral glucocorticoid therapy as described above should be initiated. Long-term therapy with methylprednisolone acetate should be avoided because the cat so treated may become cushingoid. In cats that have recurrent lesions, daily oral prednisone or prednisolone as described above is given initially. Once the lesions have resolved, prednisone or prednisolone is then given every other day at the lowest possible dosage for maintenance. For lesions that recur infrequently, methylprednisolone acetate injections can be repeated, but never more often than every 2 months.

A variety of other treatments have been tried for glucocorticoid refractory lesions. They include radiotherapy, cryosurgery, laser therapy, surgical excision, levamisole, and aurothioglucose (Solganol, Schering). However, efficacy of these forms of therapy has not been proved. Progestational compounds may also be effective but have potentially serious side effects (see section on allergic skin disease for dosage and side effects).

Acral Lick Dermatitis (Lick Granuloma)

The initiating factor for acral lick dermatitis should be identified if possible. Underlying factors include fleas, atopy, food hypersensitivity, bacterial or mycotic infection, hypothyroidism, trauma, foreign body, neoplasia, sensory neuropathy, and psychological causes (i.e., boredom). Treatment should include removing or correcting the underlying cause. Early (noninfected) lesions may resolve with topical or intralesional steroid therapy. For topical treatment, a combination of fluocinolone and DMSO (Synotic, Syntex) is applied to the lesion twice a day. To increase effectiveness, 3 ml of flunixine meglumine (Banamine Solution, Schering), a nonsteroidal anti-inflammatory agent, can be added to 8 ml of Synotic. When using Synotic, rubber gloves must be worn to prevent absorption of DMSO through human skin. Triamcinolone (Vetalog, Solvay), 1 mg/kg intralesionally, may be effective in lesions of less than 3 cm diameter. Steroids may aggravate chronic lesions especially when secondary bacterial infection is present. Even when the initiating factor is no longer present, the secondary deep pyoderma may be pruritic and cause continued self-mutilation. We perform bacterial cultures from biopsies of all chronic lesions in order to initiate appropriate antibiotic therapy. Antibiotics are continued 2 weeks past the time the lesion has completely regressed (usually 8–12 weeks minimum). For antibiotic dosages, see the section on pyoderma.

Psychological causes, if present, should be eliminated. If not possible, treatment with antianxiety drugs may be helpful. Phenobarbital, diazepam (Valium, Roche Products), or primidone (Primidone tablets, Danbury) can be tried (for dosages see Chapter 13). Progesterone therapy may also be effective. Either repositol progesterone (Depo-Provera, Upjohn) 20 mg/kg every 3 weeks or megestrol acetate (Megace, Mead-Johnson; Ovaban, Schering) 1 mg/kg PO daily with eventual tapering to the lowest possible dosage and frequency for maintenance can be tried. Progestational compounds should not be used in intact females. Another drug found effective in selective cases of acral pruritic dermatitis is naltrexone (Trexan, Dupont Pharmaceuticals). The dosage used is 2.2 mg/kg PO once or twice daily. Long-term therapy is required in most dogs to maintain remission.

Surgical excision is generally not recommended unless the lesion is very small or dehiscence is likely. Cryosurgery, radiation therapy, and acupuncture have been reported effective in some cases. Mechanical restraint using Elizabethan collars, muzzles, side braces, or bandages are rarely effective by themselves but may be useful as adjunctive treatment.

Canine Sterile Pyogranulomas

Canine sterile pyogranulomas are characterized by nonpainful, nonpruritic papules and nodules that may involve the face (especially the bridge of the nose), ear pinnae, and feet. Histologically, there is a nodular to diffuse granulomatous or pyogranulomatous dermatitis, but fungal and bacterial cultures are negative. Treatment consists of surgical excision if the lesion is solitary. For multiple or large lesions, prednisone or prednisolone 2.2–4.4 mg/kg is given PO once daily. Once the lesions resolve, alternate-day therapy with prednisone or prednisolone may be needed to maintain remission.

For steroid refractory cases, azathioprine (Imuran, Burroughs Wellcome) is administered orally at 2.2 mg/kg once daily until remission occurs and then 2.2 mg/kg every other day for maintenance. Toxic side effects include bone marrow suppression, hepatotoxicosis, increased susceptibility to infections, teratogenicity, and skin eruptions. Laboratory monitoring during azathioprine therapy is discussed in the section on autoimmune skin diseases.

Feline Psychogenic Alopecia

Before an alopecic cat is diagnosed as "psychotic," other underlying causes of pruritus must be ruled out. They include ectoparasites (fleas, cheyletiellosis, otodectes, demodicosis), atopy, food hypersensitivity, cystitis, anal sac disease, dermatophytosis, eosinophilic plaques, and neoplasia.

The treatment of feline psychogenic alopecia involves correcting the psychological cause. Causes include a new pet, baby, or adult in the household, moving to new surroundings, boredom, and boarding. Cats with secondary excoriations should be treated with glucocorticoids (see eosinophilic granuloma complex for drug regimen). If psychological causes cannot be corrected, tranquilizers and sedatives can be tried. Therapy with diazepam (Valium) 1.25–2.50 mg once or twice daily, or phenobarbital 2.2–6.6 mg/kg twice daily can be tried. If the cat becomes hyperexcitable or ataxic due to diazepam therapy, the dosage or frequency of administration should be decreased. Progestational compounds may also be effective but have potentially serious side effects in cats (see section on allergies for regimen and side effects).

SUGGESTED READINGS

Allergic Skin Disorders

Kwochka KW: Differential diagnosis of feline miliary dermatitis. In: Kirk RW, ed. Current Veterinary Therapy IX. Philadelphia: WB Saunders, 1986;538.
Muller GH, Kirk RW, Scott DW: Small Animal Dermatology, 4th ed. Philadelphia: WB Saunders, 1989.

Reedy LM, Miller WH: Allergic Skin Diseases of Dogs and Cats. Philadelphia: WB Saunders, 1989.

Rosser EJ: Antipruritic drugs. Vet Clin North Am 1988;18:1093.

Scott DW, Buerger RG: Nonsteroidal anti-inflammatory agents in the management of canine pruritus. J Am Anim Hosp Assoc 1988;24:425.

White SD: Food hypersensitivity in 30 dogs. J Am Vet Med Assoc 1986;188:695.

Pyoderma

Becker AM, Janik TA, Smith EK, et al: *Propionibacterium acnes* immunotherapy in chronic recurrent canine pyoderma: an adjunct to antibiotic therapy. J Vet Int Med 1989;3:26.

Buerger RG: Staphylococci and German shepherd pyoderma. In: Kirk RW, ed. Current Veterinary Therapy X. Philadelphia: WB Saunders, 1989;609.

Carro T, Pedersen NC, Beaman BL, Munn R: Subcutaneous abscesses and arthritis caused by a probable L-form in cats. J Am Vet Med Assoc 1989;194:1583.

Crawford MA, Foil CS: Vasculitis: clinical syndromes in small animals. Comp Contin Educ 1989;11:400.

DeBoer DJ, Moriello KA, Thomas CB, Schultz KT: The use of Staphylococcus phage lysate (SPL) as adjunct therapy for idiopathic recurrent pyoderma in the dog: a controlled study. In: Proc 5th Annual Meeting of the Am Acad of Vet Dermatol and Am College of Vet Dermatol, 1989;27 (abstract).

Giger U, Werner LL, Millichamp NJ, Gorman NT: Sulfadiazine-induced allergy in six Doberman pinschers. J Am Vet Med Assoc 1985;186:479.

Hardie EM, Barsanti JA: Treatment of canine actinomycosis. J Am Vet Med Assoc 1982;180:537.

Ihrke PJ: Antibiotic therapy in canine skin disease: dermatologic therapy (part III). Comp Contin Educ 1980;177.

Keane DP: Chronic abscesses in cats associated with an organism resembling Mycoplasma. Can Vet J 1983;24:289.

Krick SA, Scott DW: Bacterial folliculitis, furunculosis, and cellulitis in the German shepherd dog: a retrospective analysis of 17 cases. J Am Anim Hosp Assoc 1989;25:23.

Mercer HD: The comparative pharmacology of chloramphenicol. J Am Vet Med Assoc 1980;176:923.

Rosenkrantz W: Immunomodulating drugs in dermatology. In: Kirk RW, ed. Current Veterinary Therapy X. Philadelphia: WB Saunders, 1989;570.

Watson ADJ, Middleton DJ: Chloramphenicol toxicosis in cats. Am J Vet Res 1978;39:1199.

Dermatophytosis

Hay RJ: The azole antifungal drugs. J Antimicrob Chemother 1987;20:1.

Lesher JL, Smith JG: Antifungal agents in dermatology. J Am Acad Dermatol 1987;17:383.

Muller GH, Kirk RW, Scott DW: Small Animal Dermatology, 4th ed. Philadelphia: WB Saunders, 1989.

Ectoparasitism

Dryden MW, Long GR, Gaafar SM: Effects of ultrasonic flea collars on Ctenocephalides felis on cats. J Am Vet Med Assoc 1989;195:1717.

Dryden MW, Neal JJ, Bennett GW: Concepts of flea control. Comp Anim Pract 1989;19:11.

Fehrer SL, Halliwell RE: Effectiveness of Avon's Skin-So-Soft® as a flea repellent on dogs. J Am Anim Hosp Assoc 1987;23:217.

Garg RC, Donahue WA: Pharmacologic profile of methoprene, an insect growth regulator, in cattle, dogs, and cats. J Am Vet Med Assoc 1989;194:410.

Halliwell REW: Hyposensitization in the treatment of flea-bite hypersensitivity: results of a double-blind study. J Am Anim Hosp Assoc 1981;17:249.

Hooser SB, Beasley VR, Everitt JI: Effects of an insecticidal dip containing d-limonene in the cat. J Am Vet Med Assoc 1986;189:905.

Kwochka KW: Fleas and related disease. Vet Clin North Am [Small Anim Pract] 1987;17:1235.

Kwochka KW: Mites and related disease. Vet Clin North Am [Small Anim Pract] 1987;17:1263.

Kwochka KW, Kunkle GA, Foil CO: The efficacy of amitraz for generalized demodicosis in dogs: a study of two concentrations and frequencies of application. Comp Contin Educ 1985;7:8.

Schick MP, Schick RO: Understanding and implementing safe and effective flea control. J Am Anim Hosp Assoc 1986;22:421.

Seborrhea

Griffin C: *Malassezia pachydermatis* skin disorders. Vet Rep 1989;2(2):4.

Ihrke PJ, Goldschmidt MH: Vitamin-A responsive dermatosis in the dog. J Am Vet Med Assoc 1983;182:687.

Muller GH, Kirk RW, Scott DW: Small Animal Dermatology, 4th ed. Philadelphia: WB Saunders, 1989.

Parker W, Yager-Johnson JA, Hardy MH: Vitamin A responsive seborrheic dermatosis in a dog; a case report. J Am Anim Hosp Assoc 1983;19:548.

Rosser EJ, Dunstan RW, Breen PT, et al: Sebaceous adenitis with hyperkeratosis in the standard poodle: a discussion of 10 cases. J Am Anim Hosp Assoc 1987;23:341.

Scott DW: Granulomatous sebaceous adenitis in dogs. J Am Anim Hosp Assoc 1986;22:631.

Scott DW: Vitamin-A responsive dermatosis in the cocker spaniel. J Am Anim Hosp Assoc 1986;22:125.

Stewart LJ: Isotretinoin in the treatment of sebaceous adenitis in two dogs. Proc Ann Meet Am Acad Vet Dermatol 1988;8.

Otitis Externa

Paradis M: Ivermectin in small animal dermatology. In: Kirk RW, ed. Current Veterinary Therapy X. Philadelphia: WB Saunders, 1989;560.

Paul A, Tranquilli W: Ivermectin. In: Kirk RW, ed. Current Veterinary Therapy X. Philadelphia: WB Saunders, 1989;140.

Autoimmune Disease

Olivry T, Heripret D: A case of pemphigus vulgaris successfully treated with heparin. Proc Ann Meet Am Acad Vet Dermatol, 1989;60 (abstract).

Rosenkrantz W: Immunomodulating drugs in dermatology. In: Kirk RW, ed. Current Veterinary Therapy X. Philadelphia: WB Saunders, 1989;570.

Rosenkrantz WS, Griffin CE, Barr RJ: Clinical evaluation of cyclosporine in animal models with cutaneous immune-mediated disease and epitheliotropic lymphoma. J Am Anim Hosp Assoc 1989;25:377.

Scott DW: Dermatologic use of glucocorticoids—systemic and topical. Vet Clin North Am [Small Anim Pract] 1982;12:19.

Scott DW, Walton DK, Slater MR, et al: Immune-mediated dermatoses in domestic animals: ten years after. Part I. Comp Contin Educ 1987;9:424.

Scott DW, Walton DK, Slater MR, et al: Immune-mediated dermatoses in domestic animals: ten years after. Part II. Comp Contin Educ 1987;9:539.

Serra DA, White SD: Oral chrysotherapy with auranofin in dogs. Am J Vet Med Assoc 1989;194:1327.

White SD, Steward LJ, Bernstein M: Corticosteroid (methylprednisolone sodium succinate) pulse therapy in five dogs with autoimmune skin disease. J Am Vet Med Assoc 1987;191:1121.

Miscellaneous Skin Conditions

MacEwen EG, Hess PW: Evaluation of effect of immunomodulation on the feline eosinophilic granuloma complex. J Am Anim Hosp Assoc 1982;23:519.

Manning TO, Crane SW, Scheidt VJ, et al: Three cases of feline eosinophilic granuloma complex (eosinophilic ulcer) and observations on laser therapy. Semin Vet Med Surg 1987;2:206.

Muller GH, Kirk RW, Scott DW: Small Animal Dermatology, 4th ed. Philadelphia: WB Saunders, 1989.

Scott DW: Feline dermatology 1900–1978: a monograph. J Am Anim Hosp Assoc 1980;16:331.

White SD: Treatment of acral lick dermatitis with the endorphin-blocker naltrexone. Proc Ann Meet Am Acad Vet Dermatol 1988;37.

CHAPTER FOUR

Endocrinologic Disorders

Duncan Ferguson, Margarethe Hoenig, and Larry Cornelius

DIABETES MELLITUS IN DOGS AND CATS

Diabetes mellitus (DM) is a complex endocrine disorder characterized by an absolute or relative deficiency of insulin resulting in fasting hyperglycemia and potentially a variety of other metabolic disturbances. It is more common in dogs than in cats but occurs with a high enough frequency in both species that the small animal practitioner needs to be familiar with the basics of appropriate management.

Diabetes mellitus is categorized into uncomplicated and complicated forms, and treatment of the two differs considerably. Complicating disorders often present in diabetic dogs include hyperadrenocorticism, pancreatitis, ketoacidosis, and sepsis. Diabetic cats are less frequently affected by hyperadrenocorticism and pancreatitis but do become ketoacidotic with prolonged uncontrolled DM. The reproductive hormones progesterone and estrogen cause insulin resistance in both dogs and cats and may induce or worsen DM. Excessive growth hormone, due to a pituitary tumor or excessive progestins, also may cause insulin-resistant diabetes.

Treatment of Uncomplicated DM in Dogs

Standard Therapy. Most diabetic dogs require insulin injections for their entire lives. The occasional successful use of oral hypoglycemic drugs has been reported, but these agents have not been widely utilized.

The general objectives of treatment are to: 1) have the patient feel well; 2) control polyuria/polydipsia (PU/PD); 3) prevent the serious complications of DM such as ketoacidosis and (if possible) cataracts; and 4) avoid insulin-induced hypoglycemia. Factors to be considered regarding treatment are insulin, diet, and exercise, with the former two items usually being the most important.

Initial In-Hospital Treatment and Monitoring: Days 1–3. Table 4-1 outlines the first three days of treatment.

Many types of insulin are available, but only a few have been extensively evaluated in diabetic dogs and cats: regular, NPH, and PZI. Before a detailed

TABLE 4-1.   Suggested Protocol for Initial Regulation of an Uncomplicated Diabetic Dog

Days 1–3

1. 7:50 a.m.   Submit samples for CBC, biochemical profile, and urinalysis. Do blood glucose with Chemstrip bG.

2. 7:55 a.m.   Feed one-third of caloric needs.

3. 8:00 a.m.   Administer 0.5–1.0 unit NPH insulin/kg SC.

4. Noon   Measure blood glucose with Chemstrip bG.

5. 2:00 p.m.   Feed one-third of caloric needs.

6. 4:00 p.m.   Measure blood glucose with Chemstrip bG.

7. 8:00 p.m.   Measure blood glucose with Chemstrip bG. Feed one-third of caloric needs.

Do not change insulin dosage or type or feeding regimen during this initial 3-day period unless grossly unacceptable blood glucose results are obtained.

Day 4

1. 7:50 a.m.   Measure blood glucose with Chemstrip bG.

2. 7:55 a.m.   Feed one-third of caloric needs.

3. 8:00 a.m.   Adjust dosage of NPH insulin up or down (usually by 1–2 units) depending on the results of blood glucose values near the expected peak of insulin action on days 1–3 and administer SC.

4. 10:00 a.m.   Measure blood glucose every 1–2 hours until 8:00 a.m. of day 5 (24 hours total).

5. 2:00 p.m.   Feed one-third of caloric needs.

6. 8:00 p.m.   Feed one-third of caloric needs.

Day 5

1. 7:50 a.m.   Graph the insulin-glucose response curve, adjust insulin dosage, and if necessary change the frequency of administration, the type of insulin, or both. Evaluate the feeding schedule for possible changes.

discussion of the specifics of insulin treatment and monitoring, it is important to emphasize the appropriate goals one should strive to achieve. With one or two insulin injections daily, *realistic goals* are to: 1) maintain blood glucose between 60 and 180 mg/dl (preferably between 80 and 140 mg/dl) for as many of the 24 hours each day as possible (at least 16–18 hours of each day); and 2) avoid potentially serious hypoglycemia (< 60 mg/dl). Until blood glucose exceeds 180 mg/dl (approximate renal threshold), glucosuria and therefore PU/PD do not occur. Although it would be ideal to have blood glucose in the normal range 24 hours a day, it is not necessary for adequate control; if such a goal is attempted with intensive insulin treatment, it usually leads to serious hypoglycemia. The same should be said about attempts to maintain a glucose-free urine. In fact, periodic mild glucosuria when the effects of insulin are diminishing is preferred because it provides some assurance that hypogly-cemia is less likely (see below). Experience indicates that diabetic dogs do well long term when insulin therapy results in their blood glucose being controlled between about 60 and 180 mg/dl for at least 16–18 hours of each 24-hour period. At this level of control, patients feel well, PU/PD is minimized, and ketoacidosis does not occur. Cataracts may develop eventually, but this com-plication often occurs despite intensive efforts at prevention. "Tight" control of blood glucose, as is necessary in diabetic people to prevent severe vasculopathy, should not be a goal when treating diabetic dogs and cats.

Prior to beginning insulin treatment, it is best to place an indwelling venous catheter to aid in sample collection for multiple blood glucose determinations. Samples should be submitted for a complete blood count (CBC), biochemical profile, and urinalysis. Promptly after blood is obtained for blood glucose measurement and immediately before insulin administration, the patient should be fed about one-third of its daily caloric needs. Treatment is begun with NPH insulin (0.5–1.0 units/kg SC) usually around 8:00 a.m. Larger dogs should receive the smaller dose per unit of body weight and smaller dogs the larger dosage. Two additional meals, each consisting of one-third of daily calories, should be fed at 6 and 12 hours after the first meal (see below for additional information). Because it usually takes 2–3 days for a patient to adapt fully to an insulin dosage change (or to a new insulin preparation), there is no need to determine blood glucose levels every 1–2 hours (insulin-glucose response curve) during this early period. Checking blood glucose immediately prior to the morning insulin injection and at 4, 8, and 12 hours after insulin administration is adequate during this initial period. It is important to docu-ment that insulin therapy is indeed lowering blood glucose but is not causing serious hypoglycemia. Reagent "sticks" such as Chemstrip bG (Boehringer Mannheim) work well for monitoring diabetic regulation, especially when used in conjunction with accompanying digital readout meters such as the AccuChek II instrument (Boehringer Mannheim). Reagent strip methods are less expensive and more convenient than standard laboratory procedures. The insulin dosage and the feeding schedule are subject to change after evaluating multiple daily blood glucose values (insulin-glucose response curve, see below).

Daily caloric intake should be estimated on the basis of the dog's ideal body weight. Diabetic dogs are often obese, or were obese, and therefore one should avoid feeding excessive calories; body weight should be monitored carefully. Caloric requirements are approximately 40–80 cal/kg/day. If obesity is present, the calculated daily caloric requirements should be reduced by about 40% to promote weight loss. It is generally agreed that daily caloric requirements should be divided into three or more feedings as described above. Patients receiving insulin once a day should be placed on a three-meal-a-day schedule (immediately prior to insulin administration and 6 and 12 hours later). Animals on twice-daily insulin should be fed four meals each day (immediately prior to each insulin injection, midafternoon, and late evening). These feeding regimens usually lessen the magnitude of the expected postprandial blood glucose elevation observed in diabetic dogs being fed on either a once- or twice-a-day schedule.

Studies have shown that it is best to feed either a canned or dry commercial dog food, not semimoist preparations. Semimoist products should not be fed because they are higher in sucrose and cause more marked postprandial hyperglycemia. A moderately to markedly fat-restricted diet with an increased fiber content is also advised. For diabetic people, a diet consisting of 55–60% complex carbohydrates, 20% protein, and 20–25% fat is recommended. Comparable figures for dogs are not available but are probably similarly desirable. Most commercial canned and dry foods, although acceptable, do not contain ideal amounts of carbohydrates and may contain excessive fat. Semimoist foods are high in simple sugar content and should be avoided. Prescription diets w/d, r/d, and g/d (Hill's Pet Products) are all suitable, but w/d and r/d contain more fiber, which may be of benefit to slow, smooth glucose absorption from the intestine. Prescription diet r/d is markedly fat-restricted and should be used only if the dog is obese. For finicky eaters, a mixture of cooked white rice, lean chicken, fish, and canned w/d is an alternative. Care must taken to accurately estimate required calories and to feed consistent quantities at the recommended times each day.

Because the response to insulin is so variable from one patient to the next, it is not possible to generalize about the best feeding schedule. Therefore it is necessary to evaluate the insulin-glucose response curve (see Follow-Up In-Hospital Treatment and Monitoring, below) before deciding on the exact feeding schedule. It must be remembered that changes in caloric intake, both amount and timing, markedly influence insulin requirements; therefore it must be emphasized to the client that dietary control is just as important as the proper daily insulin dosage. The general rules are 1) same food in the same quantities at the same times each day and 2) no between-meal "snacks."

Follow-Up In-Hospital Treatment and Monitoring. After the initial 2- to 3-day period, a serial insulin-glucose response curve should be determined. It is accomplished by administering NPH insulin, feeding as described above, and measuring blood glucose with the Chemstrip bG system every 1–2 hours for 24 hours. It is recognized that around-the-clock blood sample procurement is laborious, but the effort is necessary if the patient's response to insulin and feeding is to be understood. Help may be available at local emergency hospitals.

Such a curve should be graphed showing insulin dosage, blood glucose values, and times of feeding (Figures 4-1 and 4-2). It can be determined from the curve if the dosage and duration of action of NPH are appropriate and if the feeding times need to be changed. A large rise in blood glucose just after a meal indicates that the effects of the last insulin injection are nearly gone. In this situation, one must consider shortening the time between insulin administration and feeding. Because of marked patient variation in response to insulin, *it is important that the insulin-glucose response curve be determined.*

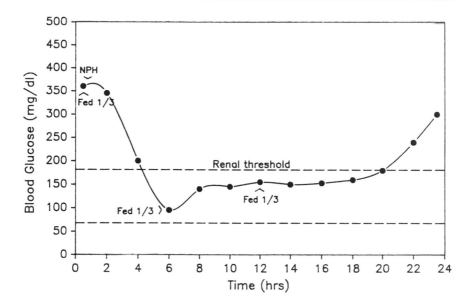

FIGURE 4-1. Adequate response to once-daily subcutaneous NPH insulin and feeding three times daily in an uncomplicated diabetic dog. Blood glucose is in the acceptable range of 60–180 mg/dl for 16–18 hours of the 24-hour period.

It is preferable to start with conservative amounts of insulin and gradually increase the dosage (usually by 1–3 units/day). Remember to wait 2–3 days between each dosage change to allow complete equilibration of the blood glucose. After the initial 24-hour insulin-glucose response curve is determined, one can generally adjust the insulin dosage by measuring blood glucose two or three times daily (prior to morning insulin administration and around the time of expected peak insulin action as determined from the curve). If adjustments are also made in the feeding schedule, it may be best to prepare a second insulin-glucose response curve. It is generally assumed that the insulin-glucose response curve does not change significantly in a particular animal, although it is still recommended that the curve be redone every 3–4 months at the time of patient recheck.

One should not attempt to "fine-tune" blood glucose in the hospital; rather, the goal should be to have the patient reasonably well regulated and then send it home. It is likely that diet and activity levels are somewhat different at home, necessitating some modification in insulin dosage.

Despite the potential "pitfalls" of monitoring a diabetic with urine glucose evaluation, the owner should be taught to collect urine for glucose and ketone measurement with Ketodiastix (Ames). Collections should be made prior to morning feeding and insulin administration and again after the owner returns home from work during the early evening. A record of results should be kept

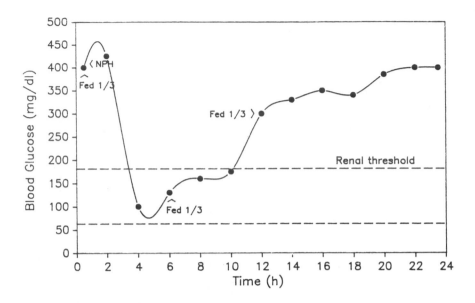

FIGURE 4-2. Inadequate response to once-daily subcutaneous NPH insulin and feeding three times daily in an uncomplicated diabetic dog. Blood glucose is in the acceptable range of 60–180 mg/dl for only 6–7 hours of the 24-hour period because of apparent rapid insulin metabolism.

in a daily log for evaluation by the veterinarian at the time of each recheck or by phone if questions arise. It is important to alert the owner to watch carefully for signs of poor regulation, such as return of PU/PD (indicating hyperglycemia) and weakness–depression–ataxia (consistent with hypoglycemia). Results of urine glucose measurement should always be considered in conjunction with clinical signs, or they may well be misleading. In our experience, it is best to inform the owner not to become unduly concerned unless the evening urine glucose is 3+ to 4+ for four or five consecutive days, or the morning urine glucose is negative for three or four straight days. Even then, if no signs of hyperglycemia or hypoglycemia are present, no change in insulin dosage is usually necessary. It is not wise for either the owner or the veterinarian to make changes in the insulin dosage or feeding regimen based solely on urine glucose and clinical signs. Appearance of ketones in the urine usually indicates longer-term poor control of diabetes. A recheck should be scheduled for such patients as soon as possible. If the owner is concerned about the results of urine glucose or ketone testing, the patient should be rechecked at the time of peak insulin action so the blood glucose can be measured. Sometimes the 24-hour insulin-glucose response curve may need to be repeated.

It may be feasible to teach selected owners to collect a drop or two of blood periodically to determine the patient's blood glucose using the Chemstrip bG method. Some calm dogs may permit sample collection from a foodpad or ear margin using a lancet. Ideally, blood glucose should be checked periodically in the morning immediately prior to insulin administration and again at the expected peak of insulin action. As described for urine glucose values, a log should be kept and the veterinarian periodically consulted. Rechecks should be scheduled at least every 3–4 months.

If the duration of action of once-daily NPH, as determined from the insulin-glucose response curve, is insufficient (< 16–18 hours daily), two options are available: 1) try a potentially longer-acting insulin (PZI); or 2) administer NPH every 12 hours. It is usually easier for the owner to deal with one insulin injection daily, and therefore I advise trying PZI subcutaneously once daily in this situation. However, as was the case for NPH, there is also marked variation in patient response to PZI; therefore one must begin anew and follow the same guidelines for PZI administration and monitoring as described for NPH, including time for equilibration to this new insulin preparation and insulin-glucose response curves. It has also been our experience that a significant number of patients show little response to reasonable doses of PZI. Although undocumented, it is possible that poor absorption of this particular form of insulin from the subcutaneous space is responsible. I have found that some of these animals do well on intramuscular injections of PZI (usually in the paralumbar muscles), but this method causes discomfort in some patients that have decreased muscle mass.

In some animals PZI has its peak effect at 7–10 hours after administration and maintains this peak effect on blood glucose until nearly 24 hours after administration. If PZI insulin is being administered in the morning, the peak action is ongoing during late night hours when the owners are likely to be sleeping. In this situation, it may be wise to feed the third and final meal just prior to the owner's bedtime. The purpose of the late night meal is to provide "insurance" against hypoglycemia while the owner is asleep. This pattern of response to PZI is not predictable and must be documented with an insulin-glucose response curve.

If the patient's response to PZI is inadequate (blood glucose not between 60 and 180 mg/dl for at least 16 hours of each day), it is unlikely that once-daily injection of any type of insulin will be successful. I then resort to multiple NPH injections: hopefully one injection every 12 hours, although some dogs, usually those less than 5 kg body weight, occasionally require three or more NPH injections for good control. The latter situation may not be feasible for the owner, and one must settle for less than ideal regulation.

For practical considerations with the owner's schedule, twice-daily NPH administration is usually advised on an every 12 hour schedule—early morning and 12 hours later, with equal doses of NPH being given each time. As was discussed above, for the "smoothest" blood glucose curve, the dog's daily caloric requirements ideally are fed in four equal-sized meals according to the following schedule: Immediately prior to each insulin injection, midafternoon,

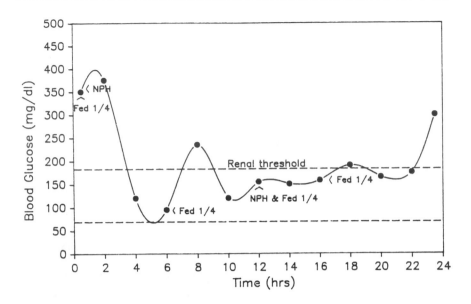

FIGURE 4-3. Adequate response to twice-daily subcutaneous NPH insulin and feeding four times daily in an uncomplicated diabetic dog. Blood glucose is in the acceptable
range of 60–180 mg/dl for 18–19 hours of the 24-hour period.

and late evening. Once again, it is necessary to document that therapeutic goals
are being achieved by obtaining an insulin-glucose response curve (Figure 4-3).

Exercise. Exercise lessens insulin requirements and should be kept fairly
constant from day to day. Exercise is not commonly a problem in the regulation of diabetic pet dogs unless the animal is used for hunting. Although
dogs are likely to exercise more at home than in the hospital, thus lowering
insulin needs, it is generally offset by the usual tendency for the patient to eat
more at home. The net result is that more insulin is commonly required in the
home environment.

It should be apparent that some diabetic dogs are time-consuming chal-
lenges to regulate, especially when they do not respond appropriately to initial
insulin regimens. It is the veterinarian's responsibility to adequately prepare
the owner for this possibility by providing good initial client education.

Alternative Therapy. There is no substitute for daily insulin injections in
most diabetic dogs. If compromises in laboratory monitoring must be made, it
may be possible to regulate the patient's blood glucose satisfactorily by starting
with a conservative insulin dosage (0.25 units/kg SC), carefully observing
clinical signs (improved attitude and appetite, decreased water consumption
and urine output, weight gain), and gradually increasing the insulin dosage as
required. Occasionally, blood glucose should be measured with Chemstrip bG

near the estimated peak insulin effect. Periodic urine glucose measurements may be helpful also. As previously discussed, the patient-to-patient variability in response to insulin makes this "rough" method of monitoring subject to serious inaccuracies. The owner should be made fully aware of the limitations of inadequate monitoring of insulin treatment before this method is used.

Investigational Therapy. Several methods of treatment for DM are currently being evaluated experimentally. Transplantation of pancreatic islet cells from normal dogs into the portal circulation of diabetic dogs shows promise, but the problem of eventual rejection has not been fully overcome. Use of the T-cell immunosuppressive drug cyclosporine during the early stages of insulin-dependent DM in people delays the onset of or in some cases prevents DM, thereby providing evidence that some forms of DM may be caused by immune-mediated mechanisms. Similar studies in dogs have not been reported. The use of small computer-programmed insulin pumps to automatically deliver specified doses of insulin subcutaneously or intravenously has been reported in diabetic people and should be feasible for some diabetic dogs. At this time no reports of their use in veterinary medicine are available.

Treatment of Uncomplicated DM in Cats

Standard Therapy. Treatment for uncomplicated DM in cats is generally similar to the methods used for dogs, although there are a few important differences. It is reported that an occasional obese diabetic cat responds to weight reduction through dietary management and does not require insulin to bring its abnormally high blood glucose back into the normal range. Dietary recommendations similar to those discussed for the diabetic dog probably apply to diabetic cats as well. Feline r/d (Hill's Pet Products) is the preferred diet. Some of these patients eventually require insulin.

A significant number of diabetic cats go through periods of spontaneous remission from their diabetic state and do not require insulin. They may stay in this state of remission for varying periods before again needing insulin to control their diabetes. When managing feline DM, it is especially important to be aware of this phenomenon and be alert for signs of insulin-induced hypoglycemia. It is also important to have the owner regularly test the cat's urine for glucose to help in the early detection of this transient nondiabetic state so that insulin treatment can be reduced or stopped altogether (see below).

The objectives of therapy are similar to those listed for diabetic dogs. Because diabetic cats rarely develop cataracts, preventing this complication with "tight" glucose control is usually not necessary.

Insulin and diet are the major factors to be considered. Exercise is usually not a major consideration affecting blood glucose control in diabetic cats.

Insulin Treatment and Monitoring. Table 4-2 presents the suggested protocol for initial treatment of the diabetic cat. It has been reported that NPH

TABLE 4-2. Suggested Protocol for Initial Regulation of an Uncomplicated Diabetic Cat

Days 1–3

1. 7:50 a.m.	Submit samples for CBC, biochemical profile, and urinalysis. Do blood glucose with Chemstrip bG.
2. 7:55 a.m.	Feed one-third of caloric needs.
3. 8:00 a.m.	Administer 1–3 units PZI insulin *per cat* SC.
4. Noon	Measure blood glucose with Chemstrip bG.
5. 2:00 p.m.	Feed one-third of caloric needs.
6. 4:00 p.m.	Measure blood glucose with Chemstrip bG.
7. 8:00 p.m.	Measure blood glucose with Chemstrip bG. Feed one-third of caloric needs.

Do not change insulin dosage or type or feeding regimen during this initial 3-day period unless grossly unacceptable blood glucose results are obtained.

Day 4

1. 7:50 a.m.	Measure blood glucose with Chemstrip bG.
2. 7:55 a.m.	Feed one-third of caloric needs.
3. 8:00 a.m.	Adjust dosage of PZI insulin up or down (usually by 0.25–0.50 unit) depending on the results of blood glucose values near the expected peak of insulin action on days 1–3. Administer PZI insulin (usually 1.25–3.50 units) SC.
4. 10:00 a.m.	Measure blood glucose every 1–2 hours until 8:00 a.m. of day 5 (24 hours total).
5. 2:00 p.m.	Feed one-third of caloric needs.
6. 8:00 p.m.	Feed one-third of caloric needs.

Day 5

1. 7:50 a.m.	Graph the insulin-glucose response curve, adjust insulin dosage, and if necessary change the frequency of administration, the type of insulin, or both. Evaluate the feeding schedule for possible changes.

insulin has too short a duration of effect in most diabetic cats; therefore PZI is the insulin of choice.

The specific goals of insulin therapy in diabetic cats are the same as those previously presented for diabetic dogs. It may be possible to achieve the major objectives (have the patient feel well, control PU/PD, prevent ketoacidosis, and avoid insulin-induced hypoglycemia) with even "looser" control of blood glucose. It is still advisable to try to keep the blood glucose in the range of 60–180 mg/dl (preferably between 80 and 140 mg/dl) for at least 16 hours of each 24-hour period. Slightly "loose" control of blood glucose, accompanied by mild to moderate glucosuria after insulin action has "worn off," is acceptable, especially in diabetic cats because of their tendency to go through periods of spontaneous remission as previously discussed. This practice allows somewhat of a safety factor against hypoglycemia.

As was the case for diabetic dogs, it is best to place an indwelling venous catheter to aid in sample collection for multiple blood glucose determinations. Samples should be collected prior to starting treatment for a CBC, biochemical profile, and urinalysis. Treatment is begun with 1–3 units of PZI SC per cat usually around 8:00 a.m. Equilibration takes 2–3 days, and the monitoring procedure is similar to that used for uncomplicated diabetic dogs, which includes obtaining an insulin-glucose response curve. One should be careful not to cause anemia by withdrawing excessive amounts of blood for multiple blood glucose determinations. Only 1 or 2 drops of blood should be used for each determination of blood glucose with Chemstrip bG. The initial 1–2 ml of blood removed from the catheter can be carefully returned to the cat through the catheter so long as the sample is obtained without contamination and the catheter is flushed with dilute heparin (1 ml heparin/dl sterile saline) after each sampling period.

Adjustments in PZI dosage should generally be made in increments of 0.25–0.50 units, although in some large, insulin-resistant cats larger daily adjustments are safe. As discussed for diabetic dogs, waiting 2–3 days for equilibration of each new dosage is best.

Accurate measurement of the small doses of insulin required for treatment of diabetic cats and small diabetic dogs is difficult, as insulin is sold only in concentrations of 40 and 100 units/ml. It is often necessary to dilute the insulin, usually 1:10, for the purpose of accurate dosing. There is controversy about the best way to dilute insulin for use in diabetic patients. It is probably best to purchase commercial diluting fluids formulated specifically to be used with certain types of insulin. The veterinarian or a pharmacist can then prepare a bottle of insulin diluted 1:10 with exact directions regarding its use for the owner. It is also reported from clinical experience that sterile physiologic saline solution can be used as the diluting fluid without apparent loss of insulin activity for up to 2 months. Some clinicians prefer to teach the owner to make a 1:10 dilution of insulin in either sterile physiologic saline or lactated Ringer's solution for each dose of insulin used. With this method, the dilution is made, the solution mixed, and the excessive insulin discarded prior to the injection. The obvious advantage is that one does not need to worry about the stability of the diluted insulin solution; however, the owner must be capable of learning the dilution technique.

The cat should be sent home for "fine-tuning" of the insulin dosage. The owner should be taught to collect urine for testing of urine glucose and ketones. Such collection can usually be accomplished by either covering the cat's regular litter with a commercial plastic sheeting such as SaranWrap or using shredded newspaper in place of the regular litter. The goals are to have the urine negative for glucose in the afternoon and slightly to moderately positive in the early morning just prior to insulin administration. As was discussed for monitoring diabetic dogs, results of urine glucose measurement should always be interpreted in conjunction with clinical signs so they are not misleading. The owner should be diligent about watching for return of PU/PD or weakness, lethargy, ataxia, and so on, possibly indicating hyperglycemia or hypoglycemia. Constantly negative urine glucose values are worrisome in diabetic cats and may indicate that the cat is in remission and does not require insulin. It is not advisable for either the owner or the veterinarian to change the cat's insulin dosage based solely on the results of the urine glucose testing. A recheck should be scheduled for blood glucose measurement at the peak time of insulin action if urine values are out of the desired range for 4–5 consecutive days or if signs compatible with hyperglycemia or hypoglycemia are seen. Otherwise the patient should be rechecked every 3–4 months and, ideally, an insulin-glucose response curve repeated.

The duration of action of PZI in cats is variable from patient to patient, and in some patients PZI must be used twice daily to achieve therapeutic objectives. As was true for dogs, PZI sometimes appears not to be well absorbed from the subcutaneous space. If the cat has sufficient muscle mass, intramuscular administration may be a useful alternative. In cats with little muscle mass, the use of subcutaneous NPH two or three times daily may be necessary.

Diet and Feeding Schedule. Obesity is often associated with DM in cats also. Therefore the goals for feeding diabetic cats are similar to those previously discussed for diabetic dogs. A fat-restricted diet with good quality protein is best. Prescription diet feline r/d (Hill's Pet Products) is recommended for obese cats. If obesity is not a problem, prescription diet feline w/d (Hill's Pet Products) can be used. Semimoist foods should not be fed to diabetic cats because of their high sucrose content.

Caloric requirements are 75–100 kcal/kg/day. If obesity is present, the number of calories fed (per kilogram) should be decreased by about 40% until ideal body weight is reached. Feeding regimens, including the number of meals fed daily and the percentage of calories fed at each meal, should be the same as previously discussed for diabetic dogs (three meals a day for cats on once-daily insulin, four meals a day for cats on twice-daily insulin). Many cats may not adhere to rigidly timed meals and may prefer ad libitum feeding. Potentially the latter "schedule" could make it more difficult to achieve satisfactory control of blood glucose; however, studies are needed to evaluate the issue of appropriate feeding schedules for diabetic cats on insulin therapy.

Alternative Treatment. As was discussed for diabetic dogs, there is usually no satisfactory alternative to daily insulin injections for diabetic cats. A possible exception is the occasional obese diabetic cat that sometimes has its body weight and blood glucose satisfactorily controlled with a low-fat high-fiber diet such as r/d (Hill's Pet Products).

If ideal laboratory monitoring is not possible, an alternative is to start with conservative dosages of PZI insulin (0.5–1.0 unit/cat/day SC) and monitor clinical signs (improved attitude and appetite, decreased water consumption and urine output, weight gain), gradually increasing the insulin dosage as required. Occasionally, blood glucose should be measured with Chemstrip bG near the expected peak insulin effect, and periodic urine glucose evaluation should be done. The owner should be made fully aware of the limitations of this method.

Treatment of Diabetic Ketoacidosis in Dogs and Cats

Diabetic ketoacidosis (DKA) occurs in both dogs and cats but is more common in dogs. DKA may result from failure to treat or from improperly treating uncomplicated DM or from superimposed complications (e.g., infection, stress, dehydration) in a previously well-regulated patient. Mild to moderate ketosis and acidosis are often seen in diabetic patients who are showing no obvious signs of ketoacidosis. Severe DKA has been defined as being present when there is a history of anorexia and depression, more than 5% dehydration, glucosuria, ketonuria, blood glucose of more than 300 mg/dl, and an arterial bicarbonate concentration of less than 10 mEq/L.

Standard Therapy of DKA with No Associated Clinical Signs. If a diabetic animal has significant ketonuria but is alert, not dehydrated, and showing no other major abnormal signs of ketoacidosis (e.g., vomiting), initial treatment is usually similar to that previously discussed for an uncomplicated diabetic (NPH or PZI insulin). If the animal is presented late in the day, good clinical judgment is required to properly assess whether insulin therapy should be begun that evening or if it can safely wait until early the next morning. It is probably best to begin insulin therapy right away if adequate monitoring of the patient's blood glucose is possible during the evening hours.

If treatment is begun during evening hours, regular insulin should be used because it has a rapid onset and short duration of action, which enable the clinician to evaluate its effects and change dosages frequently if necessary. Regular insulin should be given subcutaneously to nondehydrated patients at a dosage of 0.25–0.50 unit/kg every 6–8 hours. Blood should be obtained every 1–2 hours for blood glucose monitoring using Chemstrip bG, including a measurement just prior to each insulin injection. If the patient will eat, it should be fed just prior to each follow-up insulin injection (immediately after each blood sample is obtained for blood glucose measurement). If the animal refuses to eat, it may be necessary to reduce the dosage of insulin or skip an insulin injection. The objectives are to stop further ketone production, start ketone utilization, and stabilize the patient's metabolic status in preparation for beginning NPH or PZI insulin treatment early the next morning (see the sections above on the treatment of uncomplicated diabetic dogs and cats). It is best to allow the patient's morning blood glucose to exceed the upper normal value (preferably >200 mg/dl) so the NPH or PZI insulin regimen can be started safely.

Alternatively, many relatively "healthy" ketotic diabetic animals do not require special evening treatment and monitoring. These patients can be started on NPH or PZI insulin as previously described for the uncomplicated diabetic.

Standard Treatment of Severe DKA. Most animals with severe DKA are critically ill and require intensive treatment and monitoring, which is not available in some veterinary practices. In the latter situation, it is the veterinarian's responsibility to encourage referral to a practice with adequate resources to manage these patients.

Before beginning treatment of DKA, it is important to evaluate the patient for coexisting disorders. DKA is often precipitated by concurrent infections (urinary tract, prostatitis, pyometra), pancreatitis, and congestive heart failure, and it may be accompanied by azotemia as a result of dehydration (prerenal) or renal failure. An indwelling catheter should be placed in a jugular vein for repeated sampling of blood and measurement of central venous pressure (CVP). Samples should be submitted prior to treatment for CBC, biochemical profile, and urinalysis (preferably collected by cystocentesis). If pancreatitis is suspected, serum amylase and lipase assays should be done. Urine production should be monitored using a closed-system indwelling catheter placed in the bladder. If urinary tract infection develops subsequent to use of the indwelling catheter, the urine should be cultured and appropriate antibiotic therapy started after the catheter is removed. These steps take only a few minutes, after which treatment can proceed immediately.

Reported goals of treatment are to: 1) provide adequate amounts of insulin to normalize intermediary metabolism; 2) restore water and electrolyte losses; 3) correct acidosis; 4) identify precipitating factors in the disease process; and 5) provide a carbohydrate substrate intravenously when required to promote ketone utilization and prevent hypoglycemia as a result of insulin therapy. To lessen the risk of treatment-induced complications, it is best to slowly (over 36–48 hours) correct the abnormalities associated with DKA.

Insulin Therapy. As previously discussed, regular insulin should be used for DKA. Low-dose regimens are just as effective as high-dose methods and are associated with fewer complications.

Either of two methods of insulin administration may be used: hourly intramuscular or continuous intravenous infusion. The choice between these two methods depends on personal preferences as well as the facilities and expertise available for monitoring. Protocols for low-dose intermittent intramuscular and continuous intravenous insulin for treatment of severe DKA are shown in Tables 4-3 and 4-4. The main objective is to decrease the blood glucose concentration to the range of 200–250 mg/dl over a period of 2–8 hours (Tables 4-3 and 4-4). Intermittent subcutaneous insulin administration is not recommended because of slower, erratic absorption in dehydrated, hypotensive

TABLE 4-3. Low-Dose, Hourly Intramuscular Regular Insulin Treatment Protocol for the Management of Diabetic Ketoacidosis

1. Administer an initial dose of regular insulin (0.2 unit/kg IM).

2. Measure blood glucose hourly with Chemstrip bG/Accuchek II.

3. Administer follow-up dosages of regular insulin (0.1 unit/kg IM hourly).

    a. Ideally, the blood glucose concentration should decrease by 50–100 mg/dl/hr.

    b. The hourly insulin dosage can be increased to 0.2 unit/kg or decreased to 0.05 unit/kg as needed to maintain the ideal rate of blood glucose decline.

4. Stop hourly IM regular insulin when blood glucose decreases to 200–250 mg/dl (assuming the patient is hydrated, more alert, not vomiting, and probably willing to eat).

5. The treatment regimen then depends on the *time of day when the desired blood glucose value is attained*. The goal is to start the patient on NPH or PZI insulin early in the morning (as described for the uncomplicated diabetic—see text).

    a. Blood glucose of 200–250 mg/dl reached in the early morning hours (e.g., at 2:00 a.m. to 7:59 a.m.): Begin NPH or PZI SC around the following 8:00 a.m. to noon as for the uncomplicated diabetic.

    b. Blood glucose of 200–250 mg/dl reached in the afternoon, evening, or late nighttime hours (e.g., at 12:01 p.m. to 1:59 a.m.): Administer regular insulin SC q6h (0.5–1.0 unit/kg) and monitor blood glucose q1–2h with Chemstrip bG/Accuchek II. Begin NPH or PZI SC around the following 8:00 a.m. to noon as for the uncomplicated diabetic.

DKA patients. Assuming the patient begins to feel better and to eat and drink, subcutaneous NPH or PZI insulin should be started the next morning as described for treatment of the uncomplicated diabetic.

Fluid and Electrolyte Therapy. Adequate fluid and electrolyte replacement, administered intravenously, is important in the restoration of body fluids, including circulating blood volume. Beneficial effects include 1) improvement in cardiac output and renal blood flow; 2) correction of dehydration, electrolyte imbalance, and acidosis; and 3) lowering of blood glucose.

The choice of the intravenous fluid solution varies among clinicians. Isotonic saline (0.9%) has been recommended by some clinicians for DKA in dogs because of the reported tendency for these patients to be hyponatremic. Others prefer a more balanced electrolyte solution such as Ringer's or lactated Ringer's solution. It is likely that the quantity of fluid administered and the rate with which it is delivered are more critical than the fluid used.

Dogs and cats with DKA may be severely dehydrated (10–12%). Total fluid volume requirements are calculated by adding the estimated deficit, maintenance needs, and continuing losses (see Chapter 1). Although the total fluid deficit should be corrected slowly (over 24–48 hours), circulating blood volume (about 90 ml/kg) should be restored during the first 1–2 hours (with careful patient monitoring for any signs of fluid overload). The remaining calculated

TABLE 4-4.　Low-Dose, Continuous Intravenous Regular Insulin Infusion Treatment Protocol for the Management of Diabetic Ketoacidosis

1. Add 1 unit of *regular crystalline insulin* to each 100 ml of fluid (either lactated Ringer's or 0.9% saline) and infuse at a rate to deliver 0.5–1.0 unit of insulin/hr (50–100 ml/hr) or 0.025–0.050 unit/kg/hr. Cats and small dogs should receive the lower dosage. Use a pediatric minidrip infusion set or volumetric infusion pump.

2. Use a separate intravenous line for hydration or hydrate prior to starting insulin drip.

3. Measure blood glucose hourly with Chemstrip bG/Accuchek II.

   a. Ideally, the blood glucose concentration should decrease by 50–100 mg/dl/hr.

   b. The rate of insulin infusion can be adjusted up or down as needed.

4. Stop insulin infusion when blood glucose decreases to 200–250 mg/dl. This drop requires an average of 4 hours but varies from 2–8 hours.*

5. Convert to conventional insulin therapy (assuming the patient is hydrated, more alert, not vomiting, and probably willing to eat). The treatment regimen then depends on the *time of day when the desired blood glucose value is attained.* The goal is to start the patient on NPH or PZI insulin early in the morning (as described for the uncomplicated diabetic—see text).†

   a. Blood glucose of 200–250 mg/dl reached in the early morning hours (e.g., at 2:00 a.m. to 7:59 a.m.): Begin NPH or PZI SC around the following 8:00 a.m. to noon as for the uncomplicated diabetic.

   b. Blood glucose of 200–250 mg/dl reached in the afternoon, evening, or late nighttime hours (e.g., at 12:01 p.m. to 1:59 a.m.): Administer regular insulin SC q6h (0.5–1.0 unit/kg) and monitor blood glucose q1–2h with Chemstrip bG/Accuchek II. Begin NPH or PZI SC around the following 8:00 a.m. to noon as for the uncomplicated diabetic.

*A fresh mixture of regular crystalline insulin in lactated Ringer's or saline should be prepared if the infusion is to be continued beyond 8 hours.
†Some clinicians prefer to infuse 5% dextrose solution IV for a variable period of time to promote ketone utilization. This practice prolongs and complicates the treatment procedure, and it is not clear that survival is improved.

requirements should be administered in approximately equal hourly quantities by slower intravenous infusion. Once adequate hydration is achieved, a daily maintenance rate of 40–60 ml/kg/day should be administered in nearly equal hourly amounts over each 24-hour period (about 1.5–2.5 ml/kg/hr). In cats and small dogs, pediatric minidrip sets are necessary to adequately control the rate of fluid administration, especially if the patient has cardiopulmonary disease.

With an indwelling jugular catheter, it is helpful periodically to measure the CVP to prevent fluid overload. Urine production should be measured using an indwelling bladder catheter. This point is particularly important in critically ill patients who may be oliguric or anuric. Early recognition of oliguric renal insufficiency is essential so appropriate treatment can be administered if necessary (see Chapter 11).

Fluid requirements should be frequently reassessed and adjustments made as changes in hydration, urine output, and the severity and frequency of vomiting and diarrhea are observed.

Body potassium stores are often decreased in DKA because of anorexia, vomiting, diarrhea, and polyuria. Serum potassium may not correlate with body stores and may be normal, decreased, or increased. Insulin treatment and correction of metabolic acidosis with fluid therapy may cause shifting of potassium into body cells, thereby producing significant hypokalemia. Post-treatment hypokalemia is more likely to be of clinical significance if the patient has a low or low-normal serum potassium (< 4.0 mEq/L) prior to insulin and fluid administration. The objectives of potassium therapy are to maintain a normal serum potassium level on an acute basis and to gradually replenish body potassium stores. Supplemental potassium chloride mixed with the intravenous fluids is advised *only after it has been established that the patient is producing adequate amounts of urine*. Otherwise, fatal hyperkalemia can result. If hypokalemia is documented or strongly suspected, 30–40 mEq of potassium (usually as potassium chloride or potassium phosphate) should be added to each liter of fluid, and the rate of (intravenous) fluid administration adjusted so the rate of potassium administration does not exceed 0.5 mEq/kg/hr. Guidelines for the total daily dosage of potassium, based on the serum potassium, are shown in Table 1-5. It is best to measure serum potassium at least daily in order to assess the results of potassium therapy and make necessary adjustments. A lead II electrocardiogram may also be helpful, especially if serum potassium measurements are delayed. See Chapter 1 for additional information on treatment of hypokalemia.

Hypophosphatemia sometimes occurs in DKA, probably for reasons similar to those for hypokalemia. If documented, hypophosphatemia should be corrected slowly over a period of several hours by using potassium phosphate (2.5 mg phosphate/kg/day) instead of potassium chloride as a supplement in the intravenous fluid solution.

Other electrolyte abnormalities are usually corrected with the insulin and fluid therapy regimens described above.

Acid-Base Therapy. Most patients with DKA do not require alkalinizing agents such as bicarbonate or lactate to have their acidosis corrected, although many clinicians prefer to use the mildly alkalinizing fluid lactated Ringer's as a balanced electrolyte solution (see above discussion). Use of the strong alkalinizing drug bicarbonate may cause serious complications, such as hypokalemia, left-shifted oxyhemoglobin dissociation curve, decreased serum ionized calcium, and paradoxical cerebrospinal fluid acidosis. Therefore bicarbonate should not be used except for documented severe metabolic acidemia (serum bicarbonate < 10 mEq/L, blood pH < 7.10).

If facilities for complete arterial blood gas analysis are not available, venous total carbon dioxide (TCO_2) can be used as a substitute estimate of serum bicarbonate concentration. The bicarbonate deficit can be estimated from the formula

$$\text{Bicarbonate deficit} = 0.5 \text{ body wt. (kg)} \times (\text{normal } TCO_2 - \text{patient } TCO_2)$$

Sodium bicarbonate solution should never be given as an intravenous bolus. It is best to add 7.5% sodium bicarbonate solution to 0.45% saline and administer the estimated bicarbonate deficit slowly over a 24- to 48-hour period. Approximately half of the estimated bicarbonate deficit should be administered during the first 4–6 hours and the remaining half given during the next 24–48 hours. Venous TCO_2 should be rechecked at least once daily and appropriate adjustments made in bicarbonate supplementation. Bicarbonate administration should be stopped when the venous TCO_2 reaches the low normal range (about 16–20 mEq/L).

In addition to hourly monitoring of blood glucose (Tables 4-3 and 4-4), it is important to observe regularly the patient's mental status. Successful treatment of DKA should be associated with improvement in the animal's attitude, activity, and willingness to eat unless other serious disorders are present. Also, urine ketone levels can be checked every 4–6 hours. Although it is reassuring to see urine ketone levels decline, ketones often remain in the urine for several days despite an otherwise favorable response to treatment.

Treatment of Concurrent Disorders. As previously discussed, dogs and cats with DKA often have serious coexisting disorders such as pancreatitis and sepsis (see above discussion). In addition, iatrogenic complications may develop as a result of intense treatment (e.g., fluid overload, hypokalemia, hypoglycemia). The clinician must not "hone in" so intently on DKA that he or she forgets to evaluate and treat the "whole" patient. The prognosis is usually more closely related to the presence of serious concurrent disorders than to DKA itself.

HYPOGLYCEMIA

Hypoglycemia is the sequela to a variety of metabolic alterations. It is commonly seen in patients on insulin treatment who are improperly managed and may also be associated with enzymatic defects of the liver (e.g., storage diseases), drug administration, organic diseases (e.g., adrenocortical insufficiency, severe hepatic disease), septicemia, or with tumors secreting insulin or insulin-like substances. A functional hypoglycemia has been seen in puppies and hunting dogs and with starvation. The clinical signs of hypoglycemia are most frequently associated with its effect on the central nervous system, which is most severely affected, including mild changes such as trembling or weakness; however, in severe cases seizures may be seen and the animal may suffer permanent brain damage. In general, an acute fall in glucose concentrations is less well tolerated than a slow decline.

Standard Therapy

The treatment for hypoglycemia can be divided into two forms.

1. *Treatment of the acute hypoglycemic attack.* This treatment is aimed at rapid correction of the low blood glucose concentration and includes the administration of glucose or glucose-containing agents that increase blood glucose concentrations. The administration of glucagon, which is gluconeogenic, has also been recommended. Although glucagon promotes hepatic glycogenolysis, it also leads to insulin release from the beta cells of the pancreas and is therefore not indicated therapeutically except in diabetic dogs suffering from insulin overdose. It can, however, be used as a provocative test for the diagnosis of insulinoma.

2. *Treatment of chronic hypoglycemia.* The management of chronic hypoglycemia includes alterations of the feeding schedule and administration of glucocorticoids and agents that decrease insulin secretion or inhibit its action.

Treatment of Acute Hypoglycemia. *Administration of Glucose.* Acute hypoglycemic attacks require immediate attention. If the animal is at home, the owner should be advised to administer a glucose-containing solution (e.g., corn syrup, honey) and then immediately take the pet to the veterinarian. In a seizuring animal, the solution should be rubbed into the buccal mucosa to avoid aspiration. The effect is rapid, most animals responding within 1 minute.

The veterinarian can treat acute hypoglycemic attacks with administration of glucose at a dose of 0.5 g/kg body weight (1 ml of a 50% dextrose solution per kilogram) given slowly intravenously. This treatment can be repeated as needed, but it is preferred to maintain therapy with continuous infusion of a 5% dextrose solution. The animal's blood glucose can easily be monitored using glucose-impregnated strips (Dextrostix, Ames; Chemstrip bG, Boehringer Mannheim). The test strips can be visually inspected or accurately read with a reflectance colorimeter (e.g., Dextrometer, Ames; Accu-Chek II, Boehringer Mannheim).

Glucagon. As mentioned above, glucagon (Glucagon, Lilly) should be used only as an emergency treatment of the diabetic. It is administered intravenously or intramuscularly at a dose of 0.5–1.0 mg once in the dog or cat.

Dietary Management. Animals with hypoglycemic attacks should be fed multiple small meals during the day to ensure the availability of dietary substrates at all times. The recommended diet consists of canned or dry food high in protein content; simple sugars as they exist in many semimoist foods should be avoided.

Treatment of Chronic Hypoglycemia. *Dietary Management.* The dietary management is the same as that described for the treatment of acute hypoglycemic attacks. It should be used in all patients with chronic hypoglycemia.

Glucocorticoids. Glucocorticoids are used in cases of hyperinsulinism because of their insulin-antagonistic effect. The initial dose is 0.5 mg/kg/day given in two divided doses. This dose may have to be increased if it fails to control the hypoglycemia. The side effects are listed on page 32.

Diazoxide. Diazoxide (Proglycem, Schering) is a nondiuretic benzothiadiazine that has proved beneficial in humans not only in cases of hyperinsulinism but also in patients with hypoglycemia of other etiologies. In the dog it has been used for the medical treatment of insulinomas. Diazoxide increases blood glucose by inhibiting insulin secretion, enhancing epinephrine release, promoting hepatic glycogenolysis, and decreasing glucose uptake in liver.

The initial dose of diazoxide is 10 mg/kg body weight divided into two daily doses. This dose can be increased gradually but should not exceed 60 mg/kg/day. It is best given with a meal to reduce gastrointestinal side effects. The goal of therapy is to alleviate hypoglycemia and avoid hyperglycemia.

Investigational Therapy

Streptozotocin (Zanosar, Upjohn), an antibiotic that has been shown to be cytotoxic to beta cells, and is used frequently experimentally in animals to induce diabetes mellitus. In humans it is the most commonly used drug in patients with metastatic islet cell carcinoma. It is rarely used in dogs with insulinoma, most likely because of its severe side effects, which include renal tubular and hepatic damage. The dose used in humans is 500 mg/m^2 administered intravenously every 5 days.

HYPERADRENOCORTICISM
(CUSHING'S SYNDROME)

Hyperadrenocorticism (HC) is the result of chronic hypercortisolemia. It occurs in both dogs and cats but is much more common in dogs. Basic causes of HC are administration of pharmacologic doses of glucocorticoids (iatrogenic HC) and hypersecretion of cortisol from the adrenal cortex (spontaneous HC). Spontaneous hypersecretion of cortisol from the adrenals may be due to excessive adrenocorticotrophic hormone (ACTH) output from the pituitary gland (pituitary-dependent hyperadrenocorticism, or PDH) or overproduction of cortisol by an adrenocortical tumor (AT, adrenal-dependent hyperadrenocorticism).

The clinical course of HC is usually insidious and slowly progressive. Signs depend on the duration and magnitude of hypercortisolemia and probably on individual patient susceptibility. Common signs in affected dogs include polydipsia, polyuria, polyphagia, obesity, "pot-bellied" appearance, lethargy, bilaterally symmetric alopecia, and thinning of the skin. A variety of other signs may be seen, including muscle weakness, hepatomegaly, increased panting, hyperpigmentation, and calcinosis cutis. Also, chronic hypercortisolemia may predispose to several potentially fatal complications including acute pancreatitis, diabetes mellitus, pyelonephritis, gastrointestinal ulceration, colonic perforation, and pulmonary thrombosis. In cats, polydipsia, polyuria, polyphagia, a pendulous abdomen, alopecia, and thinning of the skin are the most frequently observed signs. Most cats with spontaneous HC are diabetic by the time a diagnosis is made. Characteristic laboratory findings include a stress leukogram, increased serum activities of alkaline phosphatase and alanine aminotransferase, mild hyperglycemia, hypercholesterolemia, decreased urine specific gravity, and evidence of urinary tract infection.

Diagnosis of HC is established by plasma cortisol testing, including ACTH stimulation and low-dose dexamethasone suppression. Differentiation of PDH from AT may require multiple diagnostic methods including plasma ACTH assay, high-dose dexamethasone suppression, and abdominal imaging procedures such as radiography, ultrasonography, computed tomography (CT scanning), and magnetic resonance imaging (MRI).

Iatrogenic Hyperadrenocorticism

Patients with iatrogenic HC often have secondary adrenal atrophy and limited ability to secrete glucocorticoids in response to stress, characterized by little or no increase in plasma cortisol secretion following ACTH administration (ACTH stimulation test). Clinical signs of iatrogenic HC are usually those of Cushing's syndrome (see above); however, sudden discontinuation of glucocorticoid administration may cause signs of glucocorticoid deficiency (lethargy, anorexia, vomiting, diarrhea, dehydration, shock) or both glucocorticoid and mineralocorticoid deficiency (Addison's disease: weakness, collapse, bradycardia, death). See the section on hypoadrenocorticism, below, for additional information.

Standard Therapy. The objective of appropriate therapy for iatrogenic HC is to initially reduce the quantity of glucocorticoid being administered, with the eventual goal being cessation of steroid treatment after sufficient return of adrenocortical responsiveness as documented by follow-up ACTH stimulation testing. Return of adequate adrenocortical response to ACTH usually occurs within 1–3 months, although it can take several months depending on the severity of adrenal atrophy. Two general approaches to treatment can be used: 1) cessation of administration of the potent glucocorticoid(s) responsible for HC and adrenal atrophy and replacement with the more physiologic product hydrocortisone (Cortef tablets, Upjohn); or 2) gradually "weaning" the patient from the potent glucocorticoid(s) responsible for the HC and adrenal atrophy.

With the first method, the offending glucocorticoid treatment is stopped, and Cortef is administered at a dosage of 0.1–0.5 mg/kg q12h PO daily (physiologic maintenance dosage). This dosage should be increased two- to fivefold during periods of stress. ACTH stimulation testing should be repeated every 1–2 months until adequate adrenal responsiveness is documented, at which time Cortef treatment should be terminated. Remember to temporarily (24 hours) withhold Cortef immediately prior to plasma cortisol measurement to prevent falsely high values. The patient should be carefully observed during this period for signs of glucocorticoid insufficiency and treated with glucocorticoids if necessary (rare).

The second treatment method involves gradually "weaning" the patient from the offending glucocorticoid(s). For example, if the animal has been receiving high dosages of prednisone daily per os, the dosage should be reduced by about 25% every 7–10 days over a period of 4–6 weeks while carefully observing the patient for signs of glucocorticoid insufficiency. If such signs appear, the dosage of prednisone must be increased temporarily. It is suggested that ACTH stimulation testing be done every 1–2 months to assess adrenocortical responsiveness in order to determine when to discontinue glucocorticoid treatment. (Remember to discontinue prednisone therapy for 24 hours immediately prior to plasma cortisol measurement.) If the patient has also been receiving injections of a repositol glucocorticoid preparation, e.g., methylprednisolone acetate (Depo-Medrol, Upjohn), these injections should be discontinued while gradually reducing the prednisone dosage as just described.

Elective anesthesia and surgery in patients with iatrogenic adrenal atrophy should be avoided. For nonelective surgical procedures, it is imperative to administer extra amounts of glucocorticoids, especially immediately prior to anesthesia and for the first 24–48 hours after surgery. A suggested protocol is as follows. On the day of surgery, administer Cortef at a dosage of 1–2 mg/kg PO before the procedure and again after the animal has fully recovered from anesthesia. In addition, administer prednisolone sodium succinate (Solu Delta Cortef, Upjohn) at a dosage of 1 mg/kg IV immediately prior to anesthesia and every 4–6 hours during the surgical procedure. Blood glucose should be monitored (Chemstrip bG, Boehringer Mannheim) every 1–2 hours during surgery and for the first few hours after surgery. If hypoglycemia occurs (blood glucose < 80 mg/dl), a 5% dextrose intravenous infusion should be started (see the section in this chapter on treatment of hypoglycemia). After 48 hours it is usually safe to once again administer only Cortef in physiologic maintenance amounts (0.1–0.5 mg/kg q12h PO).

Prognosis for iatrogenic HC is good if the problem is recognized and managed appropriately. Return of adrenocortical response to ACTH invariably occurs, although it sometimes requires several months.

Spontaneous Hyperadrenocorticism

Treatment of spontaneous HC may be medical or surgical depending on the cause (see below). Regardless of the treatment method used, considerable time and expense are involved. Thorough client education is important to make the owner aware of this situation as well as the long-term (usually lifelong) nature of the disorder and the need for regular follow-up examinations. Most patients with spontaneous HC should be treated because of the progressive characteristics of the disorder and the potentially serious, even fatal, conditions that may occur as a result of chronic hypercortisolemia (see above); however, for some mildly affected patients (especially older animals), treatment may not be considered necessary considering the time, expense, and potential side effects of therapy. Clients should be warned of possible complications associated with untreated HC and be allowed to participate in the often difficult decision not to treat. Prognosis depends on the cause and severity of spontaneous HC and on the diligence with which the veterinarian and client pursue diagnosis and management.

To adequately monitor response to therapy, prior to beginning treatment it is important to have baseline data, including the amount of daily water consumption (per kilogram body weight) and plasma cortisol values before and after ACTH administration.

Pituitary-Dependent Hyperadrenocorticism in Dogs

Pituitary-dependent hyperadrenocorticism (PDH) is most commonly caused by an ACTH-secreting microadenoma of the pituitary gland. These tumors are generally benign and slow-growing. Only occasionally do they expand and cause neurologic signs. Although surgical resection of the pituitary tumor would be ideal, the difficulty of the surgery usually precludes this approach.

Standard Therapy. The drug of choice for treatment of PDH in dogs is *o,p'*-DDD (Lysodren, Bristol). Lysodren causes necrosis of the adrenal cortex. The glucocorticoid-producing layers (zona reticularis and zona fasiculata) are more susceptible to Lysodren-induced necrosis, but the mineralocorticoid-producing zona glomerulosa also undergoes necrotic destruction if Lysodren is used in high enough doses for a sufficient period of time. In the protocol to be described in this section, the goal is to cause nearly complete destruction of the glucocorticoid-producing layers of the adrenal cortex but to preserve the mineralocorticoid-producing layer. Therapy with Lysodren is done in two phases: induction and maintenance.

Induction Therapy with Lysodren. The veterinarian may choose to treat dogs with PDH in the hospital or at home. We prefer to hospitalize all patients during the induction phase of treatment to facilitate observation and any changes required in the treatment protocol. If the patient is sent home during the induction phase, thorough client education is essential, and daily tele-phone contact with the owner to go over clinical signs and treatment compli-ance is important.

The induction dosage of Lysodren is 50 mg/kg/day PO. Some experts prefer to split the daily dosage and administer 25 mg/kg q12h PO. Feeding the patient immediately prior to Lysodren administration apparently improves absorption and is advised. There is considerable patient-to-patient variation in the length of time required for daily Lysodren treatment at the above dosage to suffi-ciently reduce glucocorticoid production (2–35 days, average 5–14 days). Careful observation (in the hospital or at home) of the patient's attitude and appetite, as well as measurement of daily water consumption, helps determine when PDH is in remission. Onset of listlessness and lethargy, decreased appetite, vomiting, and markedly decreased water consumption are consistent with glucocorticoid insufficiency and are strong indications that remission has been achieved. Whenever any of these signs are observed, Lysodren adminis-tration should be stopped and an ACTH stimulation test performed immedi-ately. Once the plasma samples for cortisol analysis have been collected, it is generally prudent to administer physiologic maintenance dosages of a short-acting glucocorticoid until the results of the ACTH stimulation test are known. Hydrocortisone (Cortef) at a dosage of 0.1–0.5 mg/kg q12h PO is preferred to prednisone. If prednisone is used, the equivalent physiologic maintenance dosage is 0.02–0.10 mg/kg q12h PO. When signs of glucocorticoid insufficiency are especially severe or if vomiting precludes the use of oral glucocorticoids, Solu Delta Cortef can be administered at an initial dosage of 1–2 mg/kg IV followed by a dosage of 0.1–0.5 mg/kg IV or SC q4–6h until improvement is seen. The treatment is then changed to oral Cortef at the previously recom-mended physiologic maintenance dosage (0.1–0.5 mg/kg PO q12h). Supple-mental glucocorticoids are not administered to patients during the induction phase of treatment unless signs of glucocorticoid deficiency are observed.

Even if the patient being treated with Lysodren has not shown abnormal clinical signs, an ACTH stimulation test should be repeated by the 10th day after beginning induction therapy. In this situation (no abnormal clinical signs), Lyso-dren treatment should be continued while awaiting plasma cortisol results, again carefully observing the patient for signs of glucocorticoid insufficiency.

What is the major goal of the induction phase of Lysodren therapy? The patient should be made functionally hypoadrenal without causing severe clinical signs of either glucocorticoid or mineralocorticoid insufficiency. Adre-nal function can be accurately assessed only by repeated ACTH stimulation testing and plasma cortisol evaluation. Normal values for plasma cortisol in dogs must be known for the particular laboratory being used. In our laboratory, normal canine baseline plasma cortisol is 0.5–4.0 μg/dl, and normal post-ACTH plasma cortisol is 8–20 μg/dl. Ideally, Lysodren-treated dogs with PDH have baseline cortisol values of less than 1.0 μg/dl and have little or no response to ACTH administration (post-ACTH plasma cortisol < 1.0 μg/dl). Plasma cortisol values of more than 4 μg/dl in dogs being treated with Lysodren are nearly always associated with eventual recurrence of signs of HC (see section on maintenance therapy below).

Little blunting of the plasma cortisol response to ACTH after 14–21 days of Lysodren therapy at the above recommended dosage (50 mg/kg/day) should arouse suspicion of misdiagnosis of an adrenal tumor.

Maintenance Therapy with Lysodren. Once the goals of induction therapy are attained, maintenance treatment with Lysodren should be initiated at a dosage of 50 mg/kg/week PO. Some authorities prefer to divide the total dose into two equal weekly dosages (25 mg/kg PO administered twice weekly). If induction therapy caused marked signs of glucocorticoid insufficiency and plasma cortisol values before and after ACTH administration were less than 1.0 μg/dl, it is preferable to supplement with Cortef (see above section) and wait about 2 weeks before beginning maintenance treatment with Lysodren. Waiting longer than 2 weeks to start maintenance therapy may result in some patients coming out of remission, thus necessitating reinduction with daily Lysodren treatment.

The requirement for concurrent usage of supplemental glucocorticoid in patients on maintenance Lysodren therapy is variable. Because the goal of Lysodren treatment for spontaneous HC is to cause sufficient destruction of the adrenal cortex to render it unresponsive to ACTH, it is not surprising that many patients "tightly" regulated on Lysodren periodically show signs of glucocorticoid insufficiency (lethargy, inappetance, vomiting, diarrhea), especially during periods of stress. For this reason we advise supplementation with Cortef at the physiologic maintenance dosage (0.1–0.5 mg/kg PO q12h) for nearly all patients on maintenance Lysodren therapy. This dosage should be increased by a factor of two- to fivefold if stress is anticipated or occurs.

If the owner is astute and observant, it may be satisfactory to send Cortef home with the patient with instructions to administer the drug only when signs of glucocorticoid insufficiency are seen. The appropriate dosage of Cortef for stressed patients showing early signs of glucocorticoid insufficiency is approximately two to five times the physiologic maintenance dosage (1.0–2.5 mg/kg q12h PO). Treatment should be continued for several days after resolution of clinical signs.

Repeating ACTH stimulation testing at *3-month intervals* is important for proper management and adequate control of PDH in dogs. Unfortunately, there is significant patient-to-patient variation in terms of the long-term response to the above Lysodren treatment regimen. Approximately 50% of all patients on the standard maintenance dosage of Lysodren (50 mg/kg/week) come out of remission at some point. Without regular ACTH stimulation testing, it is likely that a lengthy period will elapse before the owner realizes that the animal has come out of remission. Such patients should be evaluated for the presence of diseases commonly associated with chronic hypercortisolemia, e.g., diabetes mellitus and urinary tract infection. On the other hand, some patients on the standard maintenance dosage of Lysodren develop signs of glucocorticoid insufficiency, and an occasional dog (about 5% of all patients) becomes addisonian (signs of both glucocorticoid and mineralocorticoid insufficiency).

Clinical signs and ACTH stimulation test results (obtained every 3 months) determine if a change in Lysodren dosage is required. As was discussed above, dogs with PDH on Lysodren ideally should be normal clinically, have a baseline plasma cortisol of 0.5–1.0 μg/dl, and be unresponsive to ACTH (post-ACTH plasma cortisol 0.5–1.0 μg/dl). If the baseline plasma cortisol concentration exceeds the upper end of the normal range (>4 μg/dl for our laboratory) or a significant response to ACTH is found (post-ACTH plasma cortisol >4 μg/dl), Lysodren dosage should be increased (even if clinical signs of HC are not present). It is more effective to once again administer Lysodren daily (rein-duction phase, 50 mg/kg/day) than merely to increase the weekly maintenance dosage. The total length of time necessary to reinduce a patient who has come out of remission is variable. As was discussed in the section on the induction phase of Lysodren treatment, the patient should be carefully observed for signs of glucocorticoid insufficiency and Lysodren discontin-ued if these signs are seen. In any event, ACTH stimulation testing should be repeated every 5–7 days until the adrenal cortex is once again unrespon-sive. Because the patient came out of remission at the recommended Lysodren dosage of 50 mg/kg/week, it is logical to increase the maintenance dosage. It is suggested that the new maintenance dosage be increased by about 25% to 75 mg/kg/week.

By following the above guidelines for using Lysodren, it is unusual (al-though possible) to cause mineralocorticoid insufficiency. Serum sodium and potassium should be measured if mineralocorticoid insufficiency is suspected. (For additional information see the section in this chapter on the treatment of Addison's disease.) For the rare patient who becomes both glucocorticoid and mineralocorticoid deficient, Lysodren administration should be discontinued indefinitely and appropriate treatment for Addison's disease started immedi-ately. (See the section in this chapter on the treatment of Addison's disease.) Whether these patients can ever regain adrenal responsiveness to ACTH is uncertain. It is advisable to perform ACTH stimulation testing every 3–4 months to assess adrenal responsiveness. Some animals in this category eventually require Lysodren therapy again, but it will probably be a year or longer before this need occurs.

Problems caused by Lysodren treatment may occur for two reasons: 1) excessive dosage causing glucocorticoid and (rarely) mineralocorticoid defi-ciency; and 2) adverse reactions directly related to the drug itself. A few patients develop gastric irritation and vomit after receiving o,p'-DDD. If vom-iting occurs, discontinue the drug for 2–3 days, and then further divide the total daily dosage (50 mg/kg/day) into two or three equal dosages given with food. Rarely, central nervous system (CNS) toxicity, characterized by depression and ataxia, is reported following Lysodren administration. If these signs recur after cessation and readministration of Lysodren, an alternative treatment method must be considered (see below).

When should one expect to see improvement in clinical signs following treatment with Lysodren? Generally, decreased water and food consumption and urine output occur within 1–2 weeks. Activity and attitude also tend to improve quickly (within 2–4 weeks). Increased muscle strength and decreased "pot-bellied" appearance generally take 2–3 months. It may require 1–6 months for significant improvement in skin and hair changes.

Prognosis for control of signs of PDH with the standard Lysodren protocol is fair to good. It should be apparent that the more attention directed to details of treatment and monitoring by the client and veterinarian, the better the outcome is likely to be. Many dogs with PDH live good quality lives for several years on Lysodren treatment.

Alternative Therapy. Medical, surgical, and teletherapeutic alternatives to the standard Lysodren treatment protocol discussed above have been described.

High-Dose Lysodren Treatment Protocol. An interesting alternative treatment regimen in which Lysodren is used at higher dosages for a longer period has been reported. The objective of this protocol is to intentionally destroy all layers of the adrenal cortex and cause glucocorticoid and mineralocorticoid deficiencies. The patient is supplemented daily with the required amounts of glucocorticoids and mineralocorticoids.

Why would nearly complete adrenocortical destruction potentially be advantageous? Experts using this approach claim that patients with PDH are easier to manage long term with this method than with the standard Lysodren treatment protocol because they do not come out of remission for long periods (generally 1 year or more) and the need for supplemental glucocorticoid and mineralocorticoid is predictable. Expense and time required for treatment and monitoring may also be less, depending on the number of times a patient requires laboratory monitoring and either reinduction with Lysodren or treatment for glucocorticoid or mineralocorticoid insufficiency using the standard treatment regimen. Obviously, complete client cooperation and diligence are required to ensure that the patient receives daily glucocorticoid and mineralocorticoid supplementation without fail; otherwise the patient will probably show signs of Addison's disease and may die.

With this protocol, Lysodren is administered at a dosage of 50–75 mg/kg/day PO in three or four divided doses given with food for 25 days. Supplementation with hydrocortisone 1 mg/kg q12h PO and fludrocortisone (Florinef, Squibb) 0.1 mg/10 kg q12h is begun on the third day of Lysodren administration. Also, depending on the size of the dog, 1–5 g of sodium chloride is added to the food divided into at least two daily doses. One week after Lysodren administration is completed, the dosage of hydrocortisone is reduced to 0.5 mg/kg q12h PO. The purported major advantage of this protocol is the prolonged period (1–2 years) of remission attained without the need for maintenance Lysodren therapy. A few dogs had neurologic signs when, early in the development of this protocol, Lysodren was administered every 12 hours. These signs were apparently due to high plasma concentrations of *o,p'*-DDD and were alleviated by dividing the daily dosage of Lysodren into three or four doses. Other reported advantages include less risk of sudden, unexpected adrenocortical insufficiency and perhaps less expense. Further experience with large numbers of patients is needed before this protocol can be advocated for routine use.

Ketoconazole Treatment Protocol. Ketoconazole (Nizoral, Janssen) is used most commonly in dogs and cats for its antifungal properties. In addition, it has been shown that this drug reversibly inhibits both gonadal and adrenal steroid synthesis. It has fairly low toxicity, although hepatic damage is occasionally observed. Preliminary results from studies using ketoconazole in cushingoid dogs with PDH and AT confirm that it is effective (although expensive) for treating both of these forms of spontaneous HC. Ketoconazole should not be used as standard "first-line" therapy for HC. It may be useful in the following situations: 1) presence of AT, either benign or malignant for which surgery is not an option for whatever reason; 2) initial therapy for 4–8 weeks in an animal with AT to control signs of HC and better prepare the patient for adrenalectomy; 3) dogs who cannot tolerate Lysodren; and 4) as test therapy to provide evidence for or against HC in dogs with vague plasma cortisol test results.

The dosage of ketoconazole is 5 mg/kg q12h PO for 7 days; then 10 mg/kg q12h for 7–14 days; then, if necessary, 15 mg/kg q12h indefinitely. If signs of hepatic damage (icterus, increased liver enzyme activity) are observed, the drug should be discontinued, and supportive treatment with intravenous fluid therapy (lactated Ringer's solution) begun. If signs of hypocortisolism occur (lethargy, anorexia, vomiting), supplementation with glucocorticoid (Cortef) should be started (see the previous section in this chapter on induction treatment with Lysodren). An ACTH stimulation test without stopping ketoconazole administration should be done after 10–14 days of treatment (or sooner if signs of glucocorticoid insufficiency appear). The goals of ketoconazole therapy for spontaneous HC are the same as were discussed for Lysodren treatment: adrenal unresponsiveness to ACTH and clinical improvement without causing illness. Twice-daily administration of ketoconazole is necessary for efficacy because of the drug's mechanism of action (reversible enzyme inhibitor).

Bilateral Adrenalectomy for PDH. Bilateral adrenalectomy for PDH is seldom recommended because of the usual effectiveness of either Lysodren or ketoconazole, and the number and seriousness of postoperative complications (see the section on AT below for a discussion of management of postoperative complications). If surgery is anticipated, treatment with ketoconazole should be done for 4–8 weeks prior to the procedure (see the previous section on ketoconazole therapy) in order to improve the patient's anesthetic and surgical risks.

Hypophysectomy for PDH. Removal of the pituitary lesion responsible for excessive ACTH secretion has several potential advantages, including: 1) removal of the pituitary tumor, thus averting its potential to expand and cause neurologic signs; 2) elimination of the necessity for frequent reevaluation while on medical therapy; and 3) prevention of complications following bilateral adrenalectomy. Unfortunately, hypophysectomy requires specialized expertise and considerable equipment, and it is not generally used.

Radiation Therapy for PDH. Pituitary macroadenomas reportedly account for 5–10% of PDH in dogs. These tumors may grow significantly and cause severe neurologic signs (aimless pacing, apparent blindness, ataxia, circling, head-pressing) as they expand dorsally into the hypothalamus. CT scanning or MRI is required in a dog with spontaneous HC to distinguish a small pituitary lesion (microadenoma) from a large pituitary carcinoma (macroadenoma). Cobalt irradiation, occasionally used for treatment of pituitary macroadenomas, may markedly reduce the tumor size. However, ACTH secretion may continue at excessive levels, in which case the dog would still require treatment for HC. Special equipment and experience are obviously required for this mode of therapy for PDH.

Pituitary-Dependent Hyperadrenocorticism in Cats

There are few published reports on treatment of PDH in cats, and so therapeutic recommendations must be considered empiric at this time. Most cats with confirmed PDH also have diabetes mellitus (probably secondary to chronic hypercortisolemia) and require insulin therapy (see the section in this chapter on treatment of feline diabetes mellitus).

Standard Therapy. Bilateral adrenalectomy followed by glucocorticoid and mineralocorticoid supplementation is the treatment of choice for feline PDH at present. Early reports indicate that postoperative complications following bilateral adrenalectomy are not as frequent in cats as in dogs. Also, most diabetic cats with spontaneous HC no longer require insulin after adrenalectomy, a result that is also different than for diabetic dogs with spontaneous HC. Nonetheless, it is suggested that adrenalectomy and immediate postoperative care be done only by experienced specialists.

Alternative Therapy. Lysodren has been tried for feline PDH at a daily dosage of 25–50 mg/kg PO. Although it is apparently well tolerated by cats, its efficacy for feline PDH has not been consistent. Further studies are needed to determine if different dosage protocols might be more efficacious.

Investigational Therapy. Metyrapone (Metopirone, Ciba) is a drug that inhibits an enzyme system in the adrenal cortex that is required for synthesis of cortisol. (In this regard, it is similar to the effects of ketoconazole.) The suggested dosage is 65 mg q8h PO indefinitely. More experience with this drug is needed before it can be recommended for treating feline PDH.

Adrenocortical Tumors

In approximately 10–15% of dogs and cats with spontaneous HC, the cause is a cortisol-secreting adrenocortical tumor (AT). About half of these tumors are benign (unilateral adrenal adenoma), and half are malignant (carcinoma). Surgical removal is the treatment of choice whenever metastasis is not evident because it is potentially curative. If metastasis is documented or if surgery is not possible for some other reason (e.g., owner refusal, complicating condition of the patient), medical treatment is sometimes successful.

Standard Therapy for Unilateral Adrenocortical Adenomas or Carcinomas in Dog and Cats. Adrenalectomy is the treatment of choice for all unilateral adrenocortical tumors that have not metastasized. The technique for adrenalectomy can be found in standard veterinary surgery textbooks. Ketoconazole therapy for 4–8 weeks prior to adrenalectomy has been advocated for dogs with AT (see the section above, on ketoconazole treatment protocol, for dosage). The rationale is that ketoconazole interferes with the excessive cortisol synthesis, thereby lowering plasma cortisol and improving the patient's immunologic status, healing capacity, and ability to successfully undergo surgery.

With unilateral adrenal tumors, the contralateral adrenal gland atrophies owing to the negative feedback of cortisol (from the adrenal tumor) on pituitary ACTH output. Therefore careful attention must be given to glucocorticoid and, in some cases, mineralocorticoid supplementation prior to and during surgery, during the immediate postoperative period, and for several weeks until the unaffected adrenal again becomes responsive to ACTH (a few weeks to a few months). A suggested regimen is to administer Solu Delta Cortef at a dosage of 1–2 mg/kg immediately prior to induction of anesthesia and again at the completion of surgery. During the first postoperative day while stress is still present, administer Cortef (hydrocortisone) at a dosage of 2.5 mg/kg q12h PO (approximately five times the physiologic maintenance dosage). Unless there are postoperative complications, the dosage of Cortef can be tapered over a period of 7–10 days to the physiologic maintenance dosage (0.1–0.5 mg/kg q12h PO). [*Note:* Equivalent physiologic maintenance dosages are: 1) prednisone or prednisolone 0.02–0.10 mg/kg q12h; and 2) dexamethasone 0.004–0.020 mg/kg q12h.] If complications develop, the dosage of Cortef should be increased two- to fivefold (1.0–2.5 mg/kg q12h PO).

ACTH stimulation testing should be done monthly to evaluate the function of the remaining adrenal gland (remember to discontinue Cortef administration for 24 hours prior to ACTH stimulation). Once adequate response occurs, Cortef should be discontinued.

Standard Therapy of Nonresectable Adrenocortical Carcinomas and Alternative Treatment for Adrenocortical Adenomas. Lysodren is the treatment of choice for nonresectable adrenocortical carcinoma (or any adrenocortical tumor when surgery is not an option) in dogs. (*Note:* Treatment for nonresectable adrenocortical carcinoma in cats has not been described.) The goal of Lysodren therapy is to destroy all neoplastic adrenal tissue as documented by a low or undetectable basal plasma cortisol concentration and nonresponse to ACTH stimulation. As was discussed in the above section on the standard treatment of PDH in dogs, therapy with Lysodren is done in two phases: induction and maintenance.

Induction Therapy with Lysodren. The following protocol is suggested: 1) administer Lysodren at a dosage of 50–75 mg/kg/day PO for 10–14 days; if signs of glucocorticoid insufficiency (lethargy, decreased appetite, vomiting) are seen, temporarily stop Lysodren, perform an ACTH stimulation test, and begin glucocorticoid supplementation (see the section above on induction therapy with Lysodren in dogs with PDH for information on dosage); and 2) at the end of the 10- to 14-day Lysodren loading period, perform an ACTH stimulation test (if not already completed previously) to assess the efficacy of Lysodren. If plasma cortisol values (basal and post-ACTH) have decreased but are still higher than 1.0 μg/dl, daily Lysodren treatment should be continued (50–75 mg/kg/day PO) and ACTH stimulation testing done every 7–10 days until plasma cortisol values have decreased to less than 1.0 μg/dl. Once this level occurs, a weekly maintenance Lysodren treatment protocol (100–200 mg/kg/week PO) should be started.

If the above loading period of Lysodren causes little or no change in basal and post-ACTH plasma cortisol values, the daily loading dosage of o,p'-DDD should be increased to 100 mg/kg/day PO and the ACTH stimulation testing repeated at 7- to 10-day intervals. If this higher daily dosage of Lysodren is still ineffective in lowering plasma cortisol values, increase the o,p'-DDD dosage by increments of 50 mg/kg every 7–10 days until the plasma cortisol values have decreased or until signs of o,p'-DDD toxicity occur. When ACTH stimulation test results show that plasma cortisol values have decreased considerably but are still more than 1.0 μg/dl, continue to administer Lysodren daily (at the previous week's dosage) and repeat the ACTH stimulation testing every 7–10 days until basal and post-ACTH stimulation plasma cortisol values are less than 1.0 μg/dl. If direct toxicity to o,p'-DDD develops (not due to glucocorticoid insufficiency), Lysodren should be temporarily discontinued until signs improve and then reinstituted at the highest tolerated dosage until plasma cortisol levels decrease to less than 1.0 μg/dl.

Maintenance Therapy with Lysodren. Once plasma cortisol values before and after ACTH stimulation are less than 1.0 µg/dl, begin maintenance treatment with Lysodren at a dosage of 100–200 mg/kg/week PO in two divided doses a few days apart and glucocorticoid supplementation with Cortef (0.1–0.5 mg/kg PO q12h).

ACTH stimulation testing should be done in 1 month and thereafter at 3-month intervals. (Remember to discontinue Cortef supplementation for 24 hours prior to plasma cortisol measurement.) If the baseline plasma cortisol concentration has increased to the normal resting range (0.5–4.0 µg/dl) or a significant response to ACTH is found (post-ACTH plasma cortisol >4 µg/dl), the Lysodren dosage should be increased (even if clinical signs of HC are not present). It is more effective to again administer Lysodren daily (reinduction phase, 50–100 mg/kg/day) rather than merely increasing the weekly maintenance dosage. The dog should be carefully observed for signs of glucocorticoid insufficiency and Lysodren temporarily discontinued if these signs are seen. ACTH stimulation testing should be repeated every 5–7 days until the adrenal cortex is once again unresponsive (pre- and post-ACTH plasma cortisol values <1.0 µg/dl). Then the weekly maintenance dosage of Lysodren should be increased by about 25–50%, once again dividing the total weekly dose into two equal doses administered a few days apart. Subsequent Lysodren dosage adjustments are based on results of ACTH stimulation testing done at 3-month intervals, as well as on the patient's tolerance of high-dose Lysodren.

The most common side effects include anorexia, lethargy, weakness, vomiting, and diarrhea. These signs may be caused by glucocorticoid or mineralocorticoid insufficiency, or by direct toxic effects of high-dose Lysodren. When the above signs occur, to distinguish between these two possible causes temporarily stop Lysodren administration and perform a serum biochemical profile (including serum electrolytes) and an ACTH stimulation test. Appropriate treatment depends on the cause of the patient's signs. For glucocorticoid insufficiency, administer Solu Delta Cortef at a dosage of 1 mg/kg IV q6h until the patient improves and then increase the supplemental oral glucocorticoid (Cortef) dosage to five times maintenance levels for a few days (see the section above on the treatment of unilateral adrenocortical adenomas for additional information on dosage). Intravenous fluid therapy with lactated Ringer's solution may also be required. Wait about 2 weeks before resuming weekly maintenance Lysodren administration and then decrease the dosage by approximately 25%. For combined glucocorticoid and mineralocorticoid insufficiency, treat as for Addison's disease (see the section below on standard treatment of Addison's disease). Further Lysodren therapy may or may not be required for dogs with iatrogenic Addison's disease. ACTH stimulation testing should be done every 3 months in these patients to evaluate adrenal function and assess the need for resuming treatment with *o,p'*-DDD. If signs are due to direct Lysodren toxicity, provide supportive care with fluid therapy (intravenous lactated Ringer's solution) and reduce the weekly Lysodren dosage to the highest amount the patient has tolerated in the past. ACTH stimulation testing should be done every 3 months to evaluate the need for changes in Lysodren dosage.

Prognosis of Lysodren-Treated Adrenal Neoplasia. The prognosis for dogs with an adrenocortical adenoma treated with Lysodren is fair to good. Lifetime treatment with Lysodren and supplemental glucocorticoid administration are usually required, as well as regular follow-up evaluation, especially ACTH stimulation testing. Dogs with small adrenal carcinomas without metastasis usually improve with Lysodren therapy, but the response may be neither as complete nor as long-lasting as for adrenocortical adenoma. Patients with large adrenocortical carcinomas or widespread metastasis may show short-term palliation of clinical signs but invariably have a poor to grave prognosis.

HYPOADRENOCORTICISM

Adrenocortical insufficiency (hypoadrenocorticism) results from deficient production and secretion by the adrenal cortex of glucocorticoids, mineralocorticoids, or both (Addison's disease). Destruction of the adrenal cortex (primary adrenocortical insufficiency) or deficient pituitary production of ACTH (secondary adrenocortical insufficiency) can produce hypoadrenocorticism. This disorder occurs more commonly in dogs than in cats. Both iatrogenic and spontaneous forms are recognized. Iatrogenic hypoadrenocorticism may be induced by excessive Lysodren administration (see the above discussion on standard treatment of PDH) or by sudden withdrawal from glucocorticoid administration following prolonged use of pharmacologic doses (see the section above on iatrogenic hyperadrenocorticism). In cats, iatrogenic glucocorticoid insufficiency may also be caused by administration of progestogens such as medroxyprogesterone acetate (Ovaban, Schering). Pure glucocorticoid insufficiency is more prevalent with overuse of Lysodren, whereas deficiency of both glucocorticoid and mineralocorticoid (Addison's disease) is the more commonly encountered situation in patients with spontaneous adrenocortical insufficiency. The cause of spontaneous hypoadrenocorticism is uncertain. Bilateral adrenocortical atrophy is usually seen, and it is hypothesized that autoimmune destruction of the adrenal cortices is responsible.

Clinical signs of glucocorticoid insufficiency include anorexia, marked lethargy, weakness, vomiting, diarrhea, dehydration, and, in severe cases, vascular collapse and signs of shock. Microcardia may be seen on thoracic radiographs. Mineralocorticoid deficiency is associated with bradycardia, signs of shock, and in untreated cases death from cardiac standstill. Laboratory findings associated with glucocorticoid insufficiency may include increased packed cell volume, plasma total protein, and blood urea nitrogen (BUN) (due to dehydration); eosinophilia and lymphocytosis (occasionally); and hypoglycemia. Hyponatremia, hyperkalemia, and electrocardiographic abnormalities (tall, tented

T waves, prolonged PR interval, second or third degree heart block) are typical findings with mineralocorticoid deficiency.

Diagnosis is confirmed ideally by performing an ACTH stimulation test with pre- and post-ACTH plasma cortisol values prior to treatment. Usually both baseline and 2-hour post-ACTH plasma cortisol values are less than 1.0 μg/dl. In critically ill patients in which treatment delay is too risky, a presumptive diagnosis can be established by measuring only the baseline plasma cortisol (blood sample obtained prior to therapy). In patients with nonadrenal disorders, baseline plasma cortisol is usually increased (>4.0 μg/dl) due to stress of illness. Some clinicians prefer to use dexamethasone in the treatment protocol (see below) because, unlike hydrocortisone, prednisone, and prednisolone, it does not interfere with concurrent ACTH stimulation testing.

Iatrogenic Hypoadrenocorticism

Management of patients with iatrogenic adrenocortical insufficiency was discussed in the sections above on iatrogenic hyperadrenocorticism and PDH in dogs.

Spontaneous Hypoadrenocorticism

Patients with spontaneous hypoadrenocorticism often present in a collapsed state and in critical condition (addisonian crisis). Emergency treatment and intensive monitoring are essential.

Standard Treatment. Discussion of treatment can be divided into emergency measures and maintenance therapy.

Emergency Treatment. Restoring extracellular fluid volume, correcting hyponatremia and hyperkalemia, and supplying glucocorticoids and mineralocorticoids are the most important considerations of treatment. Normal saline solution (0.9%) should be administered intravenously at a rate of 40–90 ml/kg/hr until vascular volume and blood pressure improve significantly (usually 1–2 hours). A soluble glucocorticoid, e.g., Solu Delta Cortef, should be started at an initial dosage of 1–2 mg/kg IV followed by a dosage of 0.1–0.5 mg/kg IV q4–6h until improvement is seen. Alternatively, dexamethasone can be administered at a dosage of 0.5–1.0 mg/kg IV, repeated in 6–8 hours if necessary. Initial therapy should also include the potent mineralocorticoid desoxycorticosterone acetate (DOCA) (Percorten Acetate, Ciba) at a daily dosage ranging from 0.5 to 1.0 mg IM for cats and small dogs (<5 kg) and up to 5 mg IM for giant breeds. The dosage is adjusted daily based on the results of serum sodium and potassium concentrations until oral fludrocortisone acetate (Florinef, Squibb) can be initiated (usually 1 or 2 days—see the section on maintenance treatment, which follows).

If hyperkalemia is severe (serum K^+ >8.5 mEq/L) and signs of cardiotoxicity are prominent (pronounced bradycardia, absence of P waves, wide or bizarre QRS complexes), more specific measures to rapidly lower extracellular potassium concentration may be required. Administration of regular insulin (0.5 unit/kg as an IV bolus) and 2.0–3.0 g of dextrose per unit of insulin (10–15 ml of 20% dextrose per unit of insulin) rapidly causes transfer of potassium into the intracellular space and reduces plasma potassium concentration. Administer half of the 20% dextrose as an intravenous push over 10–15 minutes. Add the other half to 500 ml of 0.9% saline and infuse it over the following 4–6 hours at the rate of 40 ml/kg/hr. It is imperative that blood glucose be monitored frequently (preferably every hour) and the insulin-glucose treatment adjusted appropriately to avoid hypoglycemia. Also, the electrocardiogram (ECG) should be continually monitored for signs of improvement and the serum potassium rechecked every 4–6 hours if possible. Sodium bicarbonate also enhances the movement of potassium from extracellular to intracellular fluid and can be administered at a dosage of 1.0–2.0 mEq/kg IV over 10–20 minutes. The ECG should be carefully monitored during treatment until heart rate and rhythm improve significantly. Do not use sodium bicarbonate unless severe metabolic acidosis (TCO_2 < 10) is present. Administration of 10% calcium gluconate (0.5–1.0 ml/kg by slow intravenous push over 10–20 minutes) may be helpful because calcium ions directly inhibit the toxic effects of potassium on the heart. Although these emergency treatment procedures can be combined if absolutely necessary, risks of adverse effects increase with combination therapy.

Response to appropriate emergency treatment for Addison's disease usually occurs within hours in affected dogs, but for unknown reasons it is often delayed for 3–5 days in cats.

Maintenance Therapy. Long-term maintenance treatment for spontaneous hypoadrenocorticism consists of supplementation with both mineralocorticoid and glucocorticoid and, in some cases, addition of sodium chloride to the diet. Florinef is a potent mineralocorticoid preparation for oral use (0.1 mg/tablet). The dosage must be determined by trial and error based on periodic measurement of serum sodium and potassium. Commonly dogs with spontaneous hypoadrenocorticism require about 0.1 mg Florinef/5 kg body weight. Beginning at a somewhat lower initial dosage and gradually increasing by increments of 0.05–0.10 mg every 1–3 days (based on results of serum sodium and potassium) is advised. Once serum sodium and potassium values have stabilized in the normal range, these serum electrolytes, BUN, and creatinine should be rechecked every 3–4 months (or sooner if signs suggestive of mineralocorticoid insufficiency are observed). The expense of Florinef may be significant, especially for large dogs. Addition of sodium chloride to the diet (1–5 g daily) may permit a reduction of Florinef dosage in some patients. The usual dosage of Florinef for affected cats is 0.1 mg/day.

Almost all patients are brighter, more active, and appear to feel better when glucocorticoid supplementation is also used. Hydrocortisone tablets (Cortef) are preferred (0.1–0.5 mg/kg q12h PO), but prednisone and prednisolone are acceptable (0.02–0.10 mg/kg q12h PO). These dosages are generally adequate for physiologic maintenance, but during stressful episodes they should be increased two- to fivefold. In cats that are difficult to medicate orally, monthly injection of methylprednisolone acetate (Depo-Medrol, Upjohn) at a dosage of 10 mg/month IM is an alternative.

Occasionally patients become refractory to Florinef, or daily administration is unacceptable to the client. Administration of desoxycorticosterone pivilate (Percorten Pivilate, Ciba) at a dosage of 25–100 mg q3–4weeks IM depending on the dog's size is an alternative to Florinef. Percorten 25 mg is roughly equivalent in mineralocorticoid activity to 0.1 mg of Florinef. For cats, the suggested dosage of Percorten Pivilate is 12.5 mg/month IM.

If anesthesia and surgery are necessary for patients with spontaneous hypoadrenocorticism, increased dosages of corticosteroids and careful monitoring are required. See the section on standard treatment of iatrogenic hyperadrenocorticism for details.

Long-term prognosis for patients with spontaneous hypoadrenocorticism treated appropriately is fair to good. Regular follow-up to evaluate history, clinical signs, serum sodium and potassium, BUN, and creatinine are important to guide changes in the treatment protocol.

HYPOTHYROIDISM

Hypothyroidism is one of the more common endocrinopathies of the dog and is a rare disorder in the cat. This condition is the result of reduced thyroid hormone secretion by the thyroid glands resulting in a variety of clinical signs, the most frequent being problems relating to the skin and haircoat. More than 95% of cases of hypothyroidism appear to result from destruction of the thyroid gland itself (i.e., primary hypothyroidism). It is important to maintain a high degree of clinical suspicion for syndromes associated with thyroid insufficiency. Hypothyroidism may be the underlying cause of hematologic abnormalities, recurrent infections, musculoskeletal disorders, and gastrointestinal and reproductive abnormalities. Conversely, one should pay attention to the accurate diagnosis of this disorder, as other illnesses also influence thyroid function tests. Following careful diagnostic procedure, the treatment of affected animals with levothyroxine generally results in the complete resolution of clinical signs.

Causes (Dog)

The two most common causes of canine adult-onset primary hypothyroidism are lymphocytic thyroiditis and idiopathic atrophy of the thyroid gland, each accounting for about one-half of the cases of hypothyroidism. Other rare forms of canine hypothyroidism include iatrogenic conditions, neoplastic destruction of thyroid tissue, and congenital (or juvenile-onset) hypothyroidism (cretinism). Clinical signs of hypothyroidism generally follow the destruction of more than three-fourths of the thyroid tissue. Lymphocytic thyroiditis is an immune-mediated disease, with the frequent occurrence of circulating antibodies directed against thyroglobulin, a thyroid-specific protein. Clinical or biochemical detection of early thyroiditis is rare. Owners generally do not seek medical attention for their animals until they notice overt signs of thyroid hormone deficiency.

Idiopathic atrophy of the thyroid gland is the second major histologic form of canine primary hypothyroidism. Histologically, there is loss of thyroid parenchyma, which is most likely a primary degenerative disorder of the thyroid gland affecting individual follicular cells.

Less frequent causes of hypothyroidism include cretinism (congenital hypothyroidism), and pituitary and hypothalamic failure of thyroid-stimulating hormone (TSH) and thyrotropin-releasing hormone (TRH) release, respectively. No researcher has yet documented a selective inability to convert thyroxine (T_4) to triiodothyronine (T_3) by peripheral tissues. Disproportionately low (or high, depending on the assay system) serum T_3 concentrations are most likely the result of the anti-T_3 antibodies observed rarely in autoimmune thyroiditis.

Causes (Cat)

Congenital but not spontaneous adult-onset primary hypothyroidism has been documented in the cat. Hypothyroidism may be the uncommon sequela to the surgical or radioiodine treatment of hyperthyroidism. This condition is often transient because previously nonfunctional extracervical thyroid tissue becomes functional and restores normal thyroid hormone levels. An overdosage of antithyroid medication could also produce hypothyroidism; however, this problem appears to be uncommon with methimazole (Tapazole, Eli Lilly), the most common antithyroid medication at this time (see Hyperthyroidism).

Diagnosis

Several review articles (see Suggested Readings) summarize the available thyroid function tests. At the present time, we recommend confirmation of hypothyroidism with the thyrotropin stimulation test (Table 4-5). If necessary and available, a valid measurement of free thyroxine (FT_4) concentration may aid in the identification of reductions in serum T_4 concentration due to serum binding inhibitors. In most animals with primary hypothyroidism, the serum T_4 concentration does not respond to bovine thyrotropin (TSH). For the dog, we suggest obtaining a blood sample for serum T_4 determination, then administering 0.1 unit TSH/kg IV (maximum dose 5

TABLE 4-5.   Drugs Used to Treat or Diagnose Hypothyroidism

Drug	Trade Names	Dose and Route	
		Dog	Cat
L-Thyroxine	Synthroid (Flint)	0.02–0.04 mg/kg divided q12h or once q24h 0.5 mg/m^2 q12h or q24h, 0.1–0.2 mg IV (myxedema coma)	0.1–0.2 mg divided q12h or once q24h PO
	Soloxine (Daniels), Levothroid (Rorer) Levoid (Nutrition Control Products) Noroxine (Vortech), Thyro-Tab (Vet-A-Mix)		

Indications: Treatment of all forms of hypothyroidism

Side effects (with overdosage): Excitement, nervousness, polyuria, polydipsia, weight loss

Reference: Ferguson DC: Thyroid hormone replacement therapy. In: Kirk RW, ed. *Current Veterinary Therapy IX.* Philadelphia: WB Saunders, 1986;1018.

L-Triiodothyronine	Cytobin (Norden) Cytomel (SK&F)	4–6 μg/kg q8h	Dosage not available

Indications: Rare; treatment of hypothyroidism when conversion of T$_4$ to T$_3$ is impaired by drugs such as glucocorticoids or antithyroid agents

Side effects (with overdosage): Excitement, nervousness, polyuria, polydipsia, weight loss

Reference: Ferguson DC: Thyroid hormone replacement therapy. In: Kirk RW, ed. *Current Veterinary Therapy IX.* Philadelphia: WB Saunders, 1986;1018.

Bovine thyrotropin	Thytropar (Armour) Dermathycin (Pitman-Moore)	0.1 unit/kg IV; (max. 5 units); peak T$_4$ at 6 h); 1 unit/day IV; peak T$_4$ at 4 hr	1 unit/kg IV

Indications: Testing of thyroid functional reserve (TSH stimulation test)

Side effects: Allergic reaction (rare)

Reference: Peterson ME, Ferguson DC: Thyroid diseases. In: Ettinger S, ed. *Textbook of Veterinary Internal Medicine.* Philadelphia: WB Saunders, 1989.

Thyrotropin-releasing hormone (TRH)	Thypinone (Abbott)	0.1 mg/kg IV (peak T$_4$ at 6 hr)	0.1 mg/kg IV (peak T$_4$ at 6 hr)

Indications: Testing of thyroid functional reserve (TRH stimulation test) and/or differentiating tertiary from secondary hypothyroidism

Side effects: Salivation, urination, defecation, vomiting, miosis, tachycardia, tachypnea

Reference: Lothrop CD, Tamas PM, Fadok VA: Canine and feline thyroid function assessment with the thyrotropin-releasing hormone response test. *Am J Vet Res* 1984;45:2310.

From appendix contribution corresponding to Chapter 62 in Allen DG: *Small Animal Medicine.* Philadelphia: JB Lippincott, 1991;845.

units), followed by a blood sample at 6 hours post-TSH. In the cat, the serum T_4 increment above the baseline concentration 6 hours post-TSH administration increased up to the highest dose examined, 1 unit/kg IV. If cost is a factor, there is considerably more value in a single post-TSH T_4 determination than a baseline T_4 determination. The TSH stimulation test may be performed simultaneously with the ACTH stimulation test for hypo- or hyperadrenocorticism without significant effects on the results of either test.

Thyroid Replacement Therapy

See Table 4-5.

Therapy

The treatment of hypothyroidism is straightforward. The goal of thyroid hormone replacement therapy is the reversal of tissue hormone deficiency by mimicking the natural pattern of thyroid hormone secretion and metabolism. Furthermore, except following recrudescence of thyroid tissue after thyroidectomy, therapy is necessary for the rest of the animal's life. Considered over that time frame, the cost of accurate diagnostic tests becomes more acceptable.

Thyroid hormone preparations are classified into the following groups: 1) crude hormones prepared from animal thyroid; 2) synthetic L-thyroxine (L-T_4); 3) synthetic L-T_3; and 4) synthetic combinations of L-T_4 and L-T_3. As there are no good reasons to continue to use desiccated thyroid products, they are not discussed.

Standard Therapy. *L-Thyroxine: Preferred Therapy.* Sodium L-thyroxine is the thyroid hormone replacement product of choice. Oral forms are most commonly used. However, injectable forms are also available for the rare indication of myxedema coma (see below). Thyroxine is the treatment of choice for hypothyroidism for the following reasons: 1) L-thyroxine is the main secretory product of the thyroid gland; 2) L-thyroxine is the physiologic "prohormone," and its administration does not circumvent the cellular processes regulating the production of T_3 from T_4.

When starting an animal on a thyroid replacement product, it is recommended to start with a brand-name product with which broad experience has been obtained and use this product until a distinct clinical response has been seen. If one does not observe a clinical response after a period of at least 4–6 weeks following achievement of normal serum T_4 concentrations, the clinician should reevaluate the diagnosis.

The institution of thyroid replacement therapy despite the lack of confirmatory laboratory evidence has been proposed as a procedure to confirm the diagnosis of hypothyroidism. The major argument in defense of this practice is the cost of the diagnostic testing and the convenience for the owner. However, an incorrect diagnosis can also be expensive, and a delayed diagnosis of another disease could be detrimental. Furthermore, diagnostic procedures following a therapeutic trial may be difficult to interpret because exogenous hormone inhibits secretion of any normal thyroid tissue. One should not perform a TSH stimulation test prior to 6–8 weeks after discontinuation of replacement therapy.

The following guidelines are suggested for therapeutic trials: 1) Do not attempt a therapeutic trial until nonthyroidal illnesses have been ruled out. 2) Set *objective* criteria by which the success of the therapy can be judged. 3) Establish when the therapy will be reevaluated according to the criteria chosen. 4) Administer an appropriate dosage of L-thyroxine using a brand name preparation twice daily. 5) Decide on the next course of action if therapy is unsuccessful. 6) Be prepared to withdraw thyroid hormone to demonstrate the recurrence of signs.

The reported oral replacement doses for L-thyroxine sodium (e.g., Synthroid, Soloxine, Levothroid, Levoid, Noroxine, Thyro-Tab) range from a total dose of 0.02 to 0.04 mg/kg daily. One may calculate the L-thyroxine dose according to body surface area (0.5 mg/m^2), which is proportional to the metabolic rate. When dosed proportionate to body weight, large breed dogs have a greater tendency to have elevated serum T_4 concentrations. A subset of these animals may show signs of iatrogenic thyrotoxicosis (see below). It is common practice to administer T_4 in single or divided doses. It is recommended to start with a divided daily dose (e.g., 0.02 mg/kg q12h) until definite clinical improvement is seen. Probably after replenishment of intracellular stores, for some hypothyroid animals the dosage may be reduced to once-daily T_4 therapy as long as the average daily concentration is within the normal range. If the signs of hypothyroidism do not recur, an obvious advantage of single daily doses is the greater owner compliance. Gradual introduction of hormone is ideal, particularly in individuals with decreased ability to metabolize T_4 and increased risk to the development of thyrotoxicosis, as in hypoadrenal, aged, cardiac, or diabetic patients. In these groups, it is recommended to use divided dose protocols, and to increase the daily dose in 20–25% increments over a period of 4–8 weeks. Glucocorticoid replacement should begin prior to thyroid replacement therapy in patients with concomitant hypoadrenocorticism (e.g., iatrogenic adrenocortical suppression). This method ensures steroid replacement prior to the increase in metabolic demand for endogenous steroids, which follows correction of hypothyroidism.

The recommended treatment for feline hypothyroidism is daily administration of L-thyroxine at an initial dose of 0.1–0.2 mg/day. Complete resolution of clinical signs can usually be expected in cats with adult-onset iatrogenic hypothyroidism. However, the mental dullness and dwarfism that develop in kittens with hypothyroidism usually do not fully resolve.

Synthetic L-T₃: Rare Indications. Although T_3 can be defined as the cellular hormone, there are few valid reasons to use liothyronine (T_3) alone or in combination with L-thyroxine. T_3 "replacement" is not physiologic, and bypasses the final cellular regulatory step of 5'-deiodination of T_4. Liothyronine therapy is not appropriate in the "low T_3 syndrome" associated with nonthyroidal illness. Because of its higher oral bioavailability, T_3 may result in clinical improvement in cases of poor T_4 absorption in which post-therapy serum T_4 and T_3 concentrations are low. One of the rare theoretical indications of T_3 therapy is the simultaneous administration of drugs such as glucocorticoids, which inhibit the conversion of T_4 to T_3.

Anecdotal reports suggest that a small fraction of hypothyroid dogs do not respond to L-thyroxine therapy because they convert T_4 to T_3 poorly. T_3 or combination T_4–T_3 therapy has been recommended in these cases as an adjunct to T_4 or as sole therapy. The most likely cause of apparently low serum T_3 concentrations and normal or high T_4 concentrations following T_4 therapy is the presence of anti-T_3 antibodies. As previously discussed, this observation is an in vitro artifact invalidating serum T_3 measurements. In this siutation, the thyroxine dose should be increased until one observes a clinical response.

An oral dose regimen for L-T_3 (Cytobin, Norden; Cytomel, SmithKline & French) of 4–6 μg/kg q8h or possibly q12h appears necessary to maintain serum T_3 concentrations without high peaks, which appear to be associated with signs of thyrotoxicosis.

Commercial combinations of synthetic L-T_4 and L-T_3 containing a 4:1 mixture of T_4/T_3 has little rational basis in human or veterinary medicine. A variety of dosage schemes have been proposed, but the most common suggests dosing according to the T_4 content and division of the dose to account for the shorter serum half-life of T_3. Administration of these preparations commonly leads to low normal to normal serum T_4. Increasing the dose to normalize serum T_4 can result in high serum T_3 concentrations and can potentially result in overdosage due to the T_3 content. These preparations share the disadvantages of the T_3 preparations: increased cost, increased complexity of dosing regimens, and a higher incidence of thyrotoxic signs.

Myxedema Coma

There have been reports of "myxedema coma" in the dog. Classically, this syndrome, usually seen in elderly profoundly hypothyroid people, is characterized by severe mental obtundation terminating in coma and hypothermia. Although the presence of hypothyroidism is chronic, this critical care situation may develop rapidly following a stressful incident or illness. The lethargy of hypothyroidism may progress to stupor and coma. In addition to the common signs of hypothyroidism, the animal may manifest hypoventilation, hypotension, bradycardia, and profound hypothermia. An elevated blood PCO_2, decreased PO_2, and low plasma sodium and glucose concentrations may be documented. Often these events are triggered by an anesthetic episode, and the results can be fatal. Although the incidence is rare, one should take great care in anesthetizing or tranquilizing a dog suspected or known to be hypothyroid.

Standard Therapy

Treatment should be instituted promptly and vigorously as soon as the diagnosis is made. Treatment consists of 100–200 μg injectable sodium L-thyroxine (Synthroid Injection, Boots-Flint), passive rewarming (wrapping in blankets) and mechanical respiratory support as needed. Therapy for shock must include glucocorticoids and fluid and electrolyte replacement. Oral thyroxine therapy should be instituted when the animal stabilizes.

Side Effects of Replacement Therapy

The dog is relatively resistant to the development of thyrotoxic signs when thyroid hormone is administered orally. This resistance to iatrogenic thyrotoxicosis is the result of the dog's capacity to efficiently clear thyroid hormone via biliary and fecal excretion. Animals on replacement therapy, particularly with a T_3-containing product, can develop signs of thyrotoxicosis; however, the incidence at recommended doses is rare. Animals should be monitored for signs suggesting an overdose, including polyuria, polydipsia, nervousness, weight loss, increase in appetite, panting, and fever. The diagnosis of thyrotoxicosis is confirmed by the observation of elevated serum T_4 or T_3 concentration (or both). If toxicosis has followed L-thyroxine therapy, one should temporarily discontinue the medication until signs of toxicosis abate. Therapy can be reinstituted later at a proportionately lower dose in accordance with the degree of elevation of serum T_4 concentration produced by the original dose.

Patient Monitoring

Clinical criteria should be of utmost importance when evaluating success or failure of thyroid replacement therapy. The reversal of changes in haircoat and body weight should be assessed only after a period of 1–5 months on therapy. If clinical improvement is marginal or thyrotoxicosis is suspected, therapeutic monitoring of serum thyroid hormone concentrations, so-called post-pill testing, is appropriate to confirm the clinical suspicions. One should not attempt post-pill testing until steady-state conditions are reached, minimally 1 month after the initiation of therapy. Like the barbiturates, thyroid hormone induces the enzymes regulating its own metabolism. Elevated serum T_4 concentrations following T_4 administration and elevated serum T_3 concentrations following T_3 administration, concomitant with signs of thyrotoxicosis, confirm an overdose. The interpretation of post-pill serum thyroid hormone concentrations in cases of suspected underdosage is more complicated because it depends on the time of the sample relative to the dosing time. With once-daily L-thyroxine administration, the peak serum T_4 concentration should be in the normal to high normal range 4–8 hours after dosing and should be low normal or normal 24 hours after dosing. Because the dog is resistant to mild or transient elevations of thyroid hormone concentrations, it is usually sufficient to check the serum T_4 concentration only at 24 hours after a dose. At that time, the T_4 concentration should still be in the normal range. Although one may check serum T_4 concentrations in an animal on twice-daily L-thyroxine doses at any time, sampling is recommended just prior to a dose. This procedure results in determination of the lowest daily concentration, which should be still in the normal range. Following clinical improvement, once- or twice-yearly sampling of serum T_4 concentrations are recommended.

The measurement of serum T_3 is only rarely indicated for monitoring thyroid hormone therapy. Low serum T_3 and T_4 concentrations following T_4 administration, together with a poor clinical response, suggest an underdose or inadequate bioavailability (absorption). Low serum T_3 concentrations in the face of normal or high T_4 concentrations may be indicative of the "low T_3 syndrome" and a nonthyroidal illness or the development of anti-T_3 auto-antibodies. With liothyronine (T_3) administration, serum concentrations peak 2–3 hours after an oral dose. Serum T_4 concentrations are generally low or undetectable because T_3 inhibits pituitary TSH and any remaining thyroidal T_4 secretion.

If clinical signs of hypothyroidism persist despite the use of reasonable doses of thyroid hormone, consider the following possibilities: inadequate dosing regimen, owner noncompliance, poor gastrointestinal absorption, rapid metabolism of hormone, or that hypothyroidism is not the correct diagnosis.

Investigational Therapy

At the present time, long-acting slow release implants of thyroid hormone are being evaluated in dogs. These implants, formulated to last months after subcutaneous implantation, theoretically mimic more closely the continuous release of thyroid hormone by the thyroid gland. Another significant advantage would be that owners would then be able to avoid the necessity of once- or even twice-daily oral dosing of their pet.

Prognosis Following Treatment

Treated appropriately, the prognosis for an animal with hypothyroidism is excellent. Long-term therapy is without significant deleterious effects.

FELINE HYPERTHYROIDISM

Hyperthyroidism, caused by excessive concentrations of the circulating thyroid hormones, is now recognized as the most common endocrine disorder in the cat. The condition is almost always due to the adenomatous enlargement of the thyroid glands. Little is known about the cause of this generally benign (98–99%) and bilateral (70%) thyroid condition associated with thyroid hypersecretion. Thyroid carcinomas and therefore metastatic disease are rare (<2%). Investigators have suggested that nutritional factors and environmental factors interact to cause adenomatous thyroid changes in the cats over time. However, epidemiologic studies have not conclusively connected these postulated factors to the incidence of this disease. Circulating thyroid function stimulating immunoglobulins (TSIs), as found in human Graves' disease, do not appear to cause feline hyperthyroidism. However, greater amounts of thyroid growth stimulating immunoglobulins (TGIs) are present in the serum of affected cats. Despite the possibility of circulating stimulators, the tissue appears to function autonomously at the time of diagnosis.

Regardless of the causative factors, all of the signs of feline hyperthyroidism result from the excess of thyroid hormones. In excess, thyroid hormone increases the basal metabolic rate, increasing the oxygen and metabolic substrate demand of most tissues. Thyroid hormone excess causes the hyperactivity, restlessness, pacing, and irritability observed in many affected cats. In cats with severe or a long history of untreated hyperthyroidism, generalized muscle wasting contributes to weight loss despite increased appetite and food intake. Vomiting, diarrhea, increased frequency of defecation, and increased volume of feces are common with feline hyperthyroidism. Although the cause is unclear, about 20% of hyperthyroid cats also have periods of decreased appetite that usually alternate with periods of normal or increased appetite. This disease form is called "apathetic hyperthyroidism."

Of great diagnostic and therapeutic significance, hyperthyroidism results in a high-output cardiac state, the result of increased adrenergic stimulation and increased tissue metabolism and oxygen requirements. Volume overload results from low peripheral vascular resistance and by reflex renal mechanisms that conserve fluid. In addition, thyroid hormones act directly on heart muscle to add to the work demand of the heart. The principal cardiac compensatory mechanisms in high-output states such as hyperthyroidism are dilatation and hypertrophy. Auxiliary therapeutic measures directed at reducing the work of the heart should therefore be considered, particularly in cats with cardiomyopathy and tachycardia.

Also of relevance to therapy is the fact that hyperthyroidism is a disease of geriatric cats; the mean age of affected animals is approximately 12–13 years. Many of the signs of hyperthyroidism may be confused with primary diseases affecting a variety of organ systems, in particular the gastrointestinal, respiratory, and cardiac systems. Because the cats generally remain bright and alert and have good appetites, many hyperthyroid cats receive no medical attention for a year or more after the onset of signs. At this stage, weight loss is a common complaint, and the animal may have lost 50% of its original body weight. The most common clinical signs associated with hyperthyroidism are weight loss despite ravenous appetite, hyperactivity, polydipsia, polyuria, diarrhea, and periods of respiratory distress. Hyperthyroid cats tend to have impaired tolerance to stress.

Definitive Diagnosis

The definitive diagnosis of hyperthyroidism is, in the vast majority of cases, based on the observation of an elevated serum T_4 concentration. Serum T_3 concentrations and free T_4 concentrations are also elevated in most cases. However, cats with clinical signs of hyperthyroidism but normal or high-normal serum total T_4 concentrations have also been observed. Occasionally, when baseline serum T_4 concentrations are borderline or even normal, it is useful to employ dynamic tests of the thyroid axis, the most reliable being the T_3 suppression test (see below).

Protocol for T_3 Suppression Test. Exogenous thyroid hormone, via negative feedback inhibition, inhibits endogenous serum TSH and, secondarily, serum T_4 concentrations. In borderline cases of hyperthyroidism, it may be of value to test the thyroid for autonomy from these regulatory mechanisms. With hyperthyroidism the excess thyroid hormone secretion of the adenoma has already suppressed endogenous serum TSH secretion.

The T_3 suppression test may be performed in the following way.

1. Obtain blood for preliothyronine serum T_4 determination.
2. Administer exogenous T_3 (liothyronine; Cytomel, SmithKline & French; Cytobin, Norden) at a dose of 25 μg q8h for 2 days giving a seventh dose on the morning of the third day.
3. Obtain blood for postliothyronine serum T_4 determination 4 hours after the last T_3 dose.
4. Interpretation: Postliothyronine serum T_4 divided by preliothyronine serum T_4 concentration.

    a. Normal: <0.5 [or serum T_4 <1.5 μg/dl (20 nmol/L)].
    b. Hyperthyroid: >0.5 (usually little to no suppression).

Protocol for Thyrotropin Stimulation Test. In general, autonomously functioning adenomas do not respond to stimulation by exogenous thyrotropin. The TSH stimulation test is performed in the following way:

1. Obtain a blood sample for pre-TSH serum T_4 determination.
2. Administer 1 unit/kg IV bovine TSH (Thytropar, Pitman-Moore).

3. Obtain a blood sample for serum T_4 determination 6 hours after TSH administration.
4. Interpretation: post-TSH minus pre-TSH T_4 concentration.

    a. Normal: ≥ 2.5 μg/dl (25 ng/ml or 30 nmol/L).
    b. Hyperthyroid: < 2.5 μg/dl (25 ng/ml or 30 nmol/L).

When feasible, the T_3 suppression test is recommended over the TSH stimulation test for discrimination of borderline cases of hyperthyroidism. The T_3 suppression test, because it is performed over a longer period of time, is more reliable than TSH stimulation. Furthermore, the TSH stimulation test requires 1 day of hospitalization and bovine TSH is expensive, making its purchase difficult to justify in some practice situations.

General Considerations and Goals of Therapy

The practitioner should ask the following questions when planning therapy for hyperthyroidism:

1. Does the patient have concurrent illness that would rule out the treatment modality of surgery? Medical therapy may be indicated when the animal requires time to improve its body condition or the owners require evidence that the cat can improve with curative therapy. Anesthetic difficulties are minimized if the euthyroidism is medically induced prior to surgery.
2. Do the owners desire a definitive cure for their pet? Only radioiodine and surgery have curative potential in benign adenomatous goiter.
3. If the owners prefer lifelong medical therapy, are they likely to administer the medication faithfully? Antithyroid drugs generally must be given two or three times a day for the remainder of the animal's life.
4. Are you and your practice skilled and equipped to perform a thyroidectomy and provide appropriate follow-up care? Postoperative hypocalcemia requiring intravenous calcium therapy is not unusual.
5. Is referral to a center that provides radioiodine therapy an option? (Such therapy is available only at certain referral institutions.) Additionally, some institutions' interpretation of radiation safety rules requires a hospitalization of as long as 1–4 weeks.

Standard Therapy—Private Practice

See Table 4-6.

Medical Therapy. Medical therapy ameliorates the signs of hyperthyroidism but does not cure the condition. Unlike the use of adrenolytic drugs such as *o,p'*-DDD (Lysodren, Bristol), antithyroid drugs are not toxic to the thyroid gland and do not result in its destruction. If withdrawn, serum thyroid hormone concentrations rebound above the normal range and signs of disease may arise again.

The thiourylene drugs propylthiouracil (PTU) and methimazole (MMI, Tapazole, Lilly) are the most commonly used antithyroid drugs in cats. Both inhibit the thyroidal synthesis of hormone. Each drug initially must be administered continuously two to three times daily to maintain suppression of serum thyroid hormone concentrations. After the initiation of daily therapy, there is usually a delay of several days before a fall in serum thyroid hormone concentrations is observed. During this period, glandular hormone stores, which are unaffected by the drugs, become depleted. PTU has the additional beneficial effect of blocking the conversion of T_4 to T_3 in peripheral tissues such as the liver and kidney. The serum T_4 level may fall following both PTU and MMI therapy. However, with MMI, because of mechanisms resulting in enhanced T_3 production in peripheral tissues, serum T_3 is usually maintained within the normal range. As a result of this mechanism, it is rare to see a cat on MMI develop clinical signs of hypothyroidism.

Although historically it was initially the drug of choice, PTU has fallen out of favor because of its serious side effects. Both PTU and MMI can result in anorexia, vomiting, lethargy, and the development of positive antinuclear antibody (ANA) titers. Although both PTU and MMI cause autoimmune phenomena, PTU causes an unacceptable incidence of autoimmune hemolytic anemia and immune-mediated thrombocytopenia. These adverse effects are of particular concern in a cat eventually undergoing surgery. Therefore, PTU is no longer recommended for routine use in the hyperthyroid cat.

Methimazole is currently the antithyroid medication of choice for the cat. The administration of 5 mg three times daily generally brings the serum T_4 concentrations into the normal range within 2–3 weeks. The daily dose of MMI should then be adjusted upward or downward in 2.5-mg (one-half tablet) intervals until the serum T_4 concentration falls to within the normal range. Many cats can then be maintained on once-daily therapy because its biologic effect extends beyond its residence in the serum. The clinician should examine cats on chronic MMI therapy every 3–6 months to obtain blood for serum T_4 measurement and to monitor for signs of MMI toxicity (see below). The dose of MMI should be titrated to maintain the serum T_4 concentration in the low-normal range—generally 1–2 µg/dl (10–20 ng/ml or 10–30 nmol/L).

Adverse effects of methimazole are seen in about 15% of cats. Transient gastrointestinal upset is the most common and often resolves despite continued therapy. Pruritus around the face, ears, and neck with self-induced traumatic lesions have also been observed early in the course of therapy. This condition is glucocorticoid responsive; however, as with any drug allergy, the causative agent should be discontinued. Methimazole has more serious side effects: hepatopathy (< 10%), thrombocytopenia, and agranulocytosis. Proportionate to the dose and duration of therapy, positive serum ANA titers may

TABLE 4-6.   Drugs Used to Treat or Diagnose Hyperthyroidism in Cats

Drug	Trade Names	Dose and Route
Methimazole (MMI)	Tapazole (Lilly)	Starting: 5 mg q8h or q12h Adjust (up to daily dose of 30 mg q24h or divided) according to serum T_4 concentration

Indications: Short- or long-term medical therapy for hyperthyroidism

Side effects: Anorexia, vomiting, drug eruption, positive ANA, immune-mediated thrombocytopenia

Reference: Peterson ME, Kintzer PP, Hurvitz AI: Methimazole treatment of 262 cats with hyperthyroidism. *J Vet Int Med* 1988;2:150.

Propylthiouracil (PTU)	Propylthiouracil tablets	Starting: 50 mg q8h or q12h Adjust dose according to serum T_4 concentration

Indications: Short- or long-term medical therapy for hyperthyroidism (methimazole preferred)

Side effects: Immune-mediated hemolytic anemia and thrombocytopenia, anorexia, vomiting, lethargy, positive ANA, immune-mediated thrombocytopenia (no longer recommended due to high incidence of autoimmune phenomena)

Reference: Peterson ME: Treatment of feline hyperthyroidism. In Kirk RW, ed. *Current Veterinary Therapy X.* Philadelphia: WB Saunders, 1989;1002.

Potassium iodide	Lugol's solution SSKI (saturated solution of potassium iodide)	50–100 mg/day for 7–14 days PO (best administered in gelatin capsules)

Indications: Short-term medical therapy for severe hyperthyroidism (preoperative induction of euthyroidism)

Side effects: Excessive salivation, anorexia

Reference: Peterson ME: Treatment of feline hyperthyroidism. In: Kirk RW, ed. *Current Veterinary Therapy X.* Philadelphia: WB Saunders, 1989;1002.

Propranolol	Inderal	2.5–5.0 mg q8h PO as necessary to control heart rate 0.1 mg IV as necessary to control ventricular arrhythmias during surgery

Indications: To manage sinus tachycardia and ventricular arrhythmias; to manage hypertrophic cardiomyopathy

Side effects: Hypotension

Reference: Peterson ME: Treatment of feline hyperthyroidism. In: Kirk RW, ed. *Current Veterinary Therapy X.* Philadelphia: WB Saunders, 1989;1002.

(continued)

TABLE 4–6. *(continued)*

Drug	Trade Names	Dose and Route
Dihydrotachysterol (DHT)	Hytakerol liquid (Winthrop) tablets (Philips-Roxane)	Loading: 0.03 mg/kg/day for 3–4 days, then 0.01–0.02 mg/kg/day to maintain serum Ca in low normal range

Indications: Treatment of hypocalcemia associated with hypoparathyroidism

Side effects: Hypercalcemia, nephrocalcinosis

Reference: Peterson ME: Hypoparathyroidism. In: Kirk RW, ed. *Current Veterinary Therapy IX.* Philadelphia: WB Saunders, 1988;1039.

Drug	Trade Names	Dose and Route
Calcium chloride	Calcium chloride tablets	2 ml of 10% solution for cats with signs of hypocalcemia
	Calcium chloride (10%) (27.2 mg/ml elemental Ca)	2 ml/kg/day per IV infusion or as necessary to maintain Ca in low normal range
Calcium gluconate	Calcium gluconate tablets	Up to 750 mg/kg/day PO
	Calcium gluconate (10%) (9.3 mg/ml elemental Ca)	6–8 ml/kg/day per IV infusion or as necessary to maintain Ca in low normal range
Calcium lactate		Up to 600 mg/kg/day PO

Indications: Treatment of hypocalcemia associated with hypoparathyroidism

Side effects: Hypercalcemia, nephrocalcinosis

Reference: Peterson ME: Hypoparathyroidism. In: Kirk RW, ed. *Current Veterinary Therapy IX.* Philadelphia: WB Saunders, 1988;1039.

Drug	Trade Names	Dose and Route
Thyrotropin (bovine)	Dermathycin (Pitman-Moore)	1 unit/kg IV; serum samples at 0 and 6 hours for total T_4 measurement

Indications: Diagnosis of thyroid autonomy in feline hyperthyroidism

Side effects: Allergic reactions (rare)

Reference: Hoenig M, Ferguson DC: Assessment of thyroid functional reserve in the cat by the thyrotropin stimulation test. *Am J Vet Res* 1983;44:1229.

Drug	Trade Names	Dose and Route
Triiodothyronine	Cytomel (SK & F) Cytobin (Norden)	25 μg every 8 hours for 7 doses; serum samples for total T_4 measurement before first and after 7th dose

Indications: Diagnosis of thyroid autonomy in feline hyperthyroidism

Side effects: Exacerbation of signs of hyperthyroidism (rare)

Reference: Peterson ME, Graves TK: Triiodothyronine suppression test: an aid in the diagnosis of mild hyperthyroidism in cats. In: Proc Am Coll Vet Annual Forum, Washington, D.C., 1988;722, abstract 11.

As published in Ferguson DC, Hoenig MH: Feline hyperthyroidism. In: Allen DG, ed. *Small Animal Medicine.* Philadelphia: JB Lippincott, 1991;831.

develop. The incidence of this phenomenon is most common in cats receiving more than 15 mg/day for 6 months or more. However, no signs consistent with lupus erythematosus, e.g., skin or joint involvement, kidney disease, or hemolytic anemia, have been observed. If thrombocytopenia or agranulocytosis develops, MMI should be withdrawn and standard care for thrombocytopenia (e.g., blood transfusion) or agranulocytosis (e.g., prophylactic bactericidal antimicrobial drugs) instituted. Cross sensitivity to the thiourylene drugs MMI and PTU is common. Therefore when it develops the clinician should resort to alternative classes of antithyroid drugs (see below) or, preferably, surgery or radioiodine therapy.

Investigational Medical Therapy. Antithyroid drugs with alternative structures or actions are of particular interest for development as therapy for feline hyperthyroidism. Other classes of drugs, e.g., the iodinated radiocontrast agents, are presently under investigation in humans and cats for their antithyroid effects. These drugs act by inhibiting peripheral conversion of T_4 to T_3, blocking nuclear receptors for T_3, blocking thyroid hormone secretion, or blocking the uptake of thyroid hormones into tissue. One study showed the biliary contrast agent calcium ipodate (Oragrafin, Squibb), 15 mg/kg PO q12h, to be an effective inhibitor of the conversion of T_4 to T_3 in cats with experimental hyperthyroidism. The drug appeared to be safe, showing no hematologic, biochemical, or pathologic changes at this dose. The efficacy of this drug to serum T_4 concentrations has not been fully evaluated for spontaneous feline hyperthyroidism. However, extrapolating from the experience in humans and rats, the T_4 lowering effect is mild at best. Nonetheless, this drug, alone or together with low doses of MMI, may provide an alternative medical treatment for hyperthyroid cats.

Surgical Thyroidectomy. Surgical thyroidectomy is the only curative treatment modality open to private practitioners. Those performing this surgery should recognize that hyperthyroid cats are anesthetic and surgical risks because of their advanced age and cardiovascular and metabolic complications. For prognostic and therapeutic reasons, all cats with hyperthyroidism should be evaluated for overt cardiac disease (hypertrophic cardiomyopathy and congestive heart failure) and treated appropriately. In a series of 85 cats treated surgically at the Animal Medical Center in New York City, 8 (9.4%) died. Of these eight animals, six had had no preoperative antithyroid therapy.

With medical induction of euthyroidism, the anesthetic and surgical risks for a hyperthyroid cat are considerably reduced. The use of antithyroid drugs prior to and on the day of surgery is recommended to normalize the serum T_4 concentration. It is usually necessary to treat medically for at least 1–3 weeks. Methimazole is presently recommended as the drug of choice for preoperative preparation. If a cat has had adverse reactions to MMI or PTU, preoperative propranolol or potassium iodide (50–100 mg/day for 1–2 weeks) may be administered. To avoid the bitter taste that causes excessive salivation in cats, potassium iodide is best administered in gelatin capsules. Large amounts of iodide rapidly but transiently reduce thyroid hormone release from the thyroid gland. Even if tachycardia is not present prior to anesthesia, this therapy should be supplemented by a β-blocker such as propranolol (2.5–5.0 mg q8h 1–2 weeks before surgery) to minimize the tendency for intraoperative ventricular cardiac arrhythmias.

The reader is referred to detailed reviews by Peterson (1987) and Black and Peterson (1983) for anesthetic and surgical techniques associated with thyroidectomy in cats. The principles of the associated management are outlined here. The anesthetic plan should avoid agents that are arrhythmogenic and hypertensive because hyperthyroid cats are prone to cardiac disease, arrhythmias, and hypertension. This concern is of particular importance when the animal is still hyperthyroid. Glycopyrrolate is the antimuscarinic drug of choice because it has less effect on cardiac rate and rhythm than atropine. Premedication with a phenothiazine (e.g., acetylpromazine) serves to reduce the effect of circulating catecholamines and to counter arrhythmias induced by thiobarbiturates and inhalant anesthetics. Ketamine should be avoided because it leads to an increase in catecholamine release. Xylazine is also contraindicated because it potentiates the development of cardiac arrhythmias induced by inhalation or barbiturate anesthesia. Thiobarbiturates are the recommended induction agents because they possess antithyroid activity and do not stimulate catecholamine secretion. Methoxyflurane and halothane, although commonly used, may sensitize the heart to arrhythmias triggered by endogenous catecholamines.

Intraoperatively, the body temperature, ECG, and respiratory pattern should be monitored. With untreated hyperthyroidism, the oxygen consumption, anesthetic requirements, and risk of hypoxia are great. Ventricular arrhythmias are not uncommon. Management of such arrhythmias should include 1) an increase in the oxygen flow rate, and 2) propranolol (0.1 mg IV).

Even at surgery, it is difficult to accurately establish that a thyroid lobe is "normal." This distinction is best made by scintigraphic studies available only at referral institutions. However, establishment of the diagnosis of unilateral disease (about 30% of cases) is important because surgery is the treatment of choice. In approximately 15% of cases, bilateral disease exists; however, one gland may be only slightly enlarged and visually appear to be normal. If thyroid imaging is not available but the involvement appears unilateral at surgery, the obviously enlarged lobe should be removed while not damaging the associated external parathyroid gland or its blood supply. If the other lobe develops gross enlargement (generally within 9 months) and surgery is again necessary, the risk of hypocalcemia is small.

Most cases require bilateral thyroidectomy. The goal of bilateral thyroidectomy is to remove all thyroid tissue while maintaining viability of at least one, if not two, of the external parathyroid glands. Intracapsular and extracapsular surgical procedures have been described. The main advantage of the extracapsular technique is that, by removing the entire thyroid capsule with the thyroid lobe, the chances of recurrence are lower.

Postoperative Management. Postoperative complications of bilateral thyroidectomy include hypocalcemia (about 15% of cases), Horner's syndrome, and laryngeal paralysis due to disruption of the vagosympathetic trunk. Clinically evident hypocalcemia occurs only after all parathyroid glands have been removed or damaged. Although it may be apparent during the immediate postsurgical period, hypocalcemia may develop as late as 3 days after surgery (presumably after scar tissue starts to develop).

It is not uncommon for cats to have mild hypocalcemia (<7 mg/dl, or 1.75 mmol/L) without clinical signs. Severe hypocalcemia associated with clinical signs should be managed with intravenous calcium. Oral calcium supplementation (calcium gluconate up to 750 mg/kg/day or calcium lactate 600 mg/kg/day) may be instituted when the cat accepts oral medications. Dihydrotachysterol (Hytakerol liquid, Winthrop; tablets, Philips-Roxane), a synthetic vitamin D analogue that is active in the absence of parathyroid hormone, is the recommended form of vitamin D therapy. An oral loading dose of 0.03 mg/kg/day for 3–4 days followed by a maintenance dose of 0.01–0.02 mg/kg/day, if effective, increases the serum calcium 4–5 days after initiation of therapy. In most cases this therapy can be withdrawn after a period of weeks or months.

Monitoring Therapy after Thyroidectomy. Following successful unilateral or bilateral thyroidectomy, the serum T_4 generally falls into the subnormal range by 1–2 weeks after surgery and remain there for 2–3 months. Clinical signs of hypothyroidism rarely develop. However, after bilateral thyroidectomy, it may be wise to start thyroxine supplementation (0.1–0.2 mg daily in single or divided doses) beginning 1–2 days after surgery. In most cases, however, likely after hypertrophy of normal extracervical thyroid tissue, cats can maintain normal serum T_4 concentrations. Therefore L-thyroxine therapy eventually may be withdrawn. The serum T_4 concentration should be monitored once or twice a year. When retreatment is necessary, nonsurgical modalities are preferred because the incidence of hypoparathyroidism increases greatly with repeat operations.

Standard Therapy—Institutional Practice

Only available at referral institutions, the administration of large doses of radioiodine (^{131}I) is the most effective and least dangerous treatment for bilateral toxic goiter in the cat. Radioiodine selectivity destroys the functioning thyroid tissue without risking damage to the nearby parathyroid tissue. Iodine 131 has a half-life of 8 days and produces both gamma and beta radiation; however, the beta particles serve to produce most of the local tissue destruction. A low rate of recurrence of hyperthyroidism (underdosing) or induction of permanent hypothyroidism (overdosing) has been experienced with radioiodine treatment in cats. Therefore at many institutions cats are given a fixed dose of 1–5 mCi. In one study using a fixed dose of 4 mCi, euthyroidism was achieved in 84% when evaluated at 60 days after treatment. About one-half of the remainder were still hyperthyroxinemic, and the other half had become hypothyroxinemic but were not showing clinical signs of hypothyroidism. The low incidence of persistent hypothyroidism is possibly attributable to the hypertrophy of extracervical thyroid tissue normally present in cats. Higher radioiodine doses are employed for metastatic thyroid follicular carcinomas (1–2% of cases), with a much poorer prognosis. Following a therapeutic dose of ^{131}I, the serum T_4 and T_3 concentrations usually normalize within 1–2 weeks but may remain elevated for 6–8 weeks. Hypothyroidism is a rare long-term sequela, making thyroid replacement therapy generally unnecessary. The efficacy of radioiodine is reduced by recent antithyroid medical therapy, as these drugs reduce the long-term incorporation of iodine into the thyroid gland and reduce radioiodine's therapeutic effect. Therefore MMI should be discontinued for at least 3–7 days prior to radioiodine treatment.

Radioiodine is secreted in saliva and excreted in urine and feces of hyperthyroid cats treated with radioiodine. Therefore radiation safety precautions are extensive and radioiodine-treated cats must generally be hospitalized for periods of 1–4 weeks. Despite these disadvantages, radioiodine therapy is a noninvasive, nontoxic cure for bilateral adenomatous goiter. Furthermore, radioiodine can be administered without anesthesia or sedation, an important consideration in the elderly cat with other medical problems.

Prognosis

The prognosis for a cat with uncomplicated adenomatous goiter is excellent following most treatments. The metabolic severity of the disease may lead the owner to be skeptical of such a positive outcome. Therefore the use of antithyroid drugs may aid the owner to see improvement before committing to more expensive curative therapies such as surgery or radioiodine.

CALCIUM DISORDERS

Hypo- and hypercalcemia are metabolic disturbances that can present great diagnostic and therapeutic problems. The clinical spectrum ranges from an asymptomatic to a life-threatening disorder. Because both abnormalities can be due to a variety of causes, it is of utmost importance to perform a thorough physical examination as there are many causes that can be identified on physical examination. The diagnosis is confirmed by measuring serum calcium concentrations. When interpreting the results, the age, albumin concentration, and presence of lipemia should be taken into consideration; laboratory error should be excluded.

Standard Therapy of Hypocalcemia

Emergency Treatment of the Seizuring Animal. Diagnosis of the hypocalcemic animal must be made rapidly and treatment undertaken immediately. Intravenous calcium, at a 10% calcium gluconate (Elkins-Sinn) dose of 0.5–1.5 ml/kg, which is equal to 5–15 mg elemental calcium per kilogram, is administered to effect over 10–30 minutes. Preferably, the patient is monitored with ECG. If bradycardia develops or if a shortening of the Q-T interval is seen, the calcium infusion should be discontinued temporarily. Caution should be exerted in the hyperphosphatemic animal, as a calcium infusion may lead to the formation of calcium phosphate, resulting in mineralization of soft tissue and potential renal damage.

The calcium dose (see above) can be repeated every 6–8 hours as a bolus injection, or it can be administered slowly intravenously in saline solution as a continuous infusion at a dosage of 60–90 mg of elemental calcium/kg/day. The fluid rate is 40–60 ml/kg/day. As soon as the animal is conscious, the clinician should also begin oral maintenance therapy.

Oral Maintenance Therapy. Oral maintenance therapy with calcium and vitamin D are initiated if the serum calcium concentration is consistently less than 6.5 mg/dl. Oral calcium supplementation can be achieved with a variety of calcium salts. In the dog 1–4 g of calcium is administered in two or three divided doses per day, whereas in the cat the daily dose ranges from 0.5 to 1.0 g.

There are also a variety of vitamin D preparations. Vitamin D_2 preparations (Calciferol, Kremers-Urban; Drisdol, Winthrop; Deltalin, Lilly) are inexpensive, but they take several days before a clinical effect is seen. Because these preparations need activation by parathyroid hormone to be biologically active, they are not useful in patients with hypoparathyroidism. The daily dosage for vitamin D_2 is 4000–6000 units/kg body weight initially and is tapered with time according to the calcium concentration. The maintenance dose may be as low as 1000 units/kg once weekly. The goal of vitamin D and calcium therapy is to keep the calcium concentration at a low normal range (8.0–8.5 mg/dl). Because of the delayed effect of vitamin D_2, the animal has to be monitored frequently. The initial treatment phase is therefore best performed while the animal is hospitalized. Once the animal has been stabilized at a low normal serum calcium concentration without parenteral calcium supplementation, therapy can be continued at home and the patient should be monitored about once weekly for a few weeks to ensure a stable calcium concentration. Other vitamin D preparations raise the serum calcium concentration faster, but they are also more expensive.

Dihydrotachysterol (Dihydrotachysterol, Philips-Roxane; Hytakerol, Winthrop) is a newer, synthetic vitamin D preparation that is active in the absence of parathyroid hormone. It is used in dogs and cats with hypoparathyroidism, e.g., in hyperthyroid cats with hypoparathyroidism as a sequela of thyroidectomy. The dose is 0.03 mg/kg body weight/day PO for 3–4 days (loading dose), followed by a maintenance dose of 0.01–0.02 mg/kg/day. An increase in the serum calcium concentration can be expected within 5 days of treatment. Vitamin D is also available in its biologically active form, i.e., 1,25(OH)$_2$-vitamin D$_3$ (Rocaltrol, Roche). This compound is the fastest acting preparation available and has a short half-life; however, it is expensive and is not routinely used for veterinary medicine.

Because there is great individual variability in the response to these preparations, it is important to monitor therapy frequently. It is imperative that the owner is made aware of the clinical signs associated with hypo- and hypercalcemia, which are not uncommon complications of vitamin D therapy.

Standard Therapy of Hypercalcemia

Severe hypercalcemia requires emergency treatment to prevent mineralization of soft tissue, especially the kidney. Increased calcium has a negative effect on many cellular functions; e.g., it decreases the excitability of the heart and leads to neurologic dysfunction. Although the primary goal of therapy is correction of the cause for the hypercalcemia, which most commonly is malignancy, therapy often must be instituted without knowledge of the underlying cause. Several regimens are available for the symptomatic treatment of hypercalcemia. The degree of hypercalcemia and the clinical presentation of the patient are important factors when deciding whether and how to treat.

Administration of Fluids. The fluid of choice is 0.9% saline (normal saline) because it contains no calcium and aids in excretion of calcium in the urine. Rehydration is an important initial step that by itself usually leads to a decrease in the calcium concentration. A saline diuresis is administered intravenously in the severely hypercalcemic patient at two to three times the maintenance rate, which is 40–60 ml/kg/day. It is obvious that this regimen requires careful monitoring (auscultation of the chest, body weight, urine output, central venous pressure).

Diuretic Therapy. Frequently, saline diuresis is used in combination with the diuretic furosemide (Lasix, Hoechst-Roussel) to ensure maximal sodium diuresis. Furosemide has been administered at a dose of 5 mg/kg IV in the form of a bolus injection, followed by an intravenous infusion of 5 mg/kg/hr, which leads to a decrease in serum calcium to normal concentrations within a few hours. It is important to ensure adequate hydration when this regimen is used. Others have used an intermittent bolus administration of furosemide using 2–4 mg/kg IV twice daily. This regimen also lowers serum calcium, though at a slower rate.

Glucocorticoid Therapy. Glucocorticoids may be beneficial because they reduce intestinal calcium absorption and bone resorption; they also are calciuretic. Their use should be delayed, however, if a diagnosis has not been established, because their administration may interfere with the subsequent ability to diagnose lymphoreticular malignancies. A common dose of prednisone or prednisolone is 1 mg/kg twice daily.

EDTA Therapy. Sodium EDTA (Disodium Versenate Injection, Riker) is a calcium-chelating agent that has been used for treatment of patients with life-threatening hypercalcemia at a dose of 25–75 mg/kg/hr. EDTA is nephrotoxic and may lead to acute renal failure. Because of its severe side effects and short duration of effect (1–2 hours), EDTA should be used only in emergency situations and only for the time period necessary to decrease the calcium concentration to a less severe level. Other less dangerous treatment regimens should be instituted at the same time.

Dialysis. Hemodialysis or peritoneal dialysis with calcium-free dialysate are effective methods to lower serum calcium concentrations. Although hemodialysis is not usually available at referral centers, the method of peritoneal dialysis has been described and can be used in a hospital setting (see Suggested Reading).

Investigational Therapy. *Phosphate Therapy.* Administration of phosphate lowers serum calcium by precipitation of calcium phosphate salts and possibly by a direct inhibitory effect on bone resorption. Phosphate in humans is administered intravenously in doses up to 1.5 g of elemental phosphate during a 6- to 8-hour period. Doses in small animals are unavailable.

Indomethacin Therapy. In humans indomethacin and aspirin correct hypercalcemia caused by production of prostaglandins by tumors in some cases. Studies in small animals are not available.

Diphosphonate Therapy. Diphosphonates, analogues of pyrophosphates, effectively reduce hypercalcemia caused by malignancy. Their efficacy in small animals needs to be investigated.

DIABETES INSIPIDUS

Diabetes insipidus (DI) is caused by the deficiency of antidiuretic hormone (central DI) or by absence of a renal response to this posterior pituitary hormone (nephrogenic DI). The main presenting signs, in the absence of other conditions, are polyuria and polydipsia. Before pursuing specific tests of the urinary concentrating capability, other disorders causing polyuria (e.g., diabetes mellitus, hyperadrenocorticism, chronic renal failure, and liver failure) as well as therapy with agents such as glucocorticoids and diuretics should be ruled out. Urinalysis generally reveals a urine specific gravity of less than 1.006

and often as low as 1.001 associated with daily urine volumes of at least two times the normal range, which is 30–60 ml/kg/day. Except for occasional elevation of serum sodium concentration and a reduction in BUN concentrations due to renal loss of urea ("medullary washout"), the routine hematologic screening tests are generally not revealing except in that they aid in ruling out other disorders. If the animal presents in a dehydrated state, the plasma osmolality may be elevated (>310 mOsm/kg).

Causes

Central DI is due to the absolute deficiency of antidiuretic hormone (vasopressin, ADH). In partial central DI, some endogenous ADH secretion remains. These conditions are the result of the destruction of the supraoptic and paraventricular nuclei of the hypothalamus, which have axons terminating in the posterior pituitary. The damage may be due to head trauma, surgical transection of the pituitary stalk (usually only transient DI), or primary or metastatic tumors; most commonly in veterinary medicine, however, the cause is not known (idiopathic DI).

Nephrogenic DI results when the renal tubule is insensitive to ADH. In this condition ADH does not increase intratubular cyclic adenosine monophosphate (cAMP) concentrations, a necessary prerequisite to the increased water permeability normally induced by ADH. This abnormality of ADH responsiveness may be partial or total. Primary causes of nephrogenic diabetes are rare. However, secondary nephrogenic DI may result from pyometra, liver disease, hyperadrenocorticism, hyperthyroidism, hypercalcemic disorders, renal failure, and pyelonephritis.

Definitive Diagnosis

Diabetes insipidus is diagnosed if the urine specific gravity is dilute (< 1.008) in the face of dehydration or elevated plasma osmolality. However, not infrequently the animal presents in a hydrated state and has a normal or only slightly elevated plasma osmolality. Therefore a modified water deprivation test (see Feldman and Nelson, 1987, for the protocol) is recommended to confirm that endogenous ADH and urine osmolality do not rise in the face of moderate dehydration. After carefully monitored gradual water withdrawal over 3 days, water is completely withdrawn on the fourth day and the urine osmolality and plasma osmolality are monitored. If more than 5% dehydration is achieved and no urine concentration is observed, exogenous ADH is administered to test the ability to respond to exogenous hormone. Vasopressin can be administered in three ways in this test.

1. Aqueous ADH (vasopressin USP, Quad) 0.55 units/kg IM up to a maximum of 5 units. Urine volume and osmolality (or specific gravity) should be measured at 30, 60, and 120 minutes after administration.

2. Pitressin Tannate in Oil (Parke-Davis) 2–5 units IM. Urine volume and osmolality (or specific gravity) should then be monitored over 24–72 hours. Multiple daily doses may be necessary to establish the ability of the kidney to concentrate urine. The future availability of this product is in doubt.
3. Aqueous ADH (vasopressin USP, Quad) 1 milliunit/ml in Lactated Ringer's or 5% dextrose. This solution is then administered over 1 hour at the rate of 10 ml/kg body weight. Urine samples should be obtained at 15-minute intervals for 90 minutes following ADH administration.

In an animal with complete central DI the urine osmolality does not rise above isoosmolality (300 mOsm/kg) with dehydration, and subsequent ADH administration increases urine osmolality at least 50%. In an animal with partial central DI, the urine osmolality increases above isoosmolality and then increases an additional 10–50% following administration of exogenous ADH. Animals with nephrogenic DI do not concentrate their urine upon dehydration above isoosmolality and do not respond to exogenous ADH. Dogs with other polyuric disorders concentrate urine usually above 1000 mOsm/kg upon careful dehydration (allowing correction of medullary urea washout), and exogenous ADH does not increase urine osmolality more than an additional 10%.

Central Diabetes Insipidus

Standard Therapy. The most common treatment for central DI is the intramuscular administration of Pitressin Tannate (Parke-Davis) in oil, although the availability of this product in the future is in doubt. Pitressin is a partially purified form of ADH derived from bovine and porcine pituitary glands. Unlike aqueous ADH, this preparation has a sufficiently long duration of action to allow its use for the chronic management of DI. This preparation must be warmed and thoroughly mixed prior to intramuscular or subcutaneous administration. A dose of 5 units (2.5 units in small dogs and cats) should be administered at an interval corresponding to the onset of obvious new polyuria, usually every 36–48 hours. Immediately following a dose, in order to avoid water intoxication, dogs should not be given unlimited quantities of water. The transiently high levels of ADH prevent excretion of a free water load by the kidney and result in overhydration and possible neurologic sequelae such as cerebral edema. Cerebral edema may manifest by depression, vomiting, salivation, ataxia, muscle tremors, and convulsions. Pitressin Tannate is a relatively expensive therapy and requires considerable time and financial commitment by the owners.

Alternative Therapy. Alternative therapeutic agents for the treatment of total and partial central DI include the synthetic ADH analogues DDAVP (desmopressin acetate, USV Laboratories) and lysine-8-vasopressin (Diapid nasal spray, Sandoz Pharmaceuticals). Both of these preparations can be administered intranasally or into the conjunctival sac. The latter route appears to be better tolerated by the animals. Ocular or conjunctival irritation is a rare problem.

DDAVP has greater potency and slower metabolism than the natural ADH molecule. Furthermore, it has less vasopressor activity than Pitressin. Administration of 5–20 µg of DDAVP (2–4 drops) in single or divided doses controls polyuria in most animals. The peak drug action is seen at 2–6 hours, and its duration may last 10–27 hours. The clear advantage of this medication is that it does not require parenteral administration. However, the conjunctival route results in variable amounts of drug reaching the bloodstream and variable duration of effect even in the same patient. DDAVP is also expensive, and therefore it might be prudent to use the drug only when polyuria is observed or to avoid excessive nocturnal urine production.

Lysine-8-vasopressin (LVP) is another product available for managing DI via nasal or conjunctival administration. However, its duration of action is shorter and expense greater than the other products. As a result, it has not found much application in veterinary medicine.

Animals with central or nephrogenic DI may also be successfully managed by providing free access to water at all times and by housing the animals outdoors. Another inexpensive maneuver that reduces the urine output is restriction of dietary sodium using homemade diets or the commercial diets designed for use in congestive heart failure (e.g., Hill's h/d). Such products generally contain less than 0.1% sodium on a dry weight basis.

Investigational Therapy. Oral agents have also been used primarily as adjuncts to ADH therapy of central DI. Chlorpropamide (Diabinese, Pfizer), a sulfonylurea hypoglycemic agent used to treat non-insulin-dependent diabetes in humans, has produced inconsistent antidiuretic effects in the dog and cat. Chlorpropamide's effect is to enhance the effect of ADH on the renal tubules and collecting duct by increasing intracellular cAMP. It may also stimulate pituitary ADH release. As a result, it is effective only in the presence of sufficient endogenous ADH (partial central DI) or exogenously administered ADH. Careful chlorpropamide dosage studies have not been performed in the dog. Reported doses include 250 mg q12h and 10–40 mg/kg/day. Reduction in urinary volumes ranging from 18 to 50% have been reported. Maximal antidiuretic effects take 1–2 weeks to develop. Side effects of hypoglycemia can be minimized by frequent feedings and periodic monitoring of blood glucose concentrations.

Carbamazepine (Tegretol, Geigy Pharmaceuticals), an antiepileptic, and clofibrate (Atromid, Ayerst Laboratories), an antihyperlipidemic drug, are also effective in some cases of central DI. In contrast to the other drugs, these agents may increase ADH secretion and therefore would be rational therapy only for partial central DI. There have been no reports in the veterinary literature, however, of the use of these drugs for the successful treatment of DI.

Thiazide diuretics when used together with salt restriction may serve to potentiate the effect of exogenous or endogenous ADH (see below).

Nephrogenic Diabetes Insipidus

Standard Therapy. Treatment for nephrogenic DI should, if possible, start with correction of the underlying cause of the nephrogenic DI (hypercalcemia, renal infection, hyperadrenocorticism without a compressive pituitary tumor). Except for institution of a low sodium diet, the thiazide diuretics are the only agents shown to be effective in the treatment of nephrogenic DI.

Thiazide diuretics have a paradoxical antidiuretic effect in central and nephrogenic DI. These agents may work by reducing the reabsorption of sodium in the ascending loop of Henle, resulting in enhanced urinary sodium loss, mild reduction in plasma osmolality, and therefore diminished thirst. The reduction in water intake causes contraction of the extracellular volume, increased proximal tubular sodium reabsorption, and decreased glomerular filtration rate. The urine volume is thereby reduced without overt concentration of the urine osmolality. Hydrochlorothiazide (Hydrodiuril, Merck, Sharp & Dohme) at a dosage of 2.5–5.0 mg/kg has succeeded in reducing water intake by 50–85% in cases of ADH-resistant polyuria. Because of the kaliuretic effect of the thiazides, serum potassium should be monitored and oral potassium (Kaon Elixir, Adria) administered if the animal becomes anorexic.

Prognosis

Dogs with idiopathic or congenital central DI have a good prognosis, and some animals have received replacement therapy for as long as 10 years. The prognosis for central DI is generally poor if a known pathologic process is impairing the hypothalamic-pituitary axis. These animals may succumb to the neurologic problems that often arise. However, our limited experience includes a case of an ACTH-secreting macroadenoma of the pituitary that caused central DI and biochemical hyperadrenocorticism. The dog survived for 3 years with only DDAVP therapy, eventually succumbing after the development of signs consistent with central neurologic dysfunction. The prognosis for even partial recovery following treatment of nephrogenic DI is generally poor but ultimately depends on the underlying disease causing the disorder.

SUGGESTED READINGS

Diabetes Mellitus

Feldman EC, Nelson RW: Diabetes mellitus. In: Feldman EC, Nelson RW, eds. Canine and Feline Endocrinology and Reproduction. Philadelphia: WB Saunders, 1987;229.

Feldman EC, Nelson RW: Diabetic ketoacidosis. In: Feldman EC, Nelson RW, eds. Canine and Feline Endocrinology and Reproduction. Philadelphia: WB Saunders, 1987;274.

Nelson RW: Dietary therapy for canine diabetes mellitus. In: Kirk RW, ed. Current Veterinary Therapy X. Philadelphia: WB Saunders, 1989;1008.

Hypoglycemia

Feldman EC, Nelson RW: Hypoglycemia. In: Feldman EC, Nelson RW, eds. Canine and Feline Endocrinology and Reproduction. WB Saunders, 1987;304.

Leifer CE, Peterson ME: Hypoglycemia. Vet Clin North Am 1984;14:873.

Hyperadrenocorticism

Feldman EC, Bruyette DS, Nelson RW: Therapy for spontaneous canine hyperadreno-corticism. In: Kirk RW, ed. Current Veterinary Therapy X. Philadelphia: WB Saunders, 1989;1024.

Feldman EC, Nelson RW: Hyperadrenocorticism. In: Feldman EC, Nelson RW, eds. Canine and Feline Endocrinology and Reproduction. Philadelphia: WB Saunders, 1987;137.

Kintzer PP, Peterson ME: Mitotane (o,p'-DDD) treatment of cortisol-secreting adreno-cortical neoplasia. In: Kirk RW, ed. Current Veterinary Therapy X. Philadelphia: WB Saunders, 1989;1034.

Peterson ME: Canine hyperadrenocorticism. In: Kirk RW, ed. Current Veterinary Therapy IX. Philadelphia: WB Saunders, 1986;963.

Rijnberk A, Belshaw BE: An alternative protocol for the medical management of canine pituitary-dependent hyperadrenocorticism. Vet Rec 1988;122:486.

Rijnberk A, Belshaw BE: Treatment of pituitary-dependent hyperadrenocorticism in the dog. Vet Med Rep 1990;3:64.

Zerbe CA: Feline hyperadrenocorticism. In: Kirk RW, ed. Current Veterinary Therapy X. Philadelphia: WB Saunders, 1989;1038.

Hypoadrenocorticism

Feldman EC, Nelson RW: Hypoadrenocorticism. In: Feldman EC, Nelson RW, eds. Canine and Feline Endocrinology and Reproduction. Philadelphia: WB Saunders, 1987;195.

Greco DS, Peterson ME: Feline hypoadrenocorticism. In: Kirk RW, ed. Current Veterinary Therapy X. Philadelphia: WB Saunders, 1989;1042.

Schrader LA: Hypoadrenocorticism. In: Kirk RW, ed. Current Veterinary Therapy IX. Philadelphia: WB Saunders, 1986;972.

Hypothyroidism

Feldman EC, Nelson RW, eds. Hypothyroidism. In: Canine and Feline Endocrinology and Reproduction. Philadelphia: WB Saunders, 1987;55.

Ferguson DC: Thyroid function tests in the dog. Vet Clin North Am 1984;14:783.

Ferguson DC: Thyroid hormone replacement therapy. In: Kirk RW, ed. Current Veterinary Therapy IX. Philadelphia: WB Saunders, 1986;1018.

Ferguson DC: Effect of nonthyroidal factors on thyroid function tests in the dog. Compend Contin Educ (Small Anim) 1988;10:1365.

Ferguson DC: Hypothyroidism: Many presentations, one treatment. Small animal geriatrics: Viewpoints in veterinary medicine. Alpo Symposium proceedings 1989:30.

Ferguson DC, Hoenig MH: Hypothyroidism. In: Allen DG, ed. Small Animal Medicine. Philadelphia: JB Lippincott, 1991;831.

Panciera, DL. Canine hypothyroidism. Part II. Thyroid function tests and treatment. Compend Contin Educ (Small Anim) 1990;12:843.

Peterson ME, Ferguson DC. Thyroid diseases. In: Ettinger SJ, ed. Textbook of Veterinary Internal Medicine, 3rd ed. Philadelphia: WB Saunders, 1632–1675.

Hyperthyroidism

Black AP, Peterson ME: Thyroid biopsy and thyroidectomy. In: Bojrab MJ, ed. Current Techniques in Small Animal Surgery. Philadelphia: Lea & Febiger, 1983:388.

Feldman EC, Nelson RW, eds. Hyperthyroidism and thyroid tumors. In: Canine and Feline Endocrinology and Reproduction. Philadelphia: WB Saunders, 1987:91.

Ferguson DC. New perspectives on the etiology, diagnosis, and treatment of feline hyperthyroidism. Small animal geriatrics: Viewpoint in veterinary medicine. Alpo Symposium proceedings 1989:23.

Ferguson DC, Hoenig MH: Feline hyperthyroidism. In: Allen DG, ed. Small Animal Medicine. Philadelphia: JB Lippincott, 1991;831.

Meric SM, Rubin SI: Serum thyroxine concentrations following fixed-dose radioactive iodine treatment in hyperthyroid cats: 62 cases (1986–1989). J Am Vet Med Assoc 1990;197:621.

Peterson ME: Considerations and complications in anesthesia with pathophysiologic changes in the endocrine system. In: Short CE, ed. Veterinary Anesthesiology. Baltimore: Williams & Wilkins, 1987;251.

Peterson ME: Treatment of feline hyperthyroidism. In: Kirk RW, ed. Current Veterinary Therapy X. Philadelphia: WB Saunders, 1989;1002.

Peterson ME, Ferguson DC: Thyroid diseases. In: Ettinger SJ, ed. Textbook of Veterinary Internal Medicine, 3rd ed. Philadelphia: WB Saunders, 1989;1632.

Peterson ME, Keene B, Ferguson DC, Pipers F: Electrocardiographic findings in forty-five cats with hyperthyroidism. J Am Vet Med Assoc 1982;18:934.

Peterson ME, Kintzer PP, Cavanagh PG, et al: Feline hyperthyroidism: pretreatment clinical and laboratory evaluation of 131 cases. J Am Vet Med Assoc 1983;183:103.

Peterson ME, Kintzer PP, Hurvitz AI: Methimazole treatment of 262 cats with hyper-thyroidism. J Vet Int Med 1988;2:150.

Calcium Disorders

Feldman EC, Nelson RW: Hypocalcemia—hypoparathyroidism. In: Feldman EC, Nelson RW, eds. Canine and Feline Endocrinology and Reproduction. Philadelphia: WB Saunders, 1987;357.

Feldman EC, Nelson RW: The parathyroid gland—primary hyperparathyroidism. In: Feldman EC, Nelson RW, eds. Canine and Feline Endocrinology and Reproduction. Philadelphia: WB Saunders, 1987;328.

Kruger JM, Osborne CA, Polzin DJ: Treatment of hypercalcemia. In: Kirk RW, ed. Current Veterinary Therapy IX. Philadelphia: WB Saunders, 1986;75.

Ong SC, Shalhoub RJ, Gallagher P, et al: Effect of furosemide on experimental hypercalcemia in dogs. Proc Soc Exp Biol Med 1974;145:227.

Parker HR: Current status of peritoneal dialysis. In: Kirk RW, ed. Current Veterinary Therapy IX. Philadelphia: WB Saunders, 1980;1106.

Peterson ME: Treatment of hypoparathyroidism. J Am Vet Med Assoc 1982;181:1434.

Diabetes Insipidus

Feldman EC, Nelson RW, eds: Hyperthyroidism and thyroid tumors. In: Canine and Feline Endocrinology and Reproduction. Philadelphia: WB Saunders, 1987;1.

Ferguson DC, Biery DN: Diabetes insipidus and hyperadrenocorticism associated with elevated plasma adrenocorticotropin concentration and a hypothalamic/pituitary mass in a dog. J Am Vet Med Assoc 1988;193:835.

Joles JA, Mulnix JA: Polyuria and polydipsia. In: Kirk RW, ed. Current Veterinary Therapy VI. Philadelphia: WB Saunders, 1977;1050.

Schwartz-Porsche D: Diabetes insipidus. In Kirk RW, ed. Current Veterinary Therapy VII. Philadelphia: WB Saunders, 1980;1005.

Siegel ET: Endocrine Diseases of the Dog. Philadelphia: Lea & Febiger, 1977;43.

CHAPTER FIVE

Hematolymphatic Disorders

Margarethe Hoenig

ANEMIA AND BLOOD TRANSFUSION THERAPY

Anemia is seen with a multitude of disease processes. It can be differentiated into regenerative and nonregenerative anemia. The separation into these classes is important as it helps the examiner to diagnose the problem. Regenerative anemias are seen with blood loss or destruction of red blood cells. A regenerative anemia is characterized by a regenerative response, i.e., polychromasia and a high reticulocyte count. A response can usually be expected within the first 48–72 hours after the occurrence of blood loss or hemolysis. Nonregenerative anemias are seen with nutritional deficiencies, lack of erythropoietin, or bone marrow abnormalities.

The anemic patient needs to be thoroughly evaluated. The history should include any possible exposure of the pet to drugs or toxins. A physical examination, complete blood count including platelet count and reticulocyte count, chemical blood screen (in certain cases with bilirubin determination), fecal examination, and urinalysis are indicated. The morphology of the red blood cells should be evaluated carefully as it provides a clue as to the nature of the anemia. Other tests may include clotting profiles and tests for immune-mediated disorders (e.g., Coombs' test) or rickettsial diseases. A bone marrow examination (smear or core biopsy) is indicated in cases of nonregenerative anemias. In addition to morphologic abnormalities, the bone marrow can be evaluated for the amount of iron present using a special staining procedure.

Maintenance of Blood Donors

Eight blood group antigens have been identified in the dog: DEA 1.1, 1.2, and 3–8. Dogs used as donors for blood transfusions should be negative for antigens at both the DEA 1 loci and the DEA 7 locus because they have the greatest potential to induce antibody formation and lead to transfusion problems. It is also advantageous to use large breed dogs, because venipuncture is easier and their packed cell volume tends to be higher. In addition, a blood donor should have a gentle disposition to allow easy handling. Female donors should be spayed to eliminate the influence of reproductive hormones on blood parameters.

Only healthy, vaccinated, dewormed, and heartworm-negative animals should be used as donors. They must be kept in a clean environment, be exercised daily, and receive a well-balanced diet. In both dogs and cats, 22 ml/kg body weight can be withdrawn safely every 10 days.

Equipment Used for Blood Transfusions

Blood for transfusion is collected aseptically into special plastic bags, plastic syringes, or glass containers that contain either the anticoagulant and blood preservative acid citrate dextrose (ACD) or citrate dextrose phosphate (CDP). Plastic containers with ACD or CDP are commercially available (Fenwal Division, Baxter Health Care). The blood can be stored at 4°C for 21 days (ACD) or 28 days (CDP). A storage medium for blood has been described that keeps the erythrocyte viability above 70% for 6 weeks, but the medium is not commercially available. Heparin is frequently used as an anticoagulant in the cat. Blood cannot be stored in heparin but should be used within 48 hours because heparin does not contain dextrose and therefore does not have any preservative effect. It also leads to platelet adhesion and aggregation, making it less attractive as an anticoagulant. Blood administration sets with filters to remove blood clots and other aggregates are used for the transfusion (Fenwal Division, Baxter Health Care). These sets can also be used when blood has been collected in a plastic syringe. The transfusion set is then connected to an indwelling catheter placed in the cephalic or jugular vein (18–22 gauge) (Venocath, Abbott Laboratories; Intracath, Deseret Co.).

Standard Therapy

It is obvious that anemic patients require a variety of treatment regimens depending on the cause of the anemia. Such treatments may be as diverse as hookworm treatment and immunosuppressive therapy. This chapter covers only treatment forms directed at the site of red blood cell production, i.e., the bone marrow, and transfusion therapy.

Transfusion Therapy. Transfusion of whole blood or blood components is indicated in the anemic or bleeding patient. In the case of autoimmune hemolytic anemia it should only be used in acute life-threatening situations. Blood from a DEA 1.1, 1.2, and DEA 7 negative donor or, preferably, cross-matched blood should be used in the dog when whole blood or packed red blood cells are used. In the cat, crossmatching is not routinely required but recommended. If it is necessary to provide functional platelets or viable coagulation factors the blood needs to be fresh and transfused within approximately 8–12 hours.

Whole blood transfusion is indicated in animals with nonregenerative anemia in which the packed cell volume (PCV) has fallen to 12–15% in the dog and to 10% in the cat. It is indicated for acute hemorrhage when the PCV falls to 20%. It may also be used for the treatment of coagulation disorders or thrombocytopenia.

Packed red blood cells are indicated in anemic animals with volume overload. Packed red blood cells are prepared from whole blood by centrifugation; alternatively, they can be prepared by letting red blood cells sediment overnight, when plasma and red blood cells can be separated easily.

Plasma transfusions are indicated in animals with congenital or acquired deficiencies of coagulation factors and with hypoproteinemia. Plasma is prepared from whole blood by centrifugation or by separation of red blood cells after sedimentation overnight. If labile coagulation factors are needed, fresh frozen plasma or cryoprecipitates are used. These components are prepared by centrifugation and freezing of fresh plasma or by thawing of fresh frozen plasma and separation of the cold-precipitated material, which is rich in factor VIII, von Willebrand's factor, and fibrinogen. Plasma and cryoprecipitate can be frozen and stored at $-40°$ to $-70°C$ for up to 1 year. Conventionally, plasma has been thawed slowly in a waterbath; it has now been shown that frozen plasma can be thawed rapidly in a microwave oven without alteration in the activities of various coagulation factors. The oven was set at its highest setting (700 W), and the plasma units were irradiated for 15 thawing periods of 10 seconds each until only small pieces of ice remained. Between the thawing periods the plasma units were agitated by hand to thoroughly mix the specimens. The units were also agitated at the end until all ice dissolved.

Platelet transfusions are indicated for severe thrombocytopenia. Platelets are provided in whole blood transfusions, although the administration of whole blood may not always be desirable. It is possible to prepare platelet-rich plasma by centrifugation of whole blood for $1200 \times g$ for 2.5 minutes at 20°C. This technique is usually used only at referral centers that have the appropriate equipment. Platelets maintain their viability for only 8–12 hours.

Treatment Regimen.

1. *Whole blood.* Blood should be warmed in a 37°C waterbath or incubator to room temperature before administration. Blood is infused intravenously via an indwelling catheter. Alternatively, blood can also be administered into the bone marrow or into the abdominal cavity whenever intravenous administration is not possible. Absorption of red blood cells from the medullary cavity is rapid but takes several days when infused into the peritoneal cavity. The rate of administration of whole blood should not exceed 10 ml/kg/hr. In patients with cardiac disease, it should not exceed 4 ml/kg/hr. Generally, 2 ml of blood from a donor with a normal PCV given per kilogram body weight

raises the recipient's PCV by 1%. However, it is advisable to calculate the blood replacement volume for each animal according to the following formulas:

Dog: Ml of blood needed $= $ BW (kg) $\times$ 90 $\times$ $\frac{\text{(desired PCV} - \text{PCV of recipient)}}{\text{PCV of donor blood}}$

Cat: Ml of blood needed $= $ BW (kg) $\times$ 70 $\times$ $\frac{\text{(desired PCV} - \text{PCV of recipient)}}{\text{PCV of donor blood}}$

Example: Recipient is a 10 kg dog with a PCV of 15; the donor is a dog with a PCV of 50. The desired PCV is 25.

Ml of blood needed $= 10 \times 90 \times \frac{(25 - 15)}{50}$. The patient needs 180 ml of blood.

The goal of the blood transfusion is to raise the PCV to safe but not to normal levels. It has been recommended that the initial transfusion rate be decreased to 0.25 ml/kg during the first 30 minutes and the patient be observed carefully for any adverse reactions (urticaria, tremor, pulmonary edema, vomiting, diarrhea, urinary incontinence). Frequently, diphenhydramine hydrochloride (Benadryl Parenteral, Parke-Davis) is given prophylactically at 2 mg/kg IM about 30 minutes before transfusion to eliminate anaphylactic reactions.

2. *Packed cells.* Packed cells are administered like whole blood. The infusion rate of packed cells, however, is much slower than that of whole blood. This problem can be overcome by using a larger needle or diluting the red cells with normal saline at a 0.5:1.0 to 1:1 ratio. It can be done with a Y-infusion set (Y-blood Component Infusion Set, Fenwal Division, Baxter Health Care), which contains two openings, one for connecting with normal saline and one for blood. A 1:1 dilution ratio therefore means that normal saline and blood are administered simultaneously at the same rate.

3. *Plasma.* Plasma and fresh frozen plasma are administered intravenously at a dosage of 6–10 ml/kg as needed. For the patient whose bleeding is due to a deficiency in clotting factors, this dose is repeated at least three times daily until the bleeding is controlled. Cryoprecipitate plasma is given at a dosage of 12–20 ml/kg twice daily until the bleeding is controlled. It should be used for transfusion within 6 hours of thawing.

Bone Marrow Stimulants. *Factors Necessary for Normal Red Cell Maturation.* The bone marrow is a highly active organ that depends on certain nutrients for normal function, especially vitamin B_{12}, folate, and iron. Without them megaloblastic anemia (vitamin B_{12} and folate) or microcytic hypochromic anemia (severe iron deficiency) is seen.

Vitamin B_{12} (cyanocobalamin, Elkins-Sinn and others) is given intramuscularly or subcutaneously at a dosage of 500–1000 μg once weekly until the blood parameters return to normal, and then given monthly. Initially, the hematocrit is checked weekly and then monthly.

Folate (folic acid, Lilly and others) is given orally at a dosage of 1 mg once daily.

Iron (ferrous sulfate; ferrous gluconate tablets, American Pharmaceutical) is given orally as ferrous sulfate at a dosage of 100–200 mg once daily for 1 week, and should be administered with food. This treatment may lead to constipation, diarrhea, and discoloration of the feces. In severe cases, injectable iron (iron dextran; Imferon, Merrell Dow) may be given once at a dosage of 10–20 mg/kg IM followed by oral supplementation. An improvement in the hematocrit should be seen within 2–4 weeks.

Hormones. Anemia due to red cell hypoplasia or aplasia may be treated with hormonal therapy including androgens and glucocorticoids. In some cases of pure red cell aplasia, immunosuppressive therapy may be indicated.

Androgens stimulate erythropoiesis by increasing the concentration of erythropoietin, which subsequently stimulates hemoglobin production. Androgens are used primarily for anemias due to renal failure, bone marrow failure, and myelofibrosis. While on therapy, the animal's hematocrit should be monitored at biweekly to monthly intervals. It has been reported that oral androgen preparations may lead to hepatotoxicity, so animals on this form of treatment should have monitoring of liver enzymes. If no response is seen to a particular androgen dosage after 2–3 months, it may be advisable to increase the dose. If still no response is seen, a different preparation may be used. In general, variable success has been seen with androgen therapy for the treatment of nonregenerative anemias.

The treatment regimen includes oxymetholone (Anadrol-50, Syntex), which is administered orally at a dosage of 2.5–5.0 mg/kg daily. Alternatively, weekly intramuscular injections of nandrolone decanoate (Deca-Durabolin, Organon) at a dosage of 1–3 mg/kg may be given. As outlined above, therapy has to be continued for months before a response may be seen.

Immunosuppressive Drugs. *Glucocorticoids.* Glucocorticoids are used in anemic patients with myelophthisis, myelofibrosis, or suspected immune-mediated bone marrow hypoplasia or aplasia. They also stimulate erythropoietin production.

The treatment regimen includes prednisone or prednisolone (Prednisone or Prednisolone Tablets, Roxane), which is administered orally twice daily at a dose of 1.1–3.3 mg/kg until a response is seen and the PCV reaches the low normal range. The steroid dose is tapered over several weeks once the PCV is stable until a dose of 1.1 mg/kg is reached. The animal is kept on this dose on an alternate-day regimen for several weeks. However, therapy may be lifelong.

Other Immunosuppressive Agents. Cyclophosphamide (Cytoxan, Mead Johnson Pharmaceuticals) has been used for the treatment of pure red blood cell aplasia when glucocorticoids did not lead to a response. Cyclophosphamide can be administered in addition to glucocorticoids or by itself in cases of resistance or unacceptable side effects to steroids. The drug is administered once daily for 4 days weekly. This regimen is continued until the red blood cell count has increased to low normal and is stable.

The dose of cyclophosphamide varies with the size of the animal:

1.5 mg/kg for dogs >25 kg
2.0 mg/kg for dogs 5–25 kg
2.5 mg/kg for dogs <5 kg

Cyclophosphamide is given orally with food. It can also be administered intravenously. (For more details on the use of cyclophosphamide, see page 156.)

Splenectomy. Splenectomy should be a last resort for the treatment of chronic cases of immune-mediated hemolytic disease. It is also indicated in patients with hypersplenism that do not respond to other forms of therapy.

Investigational Therapy. *Bone Marrow Transplantation.* Bone marrow transplantation is indicated for patients with marrow failure induced by chemotherapy or radiation treatment for malignancies or when aplastic anemia occurs spontaneously. Application in the dog and cat is feasible and has already been done, although thus far only at specialized centers.

Recombinant Human Erythropoietin. Recombinant human erythropoietin (r-HuEpo; Epogen, Amgen) has been used successfully in people with nonregenerative anemia associated with chronic renal dysfunction. Nonregenerative anemias due to other disease processes may also be indications for the use of this hormone. Erythropoietin is a glycoprotein that is synthesized primarily in the kidney. The main regulator of red blood cell production, this drug has been studied in a small number of anemic dogs and cats with chronic renal failure, where it promoted erythroid hyperplasia. Its clinical efficacy is currently being tested at several hospitals. Thus far it has not been approved for use in animals. The only published dose in the dog and cat is 150 units/kg SC daily for 7 days and then three times a week. Potential side effects include anaphylactic reactions to the carrier protein, which is human albumin. In humans, hypertension, thrombocytosis, and hyperkalemia have been reported. See Chapter 11 for additional information.

AUTOIMMUNE HEMOLYTIC ANEMIA

In animals with autoimmune hemolytic anemia (AIHA), formation of autoantibodies to their own red blood cells leads to increased erythrocyte destruction. The erythrocytes may be destroyed intravascularly (intravascular hemolysis), or they may be phagocytized by cells of the reticuloendothelial system (extravascular hemolysis). The formation of antibodies against the body's own red blood cells occurs when diseases alter self-antigens or when cross-reacting antibodies are introduced, as is seen with certain malignancies. Frequently, the cause of the autodestruction remains unknown (idiopathic). AIHA is primarily caused by immunoglobulin G (IgG) and IgM antibodies, which may be optimally active at normal body temperature (warm type) or at temperatures below 30°C (cold agglutinin).

AIHA is a common disease in the dog and is frequently associated with systemic lupus erythematosus or immune-mediated or idiopathic thrombocytopenia. In the cat, the disease is uncommon and is most often seen in association with FeLV infection. The clinical signs depend on the severity of the anemia and on the rapidity of its onset. AIHA is characterized by moderate to severe anemia, leukocytosis, and there may be thrombocytopenia. Spherocytes are common. The anemia is usually responsive, and a reticulocyte production index of less than 1 is indicative of a concomitant bone marrow problem. Screening tests for AIHA should include a complete blood count, blood chemical screen, and urinalysis. Blood smears should be carefully evaluated for the presence of pathogenic organisms. Other diagnostic tests include the presence of autoagglutination that cannot be dispersed by the addition of physiologic saline at a 1:1 ratio, direct and indirect Coombs' tests, lupus erythematosus cell test, and antinuclear antibody test. A bone marrow examination is indicated if the anemia is nonregenerative. The prognosis of animals with AIHA is guarded, especially in cases complicated by other diseases; animals with the intravascular form of AIHA have generally a poor prognosis.

Standard Therapy

The treatment of AIHA is directed against red blood cell destruction and formation of autoantibodies. Intensive supportive care is important especially in patients with severe anemia of rapid onset. However, supportive therapy consisting of vitamin supplementation and adequate nutrition to aid in increased erythropoiesis should accompany any treatment. Usually AIHA is treated with glucocorticoids, however in severe cases of intravascular hemolysis or in cases in which glucocorticoids have not led to a response within the first 7 days of treatment, a more potent immunosuppressive agent is indicated in addition to glucocorticoids. As in all immune-mediated diseases, therapy must be administered over a long time period and in some cases may be lifelong. The prognosis is guarded, especially in severe cases and when the AIHA is associated with other disease processes.

Transfusion Therapy. Only animals with acute life-threatening anemias should be transfused, because the patient's antibodies may rapidly destroy the transfused red blood cells and aggravate the clinical condition of the patient. Cross-matched blood should be used, and the animal should receive dexamethasone (Decadron, Merck Sharp and Dohme; and others) intravenously at 0.5–1.0 mg/kg prior to transfusion. In general, patients with a PCV of more than 20% should not receive a blood transfusion, and frequently it is not necessary to transfuse blood until the PCV reaches 12%.

Fresh or stored blood or packed cells can be used in the treatment regimen. Only fresh blood, however, should be administered in cases with severe concomitant thrombocytopenia.

The goal of the blood transfusion is to raise the PCV to safe but not to normal levels. (For more details on blood transfusions, see pages 149–154.)

Immunosuppressive Therapy. *Glucocorticoids.* Glucocorticoids are the most frequently used drugs for the treatment of AIHA. They have immuno-suppressive and anti-inflammatory properties; and although they do not appear to decrease antibody production, they inhibit the function of leukocytes that are involved in the destruction and phagocytosis of red blood cells. Usually either prednisolone or prednisone is used for initial and maintenance (alternate-day) treatment. If dexamethasone is used initially, the therapy must be changed to a shorter-acting steroid such as prednisone or prednisolone for alternate-day treatment. The animal's hematocrit should be monitored once daily during the initial treatment period and at weekly intervals once the hematocrit is stable. Common side effects of high doses of glucocorticoids are polyuria and polydipsia, polyphagia, lethargy, weakness, elevation of liver enzymes, glucose intolerance, and poor wound healing.

The treatment regimen comprises prednisone or prednisolone (Prednisone or Prednisolone Tablets, Roxane), administered twice daily at a dose of 1.1–3.3 mg/kg PO until the PCV stabilizes in the low normal range. Frequently dexamethasone is given once initially at a dose of 0.5–1.0 mg/kg IV, and the therapy is then continued with prednisone or prednisolone (1.1–3.3 mg/kg PO twice daily). The dosage of prednisone or prednisolone is tapered over several weeks once the PCV is stable until a dose of 1.1 mg/kg is reached. The animal is kept on this dose on an alternate-day regimen for several weeks. Usually, AIHA is treated for 2–3 months before the animal is taken off the medication. However, in some animals, therapy is lifelong.

Cyclophosphamide. In some animals glucocorticoids do not lead to the desired response, and more potent immunosuppressive agents must be added to the therapy. In some cases the side effects of glucocorticoids become prohibitive, and glucocorticoids may have to be discontinued. With severe cases of AIHA, especially those with intravascular hemolysis, it is advantageous to initiate therapy with a combination of cyclophosphamide and glucocorticoid. Cyclophosphamide is an alkylating agent that inactivates DNA and prevents cell proliferation. Conversion in the liver activates this compound. It is carcinogenic and requires extreme care when handled (e.g., disposable gloves should be worn during administration of the drug). Cyclophosphamide has been implicated in the development of transitional cell carcinoma in the dog even after a short treatment period. Patients should be monitored weekly for signs of bone marrow suppression, and the drug should be discontinued when the leukocyte count decreases to less than 5000/μl.

It is important to maintain adequate hydration in animals on this drug, as dehydration seems to enhance its toxicity. Long-term cyclophosphamide treatment (over 4 months) may lead to sterile hemorrhagic cystitis. In this case, the drug should be discontinued and the cystitis should be treated with fluid therapy to induce a diuresis. While the dog is in the hospital normal saline can be administered intravenously at two to three times the maintenance dosage (which is 40–60 ml/kg/day). The owner should be instructed to add table salt to the food at home to increase the animal's water intake. Frequently, clinicians administer ampicillin (50 mg/kg in three divided doses per day) prophylactically to prevent a secondary infection of the bladder. Depending on the severity of the cystitis, it may take several weeks before it resolves. The instillation of a 1% formalin solution into the bladder has also been recommended, although this treatment regimen may lead to serious complications such as bladder fibrosis and even death.

The treatment regimen comprises cyclophosphamide (Cytoxan, Mead Johnson Pharmaceuticals), which may be administered along with glucocorticoids or by itself in cases of resistance or unacceptable side effects to steroids. The drug is administered once daily for 4 days of each week, and this regimen is continued until the red blood cell count has increased to low normal and is stable. The dose of cyclophosphamide varies with the size of the animal:

1.5 mg/kg for dogs >25 kg
2.0 mg/kg for dogs 5–25 kg
2.5 mg/kg for dogs <5 kg

Cyclophosphamide can be given orally with food or administered intravenously. When cyclophosphamide is administered in conjunction with prednisone or prednisolone (1.1 mg/kg PO daily in two divided doses), it is discontinued as soon as the hematocrit reaches low normal values; the glucocorticoid preparation is continued for several weeks, after which the dose is tapered as outlined above.

Splenectomy. Splenectomy may be of value in cases of AIHA that are unresponsive to conventional therapy. In cases mediated by the IgG class of antibodies, the spleen acts as the major site for removal of erythrocytes, and the liver functions as a coarse filter and leads to removal of red blood cells in the presence of large antibody molecules such as IgM or antigen excess. Removal of the spleen therefore may be indicated in patients with splenomegaly or in those with IgG-mediated extravascular hemolysis. Patients undergoing splenectomy should be carefully screened for pathogenic organisms such as *Haemobartonella* or *Babesia*. *Haemobartonella* can be treated with a 3-week course of oxytetracyclines (Terramycin, Pfipharmecs) 20 mg/kg PO twice daily if clinical signs of hemobartonellosis are present. This treatment does not eliminate the carrier state. *Babesia* can be treated with a single dose of imidocarb dipropionate (5 mg/kg SC or IM); however, this drug has not been approved for use in the United States.

Investigational Therapy

Plasmapheresis has been described as an adjunctive therapy for AIHA in the dog. It involves removal of plasma and replacement with fluid and whole blood. Anticoagulation is maintained with heparin. Frequently plasmapheresis is used in conjunction with immunoadsorption using *Staphylococcus*-purified protein A, which binds IgG and circulating immunocomplexes. In some cases of AIHA that did not respond to conventional therapy plasmapheresis was used in combination with low dose immunosuppressive therapy and was shown to lead to sustained remission. It has been associated with hypercoagulability and infection, complications that can be life-threatening. Plasmapheresis can be performed only at specialized centers that have the necessary equipment.

THROMBOCYTOPENIA

Thrombocytopenia is the most common cause of acquired bleeding disorders in the dog. Isolated thrombocytopenia is rare in the cat. The decrease in the number of platelets may be due to a decrease in the production by the bone marrow as it occurs associated with marrow toxicity (e.g., estrogen) or to marrow hypoplasia or aplasia. It may also be due to an increase in the consumption of platelets, which includes accelerated removal of platelets (seen in immune-mediated thrombocytopenia) or an increase in the sequestration of platelets (seen with splenomegaly). Frequently, the causes for thrombocytopenia cannot be found, and the condition is then called idiopathic thrombocytopenia (ITP). In the cat, thrombocytopenia is often secondary to FeLV infections. The clinical signs associated with thrombocytopenia vary with the severity of the condition, and hemorrhage is usually not seen until the platelet count decreases to less than 20,000/μl, assuming that there is no other concomitant coagulation problem and the animal has not received any nonsteroidal antiinflammatory drugs that interfere with platelet function.

A diagnosis is established after careful screening of the animal's coagulation system. Tests should include a complete blood count, a platelet count and assessment of platelet morphology, and careful examination of the blood for intracellular organisms, and evaluation of the intrinsic and extrinsic clotting system, fibrinogen concentration, and presence of fibrin degradation products. A bone marrow examination is valuable for assessing the thrombocytopenic animal. This procedure is usually not associated with severe bleeding. If immunomediated destruction of platelets is suspected, immunologic tests should be employed. They include antinuclear antibody determination, Coombs' test, platelet factor 3 test, rheumatoid factor determination, and an enzyme-linked immunosorbent assay for the detection of antiplatelet antibodies in the dog. In addition, bone marrow aspirate smears can be examined for the presence of antiplatelet antibodies associated with megakaryocytes. Serologic testing is indicated when rickettsial infections are suspected.

Standard Therapy

Treatment is directed toward control of bleeding and removal of the primary cause, e.g., withdrawal of a drug in drug-induced thrombocytopenia, removal of a tumor in disseminated intravascular coagulation, or appropriate treatment of a rickettsial disease. Frequently, this treatment leads to complete remission. However, if the cause cannot be determined (ITP) or removed, other measures have to be taken.

Transfusion Therapy. Transfusion therapy is indicated if the animal experiences life-threatening bleeding or needs to be prepared for emergency surgery. Whole blood, platelet-rich plasma, or platelet concentrates can be used. Platelet-rich plasma and platelet concentrates can be obtained from whole blood by centrifugation; they provide more platelets per unit volume than whole blood and may therefore be preferable in many thrombocytopenic conditions not associated with deficiencies of coagulation factors. However, they are not usually available in veterinary practice. (For details on transfusion therapy, see pages 149–154.)

The treatment regimen requires that only fresh (i.e., less than 12 hours old) whole blood or platelet preparations be used because the duration of platelet viability is short. Platelets are usually used unmatched in veterinary practice and survive only for a few hours in the circulation. The blood used for transfusion in the dog should be from DEA 1.1-, DEA 1.2-, and DEA 7-negative donors; but preferably, in the dog and cat, only matched blood should be transfused. The administration of whole blood in dogs and cats should not exceed 10 ml/kg/hr, and the animal should be watched for signs of transfusion reactions such as vomiting or urticaria. The goal of therapy is to raise the platelet count to 40,000–70,000/μl, a concentration that should be sufficient to prevent bleeding.

Immunosuppressive Therapy. *Glucocorticoids.* Glucocorticoids are used most frequently to suppress both the cells and the actions of the immune system. Glucocorticoids do not appear to decrease antibody production, but they decrease the functional capacity of monocytes and macrophages and stimulate platelet production and release from megakaryocytes; these effects lead to an increase in the circulating platelet count. In addition, glucocorticoids directly affect capillary integrity, which in itself may lead to a reduction in petechial hemorrhage.

Only glucocorticoids whose side effects and efficacy are well documented should be used. They are administered at a high dose initially until the platelet count becomes normal; the dose is then slowly decreased, and the drug is eventually given on alternate days. Usually prednisone or prednisolone is used, as these drugs can also be given on alternate days. If dexamethasone is used initially, alternate-day therapy must be continued with a short-acting glucocorticoid. Therapy should not be discontinued until the animal has been in remission for 2–3 months. If no response to the glucocorticoid is seen within the first 5 days (i.e., the platelet count does not increase to concentrations >70,000/μl), the addition of another immunosuppressive agent to the gluco-corticoid regimen becomes necessary.

The course of ITP cannot be predicted, and it is therefore difficult to provide the owner with a prognosis. According to one study, complete recovery is unlikely when recurrence of thrombocytopenia is seen over periods of more than 8 months.

The treatment regimen comprises administration of 1.1–3.3 mg/kg of pred-nisolone or prednisone (Prednisolone or Prednisone Tablets, Roxane) PO twice daily until the platelet count is in the normal or low normal range. The dosage is then tapered slowly over several weeks until a daily dose of 1.1 mg/kg is reached. The animal is kept on alternate-day therapy for several weeks. Few side effects are encountered with this low dose alternate-day therapy, and it is rarely necessary to decrease the alternate-day therapy further.

Azathioprine. Azathioprine is a purine analogue that acts as an immuno-suppressive agent by inhibiting purine biosynthesis. This action leads to the incorporation of abnormal purine bases in DNA and RNA and inhibits the proliferation of lymphocytes. It also has anti-inflammatory effects similar to those of the glucocorticoids; i.e., it inhibits the function of mononuclear cells. Azathioprine is a carcinogen and has to be handled with care (e.g., disposable gloves should be worn during administration of the drug). It is usually given in addition to glucocorticoid therapy if the response to steroid therapy by itself is inadequate.

The treatment regimen comprises azathioprine (Imuran, Burroughs Well-come) given at 3 mg/kg PO once daily (with food) initially and then tapered to a maintenance dose of 1 mg/kg on alternate days when glucocorticoids are not administered according to the schedule outlined for glucocorticoid therapy. Azathioprine is given preferably on days when glucocorticoids are not admin-istered. The animal's platelet count should be monitored daily until it reaches safe levels (>70,000/μl) and remains stable.

Cyclophosphamide. Cyclophosphamide is described in detail on page 156.

For treatment of immune-mediated thrombocytopenia, cyclophosphamide is administered in addition to glucocorticoids. It is given with food to decrease gastrointestinal side effects. The drug is administered once daily for 4 days of each week. This regimen is continued until the platelet count increases sufficiently.

The dose of cyclophosphamide varies with the size of the animal:

1.5 mg/kg for dogs >25 kg
2.0 mg/kg for dogs 5–25 kg
2.5 mg/kg for dogs <5 kg

It is the opinion of many clinicians that azathioprine may be preferable to cyclophosphamide as additional treatment to glucocorticoids because of the more severe side effects of cyclophosphamide.

Vincristine. Vincristine inhibits microtubule formation in the mitotic spindle and leads to an arrest of cells in metaphase. Its immunosuppressive effect is less than that seen with either azathioprine or cyclophosphamide. It stimulates thrombocytosis by an unknown mechanism. Because this effect is based on adequate megakaryocyte number, vincristine is not indicated if a bone marrow examination reveals a decrease in the number of megakaryocytes. Vincristine is neurotoxic, and animals should be observed for weakness or other signs of neuropathy.

The treatment regimen for vincristine (Oncovin, Lilly) requires a dose of 0.02 mg/kg IV once weekly until the platelet count is satisfactory. Not more than six to eight injections should be given to an animal. Frequently, one or two treatments of vincristine are used in combination with glucocorticoid therapy, as outlined above.

Splenectomy. The spleen phagocytizes antibody-coated platelets and produces antiplatelet antibodies. Its removal from humans has been shown to have merit in patients who do not respond to conventional therapy or in those with recurrent problems. The efficacy of splenectomy in veterinary medicine, however, seems questionable. Whereas some clinicians believe that it aids in the treatment of immune-mediated thrombocytopenia, others find it to be of little value. If splenectomy is considered, a prophylactic 3-week treatment with oxytetracyclines (Terramycin, Pfipharmecs) 20 mg/kg PO twice daily against a possible infection with *Haemobartonella canis* has been suggested.

Investigational Therapy

IgG Infusion. Intravenous IgG infusion in association with splenectomy has been used in humans. The infused IgG occupies receptors for IgG in the reticuloendothelial system and allows IgG-coated platelets to pass through without being destroyed. This reaction has not been described in veterinary medicine.

Vincristine-Loaded Platelets. Vinca alkaloids bound to platelets in vitro can be used in vivo in thrombocytopenic animals that do not respond to conventional treatment. The complex between platelets and vincristine allows direct delivery of a large amount of vincristine to macrophages, which leads to impairment of their phagocytic function or even cell death. The efficacy of this treatment regimen needs to be evaluated in a larger number of animals.

SYSTEMIC LUPUS ERYTHEMATOSUS

Systemic lupus erythematosus (SLE) is a complex disease characterized by the production of a variety of autoantibodies directed against various cells or cell components. It is therefore not surprising that this disorder can manifest in many ways. Frequently, however, blood cells, skin, serosal surfaces, kidney, muscle, and synovium are affected, leading to anemia, thrombocytopenia, vasculitis, skin eruptions, glomerulonephritis, nonerosive arthritis, and muscle weakness.

SLE has been well described in the dog. Few cases resembling SLE have been described in the cat. If an immune-mediated disease is suspected, the patient must be carefully evaluated. A thorough physical examination should be followed by a complete blood count (CBC) including platelet count, biochemical blood analysis including creatinine phosphokinase, and urinalysis. Roentgenograms of joints may be normal or may indicate soft tissue swelling. Specific tests include an LE cell preparation and fluorescent antinuclear antibody test (FANA) to test for the presence of antinuclear antibodies in the serum. Negative tests results, however, do not exclude the diagnosis. If the CBC shows abnormalities a Coombs' test and platelet factor 3 test are indicated. Arthrocentesis and biopsies for histologic and immunofluorescence testing of skin, synovia, or kidney may also be indicated. It is difficult to make a diagnosis of SLE, and frequently the clinician arrives at a tentative diagnosis merely by ruling out many other disease processes.

Standard Therapy

Immunosuppressive Agents. Immunosuppressive therapy is used for the treatment of SLE. Therapy is long term and in some cases is lifelong. Usually the treatment consists in administration of glucocorticoids; more potent immunosuppressive agents are used for refractory cases or cases in which the side effects of glucocorticoids become prohibitive. However, it has been recommended that more potent immunosuppressive drugs be added initially in SLE cases with polysystemic involvement.

Glucocorticoids. Glucocorticoids are the drugs used most frequently for the treatment of SLE because they have immunosuppressive and anti-inflammatory properties.

The treatment regimen includes prednisone or prednisolone (Prednisone or Prednisolone Tablets, Roxane), which is administered twice daily at a dose of 1.1–3.3 mg/kg PO until remission occurs. Remission should not be based only on clinical impression; it should be substantiated by finding normalized parameters that were previously abnormal. The steroid dosage is then tapered over several weeks until it reaches 1.1 mg/kg. The animal is kept on this dose on an alternate-day regimen for several weeks. Usually SLE is treated for several months before the animal is taken off the medication. However, in some patients therapy is lifelong. (For details on glucocorticoid therapy, see page 156.)

Azathioprine. Azathioprine is a thiopurine metabolite that inhibits cell proliferation by substituting abnormal bases in DNA and RNA synthesis. It also has an anti-inflammatory effect similar to that of glucocorticoids. It is usually used in addition to glucocorticoids but can be used as an alternative to glucocorticoids.

The treatment regimen is as follows. Azathioprine (Imuran, Burroughs Wellcome) is initially given at a dosage of 3 mg/kg PO once daily (with food) in combination with glucocorticoid therapy, as outlined above. If clinical improvement is observed, azathioprine is tapered to a maintenance dose of 1 mg/kg given on alternate days, whereas glucocorticoids are administered daily for another 2 weeks. If the animal still shows improvement, the glucocorticoid dose can be tapered and eventually be given on alternate days (i.e., it is given on days when azathioprine is not given and vice versa). If the animal worsens on glucocorticoid therapy alone, azathioprine should be reinstituted at a dosage necessary to keep the pet in remission. (For details on azathioprine therapy, see page 160.)

Cyclophosphamide. In some animals glucocorticoids and azathioprine do not lead to the desired response, and more potent immunosuppressive agents such as cyclophosphamide have to be added to the therapy.

This treatment regimen is as follows. Cyclophosphamide (Cytoxan, Mead Johnson Pharmaceuticals) can be administered in addition to glucocorticoids and azathioprine, in addition to glucocorticoids alone, or by itself in cases of resistance or unacceptable side effects to steroids. Frequently, it is given in addition to glucocorticoids and azathioprine if no clinical remission is achieved. The drug is administered once daily for 4 days of each week until clinical remission is achieved. The cyclophosphamide dose is then reduced by one-half and continued for another 2 weeks. If the animal is still in remission, cyclophosphamide is discontinued and the animal is kept on slowly decreasing doses of azathioprine and glucocorticoids, which eventually are administered on alternate days (see above).

The initial dose of cyclophosphamide varies with the size of the animal:

1.5 mg/kg for dogs >25 kg
2.0 mg/kg for dogs 5–25 kg
2.5 mg/kg for dogs <5 kg

Cyclophosphamide can be given orally with food or administered intravenously. (For details on cyclophosphamide, see page 156.)

Chlorambucil. Chlorambucil is an alkylating agent similar to cyclophosphamide. It interferes with cell division by crosslinking the DNA of resting and dividing cells. It is a potent immunosuppressive agent. Its major side effect is bone marrow suppression; therefore CBCs should be evaluated every 1–2 weeks while the animal is on this therapy. It may also cause alopecia.

The treatment regimen is as follows. Chlorambucil (Leukeran, Burroughs Wellcome) is administered once daily at a dose of 2 mg/m^2 PO until remission is achieved. The drug is then given on an alternate-day basis. It can be alternated with glucocorticoids on consecutive days.

Investigational Therapy

Plasmapheresis has been described as adjunctive therapy for SLE in the dog. (For details, see page 158.)

POLYCYTHEMIA

Polycythemia occurs in the dog and cat and is characterized by an increase in the red blood cell count, hemoglobin concentration, and hematocrit. Polycythemia can be primary, a myeloproliferative disorder (polycythemia vera) or secondary, a decrease in tissue oxygenation (e.g., pulmonary or cardiac disorders), increased erythropoietin concentrations (e.g., renal carcinoma, renal lymphosarcoma), or increased adrenocortical steroid concentration. A relative polycythemia is seen with dehydration.

The diagnosis of primary or secondary polycythemia can be challenging and requires careful evaluation of the patient. In addition to a thorough physical examination, CBC, blood chemical profile with blood gas analysis, and urinalysis, roentgenographic studies are indicated to exclude pulmonary, cardiac, or renal abnormalities. Further cardiac workup including electrocardiogram and echocardiogram may be indicated. Polycythemia vera is usually diagnosed by exclusion of dehydration or disorders causing secondary polycythemia. It can be confirmed by direct determination of red blood cell mass and plasma volume using radioactive sodium chromium (^{51}Cr) and ^{125}I-labeled serum albumin. In addition, serum or urine erythropoietin concentrations can be measured by bioassay. Whereas the concentrations are elevated in secondary polycythemia, they are low or undetectable in polycythemia vera. A bone marrow examination is usually not diagnostic.

Standard Therapy

The treatment of polycythemia is directed toward the primary cause of an increased red blood cell mass; however, frequently lowering the hematocrit is indicated initially before a specific therapy is begun to decrease the risk of clotting abnormalities associated with the high red blood cell mass. Specific therapy for secondary polycythemia is not discussed as it varies greatly depending on the underlying cause. The goal of the treatment for polycythemia vera is to decrease the red blood cell mass to normal concentrations in order to alleviate clinical signs. The prognosis for this disorder is guarded.

Phlebotomy. The treatment regimen for polycythemia vera includes phlebotomy, which is a safe symptomatic treatment, but it must be employed frequently to relieve clinical signs. Blood is removed at a rate of 20 ml/kg to keep the hematocrit within normal limits. The removal of blood may be difficult because of its high viscosity in polycythemia. Removal should always be accompanied by infusion of corresponding amounts of fluids using an isosmotic electrolyte solution such as lactated Ringer's solution or Normosol R, otherwise the decreased blood volume may lead to cardiovascular problems and an increased risk of thrombosis. The phlebotomy is repeated as needed (usually once or twice per month) to keep the hematocrit at a high normal range.

Hydroxyurea. Hydroxyurea (Hydrea, Squibb) has been used successfully for some cases of polycythemia. It causes reversible bone marrow suppression and inhibits DNA but not RNA synthesis. The side effects reported in the dog include reversible pancytopenia, bone marrow hypoplasia or aplasia, anorexia, vomiting, sloughing of the nails, and arrest of spermatogenesis. Complete blood counts and platelet counts must be monitored at weekly or biweekly intervals.

The treatment regimen for hydroxyurea is a loading dose of 30 mg/kg/day PO is given in divided doses for 7–10 days followed by a daily maintenance dose of 15 mg/kg. It has been suggested that this form of treatment be used together with phlebotomy.

Other Immunosuppressive Agents. Uracil mustard, chlorambucil, melphalan, and cyclophosphamide have been used for the treatment of polycythemia vera in man. Treatment protocols for the use of these drugs have not been established in the dog.

Alternative Therapy

Radioactive phosphorus (^{32}P), which leads to a reduction of bone marrow precursor cells, is a treatment for polycythemia that can be used only at referral centers. It has been associated with varying degrees of success. Of the few cases reported, one dog survived for more than 4 years, but the survival time in the others was much shorter. Treatment with ^{32}P seems to be associated with a greater risk of developing acute leukemias in humans than if chemotherapy is employed, although the survival time with this treatment seems to be longer. Complete blood counts including platelet counts should be carefully monitored in patients on this treatment.

For the treatment regimen, the ^{32}P (New England Nuclear; Amersham) is injected intravenously at 77–96 megabequerels (MBq)/m^2 (37 MBq = 1 millicurie). The intervals between retreatment depend on the response of the patient. It has been suggested that ^{32}P treatment be used in association with phlebotomy.

COAGULOPATHIES

Hemostasis, the process that arrests bleeding from injured blood vessels, depends on the dynamic interaction of coagulation events involving the blood vessel wall, platelets, coagulation factors, and fibrinolytic factors. Abnormalities in any one of these factors may lead to bleeding. Usually the first event in the arrest of bleeding is the formation of a platelet plug (primary hemostasis); permanent hemostasis is achieved through endothelialization and organization of the platelet plug involving the incorporation of fibrin, phagocytosis, and fibrinolysis (secondary hemostasis). Increased bleeding may be caused by clotting factor deficiencies or platelet abnormalities. Inherited coagulopathies include deficiencies of factor IX, XII, and XIII in the dog and cat; deficiencies of factor VII, X, and XI and von Willebrand's disease have to date been reported only in the dog. Acquired disorders of coagulation may be due to vitamin K deficiency, liver disease, and disseminated intravascular coagulation. Specific tests employed commonly to detect abnormalities in blood coagulation include one-stage prothrombin time, partial thromboplastin time, activated coagulation time, and thrombin time. In addition, assays are available to measure fibrinogen, fibrinogen degradation products, von Willebrand's factor, and various other proteins (e.g., antithrombin III) necessary for coagulation.

Standard Therapy

Vitamin K Deficiency. Vitamin K promotes the synthesis of the coagulation factors II, VII, IX, and X in the liver possibly by acting as an essential cofactor for the synthesis of enzymes that activate precursors. Major sources for vitamin K are green vegetables (vitamin K_1); it is also synthesized by bacteria in the intestines (vitamin K_2). Vitamins K_1 and K_2 are lipid-soluble and absorbed via the lymphatics. Natural vitamin K deficiency may occur in animals on oral antibiotics or with malabsorption. Dietary deficiency of vitamin K is rare. An acquired vitamin K deficiency is seen with coumarin derivatives; they interfere with the ability of vitamin K to activate clotting factor precursors because of their similarity in structure and other properties. Coumarin derivative compounds are used clinically for the treatment of thrombosis, but it is their use as rodenticides that the veterinarian must deal with most often. Accidental poisoning with coumarin derivatives is a common cause of coagulopathy in pet animals. The first generation rodenticides such as warfarin and indandione have shorter half-lives than the second generation rodenticides (brodifacoum and bromadiolone) and are less toxic. It is therefore important to identify the rodenticide in order to determine the duration of treatment.

Treatment Regimen. The preferred vitamin K preparation used for treatment is vitamin K_1 (phytonadione; AquaMephyton, Mephyton, Merck Sharp

& Dohme; Konakion, Roche; Vet-A-K₁, Professional Veterinary Laboratories). It can be administered orally, subcutaneously, intramuscularly, or intravenously. Intravenous use is discouraged because anaphylaxis may occur; intramuscular use may lead to hematomas, which may go unnoticed. The synthetic preparation of vitamin K, vitamin K_3 (menadione), is not recommended for use in the bleeding patient because it must be metabolized to be effective therapeutically. It is no longer available for veterinary use.

Vitamin K_1 leads usually to improvement of clotting parameters within 12–24 hours. Recommendations for doses of vitamin K_1 vary. A loading dose of 3 mg/kg body weight (subcutaneously) is recommended initially, followed by a daily parenteral K_1 subcutaneous or oral dose of 1 mg/kg for the first week, 0.5 mg/kg daily during the second week, and 0.25 mg/kg during the third and fourth week. Alternatively, it has also been recommended to administer a dose of 2.5 mg/kg SC initially, followed by 0.3–0.8 mg/kg PO q8h for 7 days. In case of indandione poisoning or accidental ingestion of second generation rodenticides, a dose of 0.8–1.5 mg/kg q8h PO has been recommended. Usually therapy has to be continued for 1 week in the case of warfarin poisoning, whereas 1–2 months of therapy may be necessary in the case of long-acting rodenticides.

Therapy is successful if the coagulation parameters remain normal after discontinuation of the drug. They are best monitored 2 and 4 days after the drug was discontinued. The main complication of vitamin K therapy at high concentrations is Heinz body anemia.

Liver Disease. Multiple factors lead to hemostatic abnormalities in liver disease: diminished synthesis of proteins, which leads to low concentrations of clotting factors and other proteins involved in coagulation; activated fibrinolysis; and reduced hepatic clearance of fibrin degradation products and activated coagulation factors. In addition, reduced synthesis of bile acids may lead to reduced absorption of vitamin K. Hemostasis is further compromised through abnormalities in platelet function. Because the liver is involved not only in the synthesis of coagulation factors but also in their removal, it is obvious that not only a hemorrhagic but also a thrombotic diathesis may be seen. Bleeding usually does not occur until liver disease is severe.

Treatment Regimen. The bleeding animal should receive fresh whole blood if blood cells are needed in addition to coagulation factors; platelet-rich plasma is indicated in thrombocytopenic animals, and fresh-frozen plasma should be administered to the animal with deficiency in coagulation factors only. The administration of stored blood should be avoided because of its high ammonia content. As severe liver disease is accompanied by vitamin K deficiency, all animals with a prolonged prothrombin time should receive vitamin K_1 therapy. If an effect is not seen within 24 hours, a generalized decrease in the ability of the diseased liver to produce clotting factors should be suspected. (For details on blood transfusion therapy, see pages 149–152.)

Hereditary Coagulopathies. The hereditary coagulopathies are usually treated with the administration of fresh whole blood or fresh or fresh-frozen plasma as needed. (For details on blood transfusion therapy, see pages 149–152.)

Administration of thyroid hormone or administration of the vasopressin analogue, desmopressin to patients with von Willebrand's disease has been recommended by some clinicians because both seem to increase FVIIIR:Ag in dogs, although inconsistently. Before these treatment forms are widely used, controlled studies should be performed to document their efficacy in von Willebrand's disease. As with all inherited disorders, the clinician should strongly advise the client not to use the affected animal for breeding purposes.

Disseminated Intravascular Coagulopathy. Disseminated intravascular coagulopathy (DIC), also called consumption coagulopathy and defibrination syndrome, is one of the most common coagulopathies in veterinary medicine. It occurs secondary to many diseases. DIC, as the term states, is characterized by a thrombotic diathesis. As the condition progresses, however, coagulation factors and platelets are consumed faster than they are replenished. The additional activation of the fibrinolytic pathway makes the coagulopathy worse, and finally overt bleeding ensues. The prognosis of patients with severe DIC is generally poor.

Treatment Regimen. Treatment of patients with DIC remains controversial and consists in a wide spectrum ranging from administration of fresh whole blood to administration of the anticoagulant heparin. The clinician should assess the condition of the animal carefully before making a therapeutic decision. Most importantly, the clinician should try to remove the inciting cause and ensure adequate tissue perfusion. Several treatment regimens are described:

1. *Administration of a balanced electrolyte solution to maintain tissue perfusion.* The infusion rate should cover replacement needs.

   Deficit ml = body weight (kg) × % dehydration (expressed as
       fraction: 100% = 1) + maintenance needs (60 ml/kg/day)
   Electrolyte and acid-base abnormalities should also be corrected. (For details, see Chapter 1.)

2. *Administration of fresh whole blood to replenish blood cells and coagulation factors.* The animal who is bleeding severely should receive fresh whole blood to replenish red blood cells, platelets, and factors necessary for the coagulation process. (For details on blood transfusion, see pages 149–152.)

3. *Administration of fresh, fresh-frozen, or platelet-enriched plasma to replenish coagulation factors and platelets.* (For details, see pages 151–152.)

4. *Administration of heparin.* In humans, heparin seems to be effective as an anticoagulant when used prophylactically and in the early stages of DIC. Its use in veterinary medicine is controversial, and it seems that a major factor contributing to the efficacy of heparin is the time of administration. Because

heparin exerts its effect through activation of antithrombin III, its use is not indicated in those patients in which this protein has been depleted to concentrations below 40% of normal. Its use is also not indicated in the hemorrhaging patient who suffers from thrombocytopenia and depletion of coagulation factors, or in patients who have excessive levels of platelet antiheparin factor. As the measurement of some of these factors are unavailable to the general practitioner and even at referral centers, the necessary information for a successful treatment with heparin is rarely available. In general, it has been recommended to administer fresh whole blood to maintain the platelet count at more than 30,000/μl and the fibrinogen levels at more than 50 mg/dl before administering heparin. High and low dose treatment regimens have been described ranging from 10 to 100 units/kg SC q6h. Frequently the high dose is used, administering 100 units/kg SC in the dog and 50 units/kg SC in the cat every 6 hours. The goal of therapy is to prolong the activated clotting time to 1.5–2.5 times normal.

Investigational Therapy

Infusion of antithrombin III in combination with its activator heparin has been shown to be effective in human patients with DIC. Antithrombin III concentrates are not available in veterinary medicine, however. Alternatively, a combination of fresh plasma or fresh-frozen plasma and heparin may be indicated in animals with low antithrombin III concentrations (< 75%).

SUGGESTED READINGS

Anemia and Blood Transfusion Therapy

Authement JM, Wolfsheimer KJ, Catchings S: Canine blood component therapy: product preparation, storage, and administration. J Am Anim Hosp Assoc 1987; 23:483.

Cowgill LD, Feldman B, Levy J, James K: Efficacy of recombinant human erythropoietin for anemia in dogs and cats with renal failure. Proc 8th ACVIM Forum, Washington, DC, 1990;A81.

Feldman BF: Hypoproliferative anemias and anemias caused by ineffective erythropoiesis. Vet Clin North Am 1981;11:227.

Flaharty KK, Grimm AM, Vlasses PH: Epoietin: human recombinant erythropoietin. Clin Pharmacol 1989;8:769.

Hurst TS, Turrentine MA, Johnson GS: Evaluation of microwave-thawed canine plasma for transfusion. JAVMA 1987;190:863.

Pichler ME, Turnwald GH: Blood transfusion in the dog and cat. Part I. Physiology, collection, storage and indications for whole blood therapy. Comp Contin Educ 1985;7:64.

Pichler ME, Turnwald GH: Blood transfusion in dogs and cats. Part II. Administration, adverse effects, and component therapy. Comp Contin Educ 1985;7:115.

Weiss DJ, Armstrong PJ: Nonregenerative anemias in the dog. Comp Contin Educ 1984;
    6:452.

Autoimmune Hemolytic Anemia

Harvey JW: Canine hemolytic anemias. J Am Vet Med Assoc 1980;176:970.
Matus RE, Schrader LA, Leifer CE, et al: Plasmapheresis as adjuvant therapy for
    autoimmune hemolytic anemia. J Am Vet Med Assoc 1985;186:691.
Switzer JW, Jain NC: Autoimmune hemolytic anemia in dogs and cats. Vet Clin North
    Am 1981;11:405.
Werner LL: Coombs' positive anemias in the dog and cat. Comp Contin Educ 1980;2:96.

Thrombocytopenia

Davenport DJ, Breitschwerdt EB, Carakostas MC: Platelet disorders in the dog and cat.
    Part I. Physiology and pathogenesis. Comp Contin Educ 1982;4:762.
Davenport DJ, Breitschwerdt EB, Carakostas MC: Platelet disorders in the dog and cat.
    Part II. Diagnosis and management. Comp Contin Educ 1982;4:788.
Helfand SC, Jain NC: Vincristine-loaded platelet therapy for idiopathic thrombocytope-
    nia in a dog. J Am Vet Med Assoc 1984;185:224.
Rosenthal RC: Clinical applications of Vinca alkaloids. J Am Vet Med Assoc 1981;
    179:1084.
Thomason KJ, Feldman BF: Immune-mediated thrombocytopenia: diagnosis and treat-
    ment. Comp Contin Educ 1985;7:569.

Systemic Lupus Erythematosus

Grindem CB, Johnson KH: Systemic lupus erythematosus: literature review and report
    of 42 new cases. J Am Anim Hosp Assoc 1983;19:489.
Matus RE, Gordon BR, Leifer CE, et al: Plasmapheresis in five dogs with immune-
    mediated disease. J Am Vet Med Assoc 1985;187:595.
Werner LL, Gorman NT: Immune mediated disorders of cats. Vet Clin North Am 1984;
    14:1053.

Polycythemia

Bush BM, Fankhauser R: Polycythemia vera in a bitch. J Small Anim Pract 1972;13:75.
McGrath CJ: Polycythemia vera in dogs. J Am Vet Med Assoc 1974;164:1117.
Peterson ME, Randolph JF: Diagnosis of primary polycythemia and management with
    hydroxyurea. J Am Vet Med Assoc 1982;180:415.
Wasserman LR: The treatment of polycythemia. Semin Hematol 1976;13:57.

Coagulopathies

Fogh JM, Fogh IT: Inherited coagulation disorders. Vet Clin North Am 1988;18:231.
Green RA: Hematostasis and disorders of coagulation. Vet Clin North Am 1981;11:298.

Mount ME, Feldman BF: Vitamin K and its therapeutic importance. J Am Vet Med
     Assoc 1982;180:1354.
Ruehl W, Mills C, Feldman BF: Rational therapy in disseminated intravascular coag-
     ulation. J Am Vet Med Assoc 1982;181:76.
Slappendel RJ: Disseminated intravascular coagulation. Vet Clin North Am 1988;
     18:169.

CHAPTER SIX

Cardiovascular Disorders

Gilbert Jacobs and Clay Calvert

CONGESTIVE HEART FAILURE IN DOGS AND CATS

Congestive heart failure (CHF) is the state of abnormal circulatory congestion that results from excessive salt and water retention by the kidney when the heart is unable to pump an adequate supply of blood for the metabolic needs of the body. With circulatory congestion, increased transudation of fluid from the capillaries into interstitial spaces develops. In the case of left-sided CHF, increased transudation of fluid from the pulmonary capillaries results in pulmonary edema. Cough and respiratory distress may develop, and audible pulmonary crackles can be detected on physical examination. Pulmonary edema may also be detected by x-ray examination of the thorax. Right-sided CHF results in systemic venous congestion that may be detected on physical examination as ascites, hepatomegaly, and peripheral edema. Causes of CHF include congenital cardiac abnormalities, acquired valvular insufficiency, cardiomyopathies, and pericardial diseases.

Treatment of CHF in veterinary patients is usually aimed at relieving symptoms and making the patient comfortable rather than reversing or correcting the etiology because in many instances the etiology is unknown (e.g., dilated cardiomyopathy) or corrective procedures such as valve replacement surgery are not generally available in veterinary medicine. Thus the course of CHF is usually progressive.

Standard Therapy

Diuretics, positive inotropic agents, and vasodilators form the basis for drug treatment of CHF in dogs and cats. The general objectives of treatment are to: 1) relieve clinical signs such as cough and dyspnea; 2) improve the heart's pumping performance; 3) reduce the heart's workload; and 4) control excessive salt and water retention.

Strategies for treating CHF have seven basic components: 1) restrict physical activity; 2) restrict salt intake; 3) remove the underlying cause or precipitating factors; 4) institute general measures, such as increasing the inspired oxygen concentration; 5) decrease preload; 6) increase contractility; and 7) decrease afterload. The clinician must consider the individual patient when developing treatment strategy. Each of the components of treatment may not be used initially in each patient. Ordinarily, drug treatment of CHF is not begun until the first signs attributable to cardiomegaly or CHF develop. The general strategy is to use the simplest means and then progress to more aggressive or complicated measures if signs persist or recur.

1. *Restrict physical activity.* The importance of exercise restriction cannot be overemphasized. Exercise increases cardiac work while also increasing the metabolic demands of tissues. In patients with depressed cardiac function, exercise can precipitate congestion. Clients can help to enforce exercise restriction by walking patients on a leash. Walking should be limited to the extent the patient is walked only the amount necessary for daily urinary and bowel habits. In advanced cases, patients may need to be carried outside or up and down stairs.

2. *Restrict salt intake.* Renin-angiotensin-aldosterone system activity is heightened, which encourages the kidney to retain sodium and water in patients in CHF. Thus sodium and water excretion is impaired. High dietary sodium promotes water retention, which expands blood volume, in turn promoting congestion and edema. Restricting sodium in the diet may be accomplished by using prescription diets such as k/d or h/d (Hill's Pet Products). Homemade recipes may be used (Table 6-1).

3. *Remove underlying causes or precipitating factors.* Removal of the underlying cause is the most desirable approach, but regrettably it is often impossible in veterinary patients. There are some notable exceptions. For instance, certain congenital malformations can be corrected surgically with a high level of success, such as patent ductus arteriosus. Balloon valvuloplasty has been used successfully in dogs to treat pulmonic valve stenosis. Hyperthyroidism is a common cause of CHF in older cats (usually >9 years of age). Fortunately, several treatment modalities (antithyroid drugs, thyroidectomy, radioiodine treatment) have been employed successfully in cats to accomplish long-term resolution of hyperthyroidism. Taurine deficiency has been recognized as a cause of dilated cardiomyopathy in cats. Supplementation with taurine is generally associated with marked improvement or resolution of CHF. Most commercial cat foods have now been supplemented with taurine. A dose of taurine that has been recommended in cats with dilated cardiomyopathy associated with low plasma taurine concentrations is 250 to 500 mg PO q12h. Taurine is available in health food stores. Finally, CHF due to pericardial disease may be resolved temporarily or permanently by pericardiocentesis or pericardectomy.

Specific incidents such as infections or cardiac arrhythmias can exacerbate CHF. Early recognition, prompt treatment, and, whenever possible, prevention

TABLE 6-1. Recipes for Homemade Diets for Dogs and Cats with Cardiac Disease

Low-Sodium Diet for Dogs

¼ lb lean ground beef or fresh pork   2 cups cooked rice (no salt)
1 tbsp vegetable oil   2 tsp dicalcium phosphate

Braise meat, retaining fat. Add the remaining ingredients and mix. Yield: 1 lb (0.5 kg). Give a balanced supplement that fulfills the canine minimum daily requirement for all vitamins and trace minerals.

% Moisture	68	% Potassium (dry matter)	1.4
% Protein (dry matter)	20	% Sodium (dry matter)	0.05
% Fat (dry matter)	17	ME (kcal)	660/lb as fed

Restricted Mineral and Sodium Diet for Cats

1 lb regular ground beef, cooked   ¼ lb liver
1 cup cooked rice (no salt)   1 tsp vegetable oil or animal fat
1 tsp calcium carbonate

Combine all ingredients. Yield: 1¾ lb (0.8 kg). Give a balanced supplement that fulfills the feline minimum daily requirement for all vitamins and trace minerals.

% Moisture	64	% Potassium (dry matter)	0.56
% Protein (dry matter)	40	% Sodium (dry matter)	0.16
% Fat (dry matter)	39	ME (kcal)	940/lb as fed

ME, metabolizable energy.
From Lewis LD, Morris ML, Hand ML: Small Animal Clinical Nutrition III. Topeka: Mark Morris Associates, 1987; and Ralston SL: Dietary considerations in the treatment of heart failure. In: Kirk RW, ed. Current Veterinary Therapy X. Philadelphia: WB Saunders, 1989.

are critical to successful management of CHF. At high heart rates the heart must work more and thus consume more oxygen, yet the time available for coronary blood flow is diminished, which may decrease cardiac oxygen delivery. Thus the development of tachyarrhythmias tends to further impair cardiac function. However, antiarrhythmic treatment is not indicated for all cardiac arrhythmias that develop in patients with CHF. For instance, occasional single atrial or ventricular premature depolarizations may have little effect on cardiac function. Antiarrhythmic drugs can have a negative influence on the force of cardiac contraction, or they can have proarrhythmic effects, so their use must be justifiable (see the section on treatment of arrhythmias in this chapter).

4. *Institute general measures.* Increasing the inspired oxygen concentration is indicated in patients with acute pulmonary edema. It can be accomplished by inserting and securing a nasal cannula attached to a flow meter and oxygen source. A 5 to 8 French flexible rubber tube with multiple holes in the distal 2 cm of its length is used as a nasal catheter. The catheter is inserted into the nostril to the midnasal region, approximately at the level of the second premolar. The catheter is secured with suture, and oxygen is administered at

a flow rate of 100 to 200 ml/kg/min. Ventilation is impaired when the lungs are compressed by severe pleural effusion. Physical removal of pleural fluid by percutaneous thoracocentesis can provide relief of dyspnea and may be life-saving. Morphine sulfate (0.05–0.50 mg/kg of body weight IV or IM to effect) can be considered in dogs with acute, severe pulmonary edema. The narcotic action diminishes patient anxiety, decreases the work of breathing, and decreases central sympathetic nervous system activity resulting in venodilation (preload reduction). Morphine should not be used in cats.

5. *Decrease preload.* The term preload refers to the degree of filling of the cardiac ventricles with blood. Because of excessive salt and water retention by the kidney in CHF, cardiac preload is generally high, causing circulatory congestion. Thus, reducing preload diminishes pulmonary congestion and edema, which improves pulmonary gas exchange in the lung in the case of left-sided CHF, and relieves systemic venous congestion and ascites in right-sided CHF. Preload is determined to a large degree by intravascular fluid volume and systemic venous tone (venous capacity). Logically, preload reduction may be accomplished in two ways: by decreasing intravascular fluid (diuresis) or by shifting blood away from the heart and toward peripheral venous reservoirs such as skeletal muscle and splanchnic veins (venodilation). Overzealous preload reduction, using diuresis or venodilation, can lead to signs of low cardiac output (e.g., weakness, syncope, azotemia) because of an insufficient volume of blood available for the heart to pump.

Diuretics remain the cornerstone for the pharmacologic treatment of CHF. They produce relief of presenting signs more rapidly than other oral agents. Generally, diuretic therapy should not be withdrawn after signs of congestion have been relieved. However, diuretics alone are usually unable to maintain long-term control of CHF. Most diuretics act directly on the kidney to inhibit salt and water reabsorption. Furosemide (Lasix, Hoechst-Roussel; Disal, TechAmerica) is potent and probably the most commonly used diuretic in veterinary medicine. Furosemide is useful for severe pulmonary edema associated with acute CHF or in chronic CHF. For acute, severe pulmonary edema, furosemide can be administered at a dosage of 2–4 mg/kg IV or IM, although in cats the dose probably should not exceed 2 mg/kg. The peak effect occurs in about 30 minutes, and the duration of action is about 2 hours when administered intravenously. This dose may be repeated every 6–8 hours. Preferably, the lowest dose required to control clinical signs should be used. Furosemide is begun orally when severe clinical signs such as dyspnea have abated— usually within the first 24 hours of treatment. The oral dosage is generally 1–4 mg/kg twice a day in dogs and 1 mg/kg once or twice a day in cats. In patients with chronic CHF, mild respiratory distress associated with minimal pulmonary edema, or chronic cough due to left-sided cardiomegaly, intravenous furosemide is unnecessary, and treatment can be initiated with oral furosemide. Seemingly, toxicity associated with furosemide is low, but dehydration leading to prerenal azotemia, as well as metabolic alkalosis and electrolyte imbalance, particularly hypokalemia, can occur. Hypokalemia, in turn, promotes cardiac arrhythmias and increases susceptibility to digitalis intoxication. Ototoxicity has been described in humans, and this effect is synergistic with aminoglycoside antibiotics. Ototoxicity has not been recognized in dogs or cats, but reason dictates that concomitant use of furosemide and aminoglycoside antibiotics or other potentially ototoxic antibiotics should be avoided.

Occasionally, thiazide diuretics, such as chlorothiazide (Diuril, Merck Sharp & Dohme) at 12 to 25 mg/kg PO q12h, are useful in patients that become refractory to furosemide, but our experience has been that their utility is limited for the treatment of CHF. Thiazide diuretics are less potent than furosemide in inducing diuresis, and they are often ineffective when renal perfusion is impaired, as in patients with severe CHF. Similarly, potassium-sparing diuretics, such as triamterene (Dyrenium, SmithKline) at 1–2 mg/kg PO once or twice a day, are uncommonly used in veterinary medicine. They have only mild diuretic potency and are relatively ineffective for the treatment of CHF unless combined with furosemide or a thiazide diuretic. Potassium-sparing diuretics can be used in patients that become hypokalemic because of other diuretic agents.

Nitrates are the most notable and commonly used venodilators. Studies documenting benefit and establishing dosage have not been reported for dogs or cats. Nitroglycerine ointment (Nitrol, Adria) is available as a 2% formulation for cutaneous application for absorption into the systemic circulation. The ointment should be spread over an area relatively devoid of hair; usually we clip the hair over an area on the thoracic wall. Gloves should be worn by the person treating the patient to prevent inadvertent absorption. In humans, tolerance to nitroglycerine develops frequently, often after only 24 hours of treatment. Likewise, drug susceptibility usually returns within 24 hours of discontinuance. It is unknown whether tolerance occurs when using nitroglycerine in dogs or cats. We occasionally use nitroglycerine for the immediate treatment of acute severe pulmonary edema during the first 12 to 24 hours and rarely use it for chronic CHF. The dose that has been used in cats is a ⅛ to ¼ inch ribbon of ointment every 8 hours and 0.5–1.0 inch in dogs every 8 hours.

6. *Increase contractility.* Contractility and inotropy are synonymous terms that refer to the ability of the heart to generate force. Positive inotropic drugs increase the force of cardiac contraction, thus improving the heart's pumping performance. In turn, the circulation becomes less reliant on compensatory mechanisms, e.g., increased sympathetic nervous system and renin-angiotensin-aldosterone stimulation, to maintain organ perfusion. Anticipated benefits include increased salt and water excretion by the kidney (decreased preload), decreased heart rate, and decreased peripheral vasoconstriction, all of which reduce congestion and edema. Positive inotropic drugs may be categorized as 1) intravenously administered drugs for acute inotropic support, and 2) orally administered drugs for chronic inotropic support.

Intravenous inotropic drugs are indicated for short-term inotropic support of a patient with severe ventricular dysfunction. Evidence of CHF on the basis of physical examination (pulmonary crackles) and thoracic radiography (pulmonary edema) and signs of low cardiac output heart failure (weak femoral pulses, pale mucous membranes, syncope, weakness or collapse, hypothermia, cool extremities, and azotemia) in the same patient suggest severe ventricular dysfunction. The clinical settings in which intravenous inotropic drugs have a role include acute CHF, decompensated chronic CHF (from dilated cardiomyopathy or advanced chronic mitral valve insufficiency), and severe patent ductus arteriosus during anesthesia or immediately postoperative. Also, patients with transient, severe depression of ventricular function associated with anesthesia, after cardiac arrest, or severe metabolic disturbances (e.g., sepsis, ketoacidosis) may benefit from intravenous inotropic support. For instance, dogs with compensated moderately advanced mitral valve insufficiency may develop signs of ventricular dysfunction and CHF during a metabolic crisis such as diabetic ketoacidosis. In such patients, temporary intravenous inotropic support while treating the crisis can be lifesaving.

Intravenous Positive Inotropic Drugs. *Catecholamines.* The catecholamines are most commonly used to provide short-term positive inotropic support. Dobutamine (Dobutrex, Eli Lilly) is a synthetic catecholamine and a potent positive inotrope. The half-life of dobutamine is about 2–3 minutes, which means that it must be administered by continuous intravenous infusion. The dosage is 5.0–15.0 μg/kg/min. Dobutamine is available in 250 mg vials, and once it is added to an infusion solution it must be discarded within 24 hours. Five percent dextrose as the infusion solution to minimize sodium administration is recommended. Also, because patients are in CHF, the infusion volume must be minimized: 5–25 ml/hour depending on body size. As an example, 250 mg of dobutamine added to 500 ml of 5% dextrose results in a solution containing 500 μg of dobutamine/ml. An infusion rate of 10 μg/kg/min can be achieved using an infusion volume of 1.2 ml/kg/hr. The short half-life ensures that most of the administered dobutamine is metabolized or eliminated soon (10–12 minutes) after the infusion is discontinued, and major metabolites are pharmacologically inactive. This characteristic of dobutamine is advantageous if adverse side effects develop. In our experience, such side effects have been uncommon in the dog, and we have little experience with dobutamine in cats. Side effects are generally dose-related and include tachycardia, ventricular arrhythmias especially if they were present prior to dobutamine administration, restlessness, and tremors. Also, dobutamine can facilitate atrioventricular conduction, which accelerates the ventricular response to atrial fibrillation, causing serious tachycardia. Patients treated with dobutamine are maintained on continuous infusion for 24 hours. The infusion rate is then decreased by half for the next 24 hours before discontinuing it. There is evidence in humans that the pharmacologic response to dobutamine is blunted after 24–48 hours, so there is probably little advantage in continuing dobutamine for longer than 48 hours. However, patients receiving dobutamine because of decompensated CHF require long-term inotropic support, and so oral positive inotropic drugs, e.g., digoxin, are initiated during the first 24 hours of dobutamine infusion.

Dopamine (Intropin, American Critical Care; Dopastat, Parke-Davis) is a natural catecholamine and a precursor of norepinephrine. Dopamine is similar to dobutamine in that it has a rapid onset of action and a short half-life, and thus it must be administered by continuous intravenous infusion. The dosage is 2–5 µg/kg/min in dogs and cats for the positive inotropic effect. Unlike dobutamine, at higher dosages of dopamine (> 10 µg/kg/min) intense peripheral vasoconstriction develops that increases cardiac work and impairs tissue and organ perfusion. Potential adverse side effects are similar to those for dobutamine.

Digitalis Glycosides. Digitalis glycosides are available in intravenous form, but in our opinion use of digitalis intravenously for acute positive inotropic support is rarely preferred; dobutamine and dopamine are superior for that role. Administered intravenously, digitalis has mild inotropic effects. The hemodynamic response in humans is highly variable, and the dose required to achieve inotropic effects often elicits toxic manifestations. Furthermore, the half-life of digoxin (the most commonly used form of digitalis) is relatively long (8–12 hours) compared to other drugs used for acute inotropic support. Thus if toxic side effects develop, they persist longer than with other intravenous positive inotropic agents. Occasionally, intravenous digitalis is indicated in patients with CHF decompensated because of supraventricular tachyarrhythmias.

Orally Administered Positive Inotropic Drugs. Digitalis glycosides remain the principal class of drugs used chronically for improving the heart's pumping performance. The beneficial effects of digitalis are rather slow in onset; and thus for patients with severe signs, it should be used in combination with diuretics. Digoxin and digitoxin are the two clinically used digitalis glycosides in veterinary medicine, but digoxin is used more widely. Both drugs have a similar ability to induce a positive inotropic effect in heart failure, but digoxin has greater vagal activity, which makes it the preferable drug when atrial arrhythmias complicate CHF.

Before digitalis glycosides are administered to a patient several factors must be considered:

1. Body size. Because large dogs have a lower body surface area/body weight ratio they require proportionally less digoxin than small dogs. Also, digoxin does not distribute well into fat and so the dosage must be based on estimation of lean body mass, whereas digitoxin is lipid-soluble so the dosage is unchanged.
2. Renal function. Digoxin is eliminated primarily by the kidney. Thus if renal function is impaired, elimination of digoxin is reduced promoting a rise in serum concentrations and the likelihood of toxicity. If azotemia is mild (creatinine <2.5 mg/dl), particularly if the cause is prerenal and attributable to poor cardiac function, digoxin may be used but the dosage is

reduced. Formulae for decreasing the dosage based on serum creatinine concentration may be inaccurate because there appears to be little correlation between the degree of azotemia and serum digoxin concentration in the dog. Recognizing the limitations of using formulae, a guideline for adjusting dosage in patients with azotemia is to divide the dose by the serum creatinine value. For example, if the serum creatinine concentration is 2 mg/dl, the dose of digoxin should be divided by 2. Ideally, in patients with renal dysfunction, serum digoxin concentrations should be measured 3 days after starting treatment and then once a week for the first month. The therapeutic range of serum digoxin is approximately 1.0–2.0 ng/ml and for serum digitoxin it is 15–35 ng/ml. When azotemia is moderate or severe, especially if due to primary renal causes, digitoxin should be considered because it is metabolized by the liver.

3. Serum electrolyte concentrations. The dosage of digitalis should be reduced with hypokalemia; however, guidelines for calculating dosage reduction are not available. Instead, the cause of hypokalemia should be determined and corrected.

4. Thyroid function. The dosage of digitalis should be reduced in patients with hypothyroid or hyperthyroid conditions, but in either case normal thyroid levels should be restored. Recommendations for dosage adjustment have not been published for dogs or cats, but dosage may be reduced 10–20%. Serum digitalis concentrations should be determined as a guide to dosage adjustment.

5. Drug interactions. Quinidine (Quinaglute, Berlex) and calcium channel blockers, particularly verapamil (Isoptin, Knoll; Calan, Searle) tend to increase serum digitalis concentrations. These drugs should be avoided in patients receiving digitalis, or the digitalis dosage must be decreased. We usually decrease the dosage by 25% and then periodically measure serum digoxin concentrations as a guide for dosage adjustment.

Digoxin is available as 0.125 and 0.250 mg tablets (Lanoxin, Burroughs Wellcome), 0.05 mg/ml elixir (Lanoxin), and 0.15 mg/ml elixir (Cardoxin, Evsco). Digitoxin (Crystodigin, Eli Lilly) is available in capsules (0.05, 0.10, 0.15 mg). The bioavailability of digoxin varies according to the formulation (e.g., tablet versus elixir), and the dosage recommendations for dogs and cats should be adjusted accordingly. The choice of tablet versus elixir is based on patient size, ease of administration, and convenience. Seemingly, cats are more sensitive to digoxin than are dogs, and a lower dosage is recommended. Dosing cats with digoxin is generally more difficult than dogs because of their small size. They often salivate excessively when the elixir is administered. Digitoxin should not be administered to cats because the half-life is too long. Dosage guidelines are listed in Table 6-2. These guidelines do not preclude the clinician from individualizing treatment for each patient. The clinician must realize that dosage adjustment is often necessary during the course of treatment.

TABLE 6-2. Oral Dosage Guidelines for Digoxin and Digitoxin in Dogs and Cats

Drug	Dog	Cat
Digoxin		
Tablet	0.006–0.008 mg/kg q12h[a]	0.008 mg/kg q24h[b]
Elixir (0.05 mg/ml)	0.004–0.006 mg/kg q12h	0.002–0.004 mg/kg q12h
Digitoxin	0.03 mg/kg q12h to q8h	

[a]Dogs 70–90 lb: 0.25 mg tablet a.m., 0.125 mg p.m.; 90–110 lb: 0.25 mg q12h.
[b]Cats under 10 lb give one-fourth of 0.125 mg tablet every other day.
These dosages are guidelines. Serum digitalis concentrations should be monitored periodically.

The most common adverse side effects of digitalis are gastrointestinal, particularly anorexia and vomiting. Cardiac arrhythmias and conduction disturbances of any kind can also develop. Arrhythmias may be precipitated or exacerbated by electrolyte abnormalities, especially hypokalemia, as from overzealous diuretic treatment. When digitalis intoxication is suspected, the drug should be discontinued for at least 24–48 hours or until toxic side effects abate; the serum digitalis concentration should be measured for confirmation, and precipitating causes of digitalis intoxication, such as azotemia, electrolyte abnormalities, changes in body weight, and miscommunication with the owner about the dosing regimen, should be sought.

7. *Decrease afterload.* The term *afterload* refers to the resistance to ventricular ejection of blood imposed by the degree of peripheral arterial constriction also called systemic vascular resistance. With CHF, activation of the sympathetic nervous and renin-angiotensin-aldosterone systems induces arterial constriction impeding the pumping function of the heart and increasing the workload. Arterial vasodilators lower systemic vascular resistance promoting forward ejection of blood and reducing cardiac work. Drugs that act as arterial vasodilators have in common several potentially adverse side effects, including hypotension, reflex tachycardia, and increased fluid retention. Clinical signs of hypotension include weakness, syncope, collapse, tachycardia, azotemia, and cool extremities. Increased fluid retention is probably the result of offsetting compensatory mechanisms; hypotension induces reflex sympathetic nervous system stimulation and leads to renal hypoperfusion, which increases renin-angiotensin-aldosterone activation. Thus vasoconstriction and fluid retention are enhanced, offsetting the potential beneficial effects of vasodilation. Ideally, arterial blood pressure should be monitored in patients before and during vasodilator treatment.

We use the following method to initiate oral vasodilator therapy. The patient is hospitalized, baseline evaluations are performed (Table 6-3), a vasodilator is selected, and one-half of the calculated dose is administered. The

TABLE 6-3.   Evaluation of Vasodilator Therapy

Patient Evaluation	Desired Therapeutic Response	Signs of Hypotension
Heart rate	Decreased, no change, or increased by 10–30 bpm	Tachycardia
Arterial pulse pressure	Increased intensity	Weaker or thready
Capillary refill time	Decreased	Prolonged
Attitude	Still alert	Depressed, comatose
Exercise tolerance	Improved or maintained	Weak, ataxic, syncopal
Mean arterial blood pressure (measured)	Reduced by 10–30 mm Hg	Moderate to severe hypotension
Arterial pulse pressure (systolic-diastolic)	Increased	—
Serial venous PO_2	Increased from baseline	—
Venous congestion, pulmonary edema	Reduced congestion, less dyspnea	—

From Bonagura JD, Muir WW: Vasodilator therapy. In: Kirk RW, ed. Current Veterinary Therapy IX. Philadelphia: WB Saunders, 1986.

patient is evaluated for drug effects for the first 3 hours. If no significant adverse effects are observed, a full dose is given 8–12 hours later, and the patient is again observed for adverse side effects.

There is no documentation in dogs or cats that one vasodilator is preferable over another. Based on studies of efficacy in humans, hydralazine (Apresoline, Ciba) or captopril (Capoten, Squibb) have gained the widest acceptance and use by veterinary cardiologists. Evidence in humans that captopril may prolong life in patients with CHF could prompt veterinary cardiologists to choose angiotensin-converting enzyme inhibitors as first-line vasodilators for treating CHF. Prazocin (Minipress, Pfizer) has fallen out of favor as a vasodilator for treating CHF in humans because of the frequent development of tolerance and poor clinical response.

Hydralazine is available in 10, 25, and 50 mg tablets and the dosage is 0.5–1.5 mg/kg PO twice a day in both dogs and cats. It is a potent direct-acting arteriolar smooth muscle relaxant, and clinicians must be vigilant for signs of hypotension. The diuretic dosage sometimes has to be increased because the tendency for hypotension increases fluid retention. For small dogs (<5 kg) or cats, the liquid intravenous preparation (20 mg/ml) of hydralazine can be used orally. This method permits more accurate dosing in small animals and avoids recompounding tablet formulations.

Prazocin induces vasodilation by blocking α_1-adrenergic receptors. Because these receptors are on both venous and arteriolar smooth muscle, prazocin induces venodilation and arteriolar dilation ("balanced vasodilation"). Prazocin may exhibit "first-dose effect"; the first dose may cause pronounced hypotension attributed to sudden adrenergic blockade. Accordingly, the first dose should be a low, test dose (about one-half the calculated dose). Prazocin is available only in capsules, and thus dosing is often inconvenient in dogs and cats.

By inhibiting the enzyme that converts angiotensin I to angiotensin II, angiotensin-converting enzyme (ACE) inhibitors block renin-angiotensin-aldosterone activation. This effect reduces sodium and water retention by the kidney by decreasing plasma aldosterone concentration. Venodilation and arteriolar dilation are also induced because of decreased angiotensin II, a potent vasoconstrictor. In humans, there is evidence that ACE inhibitors may attenuate progressive ventricular enlargement and prolong life in patients with CHF. Traditionally, use of ACE inhibitors was reserved for late stages of CHF refractory to conventional therapy. This therapeutic approach to CHF must be reevaluated to consider the potential advantage of ACE inhibitors early in the disease process. Captopril is the most commonly used ACE inhibitor in veterinary medicine. The dosage in dogs and cats is 0.5–1.5 mg/kg of body weight PO three times a day. In addition to hypotension, gastrointestinal side effects such as anorexia and vomiting often occur. Captopril may have direct nephrotoxic effects, and renal failure has been reported in dogs associated with captopril administration; thus urinalysis, blood urea nitrogen (BUN), and serum creatinine should be monitored periodically. Enalapril (Vasotec, Merck Sharp & Dohme) is a newer generation ACE inhibitor that seems to have fewer gastrointestinal side effects and can be administered less frequently than captopril. We have used enalapril at a dosage of 0.25–0.50 mg/kg PO once or twice a day in dogs.

Clinical Application of Treatment Strategies. Successfully treating patients with CHF while inducing minimal adverse side effects is a science and an art. We discourage rigid adherence to any single treatment protocol. No one protocol suits the needs of all patients in CHF; treatment must be tailored to the special needs of individual patients. What is a clinician to do? We espouse several principles in our approach to drug treatment of CHF.

1. Stepwise drug treatment. Use the minimal number of drugs to control clinical signs. The clinician must be concerned and ever vigilant for adverse drug reactions. Furthermore, as more drugs are added to a treatment protocol, the opportunity for unpredictable drug interactions increases.
2. Monitor response to treatment. In veterinary patients acquisition of objective hemodynamic data is difficult in general practice. Fortunately, several easily obtained clinical parameters can be monitored to evaluate treatment response. Such parameters include clinical signs (dyspnea, cough), thoracic auscultation for pulmonary crackles, abdominal palpation for ascites, evaluation of jugular venous and femoral artery pulses, and thoracic radiography.

3. Therapeutic drug monitoring. For example, serum concentrations of digitalis glycosides should be routinely determined. Blood samples should be
obtained 8–10 hours after a dose is administered. Before concluding that
digitalis treatment is ineffective in a patient, we ensure that therapeutic
concentrations of digitalis have been achieved.

It is often difficult to know when and how to intervene with cardiac drugs.
Recognizing the frequent dichotomy between symptom state (functional
class) and hemodynamic data, we find it helpful when devising individual
treatment strategies to categorize patients into one of four functional heart
failure classes adapted from the New York Heart Association classification
scheme.

Class I: These patients have heart disease but no overt evidence of heart
failure (asymptomatic). They often have a murmur and either no or mild
cardiomegaly. Treatment with cardiac drugs is not required, but the
underlying cause should be treated if possible (i.e., heartworm infection).

Class II: These patients exhibit exercise intolerance or coughing attributable
to cardiac disease (or both). Moderate cardiomegaly without congestive
heart failure is often present. Exercise and dietary salt restriction, as well
as diuretic treatment, are recommended. Then, if clinical signs are not
controlled adequately, additional cardiac drugs, such as digitalis glycosides or vasodilators, may be necessary.

Class III: These patients have signs of heart failure during normal activity.
In left heart failure, cough is usually present and can be attributed to
severe cardiomegaly, causing compression of large airways or perihilar
pulmonary edema (or both). With right heart failure, jugular distention
and hepatomegaly are often detectable. Treatment includes exercise and
dietary salt restriction, diuretics, and either a positive inotrope or a
vasodilator. It is unclear in veterinary medicine whether a positive
inotrope, such as digitalis, or vasodilators are preferable at this stage of
heart failure. Traditionally, digitalis has been used. Because the ACE
inhibiting class of vasodilators have been demonstrated to attenuate
ventricular enlargement and improve survival in people with heart failure, many veterinary cardiologists recommend ACE inhibitors for patients in class III heart failure. It is our preference to use digoxin in
patients at this stage of heart failure, especially if there are signs of low
cardiac output (e.g., syncope, weakness, hypothermia, and weak arterial
pulses) or if sustained, clinically significant supraventricular tachyarrhythmia is present. Then, if a patient's clinical signs do not resolve
sufficiently, we add a vasodilator to the treatment protocol.

Class IV: These patients exhibit signs of heart failure at rest or with minimal
activity. Exercise and dietary salt restriction, diuretics, positive inotropes
and vasodilators are generally indicated. In accordance with our philos-
ophy of stepwise drug therapy, we initiate treatment with diuretics and

oral positive inotropic agents, establish therapeutic serum concentrations (in the case of digitalis), and then initiate vasodilator therapy. In selected cases the patient's clinical condition may be so severe that we initiate positive inotropic and vasodilator therapy at the same time. Vasodilator therapy may be contraindicated in patients with right-sided CHF associated with fixed pulmonary resistance due to heartworm disease. Also, in right-sided CHF due to pericardial effusion, cardiovascular drugs are contraindicated. Instead, efforts should be directed at relieving the effusion (pericardiocentesis or pericardectomy). In advanced or acute class IV patients, heart failure may be so severe that it constitutes a medical emergency. In these patients, intravenous positive inotropic treatment is indicated, especially if low cardiac output signs are present. Other appropriate treatments include oxygen therapy, thoracocentesis for hydrothorax, and abdominocentesis for ascites.

Investigational Therapy

Bumetanide (Bumex, Roche) is structurally similar to furosemide but is more potent on a body weight basis. Pharmacokinetic and pharmacodynamic effects are similar to those of furosemide. Occasionally, a beneficial therapeutic effect is observed in human patients unresponsive to furosemide treatment. We are unaware of its use in dogs or cats on a clinical basis.

Amrinone (Inocor, Winthrop) is a positive inotrope with pronounced vasodilator activity. Its mechanism of action is not fully elucidated, but the inotropic effect is believed due to inhibition of myocardial cyclic adenosine monophosphate (cAMP) phosphodiesterase activity, which increases cellular levels of cAMP. Amrinone should be administered by constant intravenous infusion (10–20 μg/kg/min in dogs) only under close monitoring because of its potentially hypotensive effect.

Milrinone was used successfully as an investigational oral positive inotropic drug for dogs with CHF. Milrinone may become available for clinical use in dogs. It appears to have some distinct advantages over digitalis glycosides. The onset of action after oral administration is about 30 minutes; its inotropic potency appears to be greater than that of digoxin, with a wider margin of safety between therapeutic and toxic concentrations. Milrinone produces peripheral vasodilation (decreased afterload), which may further improve cardiac performance but may cause hypotension and reflex tachycardia. Also, milrinone may be arrhythmogenic, particularly in dogs with preexisting arrhythmias. The dose of milrinone recommended during the investigational trial was 0.5–1.0 mg/kg PO two or three times a day.

Several other positive inotropic drugs are undergoing investigational use in humans. Ibopamine, pirbuterol, and prenalterol are orally active sympathomimetic amines. Ibopamine has hemodynamic characteristics similar to those of dopamine. A major obstacle in the development of any β-adrenergic agonist administered continuously for long periods is tolerance to the favorable hemo-dynamic effects, similar to that seen with dobutamine or dopamine. Enoximone and piroximone appear to act by inhibiting phosphodiesterase, similar to milrinone, but they have a different chemical structure. Efficacy and long-term safety have not been studied adequately.

In humans cardiac transplantation or biventricular replacement devices (total artificial heart) are considered in selected patients with refractory, end-stage CHF. These therapeutic options are not available or practical on a clinical basis in veterinary medicine.

INFECTIVE ENDOCARDITIS IN DOGS AND CATS

Infective endocarditis is an infection of the endocardium, usually involving the cardiac valves, particularly the aortic and mitral valve in dogs. Infective endocarditis is rare in cats. In dogs, infective endocarditis is virtually always bacterial in origin. The clinical manifestations of infective endocarditis may be related to four pathogenic mechanisms: damage to the involved valve(s) by the infective process inducing valvular incompetence; embolization of thrombi compromising organ function; metastatic infection from embolization of infective thrombi; and deposition of circulating immune complexes at various sites remote from the heart.

Definitive diagnosis presents a clinical challenge, requiring clinical signs, hemogram, and biochemical findings consistent with bacteremia as well as positive blood culture results. Echocardiography has assumed a prominent role in diagnosing bacterial endocarditis because bacteremia is not always present and blood culture results are not always positive in animals with bacterial endocarditis. The prognosis of dogs with bacterial endocarditis is usually poor, particularly if the aortic valve is involved. Because of the difficulty in diagnosis and resultant delay in treatment, valvular damage is often advanced, leading to congestive heart failure.

Standard Therapy

Therapy involves long-term, intensive treatment with antimicrobial drugs, preferably based on the results of antibiotic sensitivity tests from positive blood cultures. Many animals also require treatment of cardiac (congestive heart failure and arrhythmias) and extracardiac (renal insufficiency) sequelae.

The general objectives of treatment are to: 1) resolve bacteremia, if present; 2) eliminate extracardiac sources of infection; 3) prevent further valvular damage; 4) treat cardiac complications such as CHF or arrhythmias; and 5) treat extracardiac complications. Factors to be considered during treatment are choice and route of administration of antimicrobial drugs and the extent of cardiac and extracardiac complications, if present.

Antimicrobial Treatment. Ideally, the choice of antibiotics should be based on results of bacterial isolation from blood cultures and in vitro sensitivity testing. However, blood cultures are often negative because patients were not bacteremic at the time of sampling because special handling or culture techniques required to grow some organisms (e.g., anaerobic bacteria) were not used or because of previous antibiotic therapy. In some cases the acute and critical nature of the illness demands an immediate and aggressive response before the results of blood culture are received. In such instances, the choice of antibiotic(s) must be based on known antibiotic sensitivity patterns of bacteria most commonly isolated in cases of documented bacterial endocarditis. Bactericidal antibiotics should be used. According to Calvert, *Staphylococcus aureus, Escherichia coli,* and β-hemolytic streptococci account for 70–90% of the aerobic isolates in dogs with bacteremia. Antibiotic sensitivity patterns in bacteremic dogs show that most *S. aureus* isolates are sensitive to gentamicin and to cephalosporins, whereas β-hemolytic streptococci are often resistant to gentamicin but sensitive to ampicillin or cephalosporins. Most *E. coli* strains are sensitive to gentamicin, but many are resistant to ampicillin and cephalosporins. Accordingly, if bacterial culture results are negative or if results are not yet available in a patient with suspected life-threatening bacteremia, the combinations of ampicillin and gentamicin or cephalosporin are justifiable treatment options. Anaerobic bacteria are difficult to grow in culture, but fortunately most are sensitive to ampicillin.

Sometimes the organism responsible for bacterial endocarditis can be suspected by uncovering extravascular sources of bacterial infection. For example, infection of the urinary tract may serve as a source of bacteremia, or conversely urinary tract infection or bacteriuria can occur secondary to bacteremia. Thus the results of sensitivity testing of isolates of bacteria from the urine in patients with suspected bacterial endocarditis can direct the clinician's choice of antibiotics.

For suspected bacterial endocarditis, initial antibiotic treatment should be administered intravenously in order to achieve high serum antibiotic concentrations rapidly. The following dosages may be used intravenously: ampicillin or cephalothin 20–40 mg/kg q6–8h; gentamicin 2 mg/kg q8h. Hydration must be maintained and renal function monitored because cephalothin and gentamicin are potentially nephrotoxic. Nephrotoxicity of gentamicin is aggravated by hypokalemia, dehydration, fever, and established renal insufficiency. Some of the earliest signs of gentamicin nephrotoxicity are the observation of casts, hematuria, proteinuria, and impaired ability to concentrate urine. Thus urinalysis and serum creatinine concentration should be monitored approximately every third day in patients receiving gentamicin. Intravenous antibiotic treatment should continue for 5–10 days, if possible. Oral antibiotic treatment such as ampicillin 20 mg/kg q8h and cefaclor 20 mg/kg q8h may be initiated when the patient's clinical condition and leukocyte counts suggest that the infection is under control. Treatment must be continued for at least 6–8 weeks.

Blood specimens should be cultured approximately 7 days and then 1 month after oral antibiotic treatment is discontinued.

Treatment of Cardiac Complications. Emboli from the involved cardiac valve(s) may enter the coronary circulation and lead to microinfarctions or myocarditis. Cardiac arrhythmias are apt to develop under these circumstances. If arrhythmias are frequent and rapid, clinical signs may develop; and antiarrhythmic treatment is indicated (see Treatment of Cardiac Rhythm Disturbances). In some cases, cardiac valves are damaged such that valvular incompetence develops to a degree severe enough to cause CHF (see Treatment of Congestive Heart Failure in Dogs and Cats).

Treat Predisposing Conditions and Extracardiac Complications. Urinary tract or prostatic infections, pneumonia, pyodermas, oral infections, and use of glucocorticoids reportedly predispose to bacterial endocarditis. Therefore if extracardiac infections are detected, bacterial culture and sensitivity testing should be performed. The results may provide the clinician with a basis for choosing antimicrobial therapy if blood cultures fail to grow bacteria. In some instances surgical drainage is required to eliminate the source of infection (e.g., pulmonary or prostatic abscess).

Renal insufficiency requiring treatment (see Treatment of Renal Failure) may result from renal embolization and infarction. Clinicians might logically conclude that systemic anticoagulation is appropriate therapy in dogs with bacterial endocarditis, but it has not been shown to significantly diminish embolic complications. Also, unless carefully and intensively monitored, anticoagulation therapy may result in serious bleeding episodes. We do not routinely use anticoagulation therapy in patients with bacterial endocarditis.

Alternative Therapy

There is no legitimate alternative treatment strategy that precludes long-term antimicrobial therapy, preferably based on the results of blood cultures and sensitivity testing.

Investigational Therapy

In humans, valve replacement is a logical and practical intervention when irreparable valvular damage provokes progressive cardiomegaly and CHF. Valve replacement does not preclude the clinician from eliminating bacteremia and its source, if known, because prosthetic valves can also become "infected." Replacement of the aortic valve has been attempted by some specialized veterinary centers on a clinical basis in dogs. This therapeutic option is not widely available in veterinary medicine, and series of clinical successes have not been reported.

TABLE 6-4. General Classification of Cardiac Rhythm Disturbances

Tachyarrhythmias	Bradyarrhythmias
Supraventricular	Sinus bradycardia
Atrial fibrillation	Sinoatrial arrest
Atrial tachycardia	Atrioventricular block
Atrial extrasystoles	First degree
Others	Second degree
Ventricular	Simple
Ventricular tachycardia	Advanced
Ventricular extrasystoles	Complete (third degree)
Others	Others

CARDIAC RHYTHM DISTURBANCES

To determine whether a cardiac rhythm disturbance requires therapy and what that therapy should be, the following questions must be answered:

1. What is the cardiac rhythm disturbance?
2. What is the underlying cause of the cardiac rhythm disturbance?
3. Is the cardiac rhythm disturbance benign, potentially life-threatening or life-threatening?

The first question can be answered only by an accurate electrocardiographic (ECG) assessment. It is usually accomplished by performing one or more static ECGs, by continuous ECG monitoring in an intensive care unit or during surgery, or by long-term ambulatory ECG (Holter) recording. An abbreviated classification of cardiac rhythm disturbance is presented in Table 6-4.

The underlying cause of a cardiac rhythm disturbance may be determinable by analyzing the minimum database. The minimum database should usually include an ECG, CBC, serum biochemistry profile, and urinalysis. Frequently an extended database is indicated that variably includes thoracic radiographs, echocardiographs, abdominal radiographs, blood culture results, and other special test results. The causes of cardiac rhythm disturbances are extensive and often indeterminable. Nonetheless, a search should always be made to identify underlying diseases, disorders, or drugs that could initiate or aggravate cardiac rhythm disturbances.

All cardiac rhythm disturbances should be classified as either benign, potentially life-threatening, or life-threatening. Life-threatening and potentially life-threatening cardiac rhythm disturbances are primarily restricted to complete heart block (atrioventricular block) and some ventricular tachyarrhythmias. Most cardiac rhythm disturbances are benign. Potentially life-threatening and life-threatening cardiac rhythm disturbances are complex ventricular tachyarrhythmias that are associated with dilated cardiomyopathy and subaortic stenosis. Life-threatening arrhythmias are those associated with

TABLE 6-5. Cardiac Rhythm Disturbances for Which Medical Treatment Is Indicated

Tachyarrhythmias	*Bradyarrhythmias*
Supraventricular	Symptomatic sinus bradycardia
Atrial fibrillation	Symptomatic sinoatrial arrest
Symptomatic paroxysmal atrial	Advanced second degree AV block
tachycardia	Complete AV block
Sustained atrial tachycardia	
Ventricular	
Life-threatening or potentially	
life-threatening ventricular	
tachyarrhythmias	

a prior cardiac arrest. Rapid ventricular tachycardias (> 300/minute) resulting in syncope should probably be classified as life-threatening. Atrial fibrillation and supraventricular tachycardia in patients with overt or incipient congestive heart failure may be life-threatening in that they can reduce the cardiac output significantly, thereby increasing the severity of heart failure. Most cardiac rhythm disturbances do not require treatment. Cardiac rhythm disturbances for which treatment is indicated are those associated with heart rates that are profoundly abnormal or that could result in sudden cardiac death (Table 6-5).

The classification of cardiac rhythm disturbances as life-threatening most often refers to the risk of sudden cardiac death. Most cardiac rhythm disturbances that are associated with a significant risk of sudden cardiac death are characterized by myocardial disease and impaired left-ventricular systolic function or left-ventricular outflow obstruction; they occur in dogs with dilated cardiomyopathy, especially Doberman pinschers and boxers, and in dogs with congenital subaortic stenosis. Complex ventricular tachyarrhythmias (pairs or runs of ventricular extrasystoles or ventricular tachycardia) are present in patients at increased risk of sudden cardiac death and lead to ventricular fibrillation. Syncope or prior cardiac arrest due to ventricular tachyarrhythmia dictates that the cardiac rhythm disturbance be classified as life-threatening.

Supraventricular Tachyarrhythmias

The goals of therapy vary with the type of arrhythmia. The treatment of supraventricular tachyarrhythmias involves antiarrhythmic therapy and therapy of congestive heart failure if present (see section on therapy of congestive heart failure). Drug treatment of atrial fibrillation, sustained supraventricular tachycardia, and symptomatic paroxysmal atrial tachycardia largely hinges on the underlying etiology or left-ventricular function (or both) (Table 6-6).

TABLE 6-6. Treatment of Atrial Fibrillation and Atrial Tachycardia

Cardiac Function	Arrhythmia	Treatment[a]
Poor[b]	Atrial fibrillation	Digoxin
		Digoxin *plus*
		Diltiazem *or*
		Propranolol
	Atrial tachycardia	Digoxin
Good[c]	Atrial tachycardia	Propranolol *or*
		Diltiazem *or*
		Digoxin

[a]Drug treatments listed in order of preference.
[b]Congestive heart failure present or imminent.
[c]Congestive heart failure absent and not imminent.

Atrial Fibrillation. Atrial fibrillation is always treated. The therapeutic goals are to:

1. Reduce the ventricular response rate to less than 160/minute.
2. Maintain or improve cardiac output if congestive heart failure is present.
3. Maintain or improve systemic arterial blood pressure.

Standard Therapy. Almost all patients with atrial fibrillation have serious underlying heart disease and frequently have significant ventricular dysfunction. Digoxin (Lanoxin, Burroughs Wellcome; Cardoxin, Evsco) is the treatment of choice for almost all dogs with atrial fibrillation (see Table 6-1 for dosage recommendations). Digoxin increases the vagal influence on the atrioventricular (AV) node, thus reducing conductivity and ventricular response rate.

The usual goal of adequate digitalization is to reduce the ventricular rate to less than approximately 160/minute in the hospital setting and less than 130/minute in the home environment during quiet activity. Adequate digitalization requires 3–7 days depending on the method employed. Most often, slow, oral digitalization is recommended; and approximately 7 days are required for steady-state serum concentrations to be achieved. Heart rates below 160/minute are usually not achieved in the hospital setting owing to inadequate digitalization or increased AV nodal conductivity resulting from elevated sympathetic activity. Elevated sympathetic tone is inherent in patients with overt congestive heart failure and is further enhanced by the stress and anxiety associated with the hospital environment and restraint for the ECG. However, in the home environment heart rates consistently below 160/minute can frequently be accomplished with adequate digitalization. Determination of serum digoxin levels are recommended to confirm proper dosage, as there is considerable interpatient variation in dosage and tolerated serum digoxin concentrations.

Therapeutic serum concentrations of digoxin are achieved after 2–5 days without a loading dose. To achieve therapeutic serum concentrations more rapidly, the patient's daily maintenance dosage (for dogs weighing more than 15 kg: 0.01 mg/kg daily, divided into two fractions; for smaller dogs: 0.02 mg/kg daily divided into two fractions) can be estimated and administered at 8-hour intervals for three doses followed by the maintenance schedule initiated 8–12 hours later. Rapid oral loading digitalization is not recommended because of the increased risk of toxicity and the lack of demonstrated efficacy. Although exceptions are occasionally made, intravenous digitalization is usually not recommended because those patients that potentially would benefit most from rapid reduction of heart rate are also most susceptible to the associated adverse effects of rapid digitalization, such as increased afterload and myocardial toxicity. Digoxin toxicity is indicated by alterations in appetite, partial or complete anorexia, vomiting, lethargy, diarrhea, cardiac rhythm disturbances, and possibly by profound slowing of the ventricular response. Underdigitalization is more difficult to assess, and monitoring the serum concentrations is recommended. Digoxin assay results can usually be obtained from veterinary and human laboratories within 24 hours. Recommended concentrations are 1.0–2.0 ng/ml. A 4-hour post-pill sample should be 1.5–2.0 ng/ml, and a 12-hour or trough sample should be 1.0–1.5 ng/ml.

The postdigitalization heart rate is difficult to assess in the clinic or hospital environment in dogs with atrial fibrillation. Rates are falsely elevated owing to increased sympathetic activity contributed to by the stress and excitement of an unfamiliar environment and the restraint and anxiety associated with procurement of the ECG. However, in the home environment it is virtually impossible for the client to determine the heart rate. Ambulatory recording of the ECG is a practical method of monitoring heart rate ranges in the home environment. Ambulatory recorders can be obtained on request from Biomedical Systems (Atlanta, GA) and Roche Biomedical (Burlington, NC). The recorder and recording tape are returned to the respective company for analysis. Long-term ambulatory ECG (Holter) monitoring in the home environment reveals that many dogs with atrial fibrillation and appropriate serum digoxin concentrations have heart rates of 70–90/minute during sleep and 90–130/minute during quiet activity. Rates exceeding 160/minute are uncommon with moderate activity. Severe exertion is always discouraged in dogs with congestive heart failure. These same dogs usually have in-hospital heart rates of 180–210/minute during the period immediately preceding Holter recording.

If the ventricular rate in the home environment is often in excess of 160/minute and digoxin serum concentrations are within the recommended range, additional drug therapy may be warranted. This problem is almost exclusively encountered in dogs with advanced dilated cardiomyopathy. Such patients have severe ventricular dysfunction and rely heavily on sympathetic tone for the maintenance of cardiac output and systemic blood pressure; an elevated heart rate may be the primary means of maintaining adequate cardiac output.

Alternative Therapy. Although controversial, the addition of either a β-adrenergic or calcium channel blocking drug is often recommended. These drugs reduce the conductivity of the AV node and thus reduce the number of fibrillation impulses that penetrate to the ventricular conduction system. They have the potential, however, of reducing contractility and systemic arterial vascular tone. The authors' opinion is that these drugs are often prescribed inappropriately or unnecessarily for the purpose of heart rate control in atrial fibrillation.

Propranolol (Inderal, Ayerst) is a β-adrenergic blocking drug that may be cautiously added to the treatment regimen of large dogs at a dosage of 10 mg two or three times daily. The patient must be monitored closely for deleterious effects such as weakness, evidence of hypotension, and worsening heart failure. The dosage may be increased by 10 mg/dose increments at 2-day intervals if the heart rate does not decrease. Individual dosages exceeding 30 mg are seldom required or recommended. We have observed severe deterioration of cardiac function within 24 hours of Inderal treatment in a few dogs.

Alternatively, diltiazem (Cardizem, Marion Lab.) may be cautiously added to digoxin treatment at a dosage of 0.2–0.5 mg/kg three times daily. Although diltiazem may produce less of a negative inotropic effect than propranolol, we have observed precipitation or aggravation of heart failure when excessive dosages were prescribed. Some veterinary cardiologists have initiated digoxin and diltiazem therapy simultaneously in dogs with a ventricular response to atrial fibrillation exceeding 240/minute.

An attempt to convert atrial fibrillation to sinus rhythm is reasonable in patients with new-onset atrial fibrillation and in dogs without evidence of underlying heart disease (as is seen occasionally in Irish wolfhounds). The patient should receive quinidine (Quinaglute, Berlex) at an initial dosage of approximately 8 mg/kg three times daily. The dosage should be increased by 50% every other day until either the sinus rhythm is restored or toxicity (vomiting, anorexia, weakness, diarrhea) develops. If sinus rhythm is restored, chronic quinidine therapy is maintained indefinitely at the maintenance level of 8–18 mg/kg three times daily.

Quinidine therapy is often unsuccessful and may be followed by digoxin plus propranolol 1 mg/kg three times daily or digoxin plus diltiazem (Cardizem) 1 mg/kg three times daily. This therapy is also often unsuccessful.

Occasionally dogs with congestive heart failure or severe heart enlargement that are in atrial fibrillation convert when standard therapy is employed (digoxin or digoxin plus a blocking drug).

There are exceptions to the use of digoxin as the drug of choice for atrial fibrillation in the cat. Atrial fibrillation is often associated with hypertrophic cardiomyopathy. Propranolol (2.5–5.0 mg three times daily) or diltiazem (7.5–15.0 mg three times daily) sometimes effectively reduces the ventricular rate in affected cats. Although digoxin is also effective, digoxin toxicity commonly occurs in cats, and positive inotropes are not indicated for hypertrophic cardiomyopathy.

TABLE 6-7.   Treatment of Symptomatic Paroxysmal Atrial Tachycardia and
Sustained Supraventricular Tachycardia in Dogs

Step 1: Vagotonic treatment
  A. Physical treatment
      1. Ocular pressure
      2. Gag reflex
      3. Carotid sinus massage
      4. Ice water
  B. Pharmacologic: edrophonium (Tensilon, ICN Pharmaceuticals) 0.1–0.2 mg/kg IV

Step 2: Antiarrhythmic therapy
  A. Digoxin
  B. Calcium channel blocking drug: diltiazem (Cardizem, Marion Labs.) 1 mg/kg
      PO three times daily
  C. β-Adrenergic blocking drug: propranolol (Inderal, Ayerst) 1 mg/kg PO three
      times daily

Idiopathic atrial myocarditis occurs occasionally in cats and is characterized
by atrial fibrillation with normal cardiac size and contractility. Propranolol,
diltiazem, or digoxin (one-fourth of a 0.125 mg digoxin tablet every other day)
may be prescribed.

Supraventricular Tachycardia with Overt or Incipient Heart Failure.
Standard Therapy.   Supraventricular tachycardia is common in dogs and cats.
Regardless of the underlying etiology, the initial approach to symptomatic or
sustained supraventricular tachycardia is physical or pharmacologic vagotonic
treatment (Table 6-7). Acute paroxysms of reentrant supraventricular tachycardia are often terminated by vagal maneuvers because the sinus and AV
nodal tissues contain abundant autonomic innervation. Vagal maneuvers may
terminate reentrant supraventricular tachycardia that involves the sinus or AV
node as a part of the reentrant circuit. Initially, physical vagal maneuvers are
attempted. Recommended procedures are ocular compression, gag reflex,
carotid sinus massage, and emersion of the face in cold water.

Pharmacologic vagotonic therapy can be attempted if physical maneuvers
fail. Edrophonium (Tensilon, ICN Pharmaceuticals) is a very short-acting
parasympathomimetic agent that is administered at a dose of 0.1 mg/kg IV.
Although the duration of action is less than 5 minutes, this treatment may
break supraventricular tachycardia, and resultant sinus rhythm may persist for
minutes, hours, or days. Associated side effects are salivation, weakness, and
increased intestinal peristalsis.

Regardless of the success or failure of vagal maneuvers, medical therapy is
usually initiated. Precise medical treatment is largely dependent on the presence or absence of underlying systolic ventricular dysfunction and heart failure
(Table 6-6). Digoxin is the drug of choice for patients with overt or incipient
congestive heart failure (Table 6-2). Oral digoxin therapy requires 2–4 days to

achieve therapeutic concentrations, but many dogs with supraventricular tachycardia do not require intravenous digitalization. Concomitant afterload reduction, intranasal oxygen, and placing the dog at rest may result in spontaneous conversion to, or maintenance of, sinus rhythm in the congestive heart failure patient (see Therapy of Congestive Heart Failure). Inderal (0.2–0.5 mg/kg PO three times daily) or diltiazem (0.2–0.5 mg/kg PO three times daily) should be added to the treatment regimen only in refractory instances.

Alternative Therapy. For rapid effect when supraventricular tachycardia is believed to be precipitating or aggravating congestive heart failure, digoxin is given intravenously (0.01–0.02 mg/kg, digitalization dose). About 25–50% of the digitalization dose is administered at 1- to 2-hour intervals until completion or toxicity. Digoxin toxicity resulting from intravenous administration is indicated by worsening arrhythmia or the emergence of a new arrhythmia. Hemodynamically stable patients and those with paroxysmal atrial tachycardia (PAT) with syncope can be treated with oral digoxin (Table 6-2), but the onset of action takes 2 days or more.

Supraventricular Tachycardia Without Overt or Incipient Heart Failure. *Standard Therapy.* Supraventricular tachycardia in patients without overt or incipient heart failure may be treated with either a β-adrenergic or calcium channel blocking drug or digoxin. The advantages of drugs such as oral propranolol (1 mg/kg three times daily) and diltiazem (1 mg/kg three times daily) when compared to digoxin are their rapid onset of action and wide therapeutic index. Supraventricular tachycardia frequently resolves within hours after the initiation of a blocking agent. An initial loading dosage (2 mg/kg PO) is often recommended and frequently produces a normal rhythm within 4 hours. Two days or more are required for the onset of action of orally administered digoxin. In the authors' experience, sustained rapid (>300/minute) supraventricular tachycardia is usually seen in middle sized to large dogs with no evidence of organic heart disease. Sedentary dogs are asymptomatic, whereas normally active dogs have exercise intolerance.

Medical therapy is continued indefinitely in dogs with underlying primary heart disease and for variable periods when the arrhythmia is due to other etiologies.

Complications of Treatment. Risk of toxicity always exists when digoxin is employed. Digoxin toxicity occurs more commonly in association with concomitant diuretic therapy and total body potassium depletion. If digoxin toxicity is encountered, the drug is immediately withdrawn and withheld until the signs of toxicity abate, usually 1–2 days. When toxicity resolves, the treatment regimen is reevaluated, and if necessary digoxin is reintroduced at a dosage reduction of 20–25 percent.

Calcium and β-adrenoreceptor blocking drugs can precipitate or aggravate heart failure. Should it occur, the offending drug is withdrawn.

Arrhythmias Associated with Digitalis Intoxication. When supraventricular tachycardia develops in dogs receiving a digitalis glycoside, the drug should be withdrawn immediately. Atrial tachycardia, junctional tachycardia, and PAT with block may be associated with digitalis toxicity. Junctional tachycardia is the arrhythmia most commonly associated with digitalis toxicity, and atrial tachycardia with block is nearly pathognomonic for intoxication with this drug. Appropriate treatment is withdrawal of the digitalis glycoside, reevaluation of the need for the drug, and, if appropriate, reinstitution at a decreased dosage (75–80% of the previous dosage) after toxicity has resolved.

Ventricular Tachyarrhythmias

Standard Therapy. The treatment of ventricular tachyarrhythmias is often a perplexing problem. The clinician often wonders which patient to treat and what is appropriate therapy. In veterinary medicine, antiarrhythmic therapy should be reserved for patients at risk for sudden cardiac death. This subset of patients constitutes a minority of all patients with ventricular tachyarrhythmias.

The goals of the treatment for ventricular tachyarrhythmias are to prevent sudden cardiac death while preserving cardiac output and systemic arterial blood pressure. Toxic side effects, including proarrhythmic activity, should be avoided. Cardiomyopathic Doberman pinschers and boxers and dogs with congenital subaortic stenosis often have life-threatening ventricular tachyarrhythmias with minimal left ventricular systolic dysfunction, but all dogs with advanced cardiomyopathy have severe systolic and diastolic dysfunction; therefore the use of drugs that can reduce contractility may be dangerous.

It should be kept in mind that antiarrhythmic drug therapy leaves much to be desired.

1. There is no clinical evidence that chronic antiarrhythmic drug therapy prevents sudden cardiac death.
2. All antiarrhythmic drugs have proarrhythmic potential.
3. Adverse reactions to these drugs are common.
4. Cardiac function is impaired by some agents.
5. Accurate assessment of the efficacy of maintenance therapy usually requires Holter monitoring.
6. Accurate drug dosing is important and often requires the determination of serum drug concentrations.
7. Maintenance of therapeutic serum concentrations on a chronic basis is difficult with some drugs.

Antiarrhythmic Drugs. The pharmacologic effects of antiarrhythmic drugs are varied and complex. A commonly employed classification emphasizing the primary mechanism of drug action is shown in Table 6-8. There are many more drugs available than those listed in Table 6-8, but many of the drugs have not

TABLE 6-8. Antiarrhythmic Drugs Used in Dogs

Class and Subclass	Mechanism of Action	Drugs
Class I	Membrane stabilization. Depress the fast sodium influx (channels) during phase 0 of the action potential.	
A	Prolong the action potential duration (APD).	Procainamide, quinidine
B	Decrease the APD.	Lidocaine, tocainide
C	No effect on the APD.	Ineffective or untested in dogs
Class II	Antisympathetic action. Depress the slope of phase 4 of the action potential.	β-Adrenergic blocking drugs: propranolol, metoprolol, atenolol
Class III	Prolong the APD and refractory period without depressing the slope of phase 0 of the action potential.	Amiodarone, bretyllium
Class IV	Calcium channel blocking drugs. Inhibit calcium influx during phase 2 of the action potential.	Diltiazem, verapamil, nifedipine

been used clinically in dogs or cats, have very short half-lives in dogs, or are associated with untoward effects while offering little or no advantage over more commonly employed drugs.

For the treatment of ventricular tachyarrhythmias in dogs our primary interests lie with the class I drugs and primarily propranolol of the class II group (Table 6-8). Most class I drugs have not been investigated or used extensively in cats; and because of differences in hepatic metabolism, quinidine and procainamide are not recommended. Available formulations prevent the administration of oral dosages sufficiently low enough to avoid toxicity in cats. Although there are four antiarrhythmic drug classes, the class III drugs are rarely used, and the class IV drugs are seldom used for the treatment of ventricular tachyarrhythmias.

Drug Selection. The primary objective of the treatment of ventricular tachyarrhythmias is the prevention of sudden cardiac death. Effective treatment should eliminate syncopal episodes and complex ventricular tachyarrhythmias, especially ventricular tachycardia. If syncope occurs in treated dogs, the risk of sudden cardiac death is high. The logical choices of drugs to prevent sudden cardiac death would be those with antifibrillatory activity. Although unproved in dogs and cats in the clinical setting, drugs that may have antifibrillatory activity or that may raise the ventricular fibrillation threshold are the class IB, II, and III drugs (Table 6-8). Because class III drugs have not been investigated or have received little clinical attention in dogs, the drugs of choice are lidocaine, tocainide (Tonocard, Merck) and the β-adrenergic blocking drugs, primarily propranolol. With the possible exception of ventricular tachyarrhythmias associated with subaortic stenosis, where propranolol may be the drug of choice, the class I drugs are considered the "first line" antiarrhythmic agents in dogs. Propranolol (2.5–5.0 mg three times daily) is the drug of choice for ventricular tachyarrhythmias in cats that require maintenance therapy.

Immediately Life-Threatening Ventricular Tachyarrhythmias. In the face of sustained, wide complex, rapid ventricular tachycardia and severe complex ventricular trachyarrhythmias, intravenous therapy is indicated in dogs and cats (Table 6-9). Lidocaine is the drug of choice, although tocainide is also an effective drug in dogs. The onset of action of lidocaine is faster and its duration of action and time to steady state are shorter compared to tocainide. Lidocaine is given as one to several bolus injections, each administered over 1–2 minutes. After each bolus the heart rhythm is reevaluated. A cumulative dose of 8 mg/kg over a period of 20–30 minutes should not be exceeded. Effective bolus lidocaine therapy results in significant resolution of ventricular tachyarrhythmias, which is usually maintained for only several to 15 minutes. Bolus therapy should be immediately followed by the initiation of a constant rate infusion of lidocaine. Steady-state plasma concentration is not achieved for several hours. Increasing the dosage rate of lidocaine infusion during this period should be avoided in order to prevent toxicity from developing. Instead, intermittent boluses of 1.0 mg/kg should be administered as necessary. Unless there is evidence that the arrhythmia is transient, i.e., anesthesia related, maintenance therapy should be initiated as soon as possible employing a class I agent (Tables 6-8 and 6-9).

Constant-rate infusion of lidocaine must be maintained until therapeutic serum concentrations of an orally administered drug can be achieved and maintained throughout the dosing interval. Therapeutic serum concentrations are achieved and maintained within 16 hours with tocainide (Tonocard) and procainamide HCl (Pronestyl), and 24–48 hours after sustained-release procainamide (Procan SR). Effective maintenance control of ventricular tachyarrhythmias may be achieved more rapidly when procainamide HCl (6–8 mg/kg) is injected intramuscularly every 4 hours for two or three doses. Oral procainamide treatment is begun simultaneously, and lidocaine infusion is gradually withdrawn after 8 hours.

In addition to their efficacy, lidocaine and tocainide have less negative inotropic potential than quinidine and procainamide. Thus they are the drugs of choice for dogs with overt or incipient heart failure, particularly when heart failure is the result of dilated cardiomyopathy.

Lidocaine-Resistant Ventricular Tachyarrhythmias. Some ventricular tachyarrhythmias, particularly those associated with the early phases of boxer

TABLE 6-9. Commonly Used Antiarrhythmic Drugs and Recommended Dosages

Drug Names: Generic (Proprietary)	Drug Dosage and Route
Lidocaine	*Dogs* 2 mg/kg IV bolus over 1–2 minutes; may be repeated 2–3 times over 30 minutes. Do not exceed 8 mg/kg cumulative dosage over 30–45 minutes. *Dogs* 50 μg/kg/min IV constant-rate infusion (range 40–80 μg/kg/min). Requires 2–3 hours for steady state. *Cats* 0.25–0.50 mg/kg IV given over 5 minutes.
Tocainide (Tonocard, Merck)	*Dogs* 15–20 mg/kg q8h PO. 10 mg/kg IV bolus over several minutes.
Procainamide (Pronestyl, ER Squibb & Sons)	*Dogs* 10–12 mg/kg q6h PO. 5–10 mg/kg IV over 2–5 minutes. 20–50 μg/kg/min constant-rate infusion.
Procan SR (Parke-Davis)	15–17 mg/kg q8h PO.
Quinidine (Quinaglute, Berlex)	*Dogs* 8–18 mg/kg q8h PO.
Propranolol (Inderal, Ayerst[a,b])	*Dogs* 0.5–1.0 mg/kg q8h PO. *Cats* 2.5 mg (5–8 lb) to 5 mg (>8 lb), q8–12h

[a]Generic propranolol is not recommended for the treatment of ventricular tachyarrhythmia.
[b]Propranolol for the treatment of ventricular tachyarrhythmia is seldom indicated in small breed dogs.

and Doberman pinscher cardiomyopathy and idiopathic myocarditis in puppies, do not respond to lidocaine. Procainamide is the second drug of choice. It is given by slow, intravenous push while monitoring the heart rhythm (Table 6-9). Hypotension and bradycardia are important adverse effects of intravenous procainamide therapy. Intravenous procainamide treatment is followed by constant-rate infusion or intramuscular procainamide, which is continued for 1–2 days (Table 6-9). Maintenance oral therapy is begun as soon as possible after the efficacy of intravenous therapy is evidenced and simultaneously with intramuscular therapy.

Nonimmediately Life-Threatening Ventricular Tachyarrhythmias.
If a ventricular tachyarrhythmia is not immediately life-threatening, oral antiarrhythmic therapy can be initiated. Effective control of the arrhythmia

usually occurs within 1–2 days. Control is achieved more rapidly with tocainide, short-acting quinidine (quinidine SO_4), or procainamide HCl than with sustained-action drugs such as Procan SR and quinidine gluconate (Quinaglute, Berlex). A loading dose of tocainide (40 mg/kg) often suppresses the ventricular tachyarrhythmias within 8 hours. From 24 to 48 hours may be required for efficacy with sustained-action drugs such as Quinaglute and Procan SR. To establish therapeutic blood levels more rapidly, three or four doses of procainamide HCl can be injected intramuscular at a dosage of 6–8 mg/kg q3–4h. Oral therapy is initiated concomitantly.

The primary limitation to chronic tocainide therapy is cost, so procainamide or quinidine must be used in some instances. In the authors' experience, tocainide has been effective in the short-term (up to 3 months) control of ventricular tachyarrhythmias, including those in Doberman pinschers and boxers with cardiomyopathy. Sequential Holter recordings have confirmed a 75% quantitative reduction of ventricular extrasystoles with elimination of complex ventricular tachyarrhythmias in more than 80% of treated dogs. Long-term quantitative reduction of ventricular tachyarrhythmias is more difficult to achieve with all drugs.

The maintenance treatment of severe ventricular tachyarrhythmias in cats due to hypertrophic cardiomyopathy, hyperthyroidism, or etiologies other than dilated cardiomyopathy is propranolol (1 mg/kg PO three times daily). Cats with advanced dilated cardiomyopathy usually do not require therapy for associated ventricular tachyarrhythmias.

Combined Therapy. Class I and II drugs can be combined, as can theoretically, class IA and IB drugs (Table 6-8). Class II drugs are not recommended in patients with overt or incipient congestive heart failure. Holter recording analysis has shown that the combination of class IA and IB drugs offers little or no advantage over either subclass alone. Similar findings have been reported in humans. The combination of full dose class I and II drugs in Doberman pinschers with early cardiomyopathy has been more effective than the use of class I drugs alone. Inderal may be preferred over other β-adrenergic blocking drugs because assays for plasma concentrations are available, it has membrane stabilizing activity at high dosages, and generic products may not be dependable. The maintenance of therapeutic serum concentrations of chronically administered β-blocking drugs is difficult, and severe ventricular tachyarrhythmias may occur when drug concentrations deteriorate.

Duration of Therapy. Life-threatening ventricular tachyarrhythmias and potentially life-threatening ventricular tachyarrhythmias in Doberman pinschers and boxers persist for the life of the dog. Ventricular tachyarrhythmias associated with gastric torsion and blunt myocardial contusion persist for 3–7 days. Anesthesia-related ventricular tachyarrhythmias usually persist for hours to several days. Arrhythmias associated with polysystemic, metabolic, and neoplastic disease tend to persist until the underlying etiology is resolved and often for 1–3 weeks thereafter. Idiopathic ventricular tachyarrhythmias persist for variable periods (sometimes months to years). Antiarrhythmic therapy for ventricular tachyarrhythmias associated with gastric torsion should be continued for 10–14 days. Most dogs with ventricular tachyarrhythmias resulting from myocardial contusion do not require treatment; but if treatment is prescribed, it is seldom required beyond 5–7 days. Idiopathic ventricular tachyarrhythmias should be treated for a minimum of 3 weeks, and long-term treatment may be required. Dogs with advanced cardiomyopathy whose ventricular tachyarrhythmias require treatment need extended, possibly lifelong therapy.

Antiarrhythmic drug treatment should not be withdrawn abruptly but gradually over a 2- to 3-week period while monitoring for relapse. Gradual withdrawal can be accomplished by reducing the drug dosage by 25–50% every 3–5 days. Gradual drug withdrawal is probably unnecessary when treatment is given for only a few days.

Ventricular Tachyarrhythmias Associated with Digitalis Intoxication. When ventricular tachyarrhythmias occur in association with digitalis glycoside therapy, it is important to determine if the arrhythmia is likely the result of drug toxicity. This determination is often not obvious. Careful history and observation for signs associated with digitalis toxicity are important. The detection of heart block in sinus-driven complexes supports the diagnosis of toxicity. The measurement of plasma digoxin or digitoxin concentrations may be useful, but determinations usually require 1 day or more.

If digitalis toxicity is thought to be a likely cause of the ventricular tachyarrhythmias, drug administration should be stopped for 1–2 days and the indication and dosage schedule reevaluated. Withdrawal of digitalis results in spontaneous resolution of ventricular tachyarrhythmias in one to several days. Hypokalemia, if present, should be promptly corrected.

Potentially life-threatening ventricular tachyarrhythmias may be treated with lidocaine, β-adrenergic blocking drugs, or diphenylhydantoin (Dilantin, Parke-Davis). The latter drug has not been effective in the authors' hands.

Antiarrhythmic Drug Side Effects

1. *Lidocaine.* Repeated or high-dose bolus lidocaine treatment causes central nervous system (CNS) excitability characterized by tremors, muscle rigidity, decerebration, and seizures. Less commonly, constant-rate infusion at high dosages may cause seizures; more commonly it results in drowsiness, ataxia, weakness, and tremors. Nystagmus can be seen with either bolus or constant-rate confusion of lidocaine. Diazepam (Valium, Roche) 0.25–0.50 mg/kg IV is the treatment of choice for CNS excitability caused by lidocaine.

2. *Tocainide.* Anorexia is the most common side effect associated with oral therapy. Intravenous therapy can produce signs similar to those caused by lidocaine. The range of therapeutic serum concentrations of tocainide is 4–10 mg/L with 7–10 mg/L recommended. To maintain trough serum concentrations of 6–8 mg/L in dogs with good cardiac contractility, a dosage of 20 mg/kg three times daily is required. This dosage often produces peak serum

concentrations of 11–13 mg/L at 2 hours. Anorexia may occur at serum concentrations above 10–12 mg/L. Peak serum concentrations exceeding 12 mg/L may be associated with neurotoxicity, specifically head tremor or bobbing, weakness, and ataxia. Occasionally, anorexia, lethargy, and weakness occur in dogs with peak serum concentrations of 10 mg/L. Progressive corneal endothelial dystrophy, and polyuric hyposthenuric renal failure have occurred in a number of dogs.

3. *Procainamide.* Although uncommon, oral procainamide therapy may cause anorexia, nausea, and vomiting.

4. *Quinidine.* Side effects due to oral quinidine administration are more common than with procainamide. For this reason, procainamide is often prescribed in lieu of quinidine. Anorexia, nausea, vomiting, diarrhea, and lethargy are the principal signs of toxicity.

Impending toxicity to procainamide and quinidine is indicated by an increase of the QRS duration by approximately 25% above the pretreatment duration. Heart block is also a sign of overdosage. Antiarrhythmic drugs should be given with caution in the face of significant hyperkalemia. Efficacy is reduced and the risk of toxicity increased by hypokalemia.

5. *Propranolol.* Side effects caused by propranolol are uncommon. Lethargy and bronchoconstriction are seen occasionally. Propranolol reduces the hepatic clearance of some drugs, including itself. Propranolol is contraindicated in the face of AV block greater than first degree and is relatively contraindicated in patients with congestive heart failure.

Bradyarrhythmias

Standard Therapy. The goals of bradyarrhythmic treatment are to increase the heart rate to a level adequate for the maintenance of normal activity, eliminate heart block, or circumvent complete heart block through the implantation of a pacemaker.

Clinical signs associated with bradyarrhythmias are lethargy, episodic weakness or ataxia, syncope, or seizures. Behavioral changes may result from prolonged cerebral hypoxia. Persistent bradycardia manifests as lethargy, weakness, right-sided congestive heart failure, and occasionally prerenal azotemia. Symptomatic bradycardia in dogs is most often the result of complete heart block or sinoatrial arrest. Most dogs with bradycardias are asymptomatic, and treatment is seldom prescribed. With the exceptions of heart blocks, bradycardias are uncommon in cats with normokalemia.

Sinus Bradycardia. Sinus bradycardia seldom results in overt clinical signs, and therapy is infrequently recommended. Sinus bradycardia is usually seen in brachycephalic breeds and is usually the result of exaggerated vagal tone regardless of the breed.

The administration of atropine (0.04 mg/kg IV) eliminates vagal-induced bradycardia. The sinus rate should double and normal sinus rhythm or sinus tachycardia result. Transient accentuation of the bradycardia usually occurs after intravenous or subcutaneous atropine administration, and transient first or second degree heart block may develop. This effect results from a centrally mediated increase in vagal tone. Other atropine-responsive etiologies of sinus bradycardia include increased cerebrospinal fluid pressure, cervical or thoracic tumors, obstructive jaundice, and chronic or severe respiratory disorders.

If clinical signs are associated with sinus bradycardia, the etiology should be determined and the underlying cause eliminated if possible. Drug therapy is seldom required. However, if no correctable etiology can be discovered, the patient should be given an atropine test (0.04 mg/kg IV). If atropine abolishes the bradycardia, then chronic isopropamide (Darbid, SmithKline) administration at a dosage of 0.5–1.0 mg/kg two or three times daily or propantheline (Pro-Banthine, Searle) 0.5–1.0 mg/kg three times daily can be prescribed. Dosages of these drugs of 20–40 mg two to three times daily may be used for the occasional large dog requiring treatment. Dryness of the mouth, anorexia, urine retention, gastrointestinal disturbances, and constipation are side effects that may result from these drugs.

Sinoatrial Arrest. Sinoatrial arrest is also usually associated with increased vagal tone, most often physiologic in origin in small brachycephalic dogs. Therapy is seldom required in these circumstances, and the clinical approach to this arrhythmia is identical to that for sinus bradycardia.

The "sick sinus syndrome" is a common cardiac rhythm disturbance associated with bradyarrhythmias and episodic weakness or syncope in miniature schnauzers, mostly females. This syndrome is seen in middle-aged to old dogs and is associated with sinus bradycardia, sinoatrial arrest, failure of timely escape of subsidiary pacemakers, junctional escape beats and rhythms, and in some instances paroxysmal atrial tachycardia alternating with prolonged sinoatrial arrest (tachycardia-bradycardia syndrome). Mitral valvular insufficiency is often present, and congestive heart failure may develop secondary to valvular disease. A similar syndrome may be seen in dachshunds and a few other small breeds.

Bradycardia associated with the "sick sinus syndrome" may be atropine-responsive (0.04 mg/kg IV), so chronic medical therapy may be warranted in severely affected dogs. Although most affected dogs are intermittently symptomatic, therapy may not be required as the signs are episodic, often mild, and seldom life-threatening.

Severe manifestations of sinoatrial arrest that are not improved with parasympatholytic drugs are best treated by permanent artificial pacemaker implantation.

Atrioventricular (Heart) Block. Symptomatic heart block is often associated with myocardial fibrosis in middle-aged to older brachycephalic breeds and cocker spaniels. In many instances the etiology of the conduction disturbance is unknown. Heart block may be associated with cardiomyopathies of all types, hyperkalemia, digoxin toxicity, bacterial endocarditis, and chronic doxorubicin administration. Congenital complete heart block has been reported.

Advanced (high grade) second degree and complete (third degree) AV blocks require therapy. First degree and simple second degree AV blocks are often associated with increased vagal tone or drug therapy; they do not produce symptoms, and specific treatment is unnecessary.

The long-term management of most advanced heart blocks can be accomplished only via implantation of a permanent artificial pacemaker. Initially, atropine (0.04 mg/kg IV) should be administered in an attempt to improve conduction; it may improve advanced second degree block but rarely alters complete block. If atropine improves conduction, drugs such as isopropamide or propantheline are usually useful (see Sinus Bradycardia for dosages).

When practical, pacemaker implantation is the treatment of choice for complete heart block, even if medical therapy is effective. The long-term costs, the labor associated with daily multiple administrations of a drug, and drug toxicity render medical treatment less desirable. When pacemaker implantation is not feasible because of the cost, unavailability of the device, the dog is too old, or there are concomitant medical problems, parasympatholytic therapy is indicated if the block is atropine-responsive.

If atropine is not effective and pacemaker implantation is not feasible, a trial of β-adrenergic agonist therapy is indicated. The only β-adrenergic drugs currently available for oral therapy are relative $β_2$-receptor selective. However, at high dosages these agents, e.g., metaproterenol (Alupent, Boehringer Ingelheim) and terbutaline (Brethine, Geigy) stimulate cardiac β-receptors and may increase the ventricular escape rate in complete heart block. Recommended starting dosages for these drugs is 2–3 mg/kg three times daily. The dosage is increased by 50% every other day until an increase in heart rate is achieved or toxicity develops. Adverse effects of these drugs are hyperexcitability, tachyarrhythmias, and gastrointestinal disturbances.

In the face of life-threatening complete AV block, dopamine (Intropin, American Critical Care) may be administered by constant-rate infusion (5–15 mg/kg/min) to enhance the ventricular escape rhythm. Dopamine may elicit dangerous ventricular tachyarrhythmias, particularly in dogs with underlying myocardial disease, and these ventricular trachyarrhythmias are best controlled by reducing the rate of dopamine administration by 25–50%. Isoproterenol (Isuprel, Breon) is a less desirable drug that can be administered in an attempt to increase the ventricular escape rate, but dopamine is associated with fewer ventricular tachyarrhythmias. There is no oral form of isoproterenol that has an effective duration of action. For emergencies, sublingual or rectal suppositories of isoproterenol may be used to enhance the ventricular escape rate of complete heart block. The duration for action of these modes of isoproterenol administration is less than 2 hours.

Sinoventricular Conduction. Sinoventricular conduction, a bradycardia, is associated with profound hyperkalemia due to acute hypoadrenocorticism (Addison's disease) in dogs and obstructive uropathy in dogs and cats. If not corrected, these problems can lead to idioventricular rhythm and cardiac asystole. Treatment consists in correcting the underlying hyperkalemia. Intravenous therapy with normal (0.9%) saline and appropriate treatment of the etiology are indicated. In the face of severe bradycardia associated with serum potassium concentrations exceeding 10 mEq/L, regular (crystalline) insulin (0.5 unit/kg IV) plus 2–4 g of dextrose per unit of insulin reduces hyperkalemia rapidly. About 4–8 ml of 50% dextrose (2–4 g) is added to 500 ml of normal saline and administered at a rate of approximately 20 microdrops per minute. Four grams of dextrose per unit of insulin is recommended for addisonian patients in order to avoid protracted hypoglycemia. Intravenous 10% calcium gluconate (0.5 mg/kg given slowly over 10–20 minutes accompanied by ECG monitoring) can also reverse hyperkalemic myocardial toxicity. Intravenous sodium bicarbonate (1 mEq/kg given over 15–30 minutes) also reduces serum potassium concentrations rapidly.

Persistent Atrial Standstill. Persistant atrial standstill, a bradycardia, has been seen primarily in young springer spaniels and is characterized by the absence of P waves and a junctional or ventricular escape rhythm. Pacemaker implantation is the treatment of choice. This arrhythmia has been associated with a myopathy, and heart failure due to myocardial failure may occur within a few years.

CANINE AND FELINE HEARTWORM DISEASE

Canine heartworm disease occurs in many areas and is endemic along the coast of the southeastern United States. Disease responses start at the site of the heartworms within the pulmonary arteries. Pulmonary arterial disease develops and leads to the clinical signs of coughing, dyspnea, hemoptysis, decreased exercise tolerance, congestive heart failure, and poor body condition. The pathognomonic lesion is villous myointimal proliferation on the endothelial surface of pulmonary arteries large enough to contain heartworms.

The killing of adult heartworms by thiacetarsamide treatment causes worsening of pulmonary disease. Worm fragments move distally and initiate clotting and damage to the endothelium. This endothelial damage exacerbates villous production, and blood flow becomes severely impaired. Complete obstruction of pulmonary arterial flow to the caudal lung lobes may occur. Alveolar hypoxia increases pulmonary vascular resistance (hypertension), further impeding arterial blood flow. Severe coughing, dyspnea, and even hemoptysis may develop. Within 4 to 6 weeks after adulticide treatment, the movement of heartworms away from the large pulmonary arteries permits resolution of previously described arterial surface changes.

Uncomplicated Heartworm Disease in Dogs

Standard Therapy. Thiacetarsamide sodium (Caparsolate, Abbott) is the only drug approved by the U.S. Food and Drug Administration (FDA) for the treatment of adult heartworm infection. Elimination of adult worms results in resolution of pulmonary arterial disease, except for occasional cases of severe disease with extensive chronic fibrosis.

The objectives of treatment are to:

1. Kill all or most adult heartworms
2. Avoid severe thiacetarsamide toxicity
3. Minimize postthiacetarsamide pulmonary thromboembolic complications
4. Kill all or most microfilariae, if present
5. Institute prophylactic treatment once heartworm infection is eliminated

The first step in the standard treatment of routine heartworm infection is to give an adulticide (thiacetarsamide sodium). The second step, in the face of microfilaremia, is the eradication of the microfilaria utilizing ivermectin (Ivomec, Merck). The final step is the institution of prophylactic therapy utilizing either ivermectin (Heartgard, Merck) or a diethylcarbamazine product.

Thiacetarsamide Sodium. When stored under refrigeration (2–8°C) in amber-colored sealed vials, the expiration time of thiacetarsamide is 15 months. However, when not refrigerated, the drug deteriorates rapidly and develops precipitates and a yellow-orange discoloration. Air entering the vials also contributes to more rapid deterioration.

Thiacetarsamide should be injected at intervals of not less than 6–8 hours and not more than 15 hours. The recommended dosage is 2.2 mg/kg (0.22 ml/kg) IV twice daily. Increased dosages, although possibly increasing adulticide activity, are associated with increased toxicity. It has been determined that six injections over a 3-day period are no more efficacious than four injections and result in more severe lung complications.

It should not be expected that thiacetarsamide can kill every heartworm in every treated dog. There is variation in efficacy from dog to dog. Immature worms, especially the females, are more resistant. Dogs receiving thiacetarsamide should be hospitalized throughout adulticide treatment and monitored closely. One-half to one hour before each thiacetarsamide injection, the dog should be fed and its rectal temperature determined. A urine sample should be collected and examined for bilirubinuria prior to each treatment. Anorexia and vomiting after one to three injections are an indication to abort therapy. Injections are administered in a peripheral vein as distally as feasible. Venipunctures should not be repeated at the same site, and indwelling catheters are not recommended. Intravenous catheters contribute to vein degeneration, and multiple thiacetarsamide exposures to a single site can lead to rupture of the vein. Intravenous catheters may also create a false sense of security in terms of intravenous patency. A butterfly needle facilitates the testing of venipuncture integrity. Under no circumstances should thiacetarsamide be injected unless there is 100% certainty that the vein has been appropriately cannulated. Sterile saline is first injected to ensure proper needle placement.

To determine whether adulticide treatment should be continued, prior to each treatment the dog's attitude, appetite, rectal temperature, mucous membrane color, hydration status, and bilirubinuria status are assessed, and the dog is checked for the presence or absence of vomiting. Serum liver enzyme concentrations are not used as indications of toxicity because of a lack of association with clinical toxicity. Icterus and persistent vomiting are always indications for stopping adulticide treatment. If, following initial treatment, a dog vomits only once or twice, has a normal appetite and temperature, and is not depressed, treatment is continued. A combination of any two signs (e.g., vomiting, depression, anorexia, fever, and diarrhea) are an indication to discontinue treatment. Most adverse reactions occur following the first injection. Many dogs manifesting gross bilirubinuria after one or two doses are either "sick" at the time or become "sick" after subsequent dosages. Occult bilirubinuria is a common sign of thiacetarsamide toxicity but alone is not an indication to abort therapy. Gross bilirubinuria is a warning sign, but therapy is continued if anorexia, vomiting, and lethargy are absent.

If adulticide therapy is stopped, hydration of the patient is reestablished, if necessary, and the patient discharged on a high carbohydrate, low-fat diet with instructions for restricted activity. Treatment is reinitiated in 4 weeks, and subsequent acute toxicity is unlikely.

Investigational Therapy. Melarsamine dihydrochloride (RM340, Rhone Merieux) is an investigational organic arsenical adulticide that has been studied extensively in laboratory as well as naturally infected dogs. It has a high rate (>90%) of heartworm kill and clearance. There is a high rate of antigen seroconversion 3 months after therapy.

Melarsamine has a safety margin of 2.0–2.5 times the recommended dosage regimens, although the final dosage regimen has not been determined. It is administered by deep intramuscular injection, which may be an advantage compared to thiacetarsamide sodium.

Although dithiazanine (Dizan-Pitman, Moore), levamisole (Ripercol-L, Capri), and ivermectin (Ivomec, Merck) are variably effective against microfilariae, only dithiazanine is approved by the FDA. Ivermectin is the most effective drug. Microfilaricide treatment is started 4 weeks after thiacetarsamide administration in dogs with microfilaremia.

Ivermectin is administered as a single oral dose (0.05 mg/kg) 4 weeks after thiacetarsamide. This drug also blocks reinfection by third-stage larvae, which may have occurred during the previous month. Ivermectin is diluted as 1 ml per 9 ml propylene glycol USP; this solution is then administered orally at a dosage of 1 ml/20 kg. When using this regimen, ivermectin is administered in the morning and the dog is observed throughout the day for evidence of adverse reactions (vomiting, diarrhea, lethargy, tachycardia, weakness, shock). A microfilaria concentration test is performed 3–4 weeks later; if positive, the protocol is repeated. Microfilaremia persisting after two treatments with Ivermectin is indicative of continued adult heartworm infection. Until further information and testing are available, ivermectin should not be administered to collie and collie-mix dogs.

Prevention. When microfilaremia has been eliminated, prophylactic therapy should be initiated immediately if reinfection is a potential problem. Several weeks after initiation of prophylaxis, another concentration test should be performed to detect recrudescence resulting from persisting adult heartworms. Repeating the microfilarial concentration test is most important when dithiazanine or levamasole is used as the microfilaricide. Concentration tests are then recommended at 6- or 12-month intervals.

Diethylcarbamazine (Caracide, Cyanamid) administered at 2.5–3.0 mg/kg has been tested by many investigators and consistently found to prevent adult heartworms in dogs experimentally infected with larvae. Several products are available and seem to be equally efficacious. If a dog develops microfilaremia while on a preventive program, diethylcarbamazine should be continued while the dog is being treated with the adulticide and subsequent microfilaricide. Diethylcarbamazine probably affects *Dirofilaria immitis* at the L_3–L_4 molting stage at 9–12 days after infection. Therefore it should be started prior to the mosquito season.

All dogs in endemic areas should be on a heartworm preventive program. It is recommended that it be started at the time puppy immunizations are initiated. In areas that have colder winters and in which *D. immitis* is not endemic, diethylcarbamazine may be stopped 1 month after the final frost and resumed 1 month prior to the spring mosquito season. A microfilaria concentration test should be performed on puppies at 6 months of age. Prior to the initiation of prophylaxis, dogs must test negative for microfilaremia. During the diethylcarbamazine preventive program, microfilaria concentration tests should be done at least annually and in endemic areas semiannually.

Microfilaria-positive dogs should not be given diethylcarbamazine because adverse reactions of variable severity, including death, are common consequences. Dogs with fewer than 50 microfilariae per milliliter seldom develop reactions.

Ivermectin has proved effective in preventing natural and experimental infection. The recommended oral monthly dosage is 6 μg/kg. Its advantages over diethylcarbamazine are monthly administration and lack of adverse reactions in the face of microfilaria; moreover, infectious larvae contracted up to 2 months prior to administration are eliminated.

In heartworm endemic regions, intestinal parasitism is often a concomitant problem. In these areas ivermectin prophylaxis has not been widely accepted. Instead the combination of diethylcarbamazine and oxibendazole (Filaribits Plus, Norden Laboratories) is often the preferred product.

Milbemycin oxime (Interceptor, Ciba-Geigy) is a macrolide antibiotic with a chemical structure similar to that of the avermectins, with anthelmintic activity at low concentrations. The anthelmintic activity is believed to result from disruption of invertebrate neurotransmission of γ-aminobutyric acid (GABA). Milbemycin oxime has been shown to prevent both experimental and natural *D. immitis* infection. One hundred percent efficacy has been demonstrated when administered at dosages above 0.1 mg/kg at 45 days after L_3 inoculation and at 60 and 90 days postinoculation. Adverse effects have not been reported. Milbemycin oxime, marketed for monthly administration at a dosage of approximately 0.23–0.52 mg/kg once monthly, should be a highly effective preventative. Milbemycin also effectively prevents *Ancylostoma caninum* infection when administered monthly. Adverse reactions have not been observed in collies when used as directed. Milbemycin should not be administered to microfilaremic dogs, as adverse reactions may occur in those with high microfilarial counts.

Complicated Heartworm Disease in Dogs

Standard Therapy. Approximately 10% or more of heartworm-infected dogs have clinical and radiographic evidence of severe pulmonary artery disease. Associated clinical signs include severe coughing, tachypnea, dyspnea, exercise intolerance, episodic weakness or syncope, weight loss, and ascites. The cranial and caudal lobar arteries of affected dogs are severely enlarged. The caudal lobar arteries are tortuous and have abnormal tapering.

Because platelet adhesion and activation are involved in the pathogenesis of pulmonary arterial disease, drugs that modify platelet function should be beneficial. Dogs treated with aspirin have less platelet adhesion, vascular damage, and villous proliferation than do dogs not given aspirin.

The recommended treatment for dogs with severe pulmonary arterial disease is strict cage confinement and aspirin 5 mg/kg once daily. Cage confinement and aspirin therapy must be maintained for 2–3 weeks prior to adulticide initiation, during adulticide treatment, and for 3–4 weeks posttreatment.

Aspirin. Aspirin, indicated for the treatment of severe pulmonary arterial disease, is prescribed and administered for 2 weeks or longer prior to starting adulticide therapy. It is also administered during and for 3–4 weeks after the thiacetarsamide sodium is discontinued. The severity of pulmonary arterial disease can be estimated on the basis of thoracic radiographs. Aspirin is indicated to ameliorate pulmonary arterial myointimal proliferation and thromboembolic complications before and after thiacetarsamide treatment. Aspirin inhibits platelet function and release of platelet-derived growth factor. After a period of at least 1 week of treatment, pulmonary endothelial damage begins to improve. Aspirin is not indicated for the treatment of most dogs with heartworm disease because most heartworm-infested dogs do not have severe pulmonary arterial disease. Aspirin dosages of 5–10 mg/kg/day have been shown to be effective in experimental and spontaneous infections.

Glucocorticoids. Corticosteroid hormones are indicated for the treatment of pulmonary parenchymal disease that occurs secondary to severe arterial disease and for the treatment of allergic pneumonitis. Corticosteroids, e.g., prednisone 2 mg/kg once or twice daily, are usually prescribed after the onset of clinical signs associated with parenchymal lung disease. Treatment is continued for 3–5 days until there is clinical and radiographic evidence of significant improvement. Corticosteroids are not recommended as prophylactic treatment or for clinical signs of mild parenchymal disease, e.g., occasional coughing or low-grade fever. Corticosteroid hormones are also indicated for the treatment of occult heartworm disease-associated allergic pneumonitis.

Extended corticosteroid hormone treatment exacerbates the degree of pulmonary arterial disease and thereby promotes further thromboembolism and reduced pulmonary arterial blood flow. Corticosteroids should be employed only when necessary and only until there is radiographic and clinical evidence of the resolution of parenchymal disease (usually 5–7 days). Although corticosteroid treatment during or within several days of thiacetarsamide administration may reduce the efficacy of thiacetarsamide against female worms, this effect may be relatively unimportant.

Dogs with severe pulmonary arterial disease treated with aspirin and protracted cage confinement have a higher survival rate than dogs in which this therapy is omitted. It is reported that when dogs with and without clinical right-sided congestive heart failure were treated with aspirin, cage confinement, furosemide (Lasix, Hoechst-Roussel) 1–2 mg/kg/day, and a low-sodium diet, there is no difference in survival rates.

If clinical and radiographic evidence of significant parenchymal lung disease is also present prior to adulticide treatment, prednisone 2 mg/kg once or twice daily should be administered and continued until these abnormalities resolve—usually within 5–7 days. Corticosteroid therapy is usually stopped prior to the administration of thiacetarsamide sodium because of the aforementioned effect of the glucocorticoids on the efficacy of thiacetarsamide.

Dogs with severe pulmonary arterial disease due to heartworms ideally should be hospitalized for 4–6 weeks. The platelet count and packed cell volume should be determined at the time of diagnosis and monitored periodically during the 4–6 weeks of hospitalization. Gastrointestinal bleeding due to severe thrombocytopenia or aspirin effects occurs occasionally. Aspirin, if being administered, should be stopped until there is no evidence of bleeding (melena or decreasing hematocrit). The platelet count can be increased by heparin administration (100–150 U/kg SC, T.I.D. for several days) but should not be used if there is evidence of bleeding. Vincristine (Oncovin, Eli Lilly) at a dose of 0.4 mg/kg IV (one dose) may be administered to increase the platelet count when bleeding is evident. Pulmonary arterial disease and thromboembolism may be severe enough, particularly following adulticide treatment, to cause thrombocytopenia due to platelet consumption. Heparin is recommended in the absence of hemoptysis or evidence of bleeding.

Digoxin is not recommended. It does not improve survival rates and may cause digoxin intoxication. Decreased volume of distribution due to cachexia and overestimation of lean body weight due to the effect of ascites probably account for the relatively common occurrence of digoxin toxicity.

Postadulticide Complications. *Acute Thiacetarsamide Sodium Toxicity.* Toxic reaction signs to thiacetarsamide treatment include anorexia, vomiting, depression, fever, diarrhea, tubular casts in the urine sediment, increased serum liver enzyme concentrations, icterus, and bilirubinuria, as well as death.

Thromboembolic Lung Disease. Following thiacetarsamide sodium treatment, pulmonary arterial disease is exacerbated. Extensive endothelial damage results in massive platelet adhesion, myointimal proliferation, and villous hypertrophy. Significant complications occur most frequently in dogs with preexisting severe pulmonary arterial disease. Thoracic radiographs may be useful for providing a practical estimate of pulmonary arterial disease prior to adulticide treatment.

Dead heartworms produce pulmonary thrombosis, granulomatous arteritis, perivascular edema (due to increased vascular permeability), and hemorrhage. The caudal and accessory lobes are most severely affected. Exacerbated pulmonary disease occurs 5–30 days after adulticide administration, with the greatest risk of severe thromboembolism occurring 7–17 days after treatment. Associated clinical signs include coughing, fever, dyspnea, auscultatory crackles or dullness, hemoptysis, pale mucous membranes, tachycardia, and weak pulses. A regenerative left shift may be indicated in the leukogram, and thrombocytopenia is usually present.

The recommended therapeutic steps for thromboembolic lung disease include cage confinement and corticosteroid hormone administration (prednisone 1 mg/kg PO once or twice daily). Intranasal oxygen therapy is recommended. Bronchodilator drugs such as aminophylline 2–3 mg/kg PO or IV or Theodur (Key Pharmaceuticals) 10–15 mg/kg PO twice daily are often prescribed empirically. Antibiotics are of questionable benefit unless results of transtracheal lavage cytology and microbial culture suggest a bacterial infection. Empirically, a broad-spectrum bactericidal drug such as a cephalosporin or a quinalone antibiotic is often chosen. Strict cage confinement is the most important aspect of therapy and should be continued until there is clinical and radiographic evidence of resolution of parenchymal lung disease. Judicious fluid administration, usually lactated Ringer's solution at 50–60 ml/kg daily given by constant-rate intravenous infusion over 16–24 hours, is indicated if there is evidence of decreased cardiac output (e.g., weak pulses, hypothermia, and increased toe web–rectal temperature differential). Aspirin 5 mg/kg once daily may be prescribed and should be continued for 2–3 weeks.

Drug Extravasation. If any thiacetarsamide is extravasated, the venipuncture area should be treated with topical dimethylsulfoxide (DMSO) twice daily for several days. This treatment appears to be effective for reducing inflammation, swelling, and tissue necrosis. In fact, if only a small volume of drug has been extravasated, tissue necrosis does not occur when topical DMSO is applied. If extravasation is not recognized immediately, the affected area becomes swollen, painful, and inflamed within 30 minutes to 2 hours. Topical DMSO should then be applied as soon as the problem is discovered.

Investigational Therapy. Japanese clinicians have developed a technique for retrieving adult worms utilizing a long, flexible alligator-type forceps that is passed into a jugular vein via a "cut-down" procedure and guided by fluoroscopy into the pulmonary arteries. Clinicians proficient in this technique can remove large numbers of worms during multiple incursions over a period of 15–30 minutes.

This technique holds great promise for dogs with severe pulmonary arterial disease and large worm burdens. If a few adult worms are evident (persistent microfilaremia or positive adult antigen test), when appropriate thiacetarsamide therapy can be administered following worm removal and microfilaricide treatment.

Heartworm Disease Sequelae in Dogs

Pneumonitis Associated with Occult Heartworm Disease. Approximately 10–15% of dogs with occult heartworm infections develop allergic or eosinophilic pneumonitis. Clinical signs include progressive coughing, tachypnea, dyspnea, and auscultable crackles. Cyanosis, anorexia, and mild weight loss occasionally develop. Clinical pathologic findings are variable and may include eosinophilia, basophilia, and hyperglobulinemia. Tracheal lavage cytology is usually characterized by a sterile eosinophilic exudate with some nondegenerative neutrophils and macrophages. The indirect fluorescent antibody (IFA) test for microfilarial cuticular antigen and ELISA and IFA tests for *D. immitis* adult antigens are usually positive.

Most dogs respond dramatically to corticosteroid treatment, even though the clinical signs are usually severe. Prednisone (1 mg/kg PO once or twice daily) usually brings about subjective clinical improvement within 24–36 hours. Within 48 hours, radiographic evidence of significant improvement is usual. Corticosteroid treatment is continued for 3–5 days and is then stopped 24 hours prior to adulticide therapy. Relapse during or after adulticide therapy has not been reported.

Vena Caval Syndrome. The vena caval syndrome is an acute shock-like phenomenon associated with large numbers of heartworms that obstruct venous blood return to the right ventricle. It is uncommon outside of highly endemic regions. The vast majority of affected dogs, usually 3–5 years of age (range 1.5–11.0 years), do not exhibit clinical signs of heartworm disease prior to the onset of acute illness. Typical physical examination findings include weakness, pallor, tachypnea, anorexia, hemoglobinuria, and bilirubinuria. Acute collapse with inability to stand is a common presenting sign. Death usually occurs within 24–48 hours after the onset of acute signs.

The only effective treatment of vena caval syndrome is surgical removal of some or all of the worms from the vena cava and right atrium. Surgery is performed under local anesthesia (and occasionally mild sedation) through a right jugular venotomy. If intravenous fluids are administered (usually lactated Ringer's solution), caution should be taken not to administer an excessive fluid volume (usually not to exceed 2 mg/kg/hr). See the Suggested Readings list at the end of this chapter for a reference detailing a surgical procedure for heartworm removal. Supportive care, such as fluid administration and cardiac rhythm monitoring, should be provided after surgery. Thiacetarsamide sodium is administered at the standard dose schedule after the patient's cardiovascular status, liver, and renal function have stabilized, which usually requires 5–7 days.

Azotemia. Azotemia may be detected if an appropriate minimum database is procured prior to adulticide therapy. Fortunately, primary renal failure is uncommon with heartworm disease. Mild to moderate azotemia (BUN 30–120 mg/dl) associated with a concentrated urine (specific gravity > 1.035) is common and usually of prerenal origin. Affected dogs are commonly dehydrated, and azotemia should be corrected by fluid replacement therapy prior to thiacetarsamide treatment.

Heartworm disease-induced glomerulopathy associated with a relatively concentrated urine and proteinuria may result in, or contribute to, azotemia. If severe hypoalbuminemia or the nephrotic syndrome is present, irreversible glomerular disease has probably occurred. Adulticide therapy is not indicated in dogs with the nephrotic syndrome or in dogs with severe azotemia and proteinuria. Conversely, if the BUN is 30–120 mg/dl with proteinuria, but hypoalbuminemia and the nephrotic syndrome are absent, successful adulticide therapy can be accomplished. Fluid therapy is given to improve renal function and correct azotemia (see Chapter II). If the BUN is reduced by fluid therapy (usually lactated Ringer's solution at a rate of 50–70 ml/kg daily) to less than 50 mg/dl, thiacetarsamide therapy can be initiated, and fluid therapy should be continued during and for several days after thiacetarsamide administration.

Liver Disease. The most common indication of hepatic disease in heartworm-infected dogs is increased serum alkaline phosphatase or serum alanine aminotransferase (formerly called SGPT). These abnormalities are nonspecific, and up to 10-fold pretreatment elevations of serum alkaline phosphatase or alanine aminotransferase have not been associated with acute thiacetarsamide toxicity. Likewise, increased bromsulphthalein (BSP) retention up to 15% prior to treatment has not been associated with treatment complications. Too much emphasis has been placed on the significance of increases in serum liver enzyme activities.

Hemoglobinuria. Dogs with severe pulmonary arterial disease occasionally develop hemoglobinuria, which may occur prior to or following adulticide

treatment. Associated findings include thrombocytopenia, regenerative anemia, and an inflammatory leukogram. The activated clotting time is usually
high normal or mildly prolonged.

Recommended therapy is heparin (100–200 units/kg SC three times a day)
given until hemoglobinuria is resolved and the platelet count exceeds 100,000/
μl. Because severe pulmonary arterial disease is usually present, aspirin (5
mg/kg once daily) is prescribed once the platelet count exceeds 100,000/μl and
is maintained until approximately 4 weeks after adulticide therapy.

Contraindications for Heartworm Treatment

Nephrotic Syndrome. Glomerulopathies are common sequelae to heartworm disease. These glomerulopathies are usually due to immune complex
disease but may be the result of amyloidosis. In either case, severe proteinuria,
hypoalbuminemia, hypercholesterolemia, ascites (pure transudate), and possibly peripheral edema and variable azotemia are associated with irreversible
renal disease and a grave prognosis. There is no point to heartworm treatment
in such patients.

Hepatic Failure. Dogs with severe pulmonary arterial disease due to chronic
heartworm infection occasionally develop marked hepatomegaly and icterus.
Liver enzyme activity and liver function tests are grossly abnormal in these
patients. Concomitant right-sided congestive heart failure, moderate to severe
anemia, renal failure, and hypoalbuminemia are variably present in these dogs.
These patients are not acceptable candidates for heartworm therapy.

Old Dog. Whether to treat very old dogs with subclinical or mildly clinical
heartworm disease is controversial. Dogs with moderate clinical signs of
heartworm disease should be treated, but those with severe clinical signs are
poor candidates for treatment. An alternative to adulticide therapy for the
subclinical or mildly clinical patient is aspirin (5 mg/kg daily) alone.

Feline Heartworm Disease

Feline heartworm infection is often difficult to diagnose. Microfilaremia is
usually absent at the time of presentation, and thoracic radiographic changes
are less obvious than in dogs. Enlargement of the main pulmonary artery
segment (MPA) is not radiographically visible. The caudal lobar pulmonary
arteries are often enlarged but do not appear tortuous in most instances.
Enlargement of the MPA may be demonstrated with angiography. Obstruction
of the caudal lobar pulmonary arteries may be seen on contrast and routine
radiographs and appears as a hyperlucent region in the distal caudal lung
lobes. Serologic tests that detect antigens to adult *D. immitis* may be positive,
but false-negative test results can occur if there are only one or two worms,
especially when there are no gravid female worms present.

The objectives of therapy are to eliminate adult heartworms without acute toxic thiacetarsamide reactions and without postadulticide pulmonary thromboembolic complications. Premedication with soluble corticosteroids such as prednisolone Na succinate (Solu Delta Cortef, Upjohn) at a dosage of 100 mg IV or dexamethasone sodium phosphate (Azium SP, Schering Animal Health) at a dosage of 5 mg/kg IV plus an antihistamine such as diphenhydramine (Benadryl, Parke-Davis) at a dosage of 2–4 mg/kg SC or IM followed by thiacetarsamide treatment are the components of therapy. Because most cats are amicrofilaremic, microfilaricide treatment is seldom necessary. Prophylactic treatment is seldom recommended.

Standard Therapy. Whether treatment of heartworm-infected cats is efficacious is unknown. In general, infected cats exhibiting severe or chronic cardiovascular signs should probably be treated. In the absence of clinical signs or when signs are mild and intermittent, adulticide therapy may be delayed and the patient's clinical status monitored. The recommended treatment is thiacetarsamide sodium 2.2 mg/kg IV twice daily for 2 days. Because circulating microfilariae are usually absent, evaluation of adulticide treatment is difficult. As in the dog, it should not be expected that thiacetarsamide can kill every adult worm in every infected cat. In some microfilaremic cats, repeated adulticide treatments have been required. If a serologic test for adult *D. immitis* antigens is positive prior to treatment, the test should be repeated 12 weeks or more after treatment. A positive test result indicates that retreatment is necessary.

Complications of Treatment. Some cats experience anorexia and vomiting after the first or second dosage of thiacetarsamide. These side effects warrant temporary cessation of treatment. A second attempt at thiacetarsamide administration is recommended in 2–4 weeks.

Acute fulminant pulmonary edema, pulmonary hemorrhage, and death have been observed within 2 hours after the first or second intravenous thiacetarsamide injection in some infected cats. It was not associated with pulmonary thromboembolism and probably represents an idiosyncratic or allergic drug reaction. Because of the seriousness of this potential reaction it is recommended that premedication with an antihistamine and soluble corticosteroids be given prior to each injection.

Thromboembolic complications are unpredictable and may occur 5–14 days after adulticide treatment. They are observed most commonly in cats with radiographic evidence of severe pulmonary arterial changes (e.g., enlargement, tortuosity). Acute thromboembolism in the cat is associated with an increased risk of death, compared with such reactions in dogs. Furthermore, sudden death or peracute respiratory distress may develop in cats that apparently tolerate adulticide treatment well. Aspirin administration has not been effective in reducing or preventing pulmonary arterial disease and hypertension or improving blood flow when administered at 5–10 mg/kg daily. Higher dosages may be effective, but further research is necessary.

SUGGESTED READINGS

Congestive Heart Failure

Bonagura JD, Muir WW: Vasodilator therapy. In: Kirk RW, ed. Current Veterinary Therapy IX. Philadelphia: WB Saunders, 1986;329–333.

Fitzpatrick RK, Crowe DT: Nasal oxygen administration in dogs and cats: Experimental and clinical investigations. J Am Anim Hosp Assoc 1986;22:293.

Kittleson MD: Management of heart failure: Concepts, therapeutic strategies, and drug pharmacology. In: Fox PR, ed. Canine and Feline Cardiology. New York: Churchill Livingstone, 1988;171.

Kittleson MD, Johnson LE, Pion PP: The acute hemodynamic effects of milrinone in dogs with severe idiopathic myocardial failure. J Vet Intern Med 1987;1:121.

Muir WW: Pharmacodynamics of antiarrhythmic and diuretic drugs in dogs and cats. In: Proceedings 9th Annual Kal Kan Symposium, 1985;25.

Pion PP, Kittleson MD, Rogers QR, Morris JG: Myocardial failure in cats associated with low plasma taurine: A reversible cardiomyopathy. Science 1987;237:764.

Ralston SL: Dietary considerations in the treatment of heart failure. In: Kirk RW, ed. Current Veterinary Therapy X. Philadelphia: WB Saunders, 1989;302.

Sisson DD, MacCoy DM: Treatment of congenital pulmonic stenosis in two dogs by balloon valvuloplasty. J Vet Intern Med 1988;2:92.

Smith TW, Braunwald E, Kelly RA: The management of heart failure. In: Braunwald E, ed. Heart Disease: A Textbook of Cardiovascular Medicine, 3rd ed. Philadelphia: WB Saunders, 1988;485.

Infective Endocarditis

Calvert CC, Greene CE: Cardiovascular infections. In: Greene CE, ed. Clinical Microbiology and Infectious Diseases of the Dog and Cat. Philadelphia: WB Saunders, 1984;220.

Dow SW: Bacteremia in dogs and cats. In: Kirk RW, ed. Current Veterinary Therapy X. Philadelphia: WB Saunders, 1989;1077.

Gomp RE: Bacterial endocarditis. In: Proceedings 9th Annual Kal Kan Symposium, 1985;73.

Sisson DD, Thomas WP: Bacterial endocarditis. In: Kirk RW, ed. Current Veterinary Therapy IX. Philadelphia: WB Saunders, 1986;402.

Weinstein L: Infective endocarditis. In: Braunwald E, ed. Heart Disease: A Textbook of Cardiovascular Medicine. Philadelphia: WB Saunders, 1988;1093.

Cardiac Rhythm Disturbances

Bonagura JD: Therapy of atrial arrhythmias. In: Kirk RW, ed. Current Veterinary Therapy X. Philadelphia, WB Saunders, 1989;271.

Sisson DD: Bradyarrhythmias and cardiac pacing. In: Kirk RW, ed. Current Veterinary Therapy X. Philadelphia: WB Saunders, 1989;286.

Ware WA, Hamlin RL: Therapy for ventricular arrhythmias. In: Kirk RW, ed. Current Veterinary Therapy X. Philadelphia, WB Saunders, 1989;278.

Heartworm Disease

Hribernik TM: Canine and Feline Heartworm Disease. In: Kirk RW, ed. Current Veterinary Therapy X. Philadelphia: WB Saunders, 1989;263.

Jackson RF: The vena cavae or liver failure syndrome of heartworm disease. J Am Vet Med Assoc 1969;194:384.

CHAPTER SEVEN

Respiratory Diseases

Laura Smallwood

Therapeutic success in the management of respiratory disease depends on accurate characterization of the disorder to be treated, selection of a rational therapeutic protocol, and understanding the well-defined therapeutic goals. Management is most successful when the specific etiology of a problem can be identified and appropriate therapy instituted. Unfortunately, the etiologies of many respiratory disorders in dogs and cats are either unknown or poorly understood, and therapeutic recommendations for these diseases are either empiric or symptomatic.

DISEASES OF THE UPPER AIRWAYS

Bacterial Rhinitis and Sinusitis

Bacterial rhinitis and sinusitis are rarely primary diseases in the dog and cat. Usually an underlying problem such as viral infection, nasal foreign body, neoplasia, nasopharyngeal polyp, or dental abscess exists. In cats, bacterial rhinitis is a frequent complication of feline upper respiratory tract viral infections as well as FeLV and FIV infection. In dogs, bacterial rhinitis can occur as a complication of canine distemper virus and parainfluenza virus infections.

Standard Therapy. Successful management of bacterial rhinitis depends on the identification and elimination of the underlying disease when possible. Nasal foreign bodies and polyps should be removed, and dental disease, particularly oronasal fistulas, should be treated. Broad-spectrum antibiotic therapy is recommended for treatment of the bacterial component and should be continued for 1 week after the disappearance of clinical signs. Ampicillin, amoxicillin, oral cephalosporins, and chloramphenicol have been recommended (Table 7-1). A potential side effect of chloramphenicol that may be problematic during treatment of a cat with bacterial rhinitis is drug-related anorexia. If chlamydial infection is suspected in the cat, tetracycline is recommended and should be combined with a tetracycline ophthalmic ointment. A potential side effect of tetracycline is drug-related pyrexia.

TABLE 7-1. Antibiotics Used in the Treatment of Respiratory Infections

Generic Name	Trade Name and Manufacturer	Dose
Amoxicillin		20 mg/kg q8h PO
Amoxicillin/clavulinic acid	Clavamox	20 mg/kg q8h PO
Ampicillin		20 mg/kg q8h PO 20–50 mg/kg q6–8h IV
Cephalosporins		
Cephalexin	Keflex (Dista)	20 mg/kg q8h PO
Cephradine	Velosef (Squibb)	20–40 mg/kg q8h PO
Cephalothin sodium	Keflin (Lilly)	20–40 mg/kg q6–8h IV
Cephapirin sodium	Cefadyl (Bristol-Meyers)	20–40 mg/kg q6–8h IV
Chloramphenicol		20 mg/kg q8h PO
Clindamycin	Antirobe (Upjohn)	10 mg/kg q8h PO
Gentamicin	Gentocin (Schering)	2 mg/kg q12h IM or SC
Metronidazole	Flagyl (Searle)	10–15 mg/kg q8h PO 10 mg/kg q8h IV
Tetracycline		20 mg/kg q8h PO
Trimethoprim-sulfadiazine	Tribrissen (Coopers)	14–20 mg/kg q12h PO

Additional supportive care may be necessary in the treatment of patients with primary viral infections (see Chapter 16) and should include attention to adequate hydration (see Chapter 1) and nutrition. In cats, special effort should be made to keep the nares free of dried nasal secretions because interference with olfaction can greatly reduce appetite. Intranasal decongestants have been used with some success in cats to decrease nasal discharge. Phenylephrine HCl 0.25% (Neo-Synephrine, Winthrop Pharmaceuticals), which may be administered every 4–6 hours, and 0.25% oxymethazoline (Afrin Pediatric Nose Drops, Schering), which is administered every 24 hours, have been recommended. One or two drops of the intranasal decongestant should be administered in one nostril. Treatment should be terminated after 3 days or, if signs still persist, switched to the untreated nostril. This method is recommended in order to prevent congestive rebound upon withdrawal of the decongestant.

If an underlying problem, such as a nasal foreign body or dental fistula exists, the problem must be corrected so the antibiotic therapy is successful. Fungal infections and neoplasia should be suspected in patients who respond poorly to broad-spectrum antibiotics and in whom no underlying cause for a bacterial infection can be identified.

Brachycephalic Upper Airway Obstruction

Brachycephalic upper airway obstruction is seen in the brachycephalic breeds and occurs secondary to a number of anatomic conditions in the upper airway including stenotic nares, elongation of the soft palate, and eversion of the lateral saccules. Airway obstruction in these patients occurs as the result of a vicious cycle of excitement, increased respiratory rate, and laryngeal edema secondary to widely fluctuating pressures within the laryngeal vault.

Standard Therapy. Therapy for acute respiratory distress in these patients should consist of sedation to slow respiratory rate and decrease excitement. Acepromazine maleate at a dosage of 0.05–0.10 mg/kg IM or SC may be administered for sedation. These patients should be cage-rested, and stressful diagnostics should be kept to an absolute minimum. Patients must be monitored for hyperthermia; and if the rectal temperature exceeds 105°F, temperature should be slowly lowered using fans and alcohol wetting of the footpads. Antiinflammatory doses of corticosteroids may be administered to reduce laryngeal edema. Appropriate drugs include prednisolone sodium succinate (Solu-Delta-Cortef, Upjohn) at a dosage of 1.0 mg/kg IV or IM and dexamethasone (Azium, Schering) at a dosage of 0.15 mg/kg IV or IM. Corticosteroids should be administered only as needed and should not be continued for more than 48 hours. If respiratory distress is severe and unresponsive to medical treatment, emergency tracheotomy may be necessary (see Chapter 17).

Long-term management of these patients often requires surgical intervention. Surgical techniques for correction of stenotic nares and resection of redundant palantine and pharyngeal soft tissue have been described in standard veterinary surgery textbooks.

Laryngeal Paralysis

Laryngeal paralysis is a disorder characterized by failure of the arytenoid cartilages to abduct on inspiration. Clinical signs include exercise intolerance, voice change, and possible acute inspiratory distress. The etiology of this disease is unknown, but it has been associated with damage to the recurrent laryngeal nerve, polyneuropathy, and polymyopathy. Hypothyroidism has been implicated in some cases of laryngeal paralysis associated with polyneuropathy. Patients presenting with laryngeal paralysis should be screened for hypothyroidism using the thyroid-stimulating hormone (TSH) stimulation test. The paralysis may be unilateral or bilateral, with the bilateral type causing the most severe clinical signs.

Standard Therapy. Therapy for acute respiratory distress should include sedation with acepromazine maleate at a dosage of 0.05–0.10 mg/kg IM or SC and cage rest. Antiinflammatory doses of corticosteroids should be given to reduce laryngeal edema. As with brachycephalic airway obstruction, appropriate drugs include prednisone at a dosage of 1.0 mg/kg IV or IM or dexamethasone at a dosage of 0.15 mg/kg. The patient should be monitored closely for hyperthermia; and if the rectal temperature should increase to greater than 105°F, an effort should be made to reduce body temperature with fans and wetting of the footpads with alcohol.

Thyroid replacement therapy is indicated in the patient with hypothyroidism documented by TSH stimulation test. The standard dose of levothyroxine sodium is 0.02 mg/kg PO q12h. Response to therapy has not yet been critically evaluated in this disorder, but it has been noted that some patients do not regain normal laryngeal function following replacement therapy.

Surgical intervention is the therapy of choice for long-term management of laryngeal paralysis, particularly when clinical signs are severe. Surgical procedures that have been recommended include arytenoid lateralization, partial arytenoidectomy, and ventricular cordectomy. Evidence suggests that arytenoid lateralization is a superior procedure for long-term control of clinical signs.

DISEASES OF THE LOWER AIRWAYS

Tracheal Collapse

The etiology of tracheal collapse is unknown. Tracheal collapse may occur anywhere in the trachea but is most common at the thoracic inlet. This disorder is seen most commonly in small and toy breed dogs.

Standard Therapy. Medical therapy for tracheal collapse is symptomatic. Antitussives may be used intermittently to control paroxysmal cough (Table 7-2). Hydrocodone bitartrate (Hycodan, Dupont Pharmaceuticals) is a centrally acting cough suppressant that may be administered orally at a dosage of 0.25–0.50 mg/kg q8–12h. Butorphanol tartrate (Torbutrol, Fort Dodge) is a synthetic narcotic agonist-antagonist that may be administered orally at a dosage of 0.5 mg/kg q6–12h. Butorphanol tartrate is a potent antitussive agent that is thought to act directly on the cough center of the medulla oblongata. Butorphanol tartrate is a more potent antitussive than hydrocodone bitartrate, but the clinical response varies from patient to patient. It is important to remember that the goal of antitussive therapy in the treatment of tracheal collapse is to ameliorate paroxysmal cough. It is unrealistic to expect complete elimination of the cough.

Bronchodilators have been shown to be effective in some patients with tracheal collapse. Although bronchodilators have little or no effect on the trachea itself, bronchodilation can reduce pressure changes in the airway that contribute to dynamic collapse of the trachea upon inspiration (extrathoracic tracheal collapse) or expiration (intrathoracic tracheal collapse). Bronchodilators are probably most effective in patients with coexisting bronchial disease.

TABLE 7-2. Drugs Commonly Used in the Treatment of Respiratory Disease

Generic Name	Trade Name and Manufacturer	Dose
Antitussives		
Butorphanol tartrate	Torbutrol (Fort Dodge)	0.5 mg/kg q6–12h PO Avail: 1, 5, 10 mg tablets
Hydrocodone bitartrate	Hycodan (Dupont Pharmaceuticals)	0.25–0.50 mg/kg q8–12h PO Avail: 5 mg/5 ml syrup, 5 mg tablet
Bronchodilators		
Theophylline	Theo-Dur (Key Pharmaceuticals)	20 mg/kg q12h PO Avail: 100, 200, 300, 450 mg tablets
	Slo-bid Gyrocap (Rorer Pharmaceuticals)	20 mg/kg q12h PO Avail: 50, 75, 100, 125, 200, 300 mg tablets
Terbutaline	Brethine (Geigy)	0.1 mg/kg PO q8h PO (Do not exceed 5.0 mg) Avail: 2.5, 5.0 mg tablets

Two classes of bronchodilator are available: the β-adrenergic drugs and the methylxanthines (Table 7-2). The β-adrenergic terbutaline (Brethine, Geigy) is administered at a dose of 0.1 mg/kg PO q8h not to exceed 5.0 mg per dose. A time-release form of theophylline is recommended (Theo-Dur, Key Pharmaceuticals; Slo-bid Gyrocaps, Rorer Pharmaceuticals) and should be administered at a dosage of 20 mg/kg PO q12h. Because these two classes of drugs act via different mechanisms (see Chronic Bronchitis), a combination of the two may be most efficacious. Side effects of both drugs include restlessness and hyperexcitability. If side effects occur in the patient receiving a single bronchodilator, the dose of the medication should be reduced by 25–50%. If the patient is receiving both terbutaline and theophylline, withdraw the theophylline, adjust the dose of terbutaline as needed, then add the theophylline back, adjusting the dose if signs recur. It should be noted that pharmacologic studies of terbutaline in the dog have not been published, and the recommended dosages are empirically derived from the literature on humans.

Antibiotics are *not* indicated for the routine treatment of tracheal collapse. Antibiotics *are* indicated in the treatment of tracheal collapse if bacterial tracheitis or bacterial bronchitis is strongly suspected owing to systemic signs or if documented by transtracheal wash cytology and culture. In general, bacterial contamination of the trachea is thought to be common in tracheal collapse, whereas true bacterial infection is thought to be relatively uncommon. However, if true infection is thought to exist, broad-spectrum antibiotics such as amoxicillin with clavulinic acid (Clavamox, Beecham), oral cephalosporins, or trimethoprim-sulfa (Tribrissen, Coopers) may be administered for 7–10 days. The effectiveness of any of these drugs is debatable owing to the low concentration of drug that actually reaches the airway mucosa.

Two coexisting medical conditions can complicate the management of tracheal collapse. The first is obesity, which is a common finding in the patient with tracheal collapse. Obesity decreases respiratory reserves and therefore compromises exercise tolerance, leading to breathlessness and coughing on exertion and worsening of the tracheal collapse. Weight reduction programs should be recommended for all patients with tracheal collapse or any chronic airway disease. The second complicating medical condition is dental disease. Chronic gingivitis secondary to dental tartar can provide a nidus of infection leading to pharyngitis, possible tracheitis, and exacerbation of cough. Appropriate dental prophylaxis including scaling, polishing, perioperative antibiotics, and home care is essential. Although tracheal collapse compromises a patient's status as an anesthetic candidate, untreated dental disease should be considered a greater threat to the patient's physical condition and comfort.

Acute exacerbations of tracheal collapse can be life-threatening. A vicious cycle of progressive respiratory distress and worsening tracheal collapse secondary to airway pressure changes can ensue. These patients may benefit from sedation, cage rest, and supplemental oxygen. Acepromazine maleate at a dosage of 0.05–0.10 mg/kg SC or IM may be administered. A single antiinflammatory dose of corticosteroid may be helpful for reducing airway inflammation. Appropriate drugs include prednisolone 1.0 mg/kg and dexamethasone 0.15 mg/kg. Corticosteroids should not be continued as long-term therapy, as some evidence suggests that corticosteroids can have a weakening effect on cartilagenous structures when administered chronically. If supportive therapy during the acute crisis fails, general anesthesia and tracheal intubation or tracheotomy with a tube of sufficient length to bypass the tracheal collapse may be necessary (see Chapter 17 for additional information). Patients who require this type of management have a poor prognosis for recovery without surgical intervention.

Alternative Therapy. A number of surgical procedures for the management of tracheal collapse have been described. Unfortunately, morbidity following surgery is a considerable problem. Therefore the surgical treatment of tracheal collapse at this time is generally reserved for patients with severe collapse.

Clients should be advised that tracheal collapse is a chronic airway condition that can potentially worsen with age or with concurrent disease states. The goal of therapy in these patients should be to minimize clinical signs through the judicious use of bronchodilators and cough suppressants while correcting physical problems such as obesity and dental disease that can compromise response to therapy.

Tracheal Parasites

Filaroides osleri is a parasitic organism that causes nodule-like growths in the trachea of affected dogs. Patients may present with a history of mild to moderate wheezing and cough. Diagnosis is established by the presence of larvae in tracheal washings. Occasionally, larvae are seen with Baermann analysis of feces. The characteristic nodules are easily visualized in the trachea with a bronchoscope.

Standard Therapy. A number of therapeutic protocols have been recommended for the treatment of *F. osleri*. Levamisole (Levasole, Pitman-Moore) has been used at a dosage of 7.0 mg/kg PO daily for 10–30 days. Side effects include gastrointestinal signs and restlessness. Ivermectin was used at a dosage of 2000 μg/kg once weekly for 2 months according to one report. This therapy resulted in resolution of clinical signs but incomplete resolution of the nodules.

Canine Allergic Bronchitis

Allergic bronchitis secondary to inhalant allergies has not been well documented in the dog. However, the clinical entity of allergic bronchitis has been described. These patients characteristically have a history of cough and occasionally exercise intolerance. Physical examination findings may reveal mild to moderate expiratory distress and wheezes. Radiographs typically reveal increased interstitial and peribronchial markings. Peripheral eosinophilia is variable. Allergic bronchitis is characterized by the presence of an eosinophilic exudate on transtracheal wash or bronchoalveolar lavage. Care should be taken to rule out other causes of eosinophilic infiltration including parasites and heartworm disease.

Standard Therapy. Treatment of allergic bronchitis should include elimination of potential allergens (smoke, carpet powders, aerosols) and therapy with prednisone or prednisolone at a dose of 0.5–1.0 mg/kg q12h until signs abate. It should be possible to discontinue daily therapy in 3–5 days, at which time alternate-day therapy should be instituted. The dose should be decreased to the smallest dose that controls the respiratory signs. Bronchodilators may provide symptomatic relief of bronchoconstriction but should not be used as the primary therapy. Theophylline (Theo-Dur or Slo-bid Gyrocaps) at a dosage of 20 mg/kg q12h and terbutaline (Brethine) at a dosage of 0.1 mg/kg PO q8h may both be administered orally. In many instances, therapy with corticosteroids may eventually be discontinued altogether. Injectable long-acting corticosteroids are contraindicated in the dog.

Feline Allergic Bronchitis

The cat with allergic bronchitis ("feline asthma") may present as an acute emergency in severe respiratory distress or may have a more chronic history characterized by cough and wheezing. The acute presentation must be differentiated from that associated with pleural effusion or pulmonary edema. A frequent key physical examination finding is that the patient demonstrates severe respiratory distress characterized by a labored expiratory pattern. This finding is associated with airway collapse on expiration due to bronchospasm, luminal obstruction with mucus and exudate, and edema of bronchial smooth muscle.

The cause of feline allergic bronchitis is unknown, but circumstantial evidence has implicated inhalant allergens such as kitty litter dust, aerosol sprays, carpet deodorizers, and smoke. Diagnosis depends on the demonstration of an eosinophilic exudate on transtracheal wash (obtained through a transtracheal catheter) or tracheal wash (obtained through a sterile endotracheal tube) and the diagnostic exclusion of heartworm disease and respiratory parasites.

Standard Therapy. Therapy should be aimed at stabilizing the patient's respiratory function and decreasing the inflammatory response of the airways. Cats who present in severe respiratory distress may be stabilized with an intravenous injection of prednisolone sodium succinate (Solu Delta Cortef, Upjohn) at a dosage of 10 mg/kg IV and oxygen therapy. If the patient is difficult to handle, the prednisolone may be injected intramuscularly. Handling of these patients should be kept to an absolute minimum until respiration stabilizes. If the patient fails to respond to the prednisolone sodium succinate within 30 minutes, the injection should be repeated. If the patient continues to deteriorate despite therapy, 5 mg/kg aminophylline (Elkins-Sinn) may be administered IM. Although epinephrine has been a standard recommendation in the past for the treatment of acute feline allergic bronchitis, it should be noted that this therapy can potentiate fatal cardiac arrhythmias in the hypoxic patient. In general, treatment with epinephrine should be used only as a last resort at 0.1 ml of 1:1000 dilution IM.

Antiinflammatory therapy with corticosteroids is the mainstay of chronic therapy for feline allergic bronchitis. Prednisolone at a dose of 1.0 mg/kg PO should be administered every 12 hours initially. Higher doses may be used, if necessary, to control the signs. Once clinical improvement is noted, therapy should be tapered by decreasing the frequency of administration to once daily, after which alternate-day therapy should be attempted. Tapering should be done slowly enough (every 7 days) to allow clinical evaluation of dose effectiveness. If control is maintained with alternate-day therapy, tapering the dose may be attempted. Some patients can eventually be taken off corticosteroids, whereas others suffer immediate relapse.

In the patient for which oral medication is not possible, either because the patient is fractious or the client is unable to administer tablets, injectable methylprednisolone acetate (Depo-Medrol, Upjohn) may be used as an alternative to oral prednisolone. A recommended dose is 1.0–2.0 mg/kg IM, and the injections should be given no more frequently than every 3 or 4 weeks. If no clinical signs are observed, less frequent injection or discontinuation of the medication should be attempted. Continued use of Depo-Medrol may cause signs of hyperadrenocorticism as well as adrenal atrophy and should be used with caution. Patients may become refractory to this treatment over time.

Bronchodilator therapy with oral theophylline compounds has been recommended as standard therapy in the past. However, the bronchodilator effect of theophylline has been called into question. In addition, studies involving the treatment of human asthmatics have demonstrated that, although bronchodilators may provide some symptomatic relief, inhalant corticosteroid therapy is necessary to slow the progression of the inflammatory disease occurring in the airway. Long-acting theophylline (Theo-Dur) may be administered to the cat at a dose of 10–20 mg/kg PO q24h for symptomatic relief of clinical signs, particularly in acute exacerbations. However, theophylline should not replace corticosteroid therapy in the treatment of feline allergic bronchitis.

Clients should be advised to prevent contact with potential allergens or irritants such as aerosols, carpet fresheners, and cigarette smoke. They should be advised that allergic bronchitis is a chronic, recurrent condition in most cases, and that therapy is not curative. Some patients may be weaned off corticosteroids and may not have another attack for months, whereas others require chronic medication. Recurrent attacks are common and can be potentially life-threatening.

Canine Chronic Bronchitis

Chronic bronchitis in the dog is a poorly understood entity. It is characterized by chronic irritation of the bronchial tree that results in increased mucus production and changes in bronchial architecture often leading to bronchial collapse. Mucociliary clearance is decreased in these patients and leads to decreased clearance of mucus and compromised pulmonary defense. The etiology of this disease is unknown. Affected individuals tend to be middle-aged or older and often have coexisting problems such as obesity or tracheal collapse.

The goal of therapy in chronic bronchitis is to improve airway function and, in so doing, improve the quality of the patient's life. It should be impressed on the client that chronic bronchitis is an incurable and sometimes progressive disease, and that therapy never totally resolves all of the signs.

Standard Therapy. The mainstay of recommended therapy for chronic bronchitis is bronchodilator therapy. Classically, bronchodilators are divided into two groups: β-adrenergic drugs and methylxanthines. The β-adrenergics act directly on β-receptors in bronchial smooth muscle cells to increase intracellular cyclic adenosine monophosphate (cAMP), which in turn results in bronchodilation. Theophylline derivatives were thought to act to increase cAMP also via inhibition of phosphodiesterase, which decreases breakdown of cAMP. Research indicates that this effect on phosphodiesterase occurs at concentrations far exceeding therapeutic concentrations. It is now thought that theophylline acts via other intracellular mechanisms and that the clinical effects include improved mucociliary clearance, stimulatory effects on the respiratory center, enhanced cardiac output, and enhanced diaphragmatic contraction. The bronchodilator effect of theophylline may be negligible.

Because of the different effects of the β-adrenergic drugs and the theophylline derivatives, it is a rational therapeutic approach to use the two classes of drugs in combination. Long-acting theophylline (Theo-Dur or Slo-bid Gyrocaps) is recommended and may be dosed at 20 mg/kg PO q12h. β-Adrenergics are primarily administered as inhalants in human medicine, so few oral formulations are available. Terbutaline (Brethine) is available in an oral form, and the recommended dose is 0.1 mg/kg q8h. Metaproterenol (Alupent, Boehringer Ingelheim) is an alternative drug, and the recommended dosage is 0.5 mg/kg PO q6h. It should be noted that the recommended dosages of the β-adrenergic drugs are empiric derivations of human dosages, and that pharmacodynamic studies in the dog have not been published.

Side effects associated with the use of theophylline and β-adrenergic drugs include restlessness, sleeplessness, and hyperactivity. If these side effects are observed, the dose of these medications may need to be decreased. If a patient is on both types of bronchodilator concurrently when side effects are observed, the theophylline may be withdrawn. If the signs abate, theophylline can be restarted at 25–50% the previous dose. If the signs continue, the dose of the β-adrenergic drug should be decreased by 25–50%.

Intermittent cough is a necessary mechanism in chronic bronchitis to facilitate clearance of secretions from the airways. However, in some patients cough may become paroxysmal, and in these patients intermittent and judicious use of cough suppressants is indicated. Hydrocodone bitartrate (Hycodan) at a dosage of 0.25–0.50 mg/kg PO q8–24h may be administered. Alternatively, butorphanol tartrate (Torbutrol) may be administered at a dose of 0.5–1.0 mg/kg q6–12h. Response to these two drugs seems to vary among individuals, with certain patients responding better to one than the other.

Antibiotic therapy is indicated for the treatment of chronic bronchitis only if a bacterial infection of the bronchi is suspected. Although bronchitic patients often have bacterial contamination of the airways, the frequency of bacterial infection is unknown. In humans it is known that airway infection can exacerbate preexisting bronchial disease, and it is thought that the same phenomenon can occur in dogs. Ampicillin, trimethoprim-sulfa, oral cephalosporins, and amoxicillin with clavulinic acid (Clavamox) have been recommended for treatment of airway infections. A potential problem with systemic antimicrobial therapy for airway infection is the poor penetration of these drugs into the airway mucosa (see Chapter 15). Cytology and culture and sensitivity tests from transtracheal washings are recommended prior to therapy with antibiotics. The culture of several organisms, particularly in the absence of an inflammatory tracheal wash cytology, is more consistent with airway contamination than infection.

Corticosteroids have been recommended for the treatment of chronic bronchitis in both humans and dogs; however, their use remains controversial in light of the poorly understood etiology of this disorder and inconclusive evidence of their benefit in human medicine. In one human study, an increased frequency of respiratory infections was reported in chronic bronchitis patients receiving corticosteroids. Because of the potential deleterious effects on natural defense mechanisms, corticosteroids should be used with great caution and only at antiinflammatory doses (prednisolone at 0.25–0.50 mg/kg) given on alternate days. The treatment of chronic bronchitis with corticosteroids may best be reserved for those patients who fail to respond to other treatment modalities.

Aerosol therapy may be administered to liquefy thickened secretions. NaCl 0.9% may be nebulized via an inexpensive disposable nebulizer (Airlife Misty Nebulizer, American Pharmaseal Company) connected to an oxygen source. Oxygen flow rates should be set between 3 and 5 L/minute. The patient should be nebulized for 15–30 minutes four times daily. Addition of mucolytics, e.g., acetylcysteine, to the saline has not been shown to have any added clinical benefit and may be irritating to the airways. At home, humidification of the airways should be attempted by exposing the patient to steam from the shower or by using room vaporizers. Light exercise and thoracic coupage should follow nebulization to promote removal of secretions.

Weight loss is critical to the management of the obese dog with chronic bronchitis. Abdominal and thoracic fat reduce effective lung volume, compromise reserve capacity, and predispose the patient to airway collapse. Significant improvement in respiratory signs is noted in many overweight bronchitis patients after weight loss alone.

The importance of dental hygiene in the chronic bronchitic has been debated. However, it intuitively makes sense that control of oral infection would be especially important in individuals with compromised airway defense mechanisms. Routine dental prophylaxis (scaling and polishing) should be combined with home dental care. Perioperative treatment with antibiotics is recommended. Clindamycin (Antirobe, Upjohn) 10 mg/kg PO q8h should be started 24 hours prior to the dental procedure and continued for 3 days thereafter.

Oxygen therapy may be necessary during severe exacerbations of chronic bronchitis that result in dyspnea and hypoxemia. Care should be taken during the administration of oxygen to these patients. Severe chronic bronchitis may result in chronic carbon dioxide retention, which in turn results in a respiratory drive that is no longer stimulated by carbon dioxide levels but, rather, is controlled by blood oxygen concentration. If high concentrations of oxygen are administered, the tendency of these patients is to hypoventilate. (See Chapter 17 for more information.)

Diuretics are not indicated for the treatment of chronic bronchitis unless there is coexisting congestive heart failure. Many chronic bronchitics develop pulmonary hypertension secondary to chronic hypoxemia, which eventually results in right ventricular hypertrophy or cor pulmonale. Care should be taken not to confuse these changes with those associated with congestive heart failure, especially in the patient with a mitral murmur. Furosemide (Lasix) potentially may dehydrate the patient and dry the airways, leading to thickened secretions and further compromise of mucociliary clearance.

Infectious Tracheobronchitis

Canine infectious tracheobronchitis can be caused by several viruses (canine adenovirus 2 and canine parainfluenza virus) and bacteria (i.e., *Bordetella bronchiseptica*) as well as other organisms (i.e., *Mycoplasma*). The disease is usually self-limiting, and resolution can be expected without treatment in 7–10 days in most cases. Because of the self-limiting nature of this disease, treatment is indicated only in situations where the signs are severe or persistent.

Standard Therapy. Patients with infectious tracheobronchitis may develop a severe paroxysmal cough that can potentiate airway irritation. Cough suppressants are indicated in these patients. Either hydrocodone bitartrate (Hycodan) 0.5 mg/kg PO q8–24h or butorphanol tartrate (Torbutrol) 0.5–1.0 mg/kg PO q6–12h may be administered.

Antibiotics are indicated for the treatment of infectious tracheobronchitis when hematologic or radiographic parameters suggest bacterial complications or when signs persist. Treatment should be preceded by a transtracheal wash for cytology and culture and sensitivity tests. A few antibiotics have been shown to be effective against *B. bronchiseptica* in vitro, although because of poor penetration into the airways their in vivo effectiveness is debated. Such antibiotics include tetracycline, trimethoprim-sulfonamide, oral cephalosporins, and chloramphenicol (see Table 7-1). Clinical improvement should be expected in 3–5 days, and treatment should be continued for a minimum of 7 days.

Nebulization of gentamicin has been shown to be effective for the treatment of *B. bronchiseptica* in a few studies. A dose of 2 mg/kg should be added to 0.9% NaCl and nebulized every 8 hours for up to 10 days. A disposable nebulizer (Airlife Misty Nebulizer, American Pharmaseal Company) filled with 9 ml of the 0.9% NaCl and gentamicin solution is attached to an oxygen source with the flow rate set between 3–5 L/minute. As with parenteral gentamicin, the patient should be monitored for signs of renal tubule damage. Aerosolized gentamicin should not be administered concurrently with parenteral gentamicin.

Nebulization of 0.9% NaCl alone may be useful for the treatment of tracheobronchitis. It should be performed three or four times daily for 15–30 minutes followed by thoracic coupage or light exercise to promote cough and facilitate removal of airway secretions.

Corticosteroids may decrease the severity of signs associated with infectious tracheobronchitis, and antiinflammatory doses have been recommended by some individuals. It should be noted that recovery from this disease is highly dependent on physiologic and immunologic defense mechanisms, and that corticosteroids can potentially interfere with recovery. Therefore corticosteroids should be used cautiously, if at all, for the treatment of infectious tracheobronchitis.

Intranasal vaccines against infectious tracheobronchitis are available and have been shown to protect against clinical illness. The vaccine should be administered 10–14 days prior to a potential exposure risk. Yearly boosters are recommended, but more frequent vaccination is indicated in individuals at high risk for exposure. The vaccine may offer protection within 72 hours of administration and may be useful in the face of a kennel outbreak. It is important to remember that tracheobronchitis may be caused by a number of organisms, and therefore it is possible for a vaccinated individual to develop clinical disease.

BRONCHOALVEOLAR DISEASES

Bacterial Pneumonia

Bacterial pneumonia is seldom a primary disease entity in the dog and cat but more frequently occurs secondary to other diseases. Predisposing diseases in the dog include megaesophagus, aspiration, airway foreign bodies, viral infections such as canine distemper, ciliary dyskinesia, and immunoglobulin A (IgA) deficiency. Predisposing diseases in the cat include megaesophagus, aspiration, airway foreign bodies, and viral infections such as FeLV and FIV. It is important to consider these potential underlying causes of bacterial pneumonia in any patient presented for treatment. It is particularly important to consider them in the patient who responds poorly to appropriate antibiotic therapy or who relapses after withdrawal of antibiotics.

Standard Therapy. Antibiotics are the therapy of choice for bacterial pneumonia. To select an appropriate antibiotic, it is important to identify the organism involved. Therefore prior to beginning antibiotic therapy, a transtracheal wash should be performed and the specimen submitted for cytology as well as culture and sensitivity tests. Common isolates from bacterial pneumonia in the dog include *Escherichia coli, Klebsiella, Pasteurella* spp., *Pseudomonas, Bordetella bronchiseptica,* and *Streptococcus zooepidemicus.* In the cat, *B. bronchiseptica* and *Pasteurella* spp. are common isolates. Pending culture results, trimethoprim-sulfonamide may be administered. If a gram-positive organism is suspected, cephalexin, trimethoprim-sulfonamide, or amoxicillin is indicated. If a gram-negative organism is suspected, chloramphenicol or trimethoprim-sulfonamide should be considered. If an anaerobic infection is suspected, clindamycin and metronidazole are the antibiotics of choice. Therapy should be altered on the basis of culture and sensitivity results and should be continued for 10–14 days past resolution of clinical and radiographic signs.

In the patient with evidence of generalized alveolar disease and clinical signs such as persistent fever, anorexia, and weight loss, more aggressive therapy should be considered, especially if hematologic and biochemical evidence of sepsis is present (e.g., degenerative left shift, hypoalbuminemia, elevated alkaline phosphatase, or hypoglycemia). Combination therapy with intravenous ampicillin and subcutaneous gentamicin should be considered. A parenteral cephalosporin such as cephaparin or cephalothin sodium in combination with gentamicin may be considered as an alternative. Therapy should be adjusted based on culture and sensitivity results. Gentamicin should be continued for no longer than 7–10 days, and care should be taken to keep the patient adequately hydrated and to monitor renal function throughout therapy. The other parenteral antibiotics should be continued until the patient has shown significant clinical and radiographic improvement, at which time an oral preparation of the drug may be substituted. Therapy should be continued for 10–14 days past resolution of radiographic and clinical signs.

The treatment of bacterial pneumonia requires attention not only to antibiotic therapy but to fluid and nutritional support, respiratory support, and physiotherapy. Supplemental oxygen administration is indicated in the patient with compromised respiratory function secondary to pneumonia. Because these patients often require supplemental oxygen for several days, it is necessary that it be administered either via oxygen cage, pediatric isolette, or nasal catheter. Oxygen concentration should not exceed 45% in order to avoid oxygen toxicity. Nasal catheter oxygen administration facilitates handling of the patient for treatment and monitoring and is an economic way of providing supplemental oxygen. (See Chapter 17 for additional information.)

Intravenous fluid therapy is essential for the patient with severe pneumonia to ensure adequate hydration of the patient and the airways. Dehydrated patients have airway secretions that are tenacious and difficult to clear. A balanced electrolyte solution (NaCl 0.9% or lactated Ringer's) should be administered to correct dehydration and, if necessary, to maintain normal hydration status (see Chapter 1).

Aerosol therapy combined with physiotherapy is recommended for the treatment of pneumonia to help clear secretions. Aerosolized 0.9% NaCl should be administered for 15–30 minutes four times daily using a nebulizer (Airlife Misty Nebulizer) at an oxygen flow rate of 3–5 L/minute. It should be followed by vigorous coupage or light exercise to help loosen secretions and encourage coughing. There is no proven benefit to aerosolized antibiotics over parenteral antibiotics for the treatment of bacterial pneumonia.

Environmental and nutritional support is important in the treatment of severe bacterial pneumonia. Patients should be kept warm and dry. Caloric needs, which are normally calculated at 60 kcal/kg/day, should be increased by 1.5–1.8 times in the seriously ill patient, and every effort should be made to ensure adequate caloric and protein intake.

Therapeutic response should be monitored in terms of clinical parameters, such as rectal temperature and appetite, radiographic changes, and hematologic changes. Improvement can be expected within 48–72 hours in the patient being treated with appropriate antibiotic therapy. Therapy should be continued for 10–14 days past resolution of radiographic signs. Radiographs should be reevaluated 2 weeks after discontinuation of antibiotics. If pneumonia recurs, a transtracheal wash should be performed to identify the bacteria involved and its antibiotic sensitivity, and treatment should be reinstituted. Recurrence following radiographic resolution suggests the presence of an underlying disease predisposing the patient to bacterial pneumonia. The prognosis for recovery is poor in cases of recurrent pneumonia if the underlying disease is not identified.

Aspiration Pneumonia

Aspiration pneumonia can result in a chemical pneumonitis with or without concurrent bacterial infection. Therapy in these patients should include fluid and nutritional support, aerosolization, physiotherapy, and oxygen therapy when indicated. Corticosteroids have been shown to be of no benefit in the treatment of aspiration pneumonia unless the patient presents in circulatory shock. Corticosteroids may actually interfere with the normal pulmonary defense mechanisms necessary to recovery from aspiration pneumonia. Antibiotics are not indicated in the absence of infection and do not improve clinical outcome in aseptic pneumonia. However, a transtracheal wash and culture and sensitivity tests are indicated to rule out the presence of bacterial infection.

Parasitic Diseases

A number of parasites can invade the lungs, including *Paragonimus kellicotti, Aleurostrongylus abstrusus, Capillaria aerophila*, and *Filaroides hirthi*. An inflammatory response results that may be eosinophilic. Diagnosis depends on identification of ova or larvae in transtracheal washings or by fecal flotation methods. Transtracheal wash is the more sensitive diagnostic procedure.

Standard Therapy. Occasionally, if clinical signs such as cough or respiratory distress are present, patients may benefit from treatment with prednisolone at 0.5–1.0 mg/kg PO for 3–5 days. In general, pulmonary disease accompanying parasitic infection is mild, and therapy need consist only of eliminating the parasite. Unfortunately, specific antiparasitic therapies are not well established for some pulmonary parasites.

No treatment for *Paragonimus* has been definitively established. Suggested treatments include fenbendazole (Panacur, Hoechst-Roussel) at a dosage of 25–50 mg/kg PO q12h for 10–14 days in both dogs and cats and albendazole at a dosage of 25 mg/lb PO q12h for 10–21 days in cats.

Aleurostrongylus has been reported to resolve spontaneously within 6 months in cats. Therapy is indicated, however, when evidence of pulmonary inflammation exists. Suggested therapy is fenbendazole at 25–50 mg/kg/day PO for 10–14 days.

Treatment of *Capillaria* has not been definitively established. Suggested treatment includes levamisole (Levasole) at a dosage of 8 mg/kg/day PO for 5 days and fenbendazole at a dosage of 25–50 mg/lb/day PO for 10–14 days. Levamisole should not be used in cats owing to the potential of toxic side effects.

Filaroides hirthi may be treated with albendazole at a dosage of 50 mg/kg PO q12h for 5 days. Treatment is repeated in 21 days. Fenbendazole at a dosage of 50 mg/kg/day PO for 14 days has also been recommended. *F. hirthi* has been associated with fatal superinfections in immunosuppressed dogs.

PLEURAL DISEASES

Chylothorax

Chylothorax refers to the collection of chyle in the pleural space. A prominent clinical sign is respiratory distress characterized by a rapid respiratory rate and increased inspiratory effort. Radiographic findings are consistent with free fluid in the pleural space. Thoracocentesis should be performed and fluid submitted for cytology. Chylous fluid is white to pink, and cytology may reveal lymphocytes or neutrophils. A definitive diagnosis of chylothorax may be established using the ether clearance test, which causes the chylomicrons to clear. Alternatively, triglyceride and cholesterol levels in chylous fluid may be compared to the serum levels. The triglyceride level of chyle should be higher than that in serum. Cholesterol in chylous fluid is less than or equal to the serum cholesterol level.

Underlying causes of chylothorax include thoracic duct rupture and thoracic duct obstruction secondary to neoplasia, fungal granulomas, venous thrombi, heartworm disease, and possibly congestive heart failure. In many cases, a definitive cause is not established.

Standard Therapy. Medical therapy consists of thoracocentesis to remove fluid and stabilize ventilation and dietary therapy with a low-fat diet. Prescription Diet r/d (Hill's Pet Products) is the diet of choice. Fats may be supplemented using medium-chain triglyceride (MCT) oil (Mead Johnson) at 1 ml/kg/day as these medium-chain triglycerides are absorbed directly into the portal system, bypassing the intestinal lymphatics. If repeated thoracocentesis is necessary, it is recommended that a chest tube be placed.

Alternative Therapy. If medical therapy fails, surgical therapy is recommended. Techniques for thoracic duct ligation, pleuroperitoneal shunts, and pleurovenous shunts are described in veterinary surgery textbooks. Pleurodesis represents an alternative therapy in certain cases. In general, the prognosis for the chylothorax patient in which an underlying cause for the problem cannot be identified is guarded to poor without surgical intervention.

Pyothorax

Pyothorax refers to the collection of fluid and infected material in the pleural space. Pyothorax may occur as the result of direct introduction of infection into the pleural space by penetrating trauma or extension of infection from intrathoracic structures, or it may be secondary to systemic sepsis. Clinical signs include increased respiratory rate with a pronounced inspiratory phase, fever, anorexia, and weight loss. Diagnosis is established by radiographic findings consistent with pleural effusion and analysis of thoracocentesis fluid consistent with a purulent exudate. Pleural fluid should be submitted for both aerobic and anaerobic culture and sensitivity tests. Causative organisms are numerous, and appropriate treatment depends on definitive identification.

Standard Therapy. Therapy of pyothorax requires placement of an indwelling chest tube. Placement need be only unilateral in most patients. Continuous closed-suction drainage (Plur-E-Vak, Deknatel) is ideal for continuous drainage of exudate. If continuous suction is not available, intermittent manual suction is an alternative. Unfortunately, this technique is not as effective and results in less optimal clinical resolution in some cases. Continuous or intermittent drainage should be continued until less than 2–3 ml fluid/kg/day is being removed, the fluid is free of microorganisms and degenerate neutrophils, and there is radiographic evidence of resolution of the pyothorax.

Pleural lavage has not been definitively shown to offer any therapeutic advantage over drainage alone for the treatment of pyothorax, although lavage may be helpful in certain cases. The lavage solution should consist of a balanced electrolyte solution (lactated Ringer's or NaCl 0.9%); 20 ml/kg is used for infusion. Heparin may be added to the lavage fluid at 1500 units/L of lavage solution. The fluid should be warmed to body temperature prior to lavage and then infused over a 5- to 10-minute period during which the infusion is stopped if any respiratory distress is noted. Lavage should be repeated two to three times daily and the fluid monitored for bacteria and degenerate neutrophils. Plasma protein and electrolytes should be monitored in the patient receiving pleural lavage, as they may be depleted by this procedure.

Antibiotic therapy should be initiated with a parenteral synthetic penicillin such as ampicillin at a dose of 20 mg/kg IV q6h. Other antibiotics that may be considered include cephalosporins, clindamycin, chloramphenicol, and metronidazole. If a gram-negative aerobe is suspected, either gentamicin or trimethoprim-sulfonamide should be considered. Therapy is altered based on the results of culture and sensitivity. Pleural fluid cytology and Gram stain should be repeated every 24–48 hours. A culture is repeated if bacteria continue to be present several days after initiation of therapy or if a change is noted in organism morphology. Administration of the antibiotic may be changed to the oral route when the clinical condition has improved enough to warrant removal of the tube; that antibiotic therapy is then continued for 4–6 weeks following removal of the thoracostomy tube.

After tube removal, the complete blood count and thoracic radiographs should be reevaluated every 2 weeks until antibiotics are discontinued. The prognosis for complete recovery is good in the immunocompetent patient treated aggressively with thoracic drainage and antibiotic therapy. The prognosis is poor in immunocompromised patients or those with an uncorrected underlying problem such as a thoracic foreign body. Potential adverse sequelae include restrictive pleuritis and pleural adhesions.

SUGGESTED READINGS

Diseases of the Upper Airways

Aron D: Laryngeal paralysis. In: Kirk RW, ed. Current Veterinary Therapy X. Philadelphia: WB Saunders, 1989;353.

Bedford PG: Diseases of the nose and throat. In: Ettinger SJ, ed. Textbook of Veterinary Internal Medicine. Philadelphia: WB Saunders, 1990;768.

Vaden S, Ford RB: Medical management of upper respiratory tract disease. In: Kirk RW, ed. Current Veterinary Therapy X. Philadelphia: WB Saunders, 1989;337.

Venker-van Haagen AJ: Laryngeal diseases of dogs and cats. In: Kirk RW, ed. Current Veterinary Therapy IX. Philadelphia: WB Saunders, 1986;265.

Diseases of the Lower Airways

Amis TC: Chronic bronchitis in dogs. In: Kirk RW, ed. Current Veterinary Therapy X. Philadelphia: WB Saunders, 1989;369.

Barnes PJ: A new approach to the treatment of asthma. N Engl J Med 1989;321:1517.

Bauer TG: Pulmonary hypersensitivity disorders. In: Kirk RW, ed. Current Veterinary Therapy X. Philadelphia: WB Saunders, 1989;369.

Dye J, McKiernan B, Jones S, Neft-Davis C, et al: Sustained-release theophylline pharmacokinetics in the cat. J Vet Pharmacol Therapy 1989;12:133.

Ettinger SJ, Ticer JW: Diseases of the trachea. In: Ettinger SJ, ed. Textbook of Veterinary Internal Medicine. Philadelphia: WB Saunders, 1989;795.

Fingland RB: Tracheal collapse. In: Kirk RW, ed. Current Veterinary Therapy X. Philadelphia: WB Saunders, 1989;353.

Ford RB, Vaden SL: Canine infectious tracheobronchitis. In: Greene CE, ed. Infectious Diseases of the Dog and Cat. Philadelphia: WB Saunders, 1990;259.

Hill NS: The use of theophylline in 'irreversible' chronic obstructive pulmonary disease. Arch Intern Med 1988;148:2579.

Moise NS, Spaulding GL: Feline bronchial asthma: pathogenesis, diagnostics, and therapeutic considerations. Compend Contin Educ 1981;3:1091.

Murciano D, Auclair M, Parilente, R, Aubier M: A randomized, controlled trial of theophylline in patients with severe chronic obstructive pulmonary disease. N Engl J Med 1989;320:1521.

Noone K: Pulmonary hypersensitivities. In: Kirk RW, ed. Current Veterinary Therapy IX. Philadelphia: WB Saunders, 1986;285.

Papich MG: Bronchodilator therapy. In: Kirk RW, ed. Current Veterinary Therapy IX. Philadelphia: WB Saunders, 1986;278.

Bronchoalveolar Diseases

Hawkins EC, Ettinger SJ, Suter PF: Diseases of the lower respiratory tract and pulmonary edema. In: Ettinger SJ, ed. Textbook of Veterinary Internal Medicine. Philadelphia: WB Saunders, 1989;816.

Tams TR: Pneumonia. In: Kirk RW, ed. Current Veterinary Therapy X. Philadelphia: WB Saunders, 1989;376.

Pleural Diseases

Bauer T: Mediastinal, pleural and extrapleural diseases. In: Ettinger SJ, ed. Textbook of Veterinary Internal Medicine. Philadelphia: WB Saunders, 1989;867.

Bauer T: Pyothorax. In: Kirk RW, ed. Current Veterinary Therapy IX. Philadelphia: WB Saunders, 1986;292.

Fossum TW, Birchard SJ: Chylothorax. In: Kirk RW, ed. Current Veterinary Therapy X. Philadelphia: WB Saunders, 1989;393.

Harpster NK: Chylothorax. In: Kirk RW, ed. Current Veterinary Therapy IX. Philadelphia: WB Saunders, 1986;295.

Scherding RG: Diseases of the pleura and pleural space. In: Scherding RG, ed. The Cat Diseases and Clinic Management. New York: Churchill Livingstone, 1989;819.

CHAPTER EIGHT

Diseases of the Digestive Tract

Michael D. Lorenz and Duncan C. Ferguson

VOMITING

Vomiting is caused by many disorders involving several organ systems. The pathophysiology of vomiting and its differential diagnosis have been previously described. Definitive treatment varies depending on the specific underlying cause. Before symptomatic therapy is undertaken, a sound plan for diagnosis of the specific cause must be formulated. Laboratory evaluation, including a complete blood count (CBC), serum biochemical profile, and urinalysis, made prior to any therapy, not only aids in differentiating the causes of vomiting, it provides assessment of the metabolic consequences caused by the loss of fluid, electrolytes, buffers, and calories. Furthermore, antiemetics may mask signs of a potentially fatal disorder and may delay diagnosis and definitive treatment. Symptomatic therapy should decrease further loss of fluid, electrolytes, and buffers and correct existing dehydration and electrolyte and acid-base imbalances.

Standard Therapy

With acute vomiting, confine the animal in a quiet place and withhold food and water for 24 hours. Allow the animal to lick ice cubes and drink small quantities of a carbonated beverage such as ginger ale. If dehydration is present, parenteral fluid therapy is indicated (see Chapter 1). Ringer's solution or 0.9% saline solution is used for therapy of dehydration associated with metabolic alkalosis or normal acid-base status. Lactated Ringer's solution is the fluid of choice for dehydration associated with metabolic acidosis. Although complete arterial blood gas/pH analysis is needed for thorough evaluation of most patients, plasma total CO_2 (TCO_2) is comprised mostly of bicarbonate and is a reasonable clinical substitute for measuring plasma bicarbonate. Decreased TCO_2 is associated with metabolic acidosis, and increased TCO_2 is indicative of metabolic alkalosis.

Depletion of body potassium and hypokalemia may be caused by profuse vomiting. Hypokalemia may be especially severe in alkalotic patients. If urine output is normal, potassium should be added to the fluid being used whenever vomiting is persistent and profuse and whenever hypokalemia is suspected or confirmed. The daily requirement of potassium is approximately 1–3 mEq/kg/day. Potassium at a dosage of 35 mEq/L can be safely administered subcutaneously. If this solution is given intravenously, the rate of administration should not exceed 0.5 mEq of potassium per kilogram body weight per hour. Electrocardiographic (ECG) monitoring can detect cardiotoxicity associated with intravenous potassium administration.

Antiemetics. Antiemetics should be used with caution, as they may hide clinical signs of a serious underlying disease and may have serious side effects. They are indicated when vomiting is especially profuse or protracted, leading to serious fluid, electrolyte, or acid-base disturbances. Antiemetics block one or more of the vomiting reflex pathways. Efferent pathways from peripheral receptors synapse directly on the emetic center in the medulla. Changes within the cerebrospinal fluid and pathways from the cerebrum and limbic system also directly stimulate the emetic center. Receptors are present in the chemoreceptor trigger zone (CRTZ) located in the brain stem. The CRTZ is stimulated by the vestibular system and blood-borne toxins; it stimulates receptors in the emetic center, and the vomiting reflex is initiated. The ideal antiemetic blocks activity in both the emetic center and the CRTZ without causing side effects such as depression and gastric atony. Most centrally active antiemetics interfere with the release of neurotransmitters. Acetylcholine is the primary neurotransmitter in the emetic center and in peripheral receptors. Dopamine is the primary neurotransmitter in the CRTZ.

Several classes of antiemetics are used to help control vomiting in dogs and cats. Of which, the phenothiazines and prokinetic agents are most useful. The phenothiazines antagonize dopamine and histamine and inhibit transmission in the CRTZ and emetic center. They are the most effective antiemetics used in small animals and are the initial drugs of choice. Prochlorperazine (Compazine, SmithKline Beecham) is our first choice in both dogs and cats. It is given at a dosage of 0.5 mg/kg three or four times a day intramuscularly or intravenously. Sedation and α-adrenergic receptor blockade are side effects. The administration of any phenothiazine to dehydrated or hypovolemic patients must be supported by adequate fluid therapy. Chlorpromazine (Thorazine, SmithKline Beecham) may also be used at a dosage of 0.5 mg/kg IM or IV three or four times a day. It tends to cause greater sedation than prochlorperazine.

Metoclopramide (Reglan, A.H. Robins) is a prokinetic agent that antagonizes dopamine in the CRTZ. It also sensitizes gastrointestinal smooth muscle to stimulation by acetylcholine and thus increases the tone of the lower esophageal sphincter, increases contractions of the esophagus and stomach, and promotes pyloric relaxation. Metoclopramide is useful for suppressing vomiting associated with metabolic toxins and chemotherapeutic agents. Because it helps prevent gastric atony (an important sequela in vomiting patients), metoclopramide is useful for vomiting associated with severe gastroenteritis such as parvoviral enteritis. Metoclopramide is administered at a dose of 0.2–0.4 mg/kg PO or SC three times a day. Following subcutaneous administration, the half-life may be very short and the antiemetic effects fleeting. Given by constant intravenous infusion (1.0–2.0 mg/kg/24 hr), the antiemetic effects are greatly improved. Metoclopramide may cause excitement, restlessness, and behavioral changes. It is contraindicated in epileptics and patients with gastric outlet obstruction. Metoclopramide should be given with caution to animals with renal diseases because it is primarily eliminated in the kidney. Anticholinergics diminish its effects on the gastrointestinal tract, and when given with phenothiazines, neurologic side effects may be more common. Because of the short half-life and neurologic side effects at higher doses, we prefer prochlorperazine as the immediate choice for most vomiting patients.

The anticholinergics generally act by inhibiting the effects of acetylcholine on peripheral receptors. They do not effectively cross the blood-brain barrier and thus exert little inhibition on the emetic center. Peripherally, anticholinergics inhibit smooth muscle spasm and decrease acid secretion in the stomach. Because they inhibit gastrointestinal motility, anticholinergics may contribute to vomiting by causing gastric atony. In general, any anticholinergic agent should not be used for longer than 2–3 days.

Certain antihistamines, e.g., dimenhydrinate and diphenhydramine, suppress receptors in the vestibular system and in the CRTZ. They are used to prevent vomiting and nausea associated with motion sickness and vestibular disease. We prefer oral dimenhydrinate (Dramamine, Searle) at a dosage of 25–50 mg q8h for dogs and 12.5 mg q8h for cats.

Antacids. Drugs that inhibit the release of gastric acid or neutralize acid in the stomach may be useful adjuncts when vomiting is associated with hyperacidity or gastrointestinal ulceration.

Oral antacids have limited use in vomiting patients, as retention is a problem. They neutralize gastric acid and promote the healing of gastric ulcers. Oral suspensions of magnesium or aluminum hydroxide are given at a dosage of 5 to 10 ml PO four to six times per day. Constipation, diarrhea, and interference with the absorption of other drugs are side effects.

Histamine H_2-receptor antagonists decrease the secretion of gastric acid by blocking the stimulation of histamine in the gastric mucosa. Histamine, in combination with gastrin and acetylcholine, plays a prominent role in the secretory processes for gastric acid. Two drugs, cimetidine (Tagamet, Smith-Kline Beecham) and ranitidine (Zantac, Glaxo) have been used in dogs and cats. Ranitidine has a longer half-life and is more potent. Suggested dosages are, for cimetidine, 5–10 mg/kg PO or IV q6–12h and, for ranitidine, 2 mg/kg PO or IV q8h. Both may decrease the absorption of drugs requiring a low gastric pH. Cimetidine decreases the hepatic metabolism of diazepam and in humans exerts antiandrogenic effects.

Summary. The therapy of vomiting should follow these guidelines:

1. Effectively treat the underlying cause.
2. Withhold food and water for 24 hours.
3. Correct fluid, electrolyte, and acid-base imbalances.
4. Use centrally active antiemetics. Prochlorperazine is recommended.
5. Consider other drugs only for special situations.

REGURGITATION

Regurgitation is a passive event that results in the expulsion of food or fluid from the oral or pharyngeal cavities or, most commonly, the esophagus. Regurgitation does not cause serious changes in electrolyte or acid-base status; however, dehydration and weight loss may be severe. Most frequently, regurgitation is associated with esophageal disease such as obstruction or altered motility. Aspiration pneumonia is a common sequela to chronic regurgitation.

Definite therapy varies depending on the specific cause. The morphologic causes of regurgitation, such as esophageal foreign body, stricture, neoplasia, and vascular ring anomaly are corrected with surgery. The functional causes, such as congenital or acquired megaesophagus, are usually treated medically. Therapy should be directed at the primary cause (e.g., reflux esophagitis, myasthenia gravis, and polymyositis) as well as symptomatically to aid the passage of water and food into the stomach.

Standard Therapy

With megaesophagus, attempts should be made to supply calories by feeding the animal from an elevated platform. The animal should remain in the vertical position for 10–15 minutes after eating. Chunk (kibble) foods are preferred, as they are less easily aspirated than gruels. In some cases of congenital megaesophagus, vertical feeding alone may result in control of the clinical signs.

In some cases it is necessary to place a pharyngostomy or gastrostomy tube so adequate nutrients can be delivered to the stomach. In most cases a gastrostomy tube is preferred, as fewer complications from regurgitation are encountered. Thin gruels can be prepared in a blender and administered through the gastrostomy tube to meet calculated water and caloric requirements. Feeding is continued until hopefully the primary cause is removed and the esophagus regains normal function.

Reflux Esophagitis

The reflux of small amounts of gastric fluid into the esophagus is normal in dogs and cats. This material is quickly returned to the stomach by esophageal peristalsis, and any remaining gastric acid is usually neutralized by bicarbonate present in saliva. Normal tone in the lower esophageal sphincter (LES) prevents excessive reflux of gastric or duodenal contents. Disorders that decrease tone in the LES, such as general anesthesia or hiatal hernia, and chronic vomiting are the most common causes of reflux esophagitis in dogs and cats.

With acid reflux, pepsin is the most punitive substance, causing mucosal injury. With alkaline reflux (reflux of gastroduodenal contents), pancreatic trypsin is the most harmful substance. Injury to the esophageal mucosa may cause a variety of clinical signs including salivation, anorexia, repeated attempts to swallow, and standing with the head extended. In more severe cases, regurgitation and total anorexia may occur. Signs that develop within 1–4 days of general anesthesia are especially suggestive of reflux esophagitis. If not treated effectively, reflux esophagitis may cause esophageal stricture or megaesophagus. The clinical signs are suggestive in some cases, but a definitive diagnosis is best made via endoscopic examination of the distal esophagus. In some cases gross mucosal changes are mild or absent, and mucosal biopsies may be necessary to document the correct diagnosis.

Standard Therapy. Patients should be treated with bland low-fat diets and H_2-receptor antagonists. Cimetidine (Tagamet) 5 mg/kg three times a day or ranitidine (Zantac) 2 mg/kg twice a day should be given for 2–3 weeks. The oral antacid solutions, magnesium or aluminum hydroxide, 10 ml q2–3h, may be useful in acute cases but are usually rejected by dogs and cats. Clinical signs should improve in 2 weeks. The simultaneous administration of oral antacids with H_2-receptor antagonists should be avoided as the absorption of H_2-antagonists is reduced in this situation.

Alternative Therapy. Metoclopramide (Reglan) increases the LES pressure and decreases esophageal reflux. It increases the rate of gastric emptying and distal esophageal contractions. A dose of 0.2–0.4 mg/kg two or three times a day (30 minutes before meals and at bedtime) is recommended. Metoclopramide can be given concurrently with cimetidine. Side effects are rare but include nervousness and hyperexcitability.

Sucralfate (Carafate, Marion) is an aluminum salt that binds to the surface of injured gastrointestinal mucosa to form a protective barrier that also binds bile and pepsin, preventing further damage to mucosal cells. Used primarily to treat gastric ulcers, the liquid form of sucralfate may bind to esophageal ulcers. A dosage of 1 g/30 kg four times a day is suggested. Definitive studies using sucralfate for this purpose in dogs and cats have not been published. Side effects are rare in humans treated with sucralfate.

Esophageal Strictures

Strictures may occur anywhere in the esophagus but are most common at the thoracic inlet. They may result from any insult to the esophageal mucosa that produces injury extending into the muscle layers. The ingestion of strong acid or alkali, thermal burns, foreign body trauma, and reflux esophagitis are common causes. Chronic regurgitation is the most common clinical sign. The diagnosis can be confirmed utilizing barium paste or barium meal for the standard esophagram.

Standard Therapy. Surgical removal is satisfactory in fewer than 50% of cases operated. Alternatively, esophageal dilatation using graduated dilators or balloon catheters may be tried by clinicians skilled in this technique.

After dilatation, aggressive therapy for esophagitis is undertaken. Cimetidine, 5–10 mg/kg IM or PO q8h, is given. Prednisolone, 0.5–1.0 mg/kg/day, should be given to decrease production of new scar tissue. Therapy should be continued for 2 weeks.

GASTRIC DISORDERS

Acute Gastritis

Acute gastritis, common in dogs and cats, has many potential etiologies. Frequently, the etiology is never identified, and the diagnosis of acute gastritis is warranted when the signs of gastritis (vomiting) are acute and self-limiting. The most common cause of acute gastritis is related to the ingestion of rancid or spoiled food. The ingestion of foreign materials, plants and plant toxins, and hair causes gastritis by irritating the gastric mucosa. Several drugs, e.g., the nonsteroidal antiinflammatory drugs (NSAIDs), corticosteroids (especially dexamethasone), and antibiotics such as erythromycin, may cause acute gastritis. Certain infectious agents such as coronavirus, parvovirus, canine hepatitis virus, and canine distemper virus cause acute gastritis as a component of a more extensive digestive tract inflammation. Allergic reactions to a food antigen cause repeated episodes of acute gastritis in some dogs and cats. Lastly, the reflux of duodenal fluid into the stomach (alkaline reflux gastritis) may cause recurrent vomiting episodes of bile-stained fluid.

The primary clinical signs are vomiting and drooling. The characteristics of the vomitus depend on the severity of the mucosal injury. Vomiting of food and water is associated with simple acute gastritis. Repeated episodes of vomiting yellowish-green fluid, especially in the morning, is associated with alkaline reflux gastritis. The presence of bloody vomit suggests severe ulceration of the gastric mucosa.

Standard Therapy. The recommendations for symptomatic treatment of vomiting work well for the treatment of acute gastritis. The recommendations for therapy of chronic gastritis and gastric ulcers should also be reviewed.

TABLE 8-1. Suspected Causes of Chronic Gastritis in Dogs and Cats

Exogenous factors	*Endogenous factors*
Foreign materials	Excessive gastric acid production
Toxins	Zollinger-Ellison syndrome
Dietary constituents	Systemic mastocytosis
Drugs (glucocorticoids and the	Gastroduodenal reflux
nonsteroidal antiinflammatory	Immune-mediated factors
agents)	Parasites
	Dietary antigens
	Autoimmune factors
	Hypergastrinemia

Chronic Gastritis

Chronic gastritis is classified into three categories: erosive (gastric ulcer disease), nonerosive (superficial and atrophic gastritis), and specific based on histologic changes (eosinophilic, hypertrophic, and granulomatous). The etiology of chronic gastritis is usually not determined. The suspected causes are listed in Table 8-1. Chronic gastritis is diagnosed based on the clinical signs of persistent intermittent vomiting and nausea and endoscopic examination of the stomach. The specific type of chronic gastritis is identified through histologic examination of gastric mucosal biopsies.

Chronic Atrophic Gastritis. Chronic atrophic gastritis is characterized by a thin gastric mucosa, reduction in depth and size of the gastric glands, and replacement of parietal cells with mucus-secreting cells. There are variable inflammatory infiltrates in the gastric mucosa. Chronic atrophic gastritis may predispose an animal to the development of gastric ulcers. Immunologically mediated mechanisms are suspected as the underlying cause.

Standard Therapy. The diet should be changed to a nonallergenic, low-fat, low nondigestible fiber formulation. Commercial diets (i/d, Hill's Pet Products), may be beneficial. Diets containing cottage cheese and rice are better in some cases.

To prevent back-diffusion of hydrogen ions into the damaged gastric mucosa (an event that perpetuates further mucosal damage), H_2-antagonists may be beneficial. Cimetidine 5–10 mg/kg PO q6–8h, for 3–5 weeks is recommended.

Because of the suspected immune-mediated etiology, glucocorticosteroids may seem indicated. Their effectiveness has not been demonstrated in the dog and cat for this disease, and they may contribute to the development of ulcers if not used carefully.

Alternative Therapy. Refer to the section on the therapy of gastric ulcers for alternative therapies for treatment of chronic atrophic gastritis.

Chronic Erosive Gastritis (Gastric Ulcers). Gastric ulcers may result from any condition that destroys the mucosal protective barrier, allowing acid to back-diffuse into mucosal cells. This process leads to a chain of events that eventually destroy the mucosal cell. The gut mucosal protective barrier has two basic components: the mucus-bicarbonate barrier and the mucosal cell. The mucous gel layer has lubricating and acid-neutralizing functions but is less important for protection than are the mucosal cells.

The gastric epithelial cells help prevent acid back-diffusion through three primary mechanisms: rapid epithelial cell turnover, mucosal blood flow, and prostaglandin synthesis. The rapid cell turnover protects against shear forces in the gastrointestinal tract and promotes rapid healing following injury. The gastrointestinal mucosa has a rich vascular supply and high blood flow, which are necessary for maintenance of the mucous gel layer and support of rapid cell division. Loss of blood flow in the microcirculation produces cell death, mucosal erosions, and eventually ulceration. Prostaglandins of the E type have a protective role in the gastrointestinal tract, as they inhibit gastric acid secretion, increase mucosal bicarbonate secretion, and help maintain mucosal blood flow. They stimulate the secretion and formation of the mucous gel and may stimulate epithelial turnover and migration.

Many of the suspected causes of gastric ulcers interrupt one or more components of the gut protective barrier. Table 8-2 lists the various etiologies of gastric ulcers and the proposed mechanism(s).

The diagnosis of gastric ulcers is best achieved via gastroscopy.

Standard Therapy. The standard treatment of gastric ulcers is directed at suppression of acid secretion and cytoprotection. Acid suppression is thought to be generally beneficial for promoting the healing of gastric ulcers despite the fact that excess acid secretion may not be a major factor in many dogs and cats with gastric ulcers.

Although oral antacid drugs are a mainstay for the treatment of gastric ulcers in humans, their use in dogs and cats is limited by the frequency of administration required to maintain acid suppression. Liquid preparations containing $Al(OH)_3$ and $Mg(OH)_2$ (Gelusil II liquid, Parke-Davis; Amphogel 500 liquid, Wyeth) are given at a dose of 5–10 ml five or six times a day. Mild diarrhea or constipation may be side effects. Oral antacids decrease the absorption of digoxin, tetracycline, phenothiazines, corticosteroids, and cimetidine.

Regardless of cause, histamine H_2-receptor antagonists suppress the secretion of gastric acid because histamine is the final stimulator. This effect also decreases cholinergic and gastrin stimulatory effects. The drugs most commonly used are cimetidine (Tagamet) and ranitidine (Zantac). Cimetidine (5 mg/kg q6–8h) or ranitidine (2 mg/kg q8–12h) produces effective acid suppression and promotes ulcer healing. Either drug should be given for 3–4 weeks. The potential side effects of cimetidine in humans include gynecomastia (antiandrogenic effect) and decreased sperm counts. Cimetidine may cause mild neurologic signs (confusion, abnormal behavior, excitement, seizures). In humans the side effects of ranitidine are less than those of cimetidine. Cimetidine results in increased serum concentrations of procainamide, penicillin G, erythromycin, tetracycline, morphine, lidocaine, propranolol, digitoxin, theophylline,

TABLE 8-2. Proposed Etiologies and Mechanisms for the Development of Gastric Ulcers

Etiology	Mechanism
Drugs	
Nonsteroidal antiinflammatory drugs (NSAIDs)	Reduction in mucous gel barrier Focal ischemia Decreased mucosal bicarbonate secretion Decreased mucosal cell turnover rate
Corticosteroids	Increased gastric acid production Decreased mucous gel production Decreased mucosal cell turnover rate
Hypotension/shock/sepsis/stress	Decreased blood flow in microcirculation Increased gastric acid and enzyme secretion
Duodenal-gastric reflux	Increased permeability to hydrogen ions
Metabolic diseases	
Uremia	Toxins damage mucosal cells and microcirculation Increased serum gastrin
Hepatic failure	Reduced mucosal blood flow Loss of mucous gel barrier Increased gastrin levels
Systemic mastocytosis	Increased histamine levels Increased gastric acid secretion
Zollinger-Ellison syndrome	Increased gastrin secretion Increased gastric acid production

phenytoin, carbamazepine, diazepam, and warfarin. It decreases absorption of ketoconazole. None of these interactions has been definitively shown in the dog or cat.

Alternative Therapy. Sucralfate (Carafate) is an organoprotective agent composed of aluminum hydroxide and a sulfate sucrose complex. When solubilized in gastric acid, the sulfated sucrose adheres to the damaged mucosa, creating a protective barrier to further damage from hydrochloric acid and pepsin. Sucralfate stimulates prostaglandin release and inhibits pepsin activity, increases mucous gel production, and increases bicarbonate secretion. In human studies, sucralfate promoted ulcer healing equal to the effects of H_2-receptor antagonists.

The dose of sucralfate for dogs and cats is estimated at 1 g PO q8h for large dogs (>20 kg) and 0.5 g q8h for small dogs (<20 kg). Cats should receive 0.25–0.50 g q8–12h. Other oral medications should not be given within the 2 hours following sucralfate administration. Sucralfate can be given concurrently with cimetidine or ranitidine. Constipation is an infrequent side effect.

Investigational Therapy. Two H_2-receptor antagonists have become available for use in humans. Famotidine (Pepcid, Merck) is 32 times more potent than cimetidine, and the effects last for at least 12 hours following a single oral dose. The potency of nizatidine (Axid, Lilly) is similar to that of ranitidine. Use in dogs and cats has been limited, and dosages are not currently available for these species.

Omeprazole (Losec, Merck) is a benzimidazole compound that suppresses gastric acid secretion by inhibiting the secretagogue effects of histamine, acetylcholine, and gastrin. A single dose of omeprazole can inhibit acid secretion in dogs for 3–4 days, and a single 30 mg dose can maintain complete gastric anacidity for 24 hours. It is not clinically available because the long-term side effects are not totally understood. Chronic suppression of acid secretion may cause hypergastrinemia, which produces gastric mucosal cell hyperplasia, rugal hypertrophy, and carcinoids.

Pirenzepine is an anticholinergic compound that more selectively suppresses the acetylcholine-stimulated release of gastric acid. Like other anticholinergic drugs, pirenzepine may cause side effects associated with antimuscarinic activity on the gastrointestinal tract. Hypomotility (bowel stasis, ileus, gastric atony) and decreased mucus secretion may occur. Pirenzepine has not been carefully studied in dogs and cats for the treatment of gastrointestinal ulcers, and the dosage is currently unknown.

Synthetic prostaglandins of the E type can exert a protective effect on the gastric mucosa as previously described. Misoprostol (Cytotec, Searle) is a derivative of PGE_1 and has been used in humans to treat gastrointestinal ulcers that become refractory to cimetidine. It is not licensed in the United States but is available in Canada. Misoprostol has antisecretory and cytoprotective effects. The dosage in humans is 200 µg PO q6h for 4–8 weeks. Diarrhea is the most frequent side effect.

Chronic Hypertrophic Gastritis. Chronic hypertrophic gastritis is characterized by focal, regional, or diffuse thickening of the gastric rugal folds. Histologically, glandular proliferation, cellular hyperplasia, and various inflammatory cellular infiltrates are seen. The cause is unknown, although several potential etiologies are suspected. Mucosal stimulation by histamine, gastrin, and acetylcholine may be responsible in some cases. Elevated gastrin levels are associated with renal tubular defects in Basenji dogs with gastrinomas and antral G-cell hyperplasia. Systemic mastocytoma may cause hyperplastic changes in the gastric mucosa via chronic histamine release. Pyloric outflow obstruction secondary to mucosal hyperplasia is recognized in small breeds of dogs with nervous behavioral characteristics. Genetic and neuroendocrine causes are proposed etiologies.

The clinical signs include vomiting, anorexia, abdominal pain, melena, diarrhea, and weight loss. In the Basenji dog, signs of hypoproteinemia (edema, ascites) may develop, as protein loss from the gastric mucosa (protein-losing gastropathy) can occur. Pyloric outlet obstruction causes intermittent vomiting of undigested food that may continue for months to years. The diagnosis of chronic hyperplastic gastritis is confirmed by gastroscopy and histologic evaluation of mucosal biopsies. Barium contrast radiographs of the stomach may demonstrate thickened rugal folds and pyloric outflow obstruction.

Standard Therapy. The diet should be changed to a low-fat, easily digestible formulation such as Prescription Diet i/d (Hill's Pet Products). A hypoallergenic diet may be helpful. Antral and pyloric hyperplastic disease that results in pyloric outflow obstruction must be surgically corrected. Cimetidine (5–10 mg/kg q8h) is recommended when gastric ulcers are identified. Cimetidine is also useful for hypergastrinemic conditions.

Alternative Therapy. The reader is referred to the section on treatment of gastric ulcers, as the same pharmacologic agents and principles may be used for treatment of chronic hyperplastic gastritis.

Eosinophilic Gastritis

Eosinophilic gastritis is characterized by eosinophilic cellular infiltrates in the gastric mucosa. In severe cases, eosinophilic infiltrates and fibrous tissue infiltration may occur in all layers of the gastric wall. Eosinophilic gastritis may occur in association with diffuse involvement of the gastrointestinal tract (eosinophilic gastroenteritis-colitis). The etiology is unknown, but an immunologic response by the host to parasitic or dietary antigens is most often proposed. The clinical signs include vomiting, melena, anorexia, and weight loss. Mucosal ulceration may occur. Diagnosis is based on histologic evaluation of mucosal biopsies. Associated peripheral eosinophilia and eosinophilic lymphadenitis may support the clinical diagnosis.

Standard Therapy. Affected animals should be treated with a hypoallergenic diet for 3–4 weeks. Prednisolone (0.5–1.0 mg/kg) divided twice a day is given for 2 weeks to suppress the inflammatory process. The dosage of prednisolone is then changed to 1 mg/kg every other day for 2 weeks and then decreased to 0.5 mg/kg every other day for an additional 2 weeks. At this point, prednisolone should be discontinued if the disease is in remission. Remission hopefully can be maintained through dietary control. In some cases relapse of signs may necessitate long-term glucocorticoid therapy. Cats may respond less dramatically than dogs to steroid therapy.

Alternative Therapy. The reader is referred to the section for therapy of gastrointestinal ulcers for additional strategies that may be useful in the management of refractory cases of eosinophilic gastritis or those cases with concomitant mucosal ulcers.

Investigational Therapy. Sodium cromoglycate, a mast cell stabilizer, has been used experimentally to treat inflammatory bowel disease in humans. Although its use for eosinophilic gastritis has not been described for dogs and cats, its pharmacologic action may be of some benefit in this disease. A dosage has not been established for dogs or cats.

Canine Zollinger-Ellison Syndrome (Gastrinoma)

The canine Zollinger-Ellison syndrome is caused by nonbeta islet cell tumors of the pancreas that hypersecrete the hormone gastrin. The hypersecretion of gastrin results in extreme hyperacidity of the stomach and upper small intestine. Hypertrophic gastritis, gastric and duodenal ulcers, and small intestinal malabsorption and steatorrhea may occur. Hypochloremia, hypokalemia, and hypocalcemia are associated electrolyte abnormalities. The tumor may metastasize to the liver and regional lymph nodes.

The diagnosis is based on the clinical signs of persistent vomiting, diarrhea, and gastrointestinal ulceration plus evidence of elevated gastrin levels in the presence of hyperchlorhydria. Gastric secretory testing may provide evidence to support the diagnosis. Surgical exploration of the abdomen may be needed to identify the tumor if ultrasonography is not diagnostic.

Standard Therapy. Surgical removal of the tumor provides definitive treatment; however, this option is frequently impossible because the tumor has a strong propensity to metastasize to the liver. Medical therapy is used to ameliorate the effects of hypergastrinemia. Ranitidine (2 mg/kg q12h) should be administered. Sucralfate (0.5–1.0 g q8h) should be given 2 hours after ranitidine therapy. Without total tumor excision, the long-term prognosis is poor.

Investigational Therapy. Because of its greater potency, famotidine has been useful for managing human patients with this disease. A dose of 80–480 mg/day has been used in humans. Pirenzepine, when combined with H_2-receptor antagonists, may also be useful. Neither drug has been carefully evaluated for the treatment of gastrinomas in dogs and cats. Somatostatin analogues (Sandostatin, Sandoz) may prolong remission of clinical signs when combined with cimetidine, carafate, or both. A dosage of 10–20 µg/kg SC three times a day is recommended.

Gastric Dilatation–Volvulus

Gastric dilatation–volvulus (GDV) occurs most frequently in young, large breed, deep chested dogs. It is less frequently reported in small dogs and cats. The exact etiology is unknown, but overeating, aerophagia, laxity of the gastrohepatic ligament, and gastric retention may contribute to development of the disorder. Generally, gastric dilatation precedes volvulus, but there must be a source of gas and obstruction to the removal of gas from the stomach. If not corrected, GDV results in serious fluid, acid-base, electrolyte, and coagulation disorders, with cardiovascular dysfunction. Mortality rates are high if appropriate medical and surgical treatment is not immediately undertaken.

The diagnosis of GDV is based on the clinical signs of acute retching (often nonproductive), abdominal distention, and hypotension or shock. Radiographic confirmation should be delayed until gastric distention is relieved.

Standard Therapy. The medical management of GDV is reviewed in this section. The reader is referred to other texts for specific descriptions of the surgical techniques indicated for the treatment of GDV. The progression of medical therapy is as follows.

1. Immediately relieve gastric distention by passing a large-diameter orogastric tube.
2. If decompression is not effective or the orogastric tube cannot be passed into the stomach, gastrocentesis should be performed caudal to the costal arch in the right flank. A 16-gauge needle should be used. Gastrostomy can also be used as a decompressive technique and has been effective in some institutions.
3. Once decompression is complete, cardiovascular function should improve. Intravenous infusion of lactated Ringer's solution should be started at a rate of 90 ml/kg/hr to support cardiovascular and renal functions. Prior to fluid therapy, obtain blood for baseline packed cell volume (PCV), white blood cell (WBC) count, and total protein, electrolyte, and acid-base values.
4. Intravenous potassium therapy (not more than 0.5 mEq/kg/hr) should be initiated to correct total body hypokalemia.
5. Cardiovascular function and fluid therapy should be continuously monitored by ECG.
6. Administer prednisolone sodium succinate (10 mg/kg) or dexamethasone sodium phosphate (4 mg/kg) intravenously every 4–6 hours if septic shock is suspected.
7. Administer ampicillin (10 mg/kg) intravenously every 6 hours.
8. Cardiac arrhythmias (ventricular tachyarrhythmias) are treated when they are multifocal or rapid (140 bpm) or there are signs of shock. Administer lidocaine 100 µg/kg/min IV until the arrhythmias are effectively controlled. Arrhythmias generally resolve within 2–4 days.
9. Monitor blood coagulation carefully. The activated clotting time is a useful screening test. Complete coagulation tests may be indicated when disseminated coagulopathy is suspected as a sequela to the endotoxic shock encountered in some cases of GDV.
10. Whole blood transfusions or plasma may be required before and after surgery. Early crossmatching of all GDV patients with impending shock is wise.

Alternative Therapy. The use of flunixin meglumine (Banamine, Schering) is controversial: Its antiprostaglandin activity may be beneficial in reducing hypotension associated with endotoxic shock, but it may also potentiate gastric hemorrhage and ulceration. A dose of 1.1 mg/kg IV is used in the dog, but therapy must be limited to two doses.

INTESTINAL DISORDERS

Diarrhea

Diarrhea is caused by several disorders of the gastrointestinal tract. Definitive therapy is based on finding and correcting the underlying cause. Symptomatic therapy should not be used as a substitute for a sound diagnostic plan aimed at discovering the primary cause. Symptomatic therapy may ameliorate the severity of diarrhea and decrease the severity of associated fluid, electrolyte, and acid-base imbalances. This section describes the symptomatic (pharmacologic) therapy of diarrhea regardless of the underlying etiology.

Motility Modifiers. The primary movements of the intestinal tract are mass peristalsis and rhythmic segmental contractions. Peristalsis moves ingesta aborally. Segmental contractions mix ingesta and retard its aboral movement. Segmental contractions aid digestion and absorption by slowing the gastrointestinal transit time. Peristalsis aids elimination by moving ingesta through the gastrointestinal tract. With diarrhea, segmental contractions tend to decrease in strength and frequency, which favors rapid transit of ingesta because even weak peristalsis can move ingesta a great distance. When the transit time is decreased, the absorptive capacity of the colon may be overloaded, and the fluid content of feces is greatly increased. Rapid transit decreases digestion and absorption of nutrients, which increases the osmotic gradient within the gastrointestinal lumen. Osmotically active substances greatly enhance the fluidity of feces and play a major role in the pathophysiology of diarrhea.

When motility modification is used, care must be exercised to not enhance pathophysiologic principles that contribute to diarrhea. The narcotic analgesics enhance segmental contractions and may decrease intestinal secretion of fluid and enhance fluid absorption. They reduce abdominal pain and cramping and also reduce tenesmus. They are contraindicated for infectious diarrhea and with hepatic disease.

Diphenoxylate (Lomotil, Searle) is recommended for symptomatic use in dogs at a dosage of 0.1 mg/kg PO q6–8h. Diphenoxylate can be given to cats at a dose of 0.25 mg PO twice daily. Because this drug may cause hyperactivity and respiratory depression in cats, its use should be limited to 2–3 days.

Loperamide (Imodium, Ortho Pharmaceutical) is a synthetic narcotic marketed primarily for the symptomatic control of diarrhea. It acts more promptly and lasts longer than diphenoxylate. In dogs an oral dose of 0.08 mg/kg q8h is recommended. Loperamide is not recommended for cats.

The anticholinergics decrease intestinal motility but most significantly decrease segmental contractions. Although they decrease the secretion of fluid and electrolytes, anticholinergics may actually shorten gastrointestinal transit time, an effect that favors the diarrheal state. Anticholinergics reduce tenesmus and pain associated with colonic inflammation. Chronic use of anticholinergics may cause intestinal ileus and a worsening of diarrhea. They are contraindicated with infectious enteritis.

Propantheline (Pro-Banthine, Searle) 0.25 mg/kg q8h PO reduces tenesmus and abdominal pain and enhances intestinal absorption of fluid. It can be used in dogs and cats.

Protectants, Absorbents, and Antisecretory Products. The effectiveness of kaolin and pectin in the management of diarrhea has been severely questioned in recent times. There is considerable evidence that fecal water and electrolyte content actually increase after kaolin and pectin administration. Still, there might be some beneficial effect from its coating action on the gastrointestinal mucosa.

There is some experimental and clinical evidence to support the role of salicylates in decreasing gastrointestinal secretion associated with enterotoxin release. Salicylates, perhaps through their antiprostaglandin effects, inhibit cyclic adenosine monophosphate (cAMP) and thus decrease intestinal secretion of fluid. Bismuth subsalicylate (Pepto-Bismol, Norwich-Eaton; Corrective Mixture, SmithKline Beecham) is useful in dogs and cats with hypersecretory states in the gastrointestinal tract. A dose of 2.5 ml/kg q4–6h is recommended in dogs and 1–2 ml/kg q8h is recommended for cats. Cats should be observed closely for signs of salicylate toxicity. There are few side effects associated with bismuth subsalicylate except for dark-colored stools.

Antibiotic Therapy. Unless a specific form of infectious enteritis is identified, antibiotics are not indicated for the symptomatic treatment of diarrhea. Oral aminoglycosides have been used for many years, although their use may be detrimental. Antibiotics may destroy normal gut flora that compete with pathogenic bacteria for niches on mucosal cells. When certain pathogenic bacteria attach to mucosal cells, they secrete enterotoxins that cause intestinal hypersecretion of fluid. In subsequent sections, specific uses of certain antibacterial drugs are described for appropriate diseases.

Idiopathic Hemorrhagic Gastroenteritis

Idiopathic hemorrhagic gastroenteritis (HGE) is an acute disorder of primarily young small-breed dogs. It is characterized by an acute onset of vomiting followed quickly by foul-smelling bloody diarrhea and severe hemoconcentration and hypotension. The bloody feces may have the characteristics of raspberry jam. Although tremendous mucosal hemorrhage occurs, there is little evidence of inflammation in the gastrointestinal tract wall. The lesions and clinical signs are most similar to those observed in endotoxic shock. Various etiologies have been proposed including bacterial endotoxins, immune-mediated disease, and neuroendocrine or vascular disorders. The disease is diagnosed by the typical clinical signs, markedly elevated PCV (60–80%), and absence of other diseases. The differential diagnosis should include the ingestion of toxins such as heavy metals, salmonellosis and campylobacterosis, parvoviral enteritis, and endotoxic shock.

Standard Therapy. The treatment of HGE is directed at controlling hemo-concentration and fluid loss. The etiology is unknown, and therapy is supportive because the process is generally self-limiting. Lactated Ringer's solution is given intravenously at a rapid rate (90 ml/kg/hr) until the PCV falls below 50%. The rate is then decreased to 45 ml/kg/hr for the next 24 hours. Shock doses of corticosteroids (prednisolone sodium succinate 10 mg/kg IV) should be administered if fluid therapy does not control the signs of shock. Because the permeability of the intestinal wall to gut bacteria may be increased, ampicillin 10 mg/kg q6h is given intravenously for 24 hours followed by 48 hours of oral or parenteral therapy. Food and water should be withheld for 24–48 hours; once the vomiting and diarrhea subside, bland food can be offered in small amounts two or three times a day. Centrally active antiemetics should be used with care, as they may worsen the extreme hypotension present in HGE. Their use is restricted to cases with protracted vomiting but only after the blood pressure has been stabilized with fluid therapy. Anticholinergics and narcotic analgesics are not indicated for the control of diarrhea.

HGE normally resolves within 24–48 hours followed by 2–3 days of dark, tarry feces. With prompt proper fluid therapy, the mortality associated with HGE is low. Some dogs experience multiple episodes.

Bacterial Enteritis

Although gut bacteria may play a secondary role in a variety of acute and chronic enteropathies, pathogenic enteric bacteria are not common etiologies of enteritis in dogs and cats. The bacteria most commonly identified include *Salmonella, Escherichia coli, Clostridium*, and *Campylobacter*. Bacterial enteritis is diagnosed by identifying the causative organism in feces. Caution should be exercised when interpreting fecal cultures, as the same bacteria can be isolated from asymptomatic dogs and cats.

Salmonellosis. *Salmonella* organisms produce three types of disease: purely enteric, enteric with fever, and systemic. Dogs and cats may be asymptomatic carriers of *Salmonella* and develop clinical signs following stress of another disease or therapy that compromises immune function. Salmonellosis may be acquired through nosocomial infection. *Salmonella* associated with nosocomial infection may be resistant to a variety of antibiotics. *Salmonella* organisms invade the mucosa and produce cellular damage by secreting cytotoxins. The route of exposure is fecal-oral. *Salmonella* organisms tend to attack the ileum and colon. Some strains stimulate hypersecretion as well as mucosal inflammation and necrosis. Diagnosis is based on identification of the organism in feces and correlation with the clinical signs.

Standard Therapy. The pure enteric (mucosal) form of salmonellosis is usually self-limiting, and the supportive care described for the treatment of diarrhea is recommended. When systemic signs such as fever are present, systemic antibiotics may be indicated. Trimethoprim-sulfadiazine (Tribrissen, Burroughs) 15–20 mg/kg q12h for 2 weeks is administered. Therapy at a dose of 25–30 mg/kg/day for an additional 4 weeks may help eliminate the carrier state. In some areas of the United States, *Salmonella* organisms are resistant to a variety of antibiotics, and definitive therapy should be based on results of antibiotic sensitivity tests. There is some evidence that antibiotic therapy may prolong the convalescent carrier state of this disease.

The systemic form of salmonellosis is life-threatening and associated with a high mortality rate. Vigorous therapy for endotoxemia is usually required. Antibiotics such as amikacin (Amikin, Bristol) 5 mg/kg q8h IV or IM or gentamicin (Gentocin, Schering) 2 mg/kg q8h IM are usually effective. Treatment with these antibiotics warrants close monitoring for renal toxicity.

Close attention should be given to the prevention of nosocomial infection and the zoonotic implications of the disease. Strict sanitation must be enforced. In kennel outbreaks, all dogs, human caretakers, sanitary procedures, and diets should be closely examined as possible sources of infection. The indiscriminate use of corticosteroids and antibiotics may also be contributing factors.

Campylobacteriosis. *Campylobacter jejuni* is an uncommon cause of enteric disease in dogs and cats, although it is relatively common in humans. Because of better culture techniques for isolating the organism and increased awareness by veterinarians of the disease, an increasing number of animal cases are being reported. *Campylobacter*, like *Salmonella*, invades the gastrointestinal mucosa and in humans may cause systemic disease. An enterotoxin may also be secreted, which in turn stimulates hypersecretion by the gastrointestinal mucosa.

Dogs and cats may be asymptomatic carriers of *Campylobacter* and thus are important sources of infection to humans. The role of *Campylobacter* in creating disease in dogs and cats needs further study, as there appears to be marked differences in susceptibility in these species.

A presumptive diagnosis of campylobacteriosis is based on the clinical signs plus identification of the organism in feces. *Campylobacter* is isolated on special culture media, and dark-field or phase contrast microscopy may identify typical bacteria in the feces. With both procedures, fresh feces must be used.

Standard Therapy. *Campylobacter* responds to aminoglycoside antibiotics, erythromycin, doxycycline, and chloramphenicol. When vomiting is absent, erythromycin (10 mg/kg PO q8h) is the drug of choice. Therapy should be continued for 7–10 days. If animals experience gastrointestinal side effects from erythromycin, doxycycline (Vibramycin, Pfizer) (3–5 mg/kg q12h PO or IV) is recommended. When vomiting precludes oral therapy or serious systemic signs are present, gentamicin (2 mg/kg q8h IM) is preferred. Good supportive care, as previously described, is recommended.

As with *Salmonella* infection, prevention is through good sanitation and identification of infection sources such as carrier animals and food.

Other Enteric Bacteria. Certain strains of *E. coli* and *Shigella* may cause enteric and systemic disease in dogs and cats. However, their role is not clearly understood, and a diagnosis based solely on fecal cultures must be carefully interpreted. In debilitated or stressed dogs and cats, both organisms are capable of mucosal invasion or cytopathic injury. The role of enterotoxins elaborated by these bacteria is not clear as a mechanism for diarrhea in dogs and cats.

Therapy is indicated when systemic signs are present and a culture provides presumptive evidence of infection. The aminoglycoside antibiotics are generally effective and should be given parenterally. Gentamicin 2 mg/kg q8h or amikacin 5 mg/kg q8h is recommended. Definitive therapy is based on antibiotic sensitivity tests. Good supportive care is required. Prevention is through good sanitation.

The bacterium *Yersinia enterocolitica* may cause enteric disease in dogs, and such dogs should be considered a possible reservoir for human infection. Special culture requirements exist for the growth of *Y. enterocolitica*. The antibiotic of choice is trimethoprim-sulfadiazine (15 mg/kg q12h) for 1 week. Sources of infection include water, food, and animal or human carriers.

Viral Enteritis

In susceptible dogs, three viruses are known to produce acute gastroenteritis, fever, and depression. Severity of clinical signs depends on the virus, rate of infection, degree of immunity, and secondary bacterial complications.

Of the three viruses, canine parvovirus (CPV) is the most virulent and causes the most severe disease. Clinical infections are associated with severe, often hemorrhagic vomiting and diarrhea, lymphopenia and neutropenia, multifocal myocardial necrosis (puppies less than 8 weeks of age), and immunosuppression (i.e., failure to respond to distemper vaccination). Mortality is high among neonatal puppies.

Canine coronavirus (CCV) produces clinical signs less severe than CPV. Mortality may be high among neonatal puppies, but older puppies survive when given appropriate supportive care. Infections in older animals are generally mild or inapparent. Unlike CPV, CCV rarely causes fever, and leukopenia and bloody feces are uncommon.

Rotaviruses may cause clinical signs in dogs less than 6 months of age. In general, the clinical signs are mild or subclinical.

Canine enteric viral infections are confirmed by demonstrating the virus in feces or finding a rising antibody titer in serum from convalescent animals. Good sanitation practices may help control spread of viral enteritis. Effective vaccines are available for the prevention of CPV. The effectiveness of CCV vaccines is questionable. No vaccine exists for rotavirus infection.

Feline panleukopenia virus (FPV) is a parvovirus that is especially virulent in rapidly dividing cells of the intestinal tract, bone marrow, and cerebellum. In susceptible cats, FPV produces a serious, often fatal enteritis. Clinical signs include severe vomiting, watery diarrhea, depression, anorexia, and fever. Extreme panleukopenia and dehydration are common findings. In utero infection with FPV causes cerebellar hypoplasia, and affected kittens develop nonprogressive cerebellar ataxia early in life. The diagnosis of FPV infection is made from the clinical signs and associated panleukopenia. Effective vaccines are available for the prevention of FPV infection. In fact, owing to good vaccination procedures, this disease is now rarely diagnosed in clinical practice.

Standard Therapy. Vigorous fluid therapy as described in Chapter 1 is the mainstay for therapy. Food and water is withheld until vomiting is controlled, and then easily digested food is given in small amounts several times a day.

For CPV and FPV infections, parenteral antibiotics should be given when signs of endotoxemia or severe hemorrhagic enteritis are present. Although the routine use of parenteral antibiotics is questioned for the therapy of viral enteritis, there is no evidence that their use is harmful. In addition, there is some evidence that secondary bacterial invasion of the damaged intestinal mucosa may be a factor associated with mortality. For these reasons, parenteral antibiotics effective against gram-positive anaerobes (ampicillin 10–15 mg/kg q6h IV) and gram-negative bacteria (gentamicin 2 mg/kg q8h IM) are recommended. Trimethoprim-sulfadiazine 15 mg/kg q12h IM or IV can also be used. Therapy is maintained for 5–7 days.

Centrally active antiemetics such as prochlorperazine may help control vomiting. Metoclopramide, when given by constant intravenous infusion (1.0–2.0 mg/kg/24 hr), is useful for CPV enteritis, as it has central antiemetic effects and decreases gastric atony.

Acute Colitis

The causes of acute colitis include spoiled food, bacteria, endoparasites, and the passage of abrasive foreign bodies. Clinical signs include mucoid diarrhea often containing undigested food. Tenesmus is usually present, and vomiting may occur. Colonoscopy reveals small punctate mucosal erosions or ulcers. The edges of these lesions may be friable and bleed easily. Fecal flotations and cultures should be performed to rule out parasitic and bacterial infections.

Standard Therapy. Therapy of acute colitis is directed at the underlying cause if it can be identified. Food is withheld for 24 hours, and oral glucose-electrolyte solutions (Entrolyte, SmithKline Beecham) can be given to maintain hydration. Parenteral fluid therapy with lactated Ringer's solution should be given to dehydrated patients. Trimethoprim-sulfadiazine (Tribrissen) 15 mg/kg twice a day should be given unless fecal cultures are positive for pathogenic organisms susceptible to other antibiotics. Diphenoxylate hydrochloride (0.1 mg/kg q6–8h), may relieve tenesmus and help control diarrhea. Propantheline (0.25 mg/kg q8h), is also effective in controlling tenesmus, but therapy should not exceed 48 hours. After 24 hours, a bland low-fiber diet including boiled lean hamburger or chicken plus cooked rice, pasta, or potatoes is started. Once signs are controlled, the regular diet can be gradually reinstituted.

Pseudomembranous Colitis

Pseudomembranous colitis (PMC) is an acute necrotizing disorder of the colon caused by a cytotoxin secreted by the bacterium *Clostridium difficile*. This bacteria overgrows the colon following the administration of antibiotics, especially the penicillins, cephalosporins, lincomycin, and clindamycin. It is frequently observed in laboratory animals and man but is uncommon in dogs and cats. Colonic signs generally develop 12–14 days after the start of antibiotic therapy. Colonoscopy reveals small whitish-yellow plaques that may coalesce to form a pseudomembrane. Diagnosis is based on the clinical signs of acute colitis associated with previous antibiotic therapy.

Standard Therapy. The offending antibiotic is discontinued, and vancomycin (Vancocin, Lilly) (5–12 mg/kg PO q8h) is administered to inhibit further growth of the cytotoxic clostridial organism. Supportive fluid therapy may be indicated. Motility-altering drugs are contraindicated.

Chronic Intestinal Diseases

Several diseases have been described in dogs and cats that cause chronic diarrhea associated with chronic inflammation of the small intestine or colon (or both). Most of these diseases have unknown etiologies. The inflammatory process may create abnormalities of digestion, absorption, and secretion. Therapy of the various disorders is described in the following sections. The therapy for inflammatory bowel disease is described in detail because it forms the basis for understanding the therapy of other disorders, such as intestinal malabsorption, protein-losing enteropathy, and lymphangiectasia.

Definitions. *Inflammatory Bowel Disease.* Inflammatory bowel disease (IBD) comprises a group of enteric diseases characterized by various inflammatory cell infiltrates in the mucosa and lamina propria. IBD may affect the small intestine, colon, or both regions. Lesion distribution may be focal, regional, or diffuse, and mucosal ulceration may be severe. IBD may cause malabsorption and lymphangiectasia as sequela to the chronic inflammatory process.

Malabsorption Syndrome. Intestinal malabsorption results from a variety of inflammatory processes that decrease the absorptive surface of the intestine (i.e., villous atrophy), infiltrate the gut wall inhibiting absorption, or destroy digestive enzymes in the brush border of the intestinal villi. Malabsorption should be viewed as a chronic sequela to an underlying disease and not a disease entity unto itself.

Lymphangiectasia. Intestinal lymphangiectasia describes dilatation of the lymphatics within the villi and gut wall. It is associated with intestinal malabsorption and protein-losing enteropathy. Although congenital lymphangiectasia occurs in dogs, most cases are caused by a variety of diseases that obstruct the normal flow of chyle from the intestine to the heart.

Protein-Losing Enteropathy. Protein-losing enteropathy describes a pathologic event associated with a variety of inflammatory enteric diseases whereby protein and lymphocytes are lost into the intestinal lumen. The intestinal loss of lymph is associated with IBDs but may be especially severe with lymphangiectasia.

Intestinal Bacterial Overgrowth. Intestinal bacterial overgrowth may be a sequela of several enteric diseases including pancreatic exocrine insufficiency and chronic antibiotic therapy. The overgrowth of the gut mucosa with certain enteric bacteria, especially *E. coli* and *Clostridium*, results in malabsorption through several pathologic mechanisms.

Inflammatory Bowel Disease

Inflammatory bowel disease has been described in dogs and cats. It includes a cluster of chronic enteropathies characterized by various types of inflammatory cell in the mucosa, submucosa, and lamina propria. IBD occurs in both the small and large bowels and may be regional or diffuse. The various forms of IBD recognized in dogs and cats are described in Table 8-3. The etiology of IBD is unknown, but an antigenic stimulus in the gut of a genetically primed host is a popular theory as the type and pattern of the cellular infiltrates suggest an immunologic mechanism.

Lymphocytic-Plasmacytic IBD. The characteristics of lymphocytic-plasmacytic IBD are outlined in Table 8-3. Diagnosis is based on finding the histologic lesion in mucosal biopsy specimens obtained via endoscopy or laparotomy. In the cat, disease of the small intestine is more common than the disease of the colon, which tends to predominate in dogs. Remember that small intestinal and colonic disease may coexist in the same patient.

Lymphocytic-Plasmacytic Enteritis.

1. *Standard therapy.* In both dogs and cats, the initial treatment of choice is corticosteroids. For mild to moderate disease, prednisolone at 0.5–1.0 mg/kg

TABLE 8-3. Characteristics of Inflammatory Bowel Diseases in Dogs and Cats

Specific Disease	Location	Lesion Characteristics	Proposed Etiology
Lymphocytic-plasmacytic enteropathy (LPE)	SI C	Infiltration of lamina propria with lymphocytes, plasma cells, and occasionally neutrophils; possible villous blunting and fibrosis	Food antigen Parasitic antigen Bacterial antigen
Eosinophilic enteropathy	SI C	Infiltration of mucosa with eosinophils; regional lymph nodes sometimes affected	Parasitic antigen Food antigen
Ulcerative colitis	C	Probably same as for LPE but a more severe form	See LPE
Histiocytic ulcerative colitis	C	Mucosa, submucosa, and lamina propria infiltrated with PAS-positive macrophages and other inflammatory cells	See LPE
Wheat-sensitive enteropathy (Irish setters)	Sl	Patchy villous atrophy	Failure to properly degrade gluten with subsequent hypersensitivity to gluten by-products

SI = Small intestine; C = Colon and rectum.

q12h PO is given for 2–3 weeks. For severe disease, the dosage of prednisolone is increased to 1.5–2.0 mg/kg q12h PO for 3–4 weeks. The response is generally good with a marked reduction in signs occurring within 5–7 days. If a good response occurs, the dose of prednisolone is reduced by half for an additional 2 weeks. Alternate-day prednisolone therapy is then instituted at 0.5–1.0 mg/kg for an additional 3–4 months. In some cases, corticosteroids can be withdrawn and remission maintained with dietary control.

Cats should be started immediately on low-gluten diets such as Science Diet Feline (Hill's Pet Products), Iams Feline (Iams Food Co.), or Prescription Diet c/d (Hill's Pet Products). Hypoallergenic baby food or boiled lamb or chicken can also be tried. Dietary control of signs may not be complete, but a much lower dose of corticosteroids may be needed to achieve remission.

Dogs should also receive a bland low-fiber diet or a hypoallergenic diet. Prescription Diet i/d, boiled lean hamburger and cooked rice, or cooked rice and low-fat cottage cheese are acceptable homemade diets. Prescription Diet d/d can also be tried, but occasionally this diet causes transitory diarrhea in dogs.

2. *Alternative therapy.* When corticosteroids fail to control the clinical signs or serious side effects develop, metronidazole (Flagyl, Searle) (10–20 mg/kg q8h) should be administered orally. Metronidazole has antiprotozoal activity but is used for IBD because it suppresses anaerobic bacteria in the gut and inhibits cell-mediated immune injury. Metronidazole may also suppress granuloma formation. In humans, metronidazole is effective for controlling the signs of Crohn's disease but is relatively ineffective for ulcerative colitis. Therapy must be evaluated for several weeks as the beneficial effects of metronidazole may develop slowly. Side effects associated with long-term metronidazole therapy include peripheral neuropathies and granulocytopathies.

In severe cases unresponsive to diet changes, corticosteroids or metronidazole, azathioprine (Imuran, Burroughs) 2 mg/kg PO daily is recommended based on the assumption that poorly controlled IBD results from an immune-mediated mechanism. The use of azathioprine is controversial, but studies of IBD in humans suggest that azathioprine may have a steroid-sparing effect. We recommend that prednisolone 1 mg/kg/day be used in combination with azathioprine while dietary modifications are also maintained. Side effects include bone marrow suppression and secondary infections from immune suppression.

3. *Investigational therapy.* The reader is referred to the following sections on the therapy of IBD in the colon.

Lymphocytic Plasmacytic Colitis. Lymphocytic-plasmacytic colitis is probably the most common form of ulcerative colitis in dogs and cats. The etiopathogenesis is similar to that of lymphocytic-plasmacytic enteritis and may represent chronic food antigen hypersensitivity or host response to a bacterial antigen.

1. *Standard therapy.* For mild or moderate cases, a hypoallergenic diet should be evaluated for at least 6 weeks. During the dietary trial, supportive therapy may be indicated. For acute episodes of colonic IBD, an easily digested low-fiber diet is recommended. Once clinical signs are controlled, dietary fiber should be gradually increased. Prescription diet r/d (Hill's Pet Products) is a high fiber commercially available diet. Wheat bran, 1–3 tablespoons per day, psyllium (Metamucil, Searle) 1 tablespoon per day, or high fiber wafers can also be used. High fiber diets may help control the incidence of relapse in colonic IBD.

With severe disease including acute episodes, sulfasalazine (Azulfidine, Pharmacia) therapy should be instituted. Sulfasalazine contains sulfapyridine joined to 5-aminosalicylic acid (5-ASA) by a diazo bond. When given orally, the diazo bond is broken by bacteria in the colon, releasing the two component drugs. Sulfapyridine is absorbed and excreted in the urine and has little pharmacologic activity on the bowel. 5-ASA penetrates the colonic mucosa and exerts a potent antiinflammatory effect. It inhibits the local mediators of inflammation, including prostaglandins, arachidonic acid, and leukotrienes. It may also function as a superoxide-free radical scavenger. When given orally, 5-ASA is rapidly absorbed in the upper gastrointestinal tract, and little drug is passed on to the colon. Thus sulfasalazine provides a mechanism for delivery of an effective dose of 5-ASA to the colon. Limited anti-inflammatory concentrations of 5-ASA may also exist in the distal ileum.

In dogs the initial dosage of sulfasalazine is 50 mg/kg PO q8h with a maximum dose of 1 g q8h. If the stool remains normal for 4 weeks, the dosage is decreased to 25 mg/kg q8h for an additional 3 weeks. If remission continues, the dosage is further reduced to 25 mg/kg q12h, and further reductions are made based on clinical response. Generally, continual sulfasalazine therapy is required to maintain clinical remission.

The side effects of sulfasalazine include keratoconjunctivitis sicca, granulocytopathies, drug eruptions, and lupus-like syndromes. Schirmer tear tests should be performed every 3 months to monitor tear production.

In severe cases, prednisolone (1–2 mg/kg/day) can be combined with sulfasalazine. Prednisolone may quickly suppress colonic inflammation; once signs have abated, the prednisolone is withdrawn. Remission is maintained with sulfasalazine. In some dogs chronic prednisolone therapy is necessary to maintain clinical remission.

In cats, sulfasalazine is initially given at a dosage of 15 mg/kg PO three times a day. If marked improvement does not occur within 7–10 days, prednisolone 2 mg/kg/day should be included in the regimen. With chronic therapy, cats may experience salicylate toxicity from the 5-ASA component. Remission should be attempted with prednisolone alone, or an alternative drug such as metronidazole or tylosin can be tried.

2. *Alternative therapy.* As previously discussed, metronidazole may be useful for suppressing IBD in the colon and small intestine. Tylosin (Tylan Plus, Elanco) may suppress the inflammation of IBD. In the cat, ¼ teaspoon twice a day in the food is recommended. In dogs, 1–2 teaspoons a day mixed with food is advised. There are no reported side effects with chronic tylosin therapy.

3. *Investigational therapy.* Because prolonged contact of 5-ASA with the colonic mucosa is beneficial in suppressing IBD, attempts have been made to formulate other compounds that exploit the action of 5-ASA but decrease the side effects of sulfasalazine. Formulations active in the small intestine are under development for the treatment of Crohn's disease in humans.

Topical 5-ASA preparations are used in enemas or suppositories for the treatment of distal ulcerative colitis in humans. The results are comparable to those seen with steroid enema therapy. Side effects are minimized with topical 5-ASA therapy. Dosages for dogs and cats are not available. Satisfactory retention of the drug in the colon is a problem in small animals.

Oral 5-ASA derivatives that slowly release 5-ASA in the ileum and colon are under evaluation. These compounds might be useful for IBD in the small intestine as well as the colon. One group of drugs incorporates an acrylic resin coating that slowly dissolves in a pH-dependent fashion. Eudragit-S (Asacol, Tillotts Labs) is an example. Olsalazine (Dipentum, Pharmacia Co.) contains two 5-ASA molecules arranged in a diazo bond linkage. Bacterial action in the colon liberates the two 5-ASA molecules. Dosages for these drugs in dogs and cats have not been established, and none has been released for use in the United States.

Several immunomodulatory drugs are under experimental evaluation in humans, including cyclosporin A, levamisole, and methotrexate. Cromoglycate, a mast cell stabilizer, has had limited effectiveness for ulcerative colitis. Sucralfate solutions (10%), used as an enema, may be effective for distal ulcerative colitis.

Eosinophilic Enterocolitis. Eosinophilic enterocolitis is a form of IBD characterized by eosinophilic infiltration of the lamina propria. Lesions occur in the small intestine, colon, or simultaneously in both areas. The etiology is unknown, but immune response to food or parasitic antigen is a popular theory. Visceral larval migrans may be the cause in some dogs and cats. A profound circulating eosinophilia may accompany the enteric signs. Eosinophilic infiltration of mesenteric lymph nodes may occur.

Standard Therapy. Response to oral prednisolone (2 mg/kg/day) is usually dramatic within 5–7 days. Once signs are controlled, the dose of prednisolone is reduced to 1 mg/kg/day for 2 weeks and further reduced to 1 mg/kg once every other day for 2 weeks. If no relapse occurs, the steroid therapy is discontinued.

If signs recur, prednisolone is given intermittently, and a hypoallergenic diet should be given and evaluated for 6 weeks. Fecal samples should be carefully evaluated for endoparasites.

Alternative Therapy. Recurrent cases of eosinophilic gastroenteritis may be associated with occult parasitism or visceral larval migrans. Dogs should be treated with a broad-spectrum anthelmintic such as fenbendazole (Panacur, Hoechst). In some cases, preventive therapy with oxibendazole (Filaribits Plus, SmithKline Beecham) or diethylcarbamazine-styrylpyridinium (Styrid-Caricide, American Cyanamid) may be helpful, especially if larval migrans from roundworms or hookworms is the underlying etiology.

Investigational Therapy. Ivermectin (Ivermec, Merck) 200 µg/kg once a month may be effective in dogs with disease secondary to recurrent parasite infections. Ivermectin is not currently approved for this purpose in dogs.

Histiocytic Ulcerative Colitis. Histiocytic ulcerative colitis, also known as granulomatous colitis or boxer colitis, is a form of IBD characterized by infiltration of the colonic mucosa and lamina propria with periodic acid-Schiff (PAS)-positive macrophages. The etiology of histiocytic ulcerative colitis is unknown, although the peculiar presence of macrophages suggests an infectious agent as the underlying cause. The disease was first described in young boxer dogs but has since been recognized in other breeds and rarely in cats. Histologic changes in early lesions are similar to those of lymphocytic-plasmacytic colitis. Macrophage infiltration may represent a finding associated with secondary microbial invasion of the colonic ulcers.

Standard Therapy. Sulfasalazine and corticosteroid therapy previously described for other forms of chronic colitis is the treatment of choice.

Intestinal Malabsorption Syndromes

Intestinal malabsorption may be associated with any chronic intestinal disorder that alters the absorptive capacity of the intestinal villi. Chronic small intestinal inflammation may cause villous atrophy, destruction of brush border enzymes, or mechanical obstruction to lymph flow within the villi. Ability to absorb fat may be drastically altered, as normal absorption of lipid depends on all three processes to be intact. Chronic gastrointestinal parasitism with *Giardia* and enteric bacterial overgrowth may also cause varying degrees of malabsorption.

Specific tests of gastrointestinal absorption are required to document intestinal malabsorption. A normal serum trypsin-like immunoreactivity (TLI) test can rule out pancreatic disease as the cause. Serum cobalamin levels may be decreased with ileal disease. Serum folate levels are increased with bacterial overgrowth. The absorption of D-xylose, a five-carbon sugar, may be decreased with disease of the jejunum. Significant malabsorption may be present despite normal gastrointestinal function tests. These clinical cases are presumptively diagnosed by ruling out pancreatic disease with a normal TLI test. Intestinal biopsies via endoscopy or laparotomy are needed to establish the correct diagnosis of the underlying disease process.

Standard Therapy. Definitive therapy is directed at the underlying disease. In addition, dietary therapy to improve nutrient absorption should be undertaken. The basic diet should be low in fat. Prescription diet r/d or w/d (Hill's Pet Products) are commercially available. Homemade low-fat diets also work well (Table 8-4). Care should be taken to eliminate all sources of gluten on the outside chance that gluten-induced enteropathy and malabsorption are present. An objective of dietary therapy is to decrease the osmotic load in the intestinal lumen.

Supplemental B complex and fat-soluble vitamins should be given.

TABLE 8-4. Recipe for Homemade Low-Fat Diet

Dogs	*Cats*
Boiled rice, potato, or pasta, 1 cup	Boiled chicken or lamb
Low-fat cottage cheese, 1 cup	or water-packed tuna
MCT oil, 15 ml	Provides 500+ calories exclusive of meat.

TABLE 8-5. Causes of Protein-Losing Enteropathies in Dogs and Cats

Intestinal lymphangiectasia	Acute viral enteritis
Inflammatory bowel disease	Chronic intussusception
Intestinal lymphosarcoma	Intestinal parasitism
Histoplasmosis	Gastrointestinal ulcers
Hemorrhagic gastroenteritis	

TABLE 8-6. Causes of Lymphangiectasia in Dogs and Cats

Primary lymphangiectasia (congenital lymphatic abnormalities)—rare in dogs and cats

Acquired (secondary) lymphangiectasia
  Venous hypertension
    Constrictive pericarditis
    Congestive heart failure, right-sided
    Portal hypertension
  Inflammatory bowel disease

Immunoproliferative enteropathy of Basenji dogs

Protein-Losing Enteropathy

The causes of protein-losing enteropathy (PLE) are described in Table 8-5. In PLE, both albumin and globulin are lost in near-equal amounts resulting in panhypoproteinemia. In addition to vomiting, diarrhea, and weight loss, ascites, edema, and pleural effusion may occur. There is no reliable diagnostic test for PLE in routine clinical practice. A presumptive diagnosis is made by eliminating the other causes of hypoproteinemia (liver failure, renal disease). Chromium-labeled human albumin excretion and the α_1-antitrypsin test are used in humans to detect PLE.

Intestinal Lymphangiectasia. Lymphangiectasia is pathologic dilatation of lymphatics within the intestinal mucosa and wall and the surrounding mesentery. The causes of lymphangiectasia are listed in Table 8-6. Lymphangiectasia is the major cause of PLE in dogs. Diagnosis is confirmed by histologic evaluation of gastrointestinal biopsy specimens. In addition to panhypoproteinemia, lymphopenia and hypocalcemia may be present.

Familial Immunoproliferative Enteropathy of Basenji Dogs. A familial immunoproliferative enteropathy affects Basenji dogs. It causes chronic inflammatory changes in the small intestine and lymphangiectasia. It is a progressive PLE with a relatively poor prognosis for controlling clinical signs. Diagnosis is based on the clinical signs, breed of dog, and intestinal biopsies. Hyperglobulinemia is an unusual feature of this disease.

    Standard Therapy. Dietary modification and antiinflammatory therapy are the primary components of treatment. Restriction of long-chain triglycerides in the diet decreases lymph flow and enteric protein loss. Fat reduction in the diet also decreases steatorrhea. MCTs are absorbed directly into the portal circulation, bypassing the damaged lymphatic system. MCT oil is commercially available (MCT Oil, Mead Johnson) and provides 115 kcal/teaspoon. It is added to the low-fat diet at a rate of 1–2 ml/kg body weight. The homemade diet described in Table 8-4 is low-fat and easy to make. Because this diet is not nutritionally balanced, though, supplementation with calcium, fat-soluble vitamins, and B vitamins is indicated.

The leakage of fatty acids from the dilated lymphatics produces inflammation in surrounding tissue. Prednisolone (1–3 mg/kg/day) may help control this inflammatory process as well as the inflammation associated with the underlying disease.

Chronic Bacterial Overgrowth

Intestinal bacterial overgrowth is caused by several diseases of the small intestine and pancreatic exocrine insufficiency. It can also result from achlorhydria. Any disease that decreases motility in the intestine may cause stagnant loops of bowel to develop. Bacterial growth within these areas is rapid. Bacteria deconjugate bile salts and hydroxylate fatty acids. Both compounds promote mucosal hypersecretion and watery diarrhea. Bacteria may damage brush border enzymes, resulting in intestinal malabsorption of fat, carbohydrate, and vitamin B_{12}. Intestinal bacterial overgrowth can be presumptively diagnosed when the TLI test is normal, serum folate levels are increased, and serum cobalamin levels are decreased or normal.

Standard Therapy. Chlortetracycline 20 mg/kg q8h PO is usually effective. Amoxicillin 20 mg/kg q12h PO can also be used. Signs usually resolve within 5–7 days, but therapy should be maintained for 2 weeks.

Giardiasis

Giardia are protozoal organisms that cause acute and chronic diarrhea in dogs and cats. Giardia parasitize the small intestine, and in heavy infections they cause malabsorption and maldigestion. The host immune response to the parasite produces inflammation similar to that seen with inflammatory bowel disease. Dogs and cats may be asymptomatic carriers of Giardia. Diagnosis is made by demonstrating the organism in feces. The zinc sulfate flotation procedure is the preferred technique.

Standard Therapy. Metronidazole (Flagyl, Searle) is the initial drug of choice at a dose of 65 mg/kg PO once a day for 5 days. In some cases, prolonged therapy at a dosage of 20 mg/kg twice a day may be required to eliminate the infection. Approximately 30% of Giardia isolates may be resistant to metronidazole. Side effects are minimal with short-term therapy.

Alternative Therapy. Quinacrine hydrochloride (Atabrine, Winthrop) at a dosage of 9 mg/kg PO daily for 6 days is usually effective in dogs. Side effects include occasional vomiting and rarely hepatic toxicity or bone marrow suppression.

CONSTIPATION

Colonic retention of feces caused by absent, infrequent, or difficult defecation results in constipation. When feces are retained in the colon for long periods, they become progressively drier and harder. Obstipation is extreme constipation in which the colon and rectum are so impacted that defecation cannot occur. Constipation results from several conditions that obstruct the anus or rectum, cause painful defecation, or decrease the motility of the colon or rectum. The differential diagnosis of constipation has been previously described. Although constipation can be relieved symptomatically, resolution depends on correction of the underlying cause.

Standard Therapy

Mild Constipation. Resolution is achieved with oral laxatives and high fiber diets. Oral laxatives are classified by their mechanisms of action as: 1) bulk-forming laxatives; 2) lubricant laxatives; 3) emollient laxatives; 4) osmotic laxatives; and 5) stimulant laxatives. Many compounds are available, but the bulk-forming, stimulant, and lubricant laxatives are most commonly used in dogs and cats.

Bulk-Forming Laxatives. Bulk-forming laxatives contain insoluble fiber (cellulose) or other polysaccharides. Wheat bran and psyllium contain insoluble fiber that absorbs water in the colon. This process softens feces, decreases intestinal transit time, and stimulates more frequent defecation. Wheat bran 1–5 tablespoons per meal or psyllium (Metamucil, Searle) 1–5 teaspoons per meal is recommended.

Stimulant Laxatives. Stimulant laxatives increase propulsive motility of the colon and rectum. Bisacodyl (Dulcolax, Boehringer) stimulates colonic smooth muscle and the myenteric plexus. It is effective for simple constipation, but repeated use may cause damage to the myenteric plexus. The daily dose of bisacodyl is 5 mg in cats and dogs that weigh less than 5 kg, 10 mg for dogs 5–15 kg, and 15–20 mg for dogs over 20 kg.

Lubricant Laxatives. Lubricants such as mineral oil and petrolatum soften and lubricate feces and facilitate elimination. Several products are available. Laxatone (Evsco) 1–5 ml daily PO is effective, especially for enteric hair balls in cats.

High Fiber Diets. Several high fiber diets are commercially available. Prescription Diet w/d (Hill's Pet Products) and Cycle 4 (Gaines) can be used for long-term control of simple constipation.

Severe Constipation. The immediate relief of severe constipation requires enema therapy and in some cases manual extraction of the fecal mass. In dehydrated patients, fluid therapy helps soften the stool.

Various enema solutions may be used, but warm water containing 5–10 mg of dioctyl sodium sulfosuccinate (Colace, Mead Johnson) is recommended. Colace is an emollient laxative that promotes the penetration of water into the fecal mass. The amount of enema solution is 5–10 ml/kg body weight, administered slowly through an appropriate catheter or tube. Defecation should occur within a few minutes. Enemas may be repeated as necessary to evacuate all fecal material. When constipation is associated with bone fragments in the feces, warm mineral oil slowly infused in the colon and rectum may provide additional lubrication. Mineral oil is used *after* water enemas have been tried, as mineral oil prevents the absorption of water into feces.

In some cases, enema therapy does not evacuate the colon because the fecal mass is too hard or too large for passage. In these cases, careful manual extraction should be attempted utilizing sponge forceps. The fecal mass is broken with the forceps and removed by gentle colonic irrigation. Deep sedation or general anesthesia may be required for restraint and to control pain. Appropriate supportive fluid therapy should be given.

Megacolon. Megacolon is an alteration of colonic motility that results in severe colonic dilatation. Several causes are recognized but chronic constipation, rectal obstruction, and idiopathic disease are the major causes of acquired megacolon. Idiopathic megacolon is an acquired disease of older dogs and cats. The disease is thought to be a primary colonic neuromuscular dysfunction that results in weak colonic contractions, hypomotility, and chronic fecal overloading.

Therapy for chronic constipation is undertaken. Once the impacted feces are removed, therapy is given to prevent relapses. It includes feeding a high fiber diet, use of bulk laxatives, glycerin suppositories, and intermittent enemas. Colectomy has been used to manage chronic megacolon in cats.

ENDOPARASITES

Ascariasis

Ascarid infection (roundworms) is common in dogs and cats, causing diarrhea and vomiting in young animals. Older animals generally have asymptomatic infections. Transmission is fecal-oral, transmammary, and transuterine. Diagnosis is based on finding the typical ova in fecal flotations. Ascarids have significant zoonotic implications, as visceral larval migrans is a serious disease in children.

Standard Therapy. Pyrantel pamoate (Nemex, Strongid T, Pfizer) is a safe anthelmintic that is 95% effective against ascarids and hookworms. The standard dose is 15 mg/kg PO 30 minutes after a light meal. Treatment should be repeated in 21 days.

Ascarid control in puppies and kittens should begin at 2–3 weeks of age, and treatment with pyrantel pamoate is given at 3-week intervals until 12 weeks of age.

Preventive Therapy. Diethylcarbamazine (Caricide, American Cyanamid) 6.6 mg/kg/day is effective in preventing ascarid infections. Oxibendazole (Filaribits Plus) is also effective. Good sanitation is recommended.

Ancylostomiasis

Ancylostomiasis (hookworm infection) is common in dogs and cats resulting in serious enteritis and blood loss in puppies and kittens. Mortality rates can be high when diagnosis and treatment are delayed. Transmission is fecal-oral, percutaneous, and transmammary. Diagnosis is based on finding the typical ova in standard fecal flotations. Occult infections are known to occur, so the diagnosis of hookworm infection should not be discounted when fecal flotations are negative.

Standard Therapy. Because of its efficacy and low toxicity, pyrantel pamoate is the initial anthelmintic of choice in most dogs and cats. A dose of 15 ml/kg PO is administered and repeated in 21 days. When vomiting precludes oral anthelmintic therapy, disophenol (DNP, American Cyanamid) 10 mg/kg SC can be used. The margin of safety of DNP is low (36 mg/kg is fatal), so small dogs, cats, puppies, and kittens must be weighed carefully. Butamisole (Styquin, American Cyanamid) 2.4 mg/kg is effective for hookworms and whipworms. Its use is approved for dogs, but it is contraindicated for heartworm infection, debilitated dogs, or puppies less than 8 weeks old. Both DNP and Styquin cause pain at the injection site.

Hookworm disease is associated with anemia, iron deficiency, and bloody diarrhea. In addition to anthelmintic therapy, blood transfusions, fluid therapy, and hematinic therapy may be indicated for dehydration and gastrointestinal loss of iron and hemoglobin.

Alternative Therapy. Fenbendazole (Panacur, American Hoechst) is effective against ascarids, hookworms, whipworms, *Taenia* tapeworms, and *Strongyloides*. The dosage is 50 mg/kg/day for 3 days. It is currently approved for dogs and has been safely given to cats. Toxicity is rare, but hepatotoxicity has been reported with the bendazole derivatives. Mebendazole (Telmintic, Pitman-Moore) has a spectrum of activity similar to that of fenbendazole. The dosage is 22 mg/kg in the food daily for 3 days (5 days for *Taenia* therapy). Mebendazole is approved for dogs. Occasional drug-induced acute hepatic necrosis has been reported in dogs. Milbemycin oxime (Interceptor, Ciba-Geigy) 0.5 mg/kg PO each month can control hookworm and heartworm infection simultaneously.

Trichuriasis

Trichuriasis (whipworm infection) causes acute and chronic colitis in dogs. Infections may be occult, and the absence of ova in fecal flotations does not rule out the diagnosis. Occult trichuriasis can be confirmed by finding the parasites during colonoscopy or by following the response to appropriate therapy. Transmission is fecal-oral.

Standard Therapy. Fenbendazole 50 mg/kg for 3 consecutive days is recommended. Butamisole 2.4 mg/kg SC is also effective. Dogs should be retreated in 21 and 70 days.

Tapeworms

Two major types of tapeworms cause intestinal infection in dogs and cats. *Taenia* tapeworms are transmitted by rodents and rabbits, and the *Dipylidium caninium* tapeworm is transmitted by ingestion of infected fleas. Clinical signs are generally mild; most animals remain asymptomatic.

Standard Therapy. Praziquantel (Droncit, Haver) is effective for tapeworms at a dosage of 5 mg/kg PO or IM in dogs. The dose in cats is 11 mg total for a cat weighing 1–3 lb, 22 mg total for cats weighing 3–11 lb, and 33 mg total for cats over 11 lb. Epsiprantel (Cestex, SmithKline Beecham) is also effective at a dosage of 5.5 mg/kg PO in dogs and 3.3 mg/kg PO in cats.

Alternative Therapy. Bunamide (Scolaban, Burroughs) 25–50 mg on an empty stomach is effective for *Taenia* but is only 55–90% effective on *Dipylidium*. Fenbendazole and mebendazole are effective against *Taenia* if given orally for 5 days. Febantel and praziquantel (Vercom paste, Haver) is effective for ascarids, hookworms, whipworms, and tapeworms.

Strongyloides

Strongyloides may cause acute watery diarrhea in puppies and kittens. The larvae are usually identified in feces via a Baerman apparatus or modified Baerman technique.

Standard Therapy. Fenbendazole 50 mg/kg/day for 5 days is effective. Retreatment in 30 days is recommended.

Coccidia

At least four species of *Cystoisospora* infect dogs and cats. Usually coccidia produce enteric disease in puppies and kittens or in severely stressed or immunocompromised adults. When enteric signs develop and coccidia are demonstrated in the feces, a thorough search should be undertaken for infection with other gastrointestinal parasites. Diagnosis is made by demonstrating the oocysts in feces.

Standard Therapy. Sulfadimethoxine (Bactrovet, Pitman-Moore) 50 mg/kg PO on day 1 followed by 25 mg/kg PO daily for 20 days is recommended in both dogs and cats. Treatment of any other gastrointestinal parasites is also important.

Alternative Therapy. Amprolium (Corid, Merck) is a coccidiostatic drug useful for treating puppies in large kennels. It is not approved for canine use but is effective and relatively safe. Amprolium powder (100 mg/capsule for small breed puppies and 200 mg/capsule for large breed puppies daily for 7–10 days) is given orally or mixed with food. Amprolium solution 9.6% can be mixed with drinking water at a rate of 7.8 ml/L of water for 7–10 days.

Stomatitis

Stomatitis is acute or chronic inflammation of the oral cavity. There are several etiologics, including toxic irritation, metabolic disease, viral or bacterial infection, and possibly immune-mediated disease. Poor dental hygiene is an important etiology.

Acute Ulcerative Stomatitis. Acute ulcerative stomatitis has various etiologies including immunosuppressive conditions such as hyperadrenocorticism, diabetes mellitus, and feline leukemia virus (FeLV) infection. An overgrowth of fusiform and spirochetal organisms may occur that inhibits the healing process. Bacterial cultures are generally not helpful, as they detect resident bacteria.
   Standard Therapy. The underlying cause should be treated. Symptomatic therapy includes changing the diet to a soft or bland food. Oral ulcers can be treated topically with 1% hydrogen peroxide once or twice a day. Ampicillin 10 mg/kg q8h PO may hasten healing. Dental tartar should be removed and the teeth kept clean with daily brushing.
   Alternative Therapy. Metronidazole (Flagyl, Searle) 10–15 mg/kg twice a day PO is effective when anaerobic bacteria are involved in the inflammatory process. Therapy is maintained for 10–14 days. Relapses may occur, and metronidazole therapy may be required for extended periods.

Chronic Ulcerative and Proliferative Stomatitis. Chronic ulcerative stomatitis occurs most commonly in cats and is characterized by vesicular, proliferative, or ulcerative lesions. Cellular infiltrates with lymphocytes, plasma cells, or eosinophils are common histologic findings. The cause is unknown, but an immune response to bacterial or viral antigens is suspected. Response to therapy is generally poor and unpredictable.

Standard Therapy. For lymphocytic-plasmacytic stomatitis, metronidazole 15 mg/kg PO twice a day is recommended. If no response occurs within 14 days, prednisolone 2 mg/kg/day PO should be started in conjunction with metronidazole. Therapy should be continued for 2 weeks. The dosage of prednisolone should be gradually reduced once remission is achieved.

For eosinophilic stomatitis, prednisolone 2–3 mg/kg/day PO should be given until remission is achieved. The dosage is then reduced to 2 mg/kg once every other day. Methylprednisolone acetate (Depo-Medrol, Upjohn) 15–20 mg IM every 3–4 weeks controls eosinophilic stomatitis in some cats.

SUGGESTED READINGS

Cornelius LM: Vomiting and regurgitation. In: Lorenz MD, Cornelius LW, eds. Small Animal Medical Diagnosis. Philadelphia: JB Lippincott, 1986;256.

Cornelius LM, Lorenz MD: Diarrhea. In: Lorenz MD, Cornelius LW, eds. Small Animal Medical Diagnosis. Philadelphia: JB Lippincott, 1986;268.

Cornelius LM, Roberson EL: Treatment of gastrointestinal parasitism. In: Kirk RW, ed. Current Veterinary Therapy, 9th ed. Philadelphia: WB Saunders, 1986;921.

Dimski DS: Constipation: Pathophysiology, diagnostic approach, and treatment. Semin Vet Med Surg (Small Anim) 1989;4:247.

Forrester SD, Boothe DM, Willard MD: Clinical pharmacology of antiemetic and antiulcer drugs. Semin Vet Med Surg (Small Anim) 1989;4:194.

Fossum TW: Protein-losing enteropathy. Semin Vet Med Surg (Small Anim) 1989;4:219.

Greene CE: Gastrointestinal, intra-abdominal, and hepatobiliary infections. In: Greene, CE, ed. Clinical Microbiology and Infectious Diseases of the Dog and Cat. Philadelphia: WB Saunders, 1984;247.

Leib, MS: Megaesophagus in the dog. In: Kirk RW, ed. Current Veterinary Therapy, 9th ed. Philadelphia: WB Saunders, 1986;848.

Leib MS, Hay WH, Roth L: Plasmacytic-lymphocytic colitis in dogs. In: Kirk RW, ed. Current Veterinary Therapy, 10th ed. Philadelphia: WB Saunders, 1989;939.

Lorenz MD: Constipation. In: Lorenz MD, Cornelius LM, eds. Small Animal Medical Diagnosis. Philadelphia: WB Saunders, 1986;284.

Lothrop CD: Medical treatment of neuroendocrine tumors of the gastroenteropancreatic system with somatostatin. In: Kirk RW, ed. Current Veterinary Therapy, 10th ed. Philadelphia: WB Saunders, 1989;1020.

Magne ML: Canine lymphocytic-plasmacytic enteritis. In: Kirk RW, ed. Current Veterinary Therapy, 10th ed. Philadelphia: WB Saunders, 1989;922.

Papich MG: Medical therapy for gastrointestinal ulcers. In: Kirk RW, ed. Current Veterinary Therapy, 10th ed. Philadelphia: WB Saunders, 1989;911.

Ruderman WB: Newer pharmacologic agents for the therapy of inflammatory bowel disease. Med Clin North Am 1990;74, 133.

Tams TR: Feline inflammatory bowel disease. In: Kirk RW, ed. Current Veterinary Therapy, 9th ed. Philadelphia: WB Saunders, 1986;881.

Tams TR: Reflux esophagitis. In: Kirk RW, ed. Current Veterinary Therapy, 10th ed. Philadelphia: WB Saunders, 1989;906.

Twedt DC, Magne ML: Chronic gastritis. In: Kirk RW, ed. Current Veterinary Therapy, 9th ed. Philadelphia: WB Saunders, 1986;852.

CHAPTER NINE

Liver Diseases

Larry M. Cornelius

Liver diseases are reasonably common in dogs and cats and may be life-threatening. The liver can be directly damaged by a variety of toxic and infectious agents as well as a number of metabolic, immune-mediated, or neoplastic problems, or it may be secondarily affected. The resulting acute, subacute, or chronic clinical syndromes often require therapeutic intervention. Unfortunately, liver disorders have not been as thoroughly investigated in these species as in man, and consequently therapeutic recommendations are often extrapolated from what is known about humans and may be for supportive care only; however, the availability of safer anesthetics and better liver biopsy techniques are now enhancing the veterinarian's ability to better classify and diagnose hepatic disorders and to monitor response to therapy.

The general purposes of therapy for hepatic disease are to: 1) eliminate the cause if known; 2) control or eliminate pathologic changes such as inflammation, fibrosis, and copper accumulation; 3)control complications such as septicemia, gastrointestinal bleeding, ascites, and hepatic encephalopathy; and 4) provide optimum conditions for hepatic regeneration.

ACUTE AND SUBACUTE HEPATIC FAILURE

Acute hepatic failure occurs whenever a sudden, severe insult to the liver compromises at least 70–80% of the functional hepatic mass. Acute or subacute hepatic failure may be caused by a variety of drugs, hepatotoxins, infectious agents, and metabolic disturbances (Table 9-1). Often the inciting cause cannot be determined, and the liver disorder can be categorized only by using descriptive histopathologic results (e.g., acute necrosis, hepatitis, lipidosis).

Clinical signs of acute hepatic failure (sudden onset of anorexia, depression, vomiting, diarrhea, dehydration, melena, icterus, bilirubinuria, hepatomegaly, hepatic pain, central nervous signs of hepatic encephalopathy), although generally consistent, are not diagnostic of any specific etiology, and it is often difficult to establish the precise cause. Diagnosis of acute hepatic damage is established by consideration of history and physical findings, as noted above, and typical laboratory abnormalities. Characteristic findings include increased serum enzymes [alanine aminotransferase (S-ALT, formerly SGPT) alkaline

TABLE 9-1. Causes of Acute and Subacute Hepatic Failure in Dogs and Cats

Drugs/ Hepatotoxins	Infectious/Parasitic Agents or Disorders	Metabolic Factors	Extrahepatic Disorders
Drugs	*Viral agents*	Idiopathic	Acute
Acetaminophen (cat)	ICH (adenovirus)	hepatic lipidosis	pancreatitis
Phenazopyradine (cat)	Canine herpesvirus	in cats	Acute hemolytic anemia
Thiacetarsamide	Canine acidophil hepatitis virus		Colitis
Mebendazole			(inflammatory
Oxibendazole	*Bacterial agents*		bowel disease)
Trimethoprim-sulfa	Gram-negative septicemia/ endotoxemia		
Ketoconazole (esp. cat)	Salmonella		
Halothane/ methoxyflurane	Clostridium Leptospira Bacillus		
Chemicals	piliformis (Tyzzer's		
Arsenic	disease, esp.		
Carbon tetrachloride	cats)		
Chlordane	*Fungal agents*		
Chlorinated hydrocarbons	Histoplasmosis Blastomycosis		
Dieldrin	Coccidiomycosis		
Metals: copper, iron, mercury	*Protozoal agent*		
Phosphorus	Toxoplasmosis		
Selenium			
Biologic substances	*Heartworm-associated*		
Aflatoxins (moldy grains)	*(postcaval syndrome)*		
Blue-green algae endotoxin			
Bacterial endotoxin			
Aminita mushroom toxin			

Modified from Sherding RG: Acute hepatic failure. *Vet Clin North Am* 1985;15:119.

phosphatase (SAP)] and abnormal hepatic function tests [increased serum bilirubin, abnormal clotting tests (prolonged prothrombin time, partial thromboplastin time, thrombin time, decreased fibrinogen), prolonged retention of Bromsulphalein (BSP dye), abnormal baseline ammonia or ammonia intolerance, and increased serum bile acid concentrations]. Metabolic consequences of acute hepatic failure may also include bacteremia and endotoxemia associated with hypoglycemia and disseminated intravascular coagulation (DIC), respiratory or metabolic alkalosis, and hypokalemia.

Standard Therapy. Fulminant hepatic failure is one of the most challenging disorders in clinical medicine and is associated with a high mortality rate. Ideally specific treatment of the primary cause of acute hepatic failure should be instituted as soon as possible; however, treatment is usually symptomatic and supportive because the etiology is often unknown.

Supportive Therapy. Because many drugs are capable of causing acute liver damage in a given patient, discontinuation of any suspect drug should be a high priority, which should prevent further hepatocellular damage. Also, when administering drugs to treat patients with hepatic dysfunction, one should consider the potential for altered hepatic metabolism and subsequent accumulation of the drugs. It may be necessary to avoid certain drugs that depend on the liver for elimination or to reduce their dosage. Examples include certain antibiotics (chloramphenicol, erythromycin, hetacillin, lincomycin, sulfonamides), sedatives, tranquilizers, hypnotics, anesthetics, anticonvulsants, and organophosphates.

Fluid and Electrolyte Therapy. Of special concern in the treatment of patients with acute hepatic failure are dehydration and hypovolemia, respiratory or metabolic alkalosis, hypokalemia, and hypoglycemia. Ringer's solution, a balanced electrolyte solution similar in composition to plasma, is recommended for rehydration; moreover, because of its increased chloride content, it is used to correct metabolic alkalosis. Isotonic (0.9%) saline solution is an acceptable alternative.

The volume of fluid needed is determined by estimating the percentage of dehydration (deficit needs) and accounting for maintenance requirements (40–60 ml/kg/day) and the estimated continuing losses (see Chapter 1). The rate and route of fluid administration depends on the severity of dehydration and hypovolemia. If the patient is in shock and is severely dehydrated, Ringer's solution should be administered at the rate of 90 ml/kg/hr until mucous membrane color and pulse strength improve; then the rate of fluid administration should be decreased to approximately two to three times the hourly maintenance requirements (3.4–7.5 ml/kg/hr or roughly 1.5–3.0 ml/lb/hr). Generally, one should administer about half of the estimated fluid deficit requirements during the first 4–8 hours and the remaining half during the next 16–20 hours. These figures are rough approximations, and the clinician must frequently reevaluate the patient's clinical signs of hydration and cardiopulmonary status and adjust fluid administration appropriately (see Chapter 1).

Once hydration and adequate urine production are established, it is often necessary to add extra potassium to the Ringer's solution in the form of potassium chloride (see Table 1-5). Because hyperkalemia can cause dangerous cardiotoxicity, the rate of intravenous potassium administration must be carefully controlled. A generally accepted safe rate for dogs and cats with adequate urine production is 0.5 mEq potassium/kg/hr (see Chapter 1). It is more practical in some cases to administer potassium-supplemented Ringer's solution subcutaneously (40 mEq potassium/L) because the potassium is absorbed more slowly, thus lessening the risk of serious hyperkalemia. Serum potassium should be monitored every day or two until it has stabilized in the normal range.

In some instances of fulminant hepatic failure, the patient may be in shock, in which case metabolic acidosis may be present. An alkalinizing, balanced electrolyte solution should be used in these patients (instead of Ringer's solution or 0.9% saline), but there is controversy about which fluid is best. I have had good success in correcting metabolic acidosis with lactated Ringer's solution, although theoretically the liver might not be capable of metabolizing lactate to bicarbonate, resulting in lactate accumulation and failure to alleviate acidosis. For this reason some clinicians advise adding sodium bicarbonate to either 2.5% dextrose or 0.45% saline solutions. Sodium bicarbonate should not be added to a calcium-containing solution such as lactated Ringer's because it precipitates as calcium carbonate. The estimated bicarbonate (or lactate) requirements can be calculated by using the following formula (see Chapter 1).

$$HCO_3^- \text{ deficit } = 0.5 \times \text{ body wt (kg)}$$
$$\times \text{ (normal serum } HCO_3^- - \text{ patient serum } HCO_3^-)$$

For practical purposes plasma total CO_2 (TCO_2) can be substituted for serum bicarbonate in the above formula. Estimated bicarbonate needs should be administered slowly over a 24- to 48-hour period by giving about half of the total requirements during the first 4–8 hours, 25% during the next 18–20 hours, and the remainder over the next 24 hours. Plasma bicarbonate or TCO_2 should be monitored daily and appropriate adjustments made in fluid therapy until the TCO_2 level stabilizes in the normal range.

The method of treating hypoglycemia depends on the severity of this problem (see Chapter 4). For severe hypoglycemia (blood glucose <40 mg/dl), it is better to administer 20% dextrose solution by slow intravenous bolus (about 5 ml/kg over 5–10 minutes). Blood glucose should be rechecked using one of the rapid blood glucose strip methods such as Chemstrip bG and Accuchek II blood glucose meter (Boehringer Mannheim) and the clinical signs reevaluated. If necessary the above dosage of 20% dextrose solution can be repeated until the blood glucose is in the normal range. The intravenous bolus of dextrose can be followed by a slow infusion (10–20 ml/kg/hr) of Ringer's solution to which has been added enough dextrose solution to make a final glucose concentration of 5% (e.g., add 250 ml of 20% dextrose to 750 ml of Ringer's solution). Blood glucose should be checked every 1–2 hours and the rate of glucose administration appropriately adjusted until the blood glucose has stabilized in the normal range.

Hepatic Encephalopathy

Hepatic encephalopathy (HE) is a syndrome of altered central nervous system (CNS) function associated with either severe acute or chronic hepatic failure. The precise causes of HE are not completely understood, but it is known that failure of the liver to detoxify various compounds absorbed from the intestinal tract, especially ammonia, and altered protein and amino acid metabolism play major roles in the pathogenesis.

Emergency Management of Severe HE. Intravenous fluid therapy is important to expand the extracellular space and promote diuresis, thereby lowering the blood urea nitrogen (BUN) in azotemic patients and reducing the plasma concentrations of ammonia and other toxins. Ringer's and 0.9% saline solutions are preferred. The fluid volume deficit and maintenance requirements should be estimated as described in Chapter 1. Appropriate rate of administration depends on the severity of dehydration but is usually about two to three times hourly maintenance requirements (3.4–7.5 ml/kg/hr or roughly 1.5–3.0 ml/lb/hr) for the first 4–8 hours; then the rate should be reduced to 1.5–2.0 times hourly maintenance needs (2.5–5.0 ml/kg/hr or roughly 1.0–2.5 ml/lb/hr) until the deficit volume is supplied. If hypokalemia and hypoglycemia are present, KCl and dextrose are added to the fluids as described above. Should a blood transfusion be necessary, fresh blood should be used because stored blood usually contains high concentrations of ammonia.

Cleansing enemas should be done every 4–6 hours by instilling a 1:10 dilution of warm povidone-iodine (Betadine) solution (Purdue Frederick) into the colon and draining after 10–15 minutes. The importance of multiple enemas is to decrease the urea-splitting bacterial population in the colon and reduce the concentration and absorption of ammonia and other toxins. Instillation of either neomycin (10–20 mg/kg diluted in H_2O) or lactulose (Cephulac, Merrell Dow) at a dosage of 300–450 g (200–300 ml) into the colon following evacuation of the enema solution may further reduce bacterial numbers. Lactulose is a poorly absorbed disaccharide that is fermented by colonic bacteria to acidic products that are osmotically active. Colonic acidification retards absorption of ammonia, and the increase in the number of osmotically active particles causes more rapid elimination of bacteria and toxins in feces. Management of chronic HE is discussed in a later section of this chapter.

Investigational Therapy. Infusion of branched-chain amino acid solutions to improve deranged blood amino acid ratios has been tried for acute HE in humans with variable success. These solutions are expensive and generally considered impractical for use in dogs and cats. Dopamine agonists, e.g., L-dopa and bromocriptine, have been used in human HE with some success. Purported mechanisms of action are the displacement of false neurotransmitters in the CNS and facilitation of renal ammonia excretion. I have no experience with these drugs.

Septicemia

Bacteremia and endotoxemia may complicate acute hepatic failure because of reduced hepatic reticuloendothelial function and increased intestinal bacterial proliferation and absorption. Antibiotics should be used intravenously for at least the first 48–72 hours and should include drugs effective against both gram-negative bacteria and gram-positive aerobic and anaerobic organisms. Treatment is usually begun with a combination of ampicillin 20 mg/kg q8h and gentamicin (Gentocin, Schering) 2.2 mg/kg q6–8h, and the clinical response is observed. *When using gentamicin or any systemic aminoglycoside, it is essential to maintain good hydration and monitor renal function closely* because of potential nephrotoxicity associated with use of these drugs. If the clinical response is inadequate, intravenous administration of metronidazole (Metronidazole Redi-Infusion, Elkins-Sinn) is initiated at a dosage of 10 mg/kg q8h. Metronidazole has excellent activity against a variety of pathogenic anaerobic bacteria. If the patient's clinical condition is improved after 48–72 hours, changing to oral ampicillin or metronidazole (Flagyl, Ortho) is indicated (same dosage as listed for the oral route for a total of 2 weeks of treatment). Also, administration of gentamicin should be changed to the subcutaneous route (2.2 mg/kg q12h for a total of 5–7 days of treatment).

If renal insufficiency is present or develops, gentamicin should not be used. Trimethoprim-sulfa (Septra, Burroughs Wellcome) administered slowly at a dosage of 15–20 mg/kg IV q12h is a good alternative because of its efficacy against a variety of gram-negative bacteria. It is best to use the product approved for intravenous use in humans, although it is more expensive than veterinary formulations. The latter products have been used occasionally in our hospital without noticeable adverse side effects.

Gastrointestinal Hemorrhage

Blood is a protein source for ammonia production by enteric bacteria. Intestinal bleeding should be controlled by using cimetidine (Tagamet, SmithKline & French) at a dosage of 5–8 mg/kg q8h IV or SC. Cimetidine is a histamine H_2-receptor blocker and inhibits the output of hydrochloric acid (HCl) from the stomach, thus lessening the irritative effects of HCl on upper gastrointestinal ulcers. After the patient's condition stabilizes, cimetidine can be used orally at the same dosage, and sucralfate (Caraphate, Marion Laboratories) can be added to the treatment regimen at a dosage of 0.5 g for patients weighing less than 20 kg and 1.0 g for patients weighing more than 20 kg q8h PO. Sucralfate acts by forming a protective ulcer-adherent complex and stimulating local prostaglandin synthesis, thus promoting ulcer healing.

Seizures

If seizuring occurs, check blood glucose and administer dextrose solution intravenously as previously described if the patient is hypoglycemic. Otherwise, begin treatment by using intravenous diazepam (Valium, Roche) at the lowest dosage possible to effect. Valium is administered as an intravenous bolus (3–5 mg total) and the response observed. If necessary, this dose can be repeated in 5–10 minutes, but remember to use caution because hepatic metabolism is necessary to clear diazepam, and the half-life will be prolonged. As a last resort, pentobarbital can be given intravenously *slowly and cautiously* to effect (usual dosage is 2–5 mg/kg). Barbiturates are metabolized by the liver, and their use in patients with acute hepatic failure is discouraged.

Idiopathic Hepatic Lipidosis in Cats

Idiopathic hepatic lipidosis (IHL) in cats is a syndrome characterized by persistent anorexia and marked accumulation of fat in hepatocytes, which may cause hepatic failure and death. Although the precise cause(s) are unknown, obese cats appear to be at a higher risk than nonobese cats. Stress is sometimes an initiating event. The pathophysiologic mechanisms of IHL are poorly understood, and treatment is mainly supportive.

Standard Therapy. Early diagnosis and effective fluid and caloric replacement offer the best chances for reversal of IHL. Adequate fluid and caloric intake must be ensured until the cat starts drinking and eating enough voluntarily, which often requires 1–12 weeks. Appetite stimulants can be tried and may be successful in a few cats in which IHL is diagnosed early. Several benzodiazepine compounds have been shown to stimulate appetite in animals including cats. Diazepam at a dosage of 0.05–0.15 mg/kg IV or 1.0 mg PO once or twice daily and oxazepam (Serax, Wyeth) at a dosage of 0.2–0.5 mg/kg PO once or twice daily often induce eating in anorectic cats. However, cats given these drugs usually eat only small amounts, and marked sedation and ataxia may be seen as side effects.

In most cases, the only practical method of caloric replacement is enteral administration. Methods of enteral feeding include force-feeding per os and placement of a feeding tube. Prolonged force-feeding by mouth is not recommended because of additional stress to the cat. Nasogastric intubation can be done with local anesthesia and a 5 or 6 French feeding tube (Pedi-tube, Biosearch Medical Products). Because of the feeding tube's small diameter, only fluids and liquid nutritional supplements can be administered. Commercial products designed for use in man, such as Osmolite (Ross) or Peptamen (Clinitec Nutrition), can be used for short periods of time but may cause diarrhea. Diluting such products in half with water may lessen this tendency. Better results are achieved by using a liquid nutritional supplement formulated for cats (Feline Clinicare, Pet Ag Co.). For cats with signs of HE that may be unable to tolerate the amount of protein in Feline Clinicare, Feline Renalcare (Pet Ag Co.) should be tried because it contains less protein. Fluid needs are 50–60 ml/kg/day, and caloric requirements are about 40–50 kcal/kg/day. These requirements should be met by dividing required calories into multiple administrations (six to eight tube feedings daily). At first it may be necessary to administer small amounts every 2–3 hours (5–10 ml/feeding) until the patient adapts to the tube-feeding procedure. If no vomiting occurs, progressively larger amounts per feeding can then be given, with the goal being administration of daily caloric needs in three or four feedings. Administration of metoclopramide (Reglan, A.H. Robins) at a dosage of 0.4 mg/kg SC q6–8h 30 minutes prior to feeding often improves gastric emptying and prevents vomiting. Nasogastric tubes are most useful when only a few days of caloric supplementation are needed, such as while trying to stabilize the patient prior to anesthesia for placement of a pharyngostomy or gastrostomy tube, liver biopsy, or both.

Pharyngostomy or gastrostomy tubes allow enteral administration of well-balanced commercial cat food gruels (Feline k/d, c/d, or p/d, Hill's Pet Products). The gruel is prepared using an electric blender to mix the food with sufficient water to make a slurry thin enough to be administered through the tube. For the first few days, the gruel should be administered at the rate of about 5 ml/kg six to eight times per day. If vomiting occurs, the amount administered per feeding should be reduced by half and then gradually increased over a period of a few days. The objective is to reduce the daily tube feeding frequency to three or four times per day. Reglan administration, as described above, may also help prevent vomiting.

Better success has been achieved in our hospital using gastrostomy tubes than with pharyngostomy tubes because of the persistent gagging and regurgitation sometimes seen with the latter. Cats usually tolerate the gastrostomy tube well, and complications have been minimal. Two methods for placing gastrostomy tubes have been described. If an endoscope is available, percutaneous placement can be done during general anesthesia using isoflurane (Forane, Anaquest). Otherwise, during general anesthesia, a celiotomy can be done, and a No. 16–24 Foley catheter or a mushroom-tipped catheter (C.R. Bard) can be inserted into the stomach by gastrostomy followed by gastropexy. The liver should be biopsied during this same period of general anesthesia. Tube feeding is usually done in the hospital for the first few days until it is determined that the cat is tolerating the tube and that the tube is functional and not easily plugged. The owner is usually taught to manage the tube feedings at home and should be instructed to periodically withhold tube feeding and see if the cat will eat on its own. The gastrostomy tube must be left in until the cat is eating and drinking adequate amounts voluntarily. Return of near-normal appetite is usually an indication that the feeding tube can be removed.

The best diet depends on the disease severity. If hyperammonemia or signs of HE are present, prescription diet Feline k/d (Hill's Pet Products) is recommended because of its restricted protein content, which is of high biologic value. Otherwise, prescription diets Feline c/d or p/d (Hill's Pet Products) are advised because of their moderate fat and protein levels, which appear to be well assimilated. Total caloric intake should be 40–50 kcal/kg/day, and the diet should be nutritionally balanced. Care must be used to properly liquefy the diet or the tube will become plugged. Straining the blenderized food prior to tube feeding may be advisable. B complex and fat-soluble vitamins can be mixed into the liquefied food in standard doses.

Ringer's solution is recommended (intravenously or subcutaneously) if parenteral fluids are required to help maintain hydration. Daily fluid requirements are 50–60 ml/kg.

Coagulation abnormalities may be the result of either malabsorption of vitamin K due to prolonged cholestasis or decreased hepatic synthesis of various clotting factors. If clotting function is abnormal, administration of vitamin K_1 (Aquamephyton, Merck Sharp & Dohme) at a dosage of 1–2 mg/kg SC q12h for 5–7 days) is indicated. Avoid the use of lipotropic compounds containing choline and methionine because methionine may precipitate HE in patients with hepatic insufficiency.

Send the cat home as soon as the owner can provide proper care. Although it requires a dedicated owner, it minimizes patient stress and provides the best chance for recovery from this serious disorder.

Investigational Therapy. Carnitine is a quaternary amine necessary for transport of long-chain fatty acids into mitochondria for subsequent oxidation. Its role in feline IHL is unproved, but empiric carnitine (USA International) supplementation has been tried at a dosage of 250–500 mg once daily. Carnitine is added to the gruel during the time the cat is being tube-fed. No adverse effects have been observed, and this drug is discontinued when the patient starts to eat adequately on its own.

Low doses of insulin have been recommended to help prevent lipolysis and improve hepatic secretion of very low density lipoproteins. Because of the sensitivity of cats to insulin and the potential for hypoglycemia, the use of insulin is not advised unless the cat is diabetic. Glucocorticoids are not indicated because they may worsen muscle catabolism and wasting and stimulate lipolysis, causing increased delivery of fatty acids to the liver.

TABLE 9-2.   Causes of Chronic Hepatic Failure in Dogs and Cats*

Drugs	Inflammation	Metabolic Causes	Vascular Causes
Anticonvulsants in dogs (primidone, phenytoin)	*Infectious* Leptospirosis in dogs ICH virus Canine acidophil hepatitis virus Suppurative cholangio-hepatitis FIP in cats *Noninfectious* Chronic active hepatitis in dogs (suspected autoimmune) Lobular dissecting hepatitis Lymphocytic cholangiohepatitis in cats	*Copper toxicity* Copper storage hepatitis in Bedlington terriers and West Highland white terriers *Copper-associated* hepatitis in Doberman pinschers and Skye terriers	Congenital portosystemic shunt (hepatic atrophy)

ICH = infectious canine hepatitis; FIP = feline infectious peritonitis.
*Hepatic neoplasia, primary or metastatic, may also cause signs of chronic hepatic failure, but a discussion of the treatment is beyond the scope of this chapter.

CHRONIC HEPATIC FAILURE

Chronic hepatic failure in dogs and cats is being diagnosed with increasing frequency and may be caused by drugs, hepatotoxins, infectious agents, metabolic disturbances, and autoimmune disorders (Table 9-2). As was the case for acute hepatic failure, the etiology is often idiopathic.

A tentative diagnosis of chronic hepatic insufficiency is based on history, physical examination, and laboratory, radiographic, and ultrasonographic findings. A definitive diagnosis requires liver biopsy. Animals with chronic hepatic insufficiency may be asymptomatic in the early stages of the disorder, or vague signs of lethargy, decreased appetite, weight loss, and sporadic vomiting and diarrhea may not prompt the owner to seek veterinary care until hepatic insufficiency is serious. Patients with advanced chronic hepatic disease may show polydipsia, polyuria, icterus, ascites, and signs of HE, including head-pressing, intermittent apparent blindness, stupor, coma, and seizures. Characteristic laboratory abnormalities may include persistent increases of S-ALT and other findings as were described for acute hepatic failure. A small liver is often observed radiographically; and ascites, usually a pure transudate (protein content < 2.5 g/dl), is sometimes present.

Standard Therapy. Specific treatment of the cause of chronic hepatic insufficiency (Table 9-3) is ideal, but often the cause is unknown. Early diagnosis and therapy may improve the prognosis. For example, early identification and surgical correction of a congenital portosystemic shunt often results in reversal of hepatic atrophy and restoration of hepatic function. Cirrhosis is the end result of several chronic hepatic disorders and is difficult to manage successfully. Supportive therapy for canine and feline chronic hepatic insufficiency is not well defined, and recommendations are often speculative and empiric. Discussed in the following sections are general therapeutic recommendations for various causes of chronic hepatic insufficiency. The reader is referred to Table 9-3 for treatment modalities for selected specific causes of chronic hepatic insufficiency.

Anti-inflammatory Therapy. Glucocorticoids have been used for chronic hepatitis in both dogs and cats (Table 9-3), but their use remains controversial and controlled studies have not been reported. Corticosteroids reportedly have both anti-inflammatory and antifibrotic properties, both of which should be of benefit in chronic hepatitis; however, in humans, corticosteroids are used only for immune-mediated and idiopathic chronic active hepatitis (CAH), and may worsen viral chronic hepatitis. Retrospective studies in dogs with various forms of chronic hepatitis have shown that the use of corticosteroids increased survival time threefold. Substantiation of these results with controlled prospective studies is needed because corticosteroids have a number of detrimental side effects, such as immunosuppression and increased protein catabolism.

Use of corticosteroids for canine and feline chronic hepatitis should probably be considered only for those cases in which a liver biopsy has confirmed histologic lesions consistent with immune-mediated chronic hepatitis (CAH in dogs, chronic lymphocytic cholangiohepatitis in cats) and there are no known nonimmunologic causes. Also, it is reported that glucocorticoid therapy is sometimes beneficial for copper-associated hepatitis in Doberman pinschers, but published data are limited. I occasionally use glucocorticoids for suspected immune-mediated chronic hepatitis in dogs and cats for which a hepatic biopsy cannot be performed for some reason (e.g., owner reluctance, excessive risk). The disadvantages and risks associated with such an approach should be thoroughly explained to the owner first.

Prednisolone (not prednisone, which requires hepatic activation) is recommended at an initial dosage of 1–2 mg/kg PO once daily until clinical remission is achieved. The dosage then is tapered slowly to reach a maintenance level of 0.5 mg/kg daily or on alternate days. It should always be the goal to stop steroid therapy at some point (hopefully within 3–4 months), although relapse may occur necessitating prolonged use of corticosteroids. Some patients require steroids for the rest of their lives.

TABLE 9-3. Therapy for the Most Common Disorders Causing Subacute or Chronic Hepatic Failure in Dogs and Cats*

Condition	Therapeutic Regimen	Comments
Drug-induced	Stop administration of offending drug	Most cases are reversible, but supportive care for complications of chronic hepatic insufficiency may be needed.
Infectious Suppurative cholangiohepatitis	Antibiotic for 4–6 weeks PO Prefer: Ampicillin 20 mg/kg q8h *or* Cephradine (Velosef, Squibb) 20 mg/kg q8h Alternatives: Trimethoprim-sulfa (Tribrissen, Coopers Co.) 15 mg/kg q12h *or* Metronidazole (Flagyl, Ortho) 7.5 mg/kg q8h	
	Dehydrocholic acid (Decholin, Miles Labs) 10–15 mg/kg q8h until urine bile is negative	Do not use Decholin if total biliary obstruction is suspected.
	Fluid therapy IV or SC Ringer's solution with 20 mEq K^+/L Supply deficit and maintenance needs Add B complex vitamins to fluids in standard dosages Vitamin K_1 (Aquamephyton) if coagulopathy present, 1–2 mg/kg SC q12h Enteral nutrition to supply daily caloric needs (40–50 kcal/kg/day) Appetite stimulant for a day or two Diazepam (Valium, Roche) 0.05–0.15 mg/kg q12h IV *or* Oxazepam (Serax, Wyeth) 0.2–0.5 mg/kg q12h PO	

286

TABLE 9-3. Therapy for the Most Common Disorders Causing Subacute or Chronic Hepatic Failure in Dogs and Cats (continued)

Condition	Therapeutic Regimen	Comments
	Force-feed q4–6h PO (Feline c/d or k/d, Hill's Pet Products) Nasal tube feeding q4–6h (Feline Clinicare, Pet Ag) Pharyngostomy tube feeding q4–6h (Feline c/d or k/d) Gastrostomy tube feeding (Feline c/d or k/d)	Most cases improve within 7–10 days. If response to medical treatment is poor, consider exploratory celiotomy to examine the biliary tree for possible bile sludging or choleliths. Remove by flushing, and biopsy the liver.
FIP in cats	Try immunosuppressive dosages of steroids Prednisolone 2.2 mg/kg q24h PO Supportive care as required	Prognosis is grave. Short-term improvement may be noted for a few weeks.
Inflammatory Chronic active hepatitis in dogs	Prednisolone 2 mg/kg q24h PO until clinical remission is achieved (usually about 2 weeks), then 0.5–1.0 mg/kg q24–48h for 2–3 months PO, then consider discontinuing Colchicine (West-ward) 0.03 mg/kg q24h PO indefinitely Ascorbic acid (vitamin C) 25 mg/kg q24h PO indefinitely	Recheck the dog in 2 weeks and every 1–2 months thereafter until stable. Prognosis is guarded.
Chronic lymphocytic cholangiohepatitis in cats	Treatment regimen is the same as for suppurative cholangiohepatitis *except* use immunosuppressive dosages of steroids instead of antibiotics Prednisolone 2 mg/kg q24h PO for 2 weeks, then 1–2 mg/kg q48h for 2–3 months PO, then consider discontinuing Supportive care as listed for suppurative cholangiohepatitis	Most cases show improvement within 7–10 days, but the long-term prognosis is guarded. Steroid therapy is sometimes necessary indefinitely. If response to medical treatment is poor, consider exploratory celiotomy to examine the biliary tree for possible bile sludging or choleliths. Remove by flushing, and biopsy the liver.

TABLE 9-3. Therapy for the Most Common Disorders Causing Subacute or Chronic Hepatic Failure in Dogs and Cats (continued)

Condition	Therapeutic Regimen	Comments
Metabolic Copper-toxicity hepatitis in dogs	Copper chelator indefinitely 2,2,2-Tetramine (Syprine, Merck Sharp & Dohme) 10–15 mg/kg q12h PO *or* D-Penicillamine (Cuprimine, Merck Sharp & Dohme) 10–15 mg/kg q12h PO Zinc sulfate, acetate, or gluconate indefinitely 5–10 mg/kg q12h PO Ascorbic acid (vitamin C) indefinitely 25 mg/kg q24h PO Supportive therapy as indicated	Significant "de-coppering" of the liver may require several months. Early diagnosis and treatment are important for best chances of success.
Vascular Congenital portosystemic shunt	Partial or complete ligation of the shunt if possible Protein-restricted diet may be needed (prescription diet k/d, Hill's Pet Products or homemade diet)	Prognosis with corrective surgery is fair to good. Without successful surgery, hepatic atrophy occurs leading to hepatic failure usually in a few weeks to months.

*See text for treatment of complications of hepatic insufficiency.

Monitoring should include clinical signs and laboratory testing done first at about 10–14 days after beginning corticosteroid treatment and every 2–3 months thereafter. Because glucocorticoid treatment in dogs usually causes increases in SAP and S-ALT (corticosteroid-induced hepatopathy), monitoring these enzyme activities may not be helpful. Serum albumin concentration is usually a reliable indicator of long-term hepatic function, and a favorable response to treatment should be associated with an increase in serum albumin (unless there is another coexisting disease associated with albumin loss). Ideally, the liver should be rebiopsied and its histologic appearance examined approximately 3–6 months after treatment is begun to help decide on appropriate long-term management.

In dogs with chronic hepatitis, if response to prednisolone is poor, another immunosuppressive drug, azathioprine (Imuran, Burroughs Wellcome), may be added to the steroid regimen. Combination therapy with prednisolone (0.5 mg/kg/day PO) and azathioprine (1.0 mg/kg/day PO) has been recommended. Complete blood count (CBC) and platelet counts should be checked periodically because azathioprine is reported to cause neutropenia and thrombocytopenia. Once clinical remission is achieved, both drugs may be administered on an alternate-day basis at the dosages listed above. Liver biopsy should be repeated and efforts made to discontinue treatment as described above. Use of azathioprine for feline chronic hepatitis has not been reported.

Antifibrosis Therapy. Specific antifibrosis drugs that have been used in humans with chronic hepatitis include colchicine (Colchicine tablets, Westward Pharmaceuticals), zinc gluconate, polyunsaturated phosphatidylcholine (PPC), and D-penicillamine (Cuprimine, Merck Sharp & Dohme). No controlled studies have been published proving their efficacy in dogs. Use of antifibrosis agents for hepatic fibrosis is discussed in the section on investigational therapy.

Antibiotic Therapy. Septicemia is a relatively common complication of chronic hepatic insufficiency and may be due to reduced clearance of portal antigens by the hepatic reticuloendothelial system. Antibiotics are indicated if clinical or laboratory signs compatible with sepsis are observed: severe depression; fever or hypothermia; injected, "muddy" mucous membranes; polypnea; melena; neutrophilia with left shift or neutropenia; toxic changes in neutrophils; thrombocytopenia; prolonged clotting times; hypoalbuminemia; increased SAP; and hypoglycemia. Antibiotics should not be used prophylactically for chronic hepatitis because of the potential for causing a resistant infection, the risk of undesirable side effects, and expense.

Ideally, multiple blood cultures and antibiotic sensitivity testing should be done prior to starting antibiotic administration. The most common bacterial types include gram-negative aerobes and gram-positive anaerobes. For seriously ill dogs and cats with signs of gram-negative sepsis, a combination of gentamicin 2.2 mg/kg q6–8h IV and cephapirin (Cefadyl, Bristol) 20 mg/kg q8h IV is advised. Maintenance of adequate hydration and careful monitoring of renal function are essential because of the danger of gentamicin-induced nephrotoxicity. Intravenous antibiotic therapy should be continued for 2–3 days, at which time the route should be changed to subcutaneous. Gentamicin should not be administered any longer than necessary, usually for a maximum of 7–10 days. Once the patient is improved (or in less seriously ill patients), oral antibiotic therapy with either ampicillin 20 mg/kg three times daily PO or cephradine (Velosef, Squibb) 20 mg/kg three times daily PO is recommended for an additional 10–14 days.

Antibiotics that should be avoided in chronic liver disease are chloramphenicol, erythromycin, hetacillin, lincomycin, and sulfonamides. These agents either depend on hepatic metabolism for activation or clearance, or occasionally cause liver damage.

Gastrointestinal Bleeding. Gastrointestinal bleeding in association with chronic hepatic insufficiency may be the result of intestinal ulcers caused by either portal hypertension or drug administration (glucocorticoids and nonsteroidal anti-inflammatory agents, e.g., aspirin), bacterial overgrowth in the small bowel (hemorrhagic enteritis), coagulopathies, and infestation with parasites. Chronic hemorrhage often results in iron-deficiency anemia (microcytic, hypochromic) and can cause signs of HE because blood in the gastrointestinal tract serves as a source of ammonia production.

As was discussed in the section on acute hepatic failure, histamine H_2-receptor blocking drugs are indicated in patients with hematemesis or melena. Cimetidine is recommended at a dosage of 5 mg/kg q8h SC or PO in both dogs and cats. Another useful drug for gastrointestinal ulcers in dogs is sucralfate, which acts by forming a protective ulcer-adherent complex. Sucralfate is used at a dosage of 0.5 g q6–8h PO in dogs weighing less than 20 kg and 1.0 g q6–8h PO in larger dogs (>20 kg).

The high doses of glucocorticoids often needed for animals with chronic hepatitis commonly cause gastrointestinal bleeding. In such patients it may be necessary to stop steroids for a few days, use cimetidine or sucralfate (or both), and then reinstitute steroids at a lower dose in combination with these antiulcer drugs.

Ascites. Ascites caused by chronic hepatic disease is more common in dogs than in cats. Contributing factors include portal hypertension, sodium retention, and decreased plasma oncotic pressure as a result of hypoalbuminemia. Correction of ascites is difficult unless the primary hepatic disease is controlled. Objectionable side effects often result from overly aggressive efforts to eliminate ascites. The main goal should be to control the ascites well enough that respiratory distress is prevented, patient discomfort is minimized, and renal perfusion is not compromised while treating the primary problem (chronic hepatic disease). Techniques available for control of ascites include paracentesis, cage rest, dietary sodium restriction, and use of diuretics.

Paracentesis of large amounts of ascitic fluid is not justified unless there is serious respiratory distress or unless abdominal radiography, laparoscopy, or celiotomy are to be done. Removal of large quantities of ascitic fluid may cause serious hypoalbuminemia and decreased plasma oncotic pressure, thus promoting the formation of additional ascitic fluid. Thus a vicious cycle is set up, and the patient's condition worsens.

Cage rest and feeding a sodium-restricted diet (prescription diets k/d or h/d, Hill's Pet Products, or a homemade low-sodium diet) may adequately control ascites. For patients that refuse to eat one of these diets, or if control of ascites is inadequate, careful use of diuretics that cause urinary sodium loss is recommended. A recommended protocol for diuretic therapy for ascites associated with chronic hepatitis is as follows: 1) Give spironolactone (Aldactone, Searle) 1.0 mg/kg q12h PO. 2) If adequate diuresis has not occurred after 4 days, double the dosage. 3) When diuresis is adequate, taper the spironolactone dosage to the lowest daily dosage required to control ascites. If the ascites does not respond adequately to spironolactone, add furosemide (Lasix, Hoechst-Roussel) 1 mg/kg q12h PO. Double this dosage if the ascites remains refractory. In some patients with ascites and severe hypoalbuminemia, administration of canine or feline plasma followed by intravenous furosemide may be more successful. Side effects of excessive use of furosemide include potassium depletion, dehydration, and azotemia. Excessive use of furosemide may result in hypokalemia and azotemia, each of which can precipitate HE in patients with chronic hepatic disease.

Chronic Hepatic Encephalopathy. Dietary management is important and is discussed separately in the following section.

Lactulose (Cephulac, Merrell Dow) is a nondigestible disaccharide that is metabolized by enteric bacteria to acidic products, thus acidifying the intestinal tract and increasing luminal osmolality. These effects result in decreased ammonia absorption. Lactulose is used orally at a dosage of 5 ml (3.3 g)/ 5–10 kg PO q6h with the dosage adjusted thereafter to produce two or three soft stools per day. Neomycin is sometimes advocated to reduce enteric bacterial numbers, thus lessening bacterial ammonia production. However, neomycin may damage the normal intestinal microflora and allow enteric pathogens to proliferate. There is also concern about possible excessive neomycin absorption resulting in ototoxicity and nephrotoxicity. For these reasons, I do not recommend the use of neomycin.

Gastrointestinal hemorrhage should be prevented because blood is a protein source and is converted to ammonia by enteric bacteria. Causes of such hemorrhage, e.g., intestinal parasites, should be treated, and cimetidine or sucralfate (or both) should be used as previously described.

Drugs that require the liver for elimination, e.g., sedatives, tranquilizers, hypnotics, certain intravenous anesthetics, anticonvulsants, and organophosphates, should be avoided or used carefully. Diuretics may cause dehydration, prerenal azotemia, and potassium depletion, all of which may increase blood ammonia. Lipotropic drugs contain methionine, which can worsen HE. Glucocorticoids increase body protein catabolism, which may exacerbate hyperammonemia and can cause gastrointestinal ulceration and hemorrhage.

Dietary Management. When planning a diet for a patient with chronic hepatic insufficiency, the primary concern should be to minimize the protein abnormalities that contribute to hyperammonemia and abnormal plasma amino acid ratios (excessive aromatic/branched chain). If too much protein is fed, especially meat proteins, which are high in aromatic amino acids, overproduction of ammonia may occur in the distal small bowel and colon because the normal gut microflora deaminates the amino acids. Because portosystemic shunts are present and the liver is unable to adequately convert ammonia to urea, the results are hyperammonemia and signs of HE. On the other hand, too little protein in the diet causes catabolism of body proteins associated with increased ammonia production and impaired regeneration of the liver. It is advisable to feed patients with chronic liver disease as much of their maintenance protein requirements (4.8 g/kg/day for dogs and 10 g/kg/day for cats) as they can tolerate without showing signs of HE. Dietary protein should be of high biologic value and have a high branched-chain/aromatic amino acid ratio. Avoid feeding meat; instead, feed vegetables, cottage cheese, and small amounts of egg proteins.

Easily digested carbohydrates should be used to supply most of the patient's calories; cooked white rice is an excellent carbohydrate source. It has been recommended for dogs with chronic hepatic insufficiency that only moderate amounts of fat should be in the diet because short-chain fatty acids may worsen HE; however, a deficiency of plasma fatty acids, including polyunsaturated fatty acid deficiency associated with protein-energy malnutrition, has been documented in human cirrhotic patients. Similar studies in dogs and cats are needed.

At the present time no commercial diet is ideal for dogs and cats with chronic hepatic insufficiency. Prescription diet k/d (Hill's Pet Products) has many of the desired characteristics, including reduced-quantity, high biologic value protein. Formulations for homemade diets to feed dogs with hepatic insufficiency have been published (Tables 9-4 and 9-5). Multiple feedings (three or four times a day) are recommended to maximize small intestinal digestion and absorption of dietary components and to decrease the quantity of amino acids reaching the colon, thus lessening ammonia production.

Because dogs and cats with chronic liver disease may have deficiencies of vitamins and minerals, a balanced vitamin and mineral supplement is recommended. Supplements with added copper should not be given.

Investigational Therapy. Several drugs are being evaluated for the treatment of chronic hepatitis in small animal patients.

Antifibrosis Drugs. Colchicine (Colchicine tablets, West-ward Pharmaceuticals) is an antiinflammatory and antifibrotic agent that stimulates breakdown of hepatic fibrous tissue and inhibits further production of fibrous tissue in the liver. Colchicine has been used for fibrotic liver disease in dogs at a dosage of 0.03 mg/kg once daily PO, but its use in cats has not been reported. Treatment

TABLE 9-4. Homemade Diets for Dogs with Chronic Hepatic Insufficiency*

Not Copper-Restricted Diet 1

	Oz/Batch
Instant nonfat dry milk fortified with vitamins A and D	7⅜
Blackstrap molasses	4¾
Wheat germ (raw ground if possible)	4
Bone meal (sterilized)	1³⁄₁₀
Safflower oil	3½
Lard or beef tallow	3½
Table salt (iodized)	⅜
Cornstarch	14⅕
Ascorbic acid (vitamin C)	25 mg/kg body wt/day
Choline	250 mg for dogs < 15 kg *and* 500 mg for dogs > 15 kg

Lower Copper Diet 2

	Per Batch
Low-fat cottage cheese	2 lb
Lard or beef tallow	½ lb
Safflower oil	¼ cup
Sugar	1 lb plus 3 tablespoons
Cornstarch	1 lb plus 5 tablespoons
Bone meal (sterilized)	1⅓ oz
Salt substitute (KCl), iodized	3¼ teaspoons
Table salt (iodized)	2 teaspoons
Ascorbic acid (vitamin C)	25 mg/kg/day
Choline	250 mg for dogs < 15 kg *and* 500 mg for dogs > 15 kg
Vitamin/mineral supplement (Centrum; Lederle)	One tablet daily

*Diets must be refrigerated or frozen for storage.
From Strombeck DR, Schaeffer MPH, Rogers QR: Dietary therapy for dogs with chronic hepatic insufficiency. In: Kirk RW, ed. *Current Veterinary Therapy VIII.* Philadelphia: WB Saunders, 1983;817.

is usually continued for several months or sometimes indefinitely until clinical and laboratory signs of chronic hepatic insufficiency are no longer present. Reported side effects include hemorrhagic gastroenteritis, bone marrow suppression, renal damage, myopathies, and peripheral neuropathies. I have used colchicine for several months in dogs with chronic, fibrotic hepatitis without serious side effects and have documented marked improvement in clinical signs and laboratory abnormalities. Ideally, hepatic biopsy should be repeated to help assess the need for continued colchicine administration.

Copper-Reducing Therapy. If significant hepatic accumulation of copper is found in dogs with chronic hepatitis, attempts should be made to lower hepatic copper. Measures that have been tried include reduced copper diets,

TABLE 9-5. Approximate Daily Maintenance Requirements of Homemade Diets for Dogs with Chronic Hepatic Insufficiency

Body Weight (kg)	Diet 1 (oz)	Diet 2 (oz)
4.5	3.2	4.5
9.1	5.3	7.6
13.6	7.2	10.3
15.9	8.1	11.6
20.4	9.7	14.0
25.0	11.3	16.3
36.4	15.0	21.6

From Strombeck DR, Schaeffer MPH, Rogers QR: Dietary therapy for dogs with chronic hepatic insufficiency. In: Kirk RW, ed. *Current Veterinary Therapy VIII*. Philadelphia: WB Saunders, 1983;817.

use of drugs that may interfere with copper absorption from the intestinal tract, and administration of drugs to lower liver copper.

The restriction of dietary copper probably is of little benefit in dogs with established liver disease associated with increased hepatic copper. Low-copper diets may be warranted in young dogs known to be affected with an inherited hepatic copper metabolism defect (Bedlington terrier, West Highland white terrier). Unfortunately, there are no commercial diets that are sufficiently low in hepatic copper to be recommended. Homemade diets that do not contain excess copper can be prepared (Table 9-4). Liver, shellfish, organ meats, and cereals are all high in copper content and should be avoided.

Zinc may be useful in dogs with copper-associated chronic hepatitis because it may block uptake of copper from the gastrointestinal tract. Zinc acetate, sulfate, or gluconate 5–10 mg/kg/day PO is recommended. Zinc administration should be continued in such patients indefinitely. A potential side effect of excessive administration is hemolytic anemia. It is prudent to evaluate a CBC periodically. Although zinc therapy may prevent further copper accumulation in the liver, it is doubtful that it has any effect in "de-coppering" the liver of previously affected dogs.

Ascorbic acid (vitamin C) may also inhibit intestinal copper absorption and possibly increases excretion of copper in the urine. Also, an important part of the dog's daily requirement of ascorbic acid is produced by the liver, and dogs with hepatic insufficiency are deficient in ascorbic acid when fed the amount normally found in the diet. Ascorbic acid is administered at a dose of 25 mg/kg/day PO.

Treatment with copper chelators has been helpful in abnormal hepatic copper accumulation. D-Penicillamine (Cuprimine, Merck Sharp & Dohme; Depen, Wallace) and tetramine cupretic agents have been used to chelate copper and cause its excretion in the urine, thus reducing hepatic copper content. A recommended dose of penicillamine is 10–15 mg/kg PO twice a day. D-Penicillamine acts slowly, and "de-coppering" may take months or years of treatment. Side effects such as anorexia, nausea, and vomiting occur rather often and make the use of D-penicillamine difficult. Also, some dogs develop reversible renal disease and skin eruptions while on D-penicillamine.

2,3,2-Tetramine has been shown to be an effective "de-coppering" drug with a more rapid onset of action and fewer side effects than D-penicillamine, but the drug is not available in a practical form at this time. A closely related drug, 2,2,2-tetramine (Syprine, Merck Sharp & Dohme), is available and reportedly has fewer side effects. The recommended dosage is 10–15 mg/kg PO twice a day. Unfortunately, 2,2,2-tetramine removes hepatic copper more slowly than 2,3,2-tetramine.

Hydrocholeretic Therapy. Severe cholestasis and bile inspissation occurs in some cases of chronic hepatic insufficiency, especially chronic cholangiohepatitis. Dehydrocholic acid (Decholin, Miles Pharmaceuticals) has been used empirically in both dogs and cats at a dosage of 10–15 mg/kg PO q8h to stimulate flow of watery bile and thus improve bile flow and relieve cholestasis. Use of dehydrocholic acid is continued until bilirubinuria is no longer significant. Dehydrocholic acid therapy has been associated with few side effects (occasional diarrhea) but is contraindicated if complete biliary obstruction is suspected.

Immunosuppressive Therapy. Beneficial effects of the T cell immunosuppressant cyclosporin A for autoimmune CAH in man have been reported, but no studies of its use for chronic hepatitis in dogs or cats have been published.

SUGGESTED READINGS

Black M: Hepatic detoxification of endogenously produced toxins and their importance for the pathogenesis of hepatic encephalopathy. In: Zakim D, Boyer T, eds. Hepatology: A Textbook of Liver Diseases. Philadelphia: WB Saunders, 1982;397.

Cornelius LM: Cholangiohepatitis in cats. Mod Vet Pract 1985;66:626.

Cornelius LM: Chronic hepatitis in dogs. Vet Med Rep 1989;1:328.

Cornelius LM: Fluid, electrolyte, acid-base, and nutritional management. In: Bojrab MJ, ed. Pathophysiology in Surgery. Philadelphia: Lea & Febiger, 1981;12.

Crawford MA: Schall WD, Jensen RK, et al: Chronic active hepatitis in 26 Doberman pinschers. J Am Vet Med Assoc 1985;87:1343.

Crowe DT: Enteral nutrition for critically ill or injured patients. Part 1. Compend Contin Educ Pract Vet 1986;8:603.

Crowe DT: Enteral nutrition for critically ill or injured patients. Part 2. Compend Contin Educ Pract Vet 1986;8:719.

Drazner FH: Hepatic encephalopathy in the dog. In: Kirk RW, ed. Current Veterinary Therapy VIII. Philadelphia: WB Saunders, 1983;829.

Hardy RM: Chronic hepatitis in dogs: a syndrome. Compend Contin Educ Pract Vet 1986;8:904.

Johnson SE: Acute hepatic failure. In: Kirk RW, ed. Current Veterinary Therapy IX. Philadelphia: WB Saunders, 1986;945.

Magne ML, Chiapella AM: Medical management of canine chronic hepatitis. Compend Contin Educ Pract Vet 1986;8:915.

Rogers KS, Cornelius LM: Feline icterus. Compend Contin Educ Pract Vet 1985;7:391.

Sherding RG: Hepatic encephalopathy in the dog. Compend Contin Educ Pract Vet 1979;1:55.

Strombeck DR, Miller LM, Harrold BS: Effects of corticosteroid treatment on survival time in dogs with chronic hepatitis: 151 cases. J Am Vet Med Assoc 1988;193:1109.

Strombeck DR, Schaeffer MC, Rogers QR: Dietary therapy for dogs with hepatic insufficiency. In: Kirk RW, ed. Current Veterinary Therapy VIII. Philadelphia: WB Saunders, 1980;885.

Tamms TR: Hepatic encephalopathy. Vet Clin North Am 1985;15:177.

Twedt DC: Jaundice, hepatic trauma, and hepatic encephalopathy. Vet Clin North Am 1981;11:121.

Twedt DC, Whitney EL: Management of hepatic copper toxicosis in dogs. In: Kirk RW, ed. Current Veterinary Therapy X. Philadelphia: WB Saunders, 1989;891.

CHAPTER TEN

Exocrine Pancreatic Diseases

Larry M. Cornelius

Diseases of the exocrine pancreas affect both dogs and cats but are more common in dogs. Acute and chronic pancreatic inflammatory disorders, idiopathic pancreatic atrophy, and various neoplastic disorders involving the pancreas are frequently observed by small animal practitioners.

Various classification methods have been used to describe pancreatic inflammatory disorders, but all have limitations in veterinary medicine. In dogs, sudden-onset, single episodes of pancreatic inflammation, termed acute pancreatitis, and similar multiple intermittent bouts over a longer time course, called relapsing acute pancreatitis, are much more commonly recognized than is chronic pancreatitis. The latter term is used synonymously by some veterinarians with exocrine pancreatic insufficiency (EPI), but this usage should be discouraged as EPI is the preferred terminology and is more clinically descriptive. Chronic interstitial pancreatitis, often associated with cholangiohepatitis, is the most common form of pancreatitis in cats, although acute necrotizing pancreatitis similar to that seen in dogs occasionally occurs in cats.

ACUTE PANCREATITIS

Acute pancreatitis (AP) is an inflammatory disorder of the pancreas of sudden onset. Two distinctly different forms are reported: 1) interstitial edematous pancreatitis; and 2) purulohemorrhagic, necrotic pancreatitis. It is widely believed that the interstitial edematous form is much more common and has a more benign course than does the hemorrhagic, necrotic form. The cause of AP in dogs and cats is usually idiopathic. The following are thought to be risk factors for AP in dogs: 1) obesity; 2) high fat diet; 3) chronic hypercortisolemia (use of glucocorticoids or hyperadrenocorticism); and 4) use of certain organophosphate insecticides (diazinon, cythioate). The more risk factors present in a given patient, the greater the chance of AP occurring (or recurring) in that animal.

Clinical signs of AP are nonspecific and depend on the form and severity of the inflammatory lesion. Sudden onset of lethargy, depression, anorexia, vomiting, dehydration, and signs of abdominal discomfort, often shortly after ingestion of a fatty meal, are typical signs, but variation from patient to patient is seen. Signs of sepsis and toxemia (injected sclera, prolonged capillary refilling time, fever or hypothermia, shock) may be seen with severe AP. Suspicion of AP should be especially high if these signs are observed in a dog with one or more of the risk factors above.

Definitive diagnosis of AP is difficult because clinical signs are similar to many other common diseases, there is no test specific for the disorder, and laboratory results may depend on the severity and stage of the disease at the time of sampling. Evidence must be accumulated from the history, physical examination, and laboratory data. Characteristic laboratory abnormalities include fasting chylomicronemia (milky plasma); increased plasma triglycerides; increased packed cell volume (PCV); neutrophilic leukocytosis with a left shift; increased blood urea nitrogen (BUN), serum creatinine, serum alanine aminotransferase (ALT), and alkaline phosphatase (SAP); hyperbilirubinemia; mild hyperglycemia; slightly decreased serum calcium; and increased serum amylase and lipase activities. Other electrolyte and acid-base abnormalities may occur (hypokalemia, metabolic alkalosis, or metabolic acidosis) but are variable. With sepsis or toxemia, evidence of disseminated intravascular coagulation (DIC) may be present (thrombocytopenia and prolonged clotting times). Radiographic abnormalities are not present in most cases of AP, but occasionally loss of intraabdominal contrast and displacement of intestinal loops are observed. Ultrasonography may reveal hypoechoic areas in the pancreas in cases with pancreatic abscessation.

Standard Therapy

Most animals with AP recover rapidly with routine supportive care, but in some patients the disease takes a fulminant course (5–15% of cases in humans). The primary objectives of therapy for acute pancreatitis are to: 1) eliminate the cause or risk factors if known; 2) stop the autodigestive process; and 3) stabilize the patient's clinical condition to permit resolution of inflammation and necrosis. In the vast majority of cases, these objectives can be accomplished by conservative medical measures, which are emphasized below. A few severe cases of hemorrhagic, necrotic pancreatitis require more invasive procedures, such as peritoneal lavage and celiotomy for removal and débridement of necrotic pancreatic material. Unfortunately, early prognostic factors that would permit the clinician to anticipate the animals that have severe pancreatitis or are likely to progress from mild to severe AP are not documented for dogs and cats. Therefore it is imperative that once a diagnosis of AP is suspected the veterinarian carefully observe the effects of treatment and be ready to manage the patient more intensively if response to basic therapy is inadequate.

TABLE 10-1. Standard Medical Therapy for Patients with Signs of Mild to Moderate Acute Pancreatitis

1. Stop usage of any suspect drugs such as steroids or organophosphates.
2. Give *nothing* per os (NPO) for at least 2–3 days.
3. Administer parenteral fluid and electrolyte therapy.
4. Give parenteral antibiotic therapy as needed.
   a. Trimethoprim-sulfa (Tribrissen 24%, Coopers) 15–20 mg/kg SC q12h *or*
   b. Chloramphenicol 20 mg/kg SC q8h
   c. If response is poor or if infection with anaerobic organisms is suspected:
      (1) Metronidazole (Metronidazole Redi-Infusion, Elkins-Sinn) 10 mg/kg IV q8h *or*
      (2) Clindamycin (Quad) 20 mg/kg IV q8h
5. Monitor the patient carefully.
6. If no vomiting and patient's condition is improved: Return to oral intake by offering small amounts of water followed by carbohydrates (rice, pasta, bread) or low-fat prescription diet such as r/d (Hill's Pet Products) at frequent intervals. If vomiting or depression occurs, resume NPO.
7. Recommend:
   a. Avoid or reduce exposure to suspected risk factors (obesity, high fat diet, hypercortisolemia, certain organophosphates).
   b. Strict, fat-restricted diet (suggest prescription diet r/d or w/d, Hill's Pet Products), weight control, and exercise.

Conservative Medical Therapy. The medical therapeutic regimen for AP depends on the patient's clinical condition, although it should be remembered that unpredictably rapid deterioration can occur. Careful observation of the patient is warranted in all cases.

Mild to Moderate AP. Table 10-1 outlines the basic therapeutic measures for patients with signs of mild to moderate AP. Administration of any drugs that have been incriminated as being risk factors for AP (glucocorticoids, organophosphates) should be stopped. To decrease synthesis and secretion of pancreatic enzymes, it is crucial to withhold *all* oral intake, including food, water, and medication for at least 3–4 days. Because even the sight and smell of food may stimulate pancreatic secretion, measures should be taken to avoid having the patient anywhere near food. Use of anticholinergic drugs such as atropine or other medications to decrease pancreatic secretion have not proved effective in clinical cases of AP, and I do not recommend their use. Anticholinergic agents may cause or worsen ileus, thus promoting enteric bacterial pathogen overgrowth. Routine use of nasogastric suction to decrease pancreatic secretion, as has been recommended for human AP, is usually not practical in most veterinary practices.

Parenteral fluid and electrolyte therapy should be diligently provided. It is best to place an indwelling venous catheter and slowly infuse the estimated deficit, maintenance, and continuing loss fluid volume requirements over a period of several hours (see Chapter 1). Ideally, the type of fluid used should be based on the measurement of serum electrolytes and arterial blood gases and pH (or total CO_2). If this information is not available, an acidifying, balanced polyionic solution, e.g., Ringer's solution, is recommended as metabolic alkalosis is fairly common in animals who are vomiting due to AP. After initial correction of dehydration, it is usually advisable to add at least 20 mEq of potassium to each liter of Ringer's solution to help offset potassium losses, which may be significant in patients with metabolic alkalosis. Intravenous infusion of potassium-enriched solutions must always be done with care as too rapid intravenous administration of potassium can cause dangerous hyperkalemia (see Chapter 1).

The routine use of antibiotics for AP is controversial. Most authorities agree that bacteria probably do not play a role in mild, self-limiting cases, and in such patients prophylactic antibiotic usage could encourage the development of resistant infections. In more severe cases of AP, however, sepsis is believed to be common, probably as a result of ileus and enteric bacterial overgrowth; and sometimes pancreatic abscessation is seen. Because it is often difficult to determine which patients have bacterial involvement, I recommend the routine use of parenteral antibiotics for patients with AP. If antibiotics are to be used prophylactically, they should be started early in the course of the disease in order to have the best chance of preventing infection and sepsis. The best antibiotic to use in AP is also uncertain. A blood-pancreas barrier to antibiotic penetration probably exists in the normal pancreas, but its relevance to inflamed pancreatic tissue is uncertain. In general, lipid-soluble antibiotics, e.g., trimethoprim, metronidazole, clindamycin, and chloramphenicol, are better able to cross the blood-pancreas barrier than are water-soluble agents, e.g., cephalosporins and aminoglycosides. It is most likely that gut bacteria would be the pathogens involved (gram-negative aerobic and gram-positive anaerobic organisms). I recommend starting with either trimethoprim-sulfa (Tribrissen, 24% solution, Coopers) at a dosage of 15–20 mg/kg SC q12h or chloramphenicol at a dosage of 20 mg/kg SC q8h. If response is poor, or if infection with anaerobic organisms is suspected, metronidazole (Metronidazole Redi-Infusion, Elkins-Sinn) 10 mg/kg IV q8h or clindamycin (Cleocin, Upjohn) 20 mg/kg IV q8h should be used. After the patient is started back on oral intake, the route of antibiotic administration can be changed to oral (at the same dosage). Penetration of the above antibiotics into pancreatic juice is usually good. Antibiotic therapy is generally continued for at least 2 weeks or, preferably, for 5–7 days after all abnormal signs have resolved.

The patient should be carefully observed for improvement including attitude, temperature, and lack of vomiting. Following trends in the complete blood count (CBC)— resolving of a left shift, disappearance of toxic-appearing neutrophils—may also help predict when it is safe for the animal to be started back on oral intake. When oral intake is resumed, a few milliliters of water should be offered first, and if it is tolerated without the return of vomiting and depression small amounts of a fat- and protein-restricted food can be provided.

I prefer to use prescription diet r/d (Hill's Pet Products) for this purpose, but high carbohydrate foods (boiled white rice, pasta, bread) can also be used. If vomiting or depression recurs, the animal must once again be given nothing per os (NPO) for several days and maintained with parenteral treatment. The potential role of parenteral nutrition is discussed below.

Because AP is known to be a relapsing disorder, meticulous client education is essential. Avoiding or reducing exposure to as many risk factors (obesity, high fat diet, hypercortisolemia, certain organophosphates) as possible decreases the possibility of recurrence. I emphasize the importance of a fat-restricted diet for life, weight control, and regular exercise. For obese patients, prescription diet r/d is recommended until ideal body weight is achieved, and then the slightly less fat-restricted w/d (Hill's Pet Products) is advised for long-term maintenance. If the client prefers to cook for the animal, low-fat recipes are available.

Prognosis for complete recovery from mild to moderate AP is generally excellent. Also, careful client compliance with the measures recommended above appears to markedly reduce the recurrence rate.

Severe AP. Animals with severe necrotizing AP are usually challenging to treat, and adequate facilities and help to provide intensive care are required. Shown in Table 10-2 are treatment considerations for patients with severe AP.

Shock, hypovolemic or septic, may be present at the time of initial presentation or may develop rapidly during the course of severe AP. See Chapter 17 for a discussion of shock treatment and monitoring. Use of indwelling venous catheter and rapid replacement of fluid volume are essential. Lactated Ringer's solution should be administered intravenously at a rate of 90 ml/kg for approximately 1 hour, during which time the patient is carefully monitored. Some patients with severe AP have preexisting alveolocapillary membrane damage due to high levels of circulating activated pancreatic enzymes and are more likely to develop pulmonary edema during rapid fluid infusion. If signs of fluid overload are observed (tachycardia, dyspnea, crackles), the rate of fluid administration should be reduced to 20 ml/kg/hr or less. Prednisolone sodium succinate (Solu-Delta-Cortef, Upjohn) should be administered at a dosage of 10–20 mg/kg IV. This dosage can be repeated in 6 hours if needed. Longer-term use of glucocorticoids seems ill-advised because of the potential to worsen AP.

Once the patient is no longer in shock, intravenous fluid therapy should be continued with Ringer's or lactated Ringer's solution as described previously for the patient with mild to moderate signs of AP. Special attention should be given to monitoring serum potassium and adding at least 20 mEq of potassium to each liter of fluid (see Chapter 1 and Table 1-5 for guidelines for potassium replacement). If severe anemia is present (PCV <15%), whole blood transfusion (20 ml/kg IV over 4–6 hours) may be warranted. For significant hypoalbuminemia (serum albumin <2.0 g/dl), plasma transfusion (20 ml/kg IV over 4–6 hours), is indicated. An antihistamine, e.g., pyrilamine maleate (Pyrilamine, Butler) 4–6 mg/kg IV or IM, should be administered 20–30 minutes in

TABLE 10-2. Standard Medical Therapy for Patients with Signs of Severe Acute Pancreatitis

1. Treat shock if present (see Chapter 17).
    a. Lactated Ringer's solution 90 ml/kg/hr IV for 1 hr (monitor for signs of fluid overload—see Chapter 1).
    b. Prednisolone sodium succinate (Solu-Delta-Cortef, Upjohn) 10–20 mg/kg IV. Repeat dose once at 6 hours if needed.
2. Treat dehydration (see Chapter 1). Give intravenous Ringer's solution or lactated Ringer's solution to replace deficit, for maintenance, and for continuing losses. Usually replace deficit over about 6 hours and use continuous IV drip for maintenance and continuing losses. Add 20 mEq K^+/L (as KCl) to maintenance fluids.
3. Consider plasma or whole blood transfusion.
    a. Plasma 20 ml/kg IV over 4–6 hours
    b. Whole blood 20 ml/kg IV over 4–6 hours
4. Treat DIC if present. Give heparin (50–100 IU/kg SC q8h).
5. Use antibiotics.
    a. Trimethoprim-sulfa (Septra, Burroughs Wellcome) 15–20 mg/kg IV q12h.
    b. Consider addition of metronidazole (Metronidazole Redi-Infusion, Elkins-Sinn), 10 mg/kg IV q8h.
6. Consider H_2-receptor blocker for GI ulceration or bleeding. Give cimetidine (Tagamet, SmithKline & French) 5–7 mg/kg IV q8h.
7. Consider analgesic for severe pain.
    a. Butorphanol (Torbugesic, Fort Dodge) 0.4 mg/kg IM q6h *or*
    b. Pentazocine (Talwin, Winthrop) 0.5–1.0 mg/kg IM q6h
8. Monitor the patient carefully.
9. Give *nothing* per os (NPO) for at least 5–7 days.
10. If no vomiting and patient's condition is improved, return to oral intake by offering small amounts of water followed by carbohydrates (rice, pasta, bread) or low-fat prescription diet such as r/d (Hill's Pet Products) at frequent intervals. If vomiting or depression occurs, resume NPO.
11. Recommend:
    a. Avoid or reduce exposure to suspected risk factors (obesity, high fat diet, hypercortisolemia, certain organophosphates).
    b. Prescribe strict, fat-restricted diet (suggest prescription diet r/d or w/d, Hill's Pet Products), weight control, and exercise.

advance of whole blood or plasma transfusion. Another potential advantage of whole blood and plasma transfusion for patients with AP is the restoration of plasma protease-binding protein (α-macroglobulin). See Chapters 5 and 17 for details of blood and plasma transfusion.

Chronic disseminated intravascular coagulation (DIC) is relatively common in severe AP, and the treatment of choice is low-dose heparin 50–100 IU/kg SC q8h. The activated clotting time (ACT) and platelet count should be monitored every day or two. The goal is to normalize the platelet count without causing a significant increase in ACT. When DIC is no longer a problem, the heparin dosage should be tapered off slowly over 3–5 days (reduce the heparin dosage by about 25% per day). Sudden stoppage of heparin administration can cause rebound hypercoagulation and return of DIC. See Chapter 17 for further information on the treatment of DIC.

Use of parenteral antibiotics is warranted in all cases of severe AP. As previously discussed, sepsis is believed to be common, probably as a result of ileus and enteric bacterial overgrowth, and sometimes pancreatic abscessation. Trimethoprim-sulfa (Septra, Burroughs Wellcome) 15–20 mg/kg IV q12h is a good choice because it has a fairly broad spectrum (gram-negative aerobes and gram-positive anaerobes) and is relatively safe. It is used as a substitute for aminoglycosides in patients at high risk for nephrotoxicity caused by amino-glycoside administration. If response is poor or if infection with resistant anaerobic organisms is suspected, metronidazole at a dosage of 10 mg/kg q8h IV should be used. As discussed for patients with mild to moderate AP, after the patient is started back on oral intake the route of antibiotic administration can be changed to oral.

If gastrointestinal ulceration and bleeding characterized by melena are present, H_2-receptor blockers such as cimetidine (Tagamet, SmithKline & French) 5–7 mg/kg IV q8h reduce gastric HC1 output and are helpful. Once the patient is hydrated, the route of administration can be changed to intramuscular.

Use of analgesics is debatable because of the potential for some of these drugs—morphine or meperidine (Demerol, Wyeth)—to cause spasm of the pancreatic duct sphincter and potentially worsening pancreatitis. Butorphanol (Torbugesic, Fort Dodge) 0.4 mg/kg IM q6h or pentazocine (Talwin, Winthrop) 0.5–1.0 mg/kg IM q6h are now recommended for severe abdominal pain in patients with AP and apparently do not cause pancreatic duct spasm. Nevertheless, I recommend use of analgesics only for pancreatitis patients in obvious pain.

Monitoring of patients with severe AP in an intensive care setting is important. Careful attention to fluid and electrolyte input and hydration requires logging the fluid volume delivery every 4–6 hours, checking the pulse, capillary refilling time and skin turgor frequently. Central venous pressure can be measured to help assess adequacy of fluid volume administration. Serum electrolytes (especially potassium) and acid-base status (particularly serum TCO_2) should be checked at least every 2 or 3 days until the patient is stable. See Chapters 1 and 17 for further details regarding monitoring of fluid, electrolytes, and acid-base therapy in critically ill patients. Monitoring for clinical improvement, return to oral intake, and long-term management should be done as was discussed above for animals with mild to moderate AP.

Prognosis for recovery from severe AP is guarded to poor. In humans, severe acute hemorrhagic pancreatitis is associated with an overall mortality rate of 80–90%, and there is little reason to believe that the mortality rate is less for canine and feline patients.

Surgical Therapy. The role of surgical therapy for patients with AP is unclear and remains an area of controversy in both human and veterinary medicine. It is generally agreed that surgery is not indicated as a therapeutic modality for

TABLE 10-3. Considerations for Exploratory Celiotomy and Surgical Therapy for Patients with Signs of Acute Pancreatitis

1. Surgery is not indicated for most patients with AP (mild to moderate signs that respond to conservative medical therapy).
2. Surgery is sometimes indicated for:
   a. Patients with severe signs of AP including signs of sepsis/toxemia and icterus associated with probable bile duct obstruction.
   b. Patients in which conservative medical therapy is not helping or relapse of severe signs occurs. Timing of surgery depends on the clinical course and judgment of the clinician. Varies from a day or two after initiation of medical treatment to 2–3 weeks.
3. Surgery is usually indicated in patients for which there is a high index of suspicion of pancreatic abscess (ultrasonography, CT scan, other clinical and laboratory findings).

patients with signs of mild to moderate AP (the vast majority of patients). However, it is worth noting that exploratory celiotomy may be useful for differentiating mild to moderate AP from other conditions that produce signs of an acute abdomen for which surgery is the treatment of choice. In humans, it has been established that surgery is indicated for severe pancreatic necrosis and pancreatic abscessation. The difficulty lies in accurately assessing which patients with severe signs of AP actually have these conditions. This distinction is crucial because surgical intervention is obviously invasive and expensive, and it likely worsens the condition of patients with severe AP who do not have a surgically treatable pancreatic problem. Abdominal ultrasonography, computed tomography (CT) scanning, and image-guided needle aspiration of the pancreas are helpful in identifying severe pancreatic necrosis and abscessation in human patients. These diagnostic tools are not yet available to most veterinarians, and their usefulness in animals with pancreatitis has not been thoroughly evaluated.

What then are rational recommendations for surgery for dogs and cats with AP? Shown in Table 10-3 are guidelines for considering exploratory celiotomy in patients with severe signs of AP. It is obvious that many of the listed criteria are highly subjective. Consultation and dialogue between experts in both medicine and surgery are likely to provide a better informed judgment in difficult cases.

A description of surgical procedures used for patients with AP is beyond the scope of this chapter. Surgery for AP should be attempted only by veterinarians with special expertise in difficult abdominal soft tissue procedures. General considerations are resection and débridement of necrotic tissue, drainage of abscessed areas, and thorough lavage of the peritoneal cavity. Placement of drains for more prolonged peritoneal lavage is sometimes successful, but contamination and secondary bacterial peritonitis are complications that may occur.

Investigational Therapy

Research into the causes and pathophysiology of AP in man has led to trials with several drugs. Medications discussed below are either not yet available for clinical use or cannot be recommended yet for dogs and cats with AP. However, further studies may document the effectiveness of some of these drugs.

Advances in the understanding of cellular events in pancreatic acinar cells during the early stages of AP have incriminated abnormal transport and secretion of precursors of active pancreatic enzymes causing their intracellular activation. With this increased understanding, new therapeutic modalities are being tried and offer hope for more specific treatment of AP in the future. Most of these trials have been in experimental models of AP, many in dogs.

Drugs to Decrease Pancreatic Secretion. A number of antisecretory agents have been evaluated, including atropine, acetozolamide, glucagon, calcitonin, and somatostatin analogues. The consensus at this time is that these drugs have no proved benefit in clinical cases of AP.

Enzyme-Inhibiting Drugs. Aprotinin is a protease inhibitor that has been used for AP with limited success. More recent studies have shown that the low molecular weight potent protease inhibitors gabexate mesilate (FOY) and camostate (FOY 305) help prevent co-localization of pancreatic acinar cell lysosomal enzymes with digestive enzymes, thereby reducing intraacinar cell activation of digestive enzymes. Clinical trials are needed to further evaluate these promising new agents. It is also known that protease inhibitors are helpful in preventing the sequence of intravascular events of DIC. Because severe AP often is associated with DIC, protease-inhibiting drugs may be doubly useful. Dicalcium EDTA has been used in humans with AP for its phospholipase-inhibiting effects.

Cholecystokinin-Receptor Blocking Drugs. Some work has highlighted the importance of the pancreatic stimulatory hormone cholecystokinin (CCK), which is produced by the small intestinal mucosa, as an important contributory factor in some forms of AP. Potent synthetic drugs have been developed that block CCK receptors in the pancreas, and these CCK receptor blockers markedly improve survival of patients with some forms of experimental AP.

Drugs to Maintain Circulation. β-Adrenergic receptor agonist drugs such as terbutaline (Brethine, Geigy) and isoproterenol (Isuprel, Winthrop) have been shown to inhibit the increased microvascular permeability induced by histamine and other vasoactive substances released during the course of experimental AP. Terbutaline also inhibits pancreatic secretion. For these reasons, it is possible that terbutaline and other β-adrenergic agonists may be useful to help prevent progression from edematous pancreatitis to hemorrhagic, necrotic pancreatitis.

Agents that have been demonstrated to have efficacy for maintenance of pancreatic microcirculation during experimental AP are albumin, dextran solution, and hetastarch solution. The latter two are carbohydrate macromolecular solutions that are administered in conjunction with crystalloids such as Ringer's or lactated Ringer's solution. Their usefulness is related to their large molecular size and subsequent entrapment in the vascular space rather than rapid diffusion into the extravascular compartment typical of crystalloids. Clinical trials are needed to determine their value for AP.

Other studies have documented increases in pituitary-origin β-endorphin in plasma of dogs with experimentally induced AP accompanied by decreases in systemic blood pressure, pulse pressure, and cardiac output. The opiate antagonist naloxone (Narcon, DuPont), normalizes the above parameters and may be effective for treatment of severe AP associated with hypotension or shock.

Oxygen-Derived Free Radical Scavengers. Oxygen-derived free radicals play an important role in the pathogenesis of some forms of experimental canine AP. Drugs such as allopurinol (Zyloprim, Burroughs Wellcome), superoxide dismutase, and catalase, which "scavenge" excess free radicals, are reported to be beneficial when administered prior to the initiation of experimental AP. Their value in clinical cases of AP is uncertain.

Prostaglandins. Studies have shown that the cytoprotective effects of prostaglandins are not restricted to the gastrointestinal mucosa. Prostaglandin E_2 has been shown to stabilize pancreatic acinar cell membranes and prevent release of activated digestive enzymes in experimental AP and in clinical cases of AP in man. Studies are needed to evaluate the role of prostaglandins in treating AP in animals. As an interesting side note, this understanding of the potentially helpful membrane-stabilizing effects of prostaglandins should call into question the use of prostaglandin-inhibiting drugs, e.g., flunixin meglamine (Banamine, Schering), sometimes used by veterinarians for the treatment of AP.

Lipid-Lowering Drugs. The important role of high fat diet, hyperlipidemia, and obesity in the pathogenesis of AP in dogs has been described. Seemingly, these risk factors may play a greater role in canine AP than in the human disease, in which alcoholic pancreatitis and biliary tract disease associated with cholelithiasis are the more important hazards. The benefits of a fat-restricted diet and weight loss have been emphasized. In some patients, especially in those breeds known to have an increased prevalence of circulating lipoprotein abnormalities and hyperlipidemia (miniature Schnauzer), diet control and exercise may not adequately control blood lipids. A number of lipid-lowering drugs are now available because of the importance of hypercholesterolemia and hyperlipidemia in the pathogenesis of coronary artery disease in man. Drugs such as gemfibrozil (Lopid, Parke-Davis) and nicotinic acid (niacin), which decrease levels of fasting chylomicrons, may be useful in some cases of

AP in obese, hyperlipidemic patients. Lipid-lowering drugs should not be used until it has been shown that strict diet and weight control are ineffective.

Total Parenteral Nutrition. AP induces a hypermetabolic state and thus an increased need for caloric support in conjunction with a decreased ability of the gastrointestinal tract to function effectively. Thus parenteral nutrition has become a standard part of therapy in the treatment of human AP. There is still controversy about its safety and efficacy, but some work indicates that markedly increased mortality occurs in association with negative nitrogen balance. Sources of calories for parenteral nutrition include both hypertonic glucose and lipid emulsions. Lipids are generally not used in those patients with AP accompanied by hyperlipidemia. Expense and catheter-associated sepsis are significant problems. The role of parenteral nutrition needs to be studied in canine and feline patients with AP. I would be reluctant to infuse lipid-based solutions because of the common occurrence of hyperchylomicronemia in canine AP patients.

Peritoneal Lavage. Results of peritoneal lavage therapy for severe AP in both humans and dogs have been controversial. In theory, peritoneal lavage helps remove activated pancreatic enzymes and toxic products from the peritoneal cavity, thus decreasing their absorption. Also, peritoneal lavage reportedly decreases pain and vomiting. In reality, the benefits of this procedure are not clear. It is an invasive procedure often associated with serious side effects such as peritonitis, sepsis, and hypoalbuminemia. Peritoneal lavage therapy must be done multiple times daily using special peritoneal dialysis catheters. It is labor-intensive and expensive. For these reasons, I do not advocate this treatment modality at this time. Further controlled studies to document its efficacy are needed.

CHRONIC PANCREATITIS

Chronic pancreatitis is an insidious, progressive inflammatory disorder usually characterized clinically by: 1) intermittent episodes of nonspecific gastrointestinal signs such as anorexia, vomiting, abdominal pain, diarrhea, and weight loss; or 2) a relatively asymptomatic course until late in the progression of the disease when signs of exocrine pancreatic insufficiency (EPI) (see section on EPI below) and, less commonly, diabetes mellitus occur. Icterus may ensue 1) as a result of constriction of the common bile duct by fibrous tissue and adhesions involving the pancreas or 2) owing to associated hepatobiliary inflammation (cholangiohepatitis—see Chapter 9). A mass in the pancreatic area is often found by abdominal palpation or imaging procedures (radiography, ultrasonography, CT scanning). Serum amylase and lipase are often normal, perhaps because most pancreatic acinar cells have been destroyed by the time the animal is presented for evaluation. Confirmation of chronic pancreatitis requires celiotomy and pancreatic biopsy. Chronic interstitial pancreatitis is often noted in cats in association with cholangiohepatitis, but the clinical significance is uncertain.

Standard Therapy

It should be understood that the clinical diagnosis for this chronic, intermittent gastrointestinal syndrome is relapsing acute pancreatitis, and it is usually managed as described in the previous section on acute pancreatitis. When a pancreatic mass is found, especially in an icteric patient, and response to medical treatment is poor, celiotomy should be performed to establish a definitive diagnosis and surgically treat the condition. Cholecystoduodenostomy has been reported to be an effective means of biliary decompression for patients with chronic pancreatitis and common bile duct obstruction. It is suggested that hepatic biopsy also be performed during the same surgical event.

During the surgical routine, consideration should be given to placement of a jejunostomy tube for the administration of enteral nutrition. Nutrients instilled into the jejunum cause less stimulation of pancreatic enzyme secretion (see Suggested Readings for a reference on enteral nutrition). When a patient is able to tolerate oral feeding, the jejunostomy tube is removed. Further discussion of surgical procedures for chronic pancreatitis is beyond the scope of this chapter.

Investigational Therapy

In humans with chronic pancreatitis, intractable abdominal pain is a major problem. Administration of pancreatic enzyme supplements orally often helps alleviate abdominal pain, probably because oral pancreatic enzyme administration reduces secretion of pancreatic enzymes from the inflamed pancreas by negative feedback inhibition. It is reported that this negative feedback mechanism is not present in dogs, and thus it is doubtful that pancreatic enzyme therapy would be beneficial.

EXOCRINE PANCREATIC INSUFFICIENCY

Exocrine pancreatic insufficiency occurs whenever secretion of pancreatic digestive enzymes is inadequate for proper digestion and absorption of nutrients from the small bowel. EPI is more common in dogs than in cats. Characteristic clinical signs include chronic, progressive weight loss, often to the point of severe emaciation, usually associated with an increased or voracious appetite, diarrhea or large amounts of semiformed malodorous feces, and often pica or coprophagia. Usual causes of EPI are idiopathic pancreatic acinar atrophy and multiple episodes of relapsing acute pancreatitis (chronic pancreatitis). Pancreatic acinar atrophy is the most common cause of EPI in dogs and is most commonly reported in young German shepherd dogs. Chronic pancreatitis accounts for most cases of EPI in cats. EPI is accompanied by bacterial overgrowth in the small bowel in some cases. Occasionally, diabetes mellitus results from loss of pancreatic islet cells, and characteristic signs are seen (polydipsia, polyuria, cataracts).

Diagnosis of EPI is based on a typical history, clinical findings, and laboratory test results. The most sensitive and specific test for EPI is the serum trypsin-like immunoreactivity (TLI) assay. Low serum TLI usually indicates inadequate production of trypsinogen by pancreatic acinar cells. Other tests that may be of value include serum folate and cobalamin (used to help rule out bacterial overgrowth in the small bowel), combined BT-PABA/D-xylose, and fecal proteolytic activity. Older tests such as examination of feces for fat, starch, and muscle, and x-ray film digestion to assess fecal protease activity are sometimes used as practical screening tests, but they lack adequate sensitivity and specificity.

Standard Therapy

The objectives of treatment for EPI are to improve the patient's nutritional status (achieving weight gain) and to modify the characteristics of the stool (lessening fecal volume and stopping diarrhea). Components of therapy may include one or more of the following: 1) pancreatic enzymes; 2) highly digestible, low fiber diet; 3) H_2-receptor blocker; 4) antibiotic; and 5) cobalamin and vitamin E (tocopherol).

The basic treatment of EPI is supplementation of pancreatic digestive enzymes (from ox or pig pancreas) per os. Forms of commercial pancreatic enzyme products available are powders, tablets (some of which are enteric-coated), and granules. A reputable powdered form of pancreatin should be used because enzyme content and bioavailability vary significantly, and studies have shown that the enteric-coated products are often ineffective in animals. Several good-quality commercial products are available, including Viokase-V (A.H. Robins) and Pancrezyme (Daniel's Pharmaceuticals). Starting dosage is 2 teaspoons/20 kg body weight mixed with food. Incubation of the enzymes with food prior to feeding does not improve digestion of nutrients.

If the patient is on a good commercial maintenance food, diet change may be unnecessary. It has been shown that fiber interferes with the digestive action of pancreatic enzymes; therefore if response to pancreatic enzymes is inadequate, a low fiber, highly digestible diet, such as prescription diet i/d (Hill's Pet Products) should be tried. Feeding animals with EPI approximately 10–15% more calories than usually required is advisable, as nutrient assimilation is not normalized. Addition to the food of medium-chain triglyceride (MCT) oil at a dosage of ¼ to 4 teaspoons daily can be used as an additional source of calories. Some MCTs are absorbed intact into the portal circulation, and their hydrolysis by lipase proceeds much faster than that of long-chain triglycerides. Calories should be divided into two or three daily feedings (with addition of pancreatic enzyme powder) in order to improve nutrient utilization.

Body weight ought to be checked weekly and stool consistency observed. Expected weight gain should be 0.5–1.0 kg/week, although it may take 2–3 weeks for significant weight gain to be noticed by the client. Diarrhea is usually alleviated within a few days. Because pancreatic enzyme products are relatively expensive, it is a good idea to try to titrate the dosage downward once the animal has regained desired body condition. Increasing the dosage of the enzyme above the recommended amount of 2 teaspoons/20 kg seldom results in improved response.

Gastric acid destroys much of the administered pancreatic enzyme activity before it reaches its site of action in the duodenum. It has been shown that treatment with H_2-receptor blocking drugs, which decrease gastric HCl production, improves the response to oral pancreatic enzyme supplementation. Because H_2-receptor blockers add significantly to the cost of therapy, their use is advocated only for those animals that do not respond to enzyme supplementation and dietary management alone. Cimetidine can be tried at a dosage of 5–7 mg/kg PO q8h.

Studies have shown that many dogs with EPI have associated intestinal bacterial overgrowth with either gram-negative aerobes or gram-positive anaerobes, or both. This situation may result in failure to respond to the regimen described above. In such patients, it is suggested that a therapeutic trial with one of the following antibiotics, given orally, be initiated: 1) oxytetracycline (Terramycin, Pfizer) 10 mg/kg q12h; 2) metronidazole (Flagyl, Ortho) 10–15 mg/kg q8h; or tylosin (Tylan, Elanco) 7–10 mg/kg q8h. Treatment should be continued for 1–4 weeks.

Cobalamin malabsorption and decreased serum cobalamin levels are reported in some dogs with EPI, but associated clinical abnormalities have not been documented. Some authors suggest administration of 250 μg of cobalamin SC once weekly until serum cobalamin concentration is normal. Also, fat malabsorption may cause vitamin E (tocopherol) deficiency. Although clinical signs of tocopherol deficiency in patients with EPI have not been reported, administration of tocopherol (400–500 IU PO given once daily with food) has been advised by some.

Most patients show an appropriate response to the treatment outlined above. Prognosis for weight gain and control of polyphagia and diarrhea is usually good. Treatment usually must be lifelong, and expense may be a limiting factor, especially for large dogs. Substitution of chopped, raw ox or pig pancreas (3–4 oz/20 kg body weight) obtained from a slaughterhouse for commercial pancreatic enzyme powder has been used successfully in some patients with EPI as a less expensive alternative. Pancreas can be frozen at −20°C for at least 3 months without significant loss of enzyme activity. Some authors suggest withdrawing enzyme supplementation every 6 months as a trial to see if the patient needs continued treatment.

It has been reported that lymphocytic-plasmacytic enteritis coexists with EPI in some of the dogs that respond poorly to standard treatment. Preferably, this condition should be documented by intestinal mucosal biopsies prior to treatment. Use of glucocorticoids (prednisone 0.5–1.0 mg/kg/day PO) may be indicated for treatment of lymphocytic-plasmacytic enteritis (see Chapter 8).

Not all patients respond to treatment. In long-standing cases, secondary changes in the intestinal mucosa may not be reversible.

Investigational Therapy

Efforts to improve pancreatic enzyme supplementation therapy for EPI are being made. One approach has been to convert pancreatic extracts into microspheres coated with a pH-sensitive layer that resists breakdown by gastric acid. This condition allows pancreatic enzymes to remain intact until they reach the desired site of action in the duodenum. A second avenue offering promise for improvement is the use of acid-resistant fungal lipases. Both methods need further evaluation in animals with EPI before routine use can be advocated.

EXOCRINE PANCREATIC NEOPLASIA

Neoplasia of the exocrine pancreas occurs relatively infrequently in dogs and cats. Pancreatic adenocarcinoma may originate from either acinar or duct cells and often mimics acute pancreatitis, which is poorly responsive to medical therapy. Icterus and EPI may be present owing to obstruction of biliary and pancreatic ducts. Unfortunately, the disease tends to be well advanced with regional or systemic metastasis prior to definitive diagnosis obtained by pancreatic biopsy. Only palliative treatment is available (combination of surgical resection and chemotherapy). Other references should be consulted for discussion of therapy.

SUGGESTED READINGS

Bradley EL: Antibiotics in acute pancreatitis: Current status and future directions. Am J Surg 1989;158:472.

Cribb AE, Burgerner DC, Riemann KA: Bile duct obstruction secondary to chronic pancreatitis in seven dogs. Can Vet J 1988;29:654.

Goebell H, Singer MV: Acute pancreatitis: Standards of conservative treatment. In: Beger HG, Buchler M, eds. Acute Pancreatitis: Research and Clinical Management. Berlin: Springer-Verlag, 1987:259.

Gomez G, Townsend CM, Green D, et al: Involvement of cholecystokinin receptors in the adverse effect of glucocorticoids on diet-induced necrotizing pancreatitis. Surgery 1989;106:230.

Mayer AD, McMahon MJ, Cornfield AP, et al: Controlled clinical trial of peritoneal lavage for the treatment of severe acute pancreatitis. N Engl J Med 1985;312:399.

Salisbury SK, Lantz GC, Nelson RW, et al: Pancreatic abscess in dogs: Six cases (1978–1986). JAVMA 1988;193:1104.

Sitzmann JV, Steinborn PA, Zinner MJ, et al: Total parenteral nutrition and alternate energy substrates in treatment of severe acute pancreatitis. Surg Gynecol Obstet 1989;168:311.

Wheeler SL, McGuire BH: Enteral nutritional support. In: Kirk RW, ed. Current Veterinary Therapy X. Philadelphia: WB Saunders, 1989;30.

Williams DA: Exocrine pancreatic disease. In: Ettinger SJ, ed. Textbook of Veterinary Internal Medicine. Philadelphia: WB Saunders, 1989;1528.

CHAPTER ELEVEN

Urogenital Disorders

Scott A. Brown

AZOTEMIA

Azotemia is defined as the accumulation of nitrogenous wastes within the bloodstream and is generally recognized as elevated values for serum creatinine (SCr) and blood urea nitrogen (BUN). *Uremia* is defined as the presence of azotemia plus clinical signs (e.g., inappetance or vomiting). Although a reduction of urinary clearance of nitrogenous wastes is usually the mechanism responsible for their accumulation, the treatment of azotemia depends on the cause, which may be prerenal, renal, or postrenal. *Prerenal azotemia* is due to inadequate renal perfusion pressure (e.g., systemic hypotension), greatly elevated plasma protein concentration, or increased protein catabolism. *Renal azotemia* is caused by renal dysfunction leading to retention of nitrogenous wastes. *Postrenal azotemia* may be due to obstruction of urine outflow or rupture of the lower urinary tract.

Prerenal Azotemia

Decreased renal perfusion pressure may be due to internal or external loss of whole blood or fluid from the body (e.g., hemorrhage, protracted diarrhea, or polyuria without adequate water intake) or cardiovascular system failure (e.g., congestive heart failure, sepsis, shock, or hypoadrenocorticism). Differentiating prerenal from renal azotemia is often difficult. In many cases of prerenal azotemia, other clinical signs are indicative of a prerenal cause. Many of the common causes of prerenal azotemia (e.g., dehydration) also are a stimulus for the production of concentrated urine. In dogs, an intact ability to produce concentrated urine (specific gravity > 1.030) suggests that azotemia is more likely prerenal than renal. This situation is not true in cats, where urinary concentrating ability may be retained in the presence of renal azotemia. The presence of dilute urine in an azotemic patient, however, does not guarantee that the cause is renal, as some prerenal factors impair the urine concentrating ability, e.g., hypercalcemia, diabetes insipidus, diabetes mellitus, hypo- or hyperadrenocorticism, and hepatic failure.

The purpose of therapy for prerenal azotemia is to resolve the prerenal factor, most often with fluid administration. This action should restore adequate kidney function to eliminate retained nitrogenous wastes. Some specific therapy for electrolyte and acid-base abnormalities may be required during the intervening time.

Standard Therapy. Standard treatment for prerenal azotemia is supportive, consisting of fluid and electrolyte therapy. Specific therapy, based on the cause of the azotemia, should also be instituted, where appropriate.

Choice of Fluids. A balanced isotonic, polyionic solution, such as lactated Ringer's is generally preferred.* Serum electrolyte concentrations should be measured and the addition of 10–30 mEq KCl to each liter of fluid is indicated in normokalemic or hypokalemic patients. A specific primary disease may be best treated with other electrolyte solutions, e.g., normal saline for patients with hypoadrenocorticism.

Route of Fluid Administration. The route of administration depends to some extent on the degree of azotemia and the primary or other concurrent diseases. With the noteworthy exception of patients with congestive heart failure, rapid correction of prerenal azotemia is generally desirable. Consequently, the intravenous route of administration is preferred because it ensures rapid assimilation of fluids. For some causes of prerenal azotemia, e.g., hypoadrenocorticism, intravenous fluid administration is a requirement. The presence of uremia necessitates the intravenous route. In cases of mild azotemia, the subcutaneous route for fluid administration may be satisfactory for short-term therapy. Oral fluid administration is acceptable in cases of mild azotemia where neither gastrointestinal dysfunction nor severity of illness preclude the use of this route. However, a parenteral route is nearly always preferred.

Rate of Fluid Administration. The first goal of fluid therapy for prerenal azotemia is to correct dehydration. Dehydration can be estimated on the basis of clinical observations (see Table 1-1). A formula for determining the volume of fluid necessary for correction of dehydration is:

$$\text{Volume to correct dehydration (liters)} =$$
$$(\% \text{ dehydrated}) \times \text{body wt. (kg)}$$

For example, an azotemic dog weighing 20 pounds with anorexia and mildly decreased skin turgor may be judged to be 8% dehydrated (see Table 1-1). To determine fluid requirements, body weight must first be converted to kilograms:

$$[20 \text{ lb} \times (1 \text{ kg}/2.2 \text{ lb})] = 9.1 \text{ kg}$$

The fluid requirement for correction of dehydration would be:

$$8\% \times 9.1 \text{ kg} = 0.08 \times 9.1 \text{ kg} = 0.73 \text{ L} (730 \text{ ml})$$

This quantity of fluid only corrects dehydration; it does not take into account ongoing losses (e.g., vomiting) or daily maintenance requirements (40–60 ml/kg/day). Thus the total volume for 24 hours of therapy is equal to the volume necessary to correct dehydration plus 40–60 ml/kg/day plus estimates of

---

*Throughout this chapter, where lactated Ringer's solution is recommended, other balanced, isotonic, electrolyte solutions may be substituted.

ongoing losses. One-half of this total volume should be administered over the initial 2–6 hours, with the rest given over the subsequent 18–22 hours.

For example, maintenance fluid for the above 20 lb. (9.1 kg) dog would be:

$$50 \text{ ml/kg} \times 9.1 \text{ kg} = 455 \text{ ml in 24 hours}$$

Hence total fluid requirement for the first 24 hours of therapy would be:

$$730 \text{ ml (correct dehydration)} + 455 \text{ ml (maintenance)} = 1185 \text{ ml}$$

One-half of this amount (approximately 600 ml) could be administered as intravenous lactated Ringer's solution during the first 6 hours of therapy at a rate of 100 ml/hour IV) with the remaining 600 ml at a rate of 33 ml/hour IV delivered over the subsequent 18 hours. Potassium should be added (here to the lactated Ringer's solution) at the amount of 10–30 mEq/L unless the animal is hyperkalemic. Potassium should not be delivered at a rate that exceeds 0.5 mEq/kg/hr.

Monitoring Therapy. The SCr or BUN (or both) and serum electrolytes should be measured daily. Animals with azotemia due to simple prerenal factors should have a resolution of azotemia within 3–5 days. If it does not resolve, further diagnostic evaluation of the patient should be considered.

It should not be assumed that dehydration has been completely corrected within the first day of therapy. The degree of dehydration should be reestimated each day and the above calculations repeated.

One of the most common errors during therapy for azotemic patients is inadequate supplementation of fluids with potassium, leading to the development of hypokalemia. Unless the patient is hyperkalemic, maintenance fluids for azotemic animals should be supplemented with 10–30 mEq K^+/L, and serum potassium should be measured every 24–48 hours during aggressive fluid therapy. If hypokalemia develops, fluids should be supplemented with additional potassium chloride (see Table 1-5). However, the rate of intravenous potassium administration should not exceed 0.5 mEq/kg/hr.

The degree of azotemia (SCr and BUN) should be assessed daily. On appropriate fluid therapy, azotemia due to uncomplicated prerenal factors should be completely resolved within 3–5 days. If the level of azotemia does not improve by day 3, the fluid therapy should be carefully reevaluated; and other concurrent diseases, including the possibility of postrenal or renal components to the azotemia, should be explored.

Prognosis. The prognosis for recovery from prerenal azotemia depends on the cause. If the primary cause is resolved, animals with prerenal azotemia have a good prognosis.

Classification of Renal Azotemia

Azotemia of renal origin is due to renal dysfunction, leading to retention of nitrogenous wastes. Onset of azotemia from renal dysfunction is generally not seen unless the glomerular filtration rate (GFR) and number of functional neph-rons are less than 25% of normal. A therapeutic classification system based on urine production (oliguric versus polyuric) and the presence or absence of clinical signs (uremia versus azotemia) is useful and is employed here.

Renal dysfunction may also be classified as acute (occurring over less than 2 weeks) or chronic. This classification system is useful prognostically, as animals with acute renal failure have a greater potential for reversibility of damage to nephrons, whereas compensatory renal hypertrophy is often al-ready exhausted in patients with chronic renal failure.

Polyuric, Azotemic Renal Failure

Standard Therapy. *Supportive Care.* Many components of therapy must be administered by the owner, and they should be carefully counseled in these matters. Adequate fresh water should be provided at all times, and care should be taken to avoid prerenal insults (e.g., hot temperatures where evaporation associated with panting may lead to dehydration). The patient should receive a balanced supplement containing both the B vitamins and vitamin C. Glu-cocorticoids, tetracycline, and nephrotoxic medications (e.g., aminoglycosides) should be avoided.

Dietary Energy, Protein, and Phosphate Intake. The most important goal of dietary therapy is to provide adequate caloric intake to maintain body weight. Although it is initially approximately 60–100 kcal/kg/day, a chart of monthly values for body weight maintained by the client at home is the preferred method to assess adequacy of caloric intake.

The diet utilized at home should be low in phosphate. The necessity for protein restriction in early renal failure is controversial; however, in practice, diets restricted in protein will also be low in phosphorus. Examples of such diets include canine and feline k/d (Hill's Pet Products). Other commercial low phosphorus/low protein diets are available and are preferable to homemade low protein, low phosphate diets. Severe protein restriction causes nutritional deficiencies, particularly in cats, and may predispose to the development of hypoalbuminemia and hypercoagulation syndromes in dogs. The BUN may be used as an index of owner compliance with the low protein diet. Unexplained increases in BUN that are not accompanied by an increase in SCr are likely due to an owner supplementing the pet's diet with additional protein.

A low phosphate diet is employed to reduce the degree of hyperphos-phatemia and associated hyperparathyroidism. Serum phosphate can be used to approximate the adequacy of dietary phosphate restriction. If 3–4 weeks of dietary phosphate restriction does not normalize serum phosphate concentra-tion, aluminum-containing phosphate binders (e.g., Alternagel, Stuart; Am-phojel, Wyeth; Basaljel, Wyeth) may provide additional control of serum phosphate concentration. Calcium carbonate and calcium citrate have been used as phosphate binders, but they may produce hypercalcemia in dogs and cats and should be used cautiously while monitoring plasma calcium. An initial oral dose of phosphate binders containing aluminum or calcium (30 mg/kg every 8 hours) with meals should be administered for 2 weeks, with the dose doubled if the serum phosphate remains unchanged. Phosphate binders are administered to effect with doses individualized. Binders should be discontinued if they do not lower serum phosphate concentration when evaluated in this manner.

Management of Disorders of Calcium Homeostasis. Terminally, hypocalcemia may develop in dogs with renal failure. It should not be treated with calcium supplementation, as ionized calcium concentrations are almost always adequate to prevent hypocalcemic tetany. In any case, control of hyperphosphatemia with dietary phosphate restriction and phosphate binders is the appropriate first step.

Mild hypercalcemia may develop in dogs with acute renal failure or in young dogs with chronic renal failure, possibly due to a resetting of a normal parathyroid gland. Therapy is generally not necessary in this case. However, distinguishing this cause of hypercalcemia from other more serious causes (e.g., lymphosarcoma, other neoplastic processes, or primary hyperparathyroidism) requires that appropriate diagnostic tests be performed.

If an animal is markedly hypercalcemic (serum calcium concentration 2 mg/dl or more above the normal range), therapy for hypercalemia should be instituted promptly; this condition should be considered a medical emergency if the serum calcium concentration exceeds 15 mg/dl. Therapy should be sequential and initially include lactated Ringer's solution to correct dehydration plus 5 ml/kg/hr for the first 3–6 hours. If the serum calcium has not been reduced significantly or if the value still exceeds 15 mg/dl, furosemide (Lasix, Hoechst-Roussel) should be administered at a dosage of 2.0–4.0 mg/kg PO q8h. This loop diuretic enhances urinary excretion of calcium. Thiazide diuretics, such as hydrochlorothiazide, should be avoided, as they may reduce renal clearance of calcium, potentially worsening hypercalcemia.

If further lowering of plasma calcium concentration is needed, glucocorticoids (prednisone or prednisolone) can be administered orally or parenterally at a dosage of 1.0–3.0 mg/kg q12h. Glucocorticoids limit bone resorption, inhibit gut absorption of calcium, enhance renal excretion of calcium, and may be cytolytic in cases of lymphosarcoma. Consequently, steroid therapy should not be attempted unless appropriate diagnostic tests for lymphosarcoma have already been performed. Other symptomatic therapy, such as calcitonin, mithramicin, or diphosphonates to inhibit bone demineralization or low calcium diets (e.g., prescription diet k/d) to reduce gut absorption of calcium, are generally not necessary. Specific therapy, such as parathyroidectomy in refractory cases of primary hyperparathyroidism, surgical resection of other tumors, or chemotherapy for lymphosarcoma, depend on the results of diagnostic tests.

Hypercalcemia produces polyuria through interference with the action of antidiuretic hormone in the urine-concentrating mechanism. Consequently, attention to the delivery of adequate quantities of fluid is important. Hypercalcemia causes azotemia through renal vasoconstriction and nephrocalcinosis. All of these effects of hypercalcemia, except nephrocalcinosis, are readily reversible. Marked hypercalcemia is more often a cause of azotemia than a consequence. The prognosis for hypercalcemic nephropathy depends on the degree and time course of the hypercalcemia. Considerable improvement in the level of azotemia can be expected, although some residual renal damage from nephrocalcinosis should be anticipated.

Sodium Intake and Systemic Hypertension. Systemic hypertension may be observed in animals with renal disease. Monitoring systemic arterial pressure is difficult in dogs and cats, although some instruments for indirect measurement of blood pressure are available (e.g., Ultrasonic Doppler Flow Detector, Parks Electronics Laboratory; Dinamap Research Monitor, Critikon). The systemic arterial pressure is labile and may be altered by anxiety associated with the measurement process, and this effect can be pronounced in dogs and cats. Consequently, care should be taken to measure the systemic arterial pressure in a quiet, relaxed state. Multiple sequential measurements should be obtained and averaged. Each veterinary clinician utilizing a method to measure systemic blood pressure should obtain measurements in 10 or more normal animals to develop a "normal" range. Systemic hypertension in dogs has been reported to be a systolic pressure in excess of 180 mm Hg, a diastolic pressure in excess of 95 mm Hg, or both. Similar maximal normal values are difficult to determine for the cat, but values in excess of 200/145 mm Hg have been suggested.

Animals with renal disease, Cushing's syndrome, or hyperthyroidism should undergo careful retinal evaluation at each examination as ocular lesions caused by systemic hypertension may be diagnosed. These lesions would include dilated, tortuous vessels and serous or hemorrhagic exudates. The presence of these lesions necessitates therapy for systemic hypertension.

Therapy for systemic hypertension should be based on blood pressure measurements. Response to treatment can be measured monthly in patients without complications and without severe hypertension. However, in dogs and cats with severe hypertension or ocular manifestations of systemic hypertension (or both), pharmacologic and dietary intervention should be instituted promptly and the response to therapy assessed with blood pressure measurements in 3–5 days or sooner. Potential side effects of antihypertensive therapy include systemic hypotension, syncope, and prerenal azotemia. These side effects are more likely in animals in which therapy is not based on measurement of blood pressure. Pharmacologic therapy should be instituted with the patient hospitalized, as systemic hypotension necessitating withdrawal of drug may develop during the first 1–3 days of therapy.

Appropriate therapy of systemic hypertension should be instituted sequentially and is based on assessment of systemic blood pressure. The usual sequence of therapy is: 1) dietary sodium restriction; 2) dietary sodium restriction plus diuretic therapy; and 3) dietary sodium restriction plus diuretic therapy plus adrenergic inhibitors or vasodilators.

The interaction between dietary sodium intake and systemic hypertension remains an important consideration. Commercial dry dog foods generally contain 0.5–0.7% sodium, which may contribute to the development of systemic hypertension in animals with renal failure. Appropriate sodium intake for dogs with azotemic renal failure or systemic hypertension is probably 0.1–0.4%. A variety of diets are available that meet this level of restriction (e.g., Hill's prescription diets h/d, k/d, and u/d). The transition from normal to low sodium diet should be accomplished gradually, with mixing of the two foods for 7–14 days to allow accommodation, which is considerably slower in dogs with renal failure. Sudden reductions of sodium intake may lead to extracellular volume contraction and worsening of azotemia due to this prerenal factor. In addition, sudden or severe sodium restriction may worsen metabolic acidosis. In contrast, dietary supplementation with sodium should be avoided, as sudden increases in sodium intake cause extracellular volume expansion and may lead to systemic hypertension or peripheral edema.

Thiazides, which are the first choice for diuretic therapy in hypertensive animals, include chlorothiazide (Diuril, Merck) at a dosage of 20–40 mg/kg q12–24h, or hydrochlorothiazide (Hydrodiuril, Merck Sharp & Dohme) at 2–4 mg/kg q12–24h. If this regimen is ineffective, furosemide (Lasix, Hoechst-Roussel) at a dosage of 2–4 mg/kg q12h may be tried.

Adrenergic inhibitors such as propranolol (Inderal, Ayerst) at a dosage of 0.2–1.0 mg/kg PO q8–12h in dogs and 2.5–10.0 mg PO q8–12h in cats may be helpful. Prazosin (Minipress, Pfizer) at a dosage of 1 mg/15 kg PO q12h may be effective in dogs (0.25–1.0 mg PO q12h in cats) with renal disease and coexistent systemic hypertension.

Vasodilators, including angiotensin-converting enzyme (ACE) inhibitors such as captopril (Capoten, Squibb) or calcium channel blocking agents such as verapamil (Isoptin, Knoll) or nifedipine (Procardia, Pfizer) may lower systemic resistance and restore normal blood pressure. Because of their apparent abilities to preferentially lower glomerular capillary hydrostatic pressure and to reduce glomerular hypertrophy, captopril and other ACE inhibitors such as enalapril (Vasotec, Merck) are theoretically superior to other antihypertensive agents in patients with coexisting renal azotemia. The dosage for captopril is 0.5–2.0 mg/kg q8–12h for dogs and cats. Calcium channel blockers have not been carefully evaluated as therapy for hypertension in animals.

Management of Electrolyte Imbalances. Hypokalemia and metabolic acidosis may be present, and each may be exacerbated by the use of certain diets intended for use in these patients. If hypokalemia develops in a polyuric, azotemic patient, oral potassium supplementation can be utilized to supply 1–6 mEq potassium/kg/day. Available preparations include oral tablets (Urocit-K, Mission Pharmacal), elixirs (Kaon, Adria Laboratories), or powders (Tumil-K, Daniels Pharmaceuticals). The hypokalemic cat with muscle weakness (hypokalemic polymyopathy) may suffer severe hypokalemia if treated with parenteral fluids, and oral potassium supplementation is preferred in these cats (see Chapter 1), unless they are uremic.

Acidemia should be treated if the total CO_2 (TCO_2) concentration falls below 15 mmol/L, utilizing sodium bicarbonate at an initial oral dosage of 10 mg/kg three times daily. (One teaspoon of baking soda is approximately 4000 mg of sodium bicarbonate.) Potassium citrate (Urocit-K, Mission Pharmacal) is an alternative alkalinizing agent that can be administered at an initial dosage of 35 mg/kg PO three times daily. The dosage of alkalinizing agents should generally be increased to be effective. However, sodium bicarbonate should be avoided in hypertensive patients, and potassium citrate worsens hyperkalemia, though this is not usually present in polyuric patients. Serum electrolytes and TCO_2 should be reevaluated 2 weeks after institution of alkalinizing therapy and appropriate adjustment in dosage made at that time. Alkalinizing agents should be given to effect, with a goal of TCO_2 between 15 and 25 mmol/L. Complete correction of arterial pH is not desirable, as respiratory compensations may mask the use of excessive dosages.

Monitoring Therapy. Thorough, regular evaluations, rather than waiting for the onset of uremia, is the appropriate therapeutic plan for improving the prognosis in these patients. The polyuric azotemic animal should be evaluated every 2–4 months if stable and more frequently if changes in metabolic status are identified. The physical examination should include a thorough fundic evaluation. The assessment includes a complete blood count (CBC), urinalysis ($\pm$ urine culture), BUN, SCr, calcium, phosphorus, electrolytes (including TCO_2 or HCO_3^-), body weight, and a review of dietary intake. If appropriate equipment is available, systemic blood pressure should be assessed at each visit. Frequency of assessment should increase with increasing degree of azotemia and anytime the patient's metabolic status changes. In those patients who become nonazotemic after suffering acute renal failure, annual reevaluation may be adequate. Because animals with abnormalities of the urinary tract may be prone to the development of urinary tract infections, a urine culture should be performed every 6–12 months, regardless of the results of the urinalysis.

Assessment of azotemia deserves special attention. Dietary protein is metabolized to a wide variety of molecules, referred to as middle molecules, which are responsible for the clinical signs of uremia. Although BUN is not a uremic toxin, the concentration of urea in the blood is well correlated with the level of uremic toxins. A low protein diet preferentially lowers BUN levels. A sudden increase in BUN unaccompanied by an elevation in SCr offers useful information. The most likely causes are prerenal, and they include dietary noncompliance, gastrointestinal hemorrhage, and glucocorticoid or tetracycline administration.

In contrast to BUN, SCr is better correlated with renal function (GFR) and should be measured for the purpose of assessing changes in the GFR. A graph of the inverse of SCr (1/SCr) on the y-axis versus time (months) on the x-axis reveals a linear plot in some azotemic patients, which is helpful for predicting the outcome and benefits of changes in therapy if measurements are made frequently enough. Unfortunately, in many patients this plot is not linear and may not be helpful.

Prognosis for Polyuric, Azotemic Renal Failure. The goal of therapy of animals in this category is to prevent or reduce further exacerbations of renal disease. As noted above, a plot of the inverse of creatinine (1/SCr) versus time may reveal a linear pattern of declining renal function that should be used to predict prognosis and to assess the effects of therapy on the course of renal disease in the individual patient. However, the pattern of change in renal function is often not linear; and although some patients have a progressive course of renal disease, the prognosis for patients in this category varies widely. The prognosis for long-term survival of cats with azotemic renal disease appears to be better than that for dogs. The prognosis for hypertensive animals is worse than that for normotensive ones. In both species, however, regular medical attention maximizes survival and improves the quality of life.

Investigational Therapy. *Recombinant Erythropoietin.* Anemia of renal failure often results in hematocrit values of 20–30%. In animals at the low end of this range, anemia may contribute to the clinical signs of lethargy and weakness. A major contributor to this anemia is a lack of renal production of erythropoietin. Recombinant erythropoietin (Epogen, Amgen) at a dosage of 50–100 units/kg SC daily for 7 days followed by 50–100 units/kg SC three times weekly thereafter usually increases the hematocrit value in dogs and cats that have anemia due to chronic renal disease. It may be preferable to start at the lower end of the dosage range, especially in cats. Hematocrit should initially be monitored every 5–7 days during this therapy, as the rise in hematocrit often is dramatic. Once a stable hematocrit value is obtained, the frequency of evaluations can be reduced somewhat, although never less often than monthly. Because polycythemia may develop with therapy, recombinant erythropoietin should be reserved for patients with a hematocrit value of less than 20%. An appropriate goal is 30–35%. A normal hematocrit is not to be sought, and the dosage should be reduced if it is attained. Most animals have a dramatic response to this therapy, including an increase in appetite, exercise tolerance, and an improved attitude. Disadvantages include cost and the necessity for lifelong therapy. Potential side effects include the development of life-threatening polycythemia, systemic or intrarenal hypertension, and allergic reactions to the vehicle. In rare cases, an adverse response to the recombinant human erythropoietin can produce severe life-threatening non-regenerative anemia. This agent does not increase hematocrit in the presence of anemias due to other causes, such as iron lack from chronic hematuria.

Calcitriol. In dogs, phosphate imbalance and reduced renal hydroxylation of 1-hydroxyvitamin D_3 contribute to the genesis of renal secondary hyperparathyroidism. Particularly in young dogs, hyperparathyroidism may lead to renal osteodystrophy and severe mandibular decalcification ("rubber jaw"). Control of hyperphosphatemia may not prevent renal secondary hyper-parathyroidism, and supplementation with 1,25-dihydroxyvitamin D (Rocal-trol, Hoffman-LaRoche) may be beneficial in the control of renal secondary hyperparathyroidism. This therapy is currently investigational, and dosages of 1.82–3.85 ng/kg/day PO in one daily dose have been employed to reduce the degree of renal secondary hyperparathyroidism. The long-term benefits of this therapy are not yet proved. In addition, because vitamin D enhances gut absorption of calcium and phosphorus, hypercalcemia and hyperphosphatemia may develop; and this medication should not be given with food.

Polyuric, Uremic Renal Failure

Standard Therapy. *Fluid Therapy.* An intravenous catheter, preferably in a central vein (e.g., jugular catheter) is preferred for treatment of these patients. Immediate fluid therapy is aimed at correcting dehydration and supplying maintenance needs (see Chapter 1 or section in this chapter on prerenal azotemia). It should be accomplished within the first 3–6 hours of therapy.

Osmotic Diuresis. Osmotic diuresis utilizing dextrose may be utilized to reduce the level of uremic toxins, supply caloric support, and (mildly) increase GFR. This therapy is appropriate for any uremic patient that does not have compromised cardiovascular function or evidence of systemic hypertension. However, osmotic diuresis should not be instituted if a patient is dehydrated or hypokalemic.

For osmotic diuresis, hypertonic dextrose solution (10%) should be administered through a central venous line at a dosage of 20–30 ml/kg given over 2–3 hours and repeated every 8–12 hours. The dextrose solution should not be considered in the daily calculations of fluid needs, and lactated Ringer's solution should be used during the intervening periods to correct dehydration and supply maintenance needs. Unless the patient is hyperkalemic, the lactated Ringer's solution should be supplemented with 10–30 mEq potassium per liter.

Inasmuch as daily caloric needs are approximately 60 kcal/kg and 10% dextrose contains 0.4 kcal/ml, osmotic diuresis at a rate of 30 ml/kg q8h would potentially supply more than one-third of daily caloric needs:

$$(0.4 \text{ kcal/ml}) \times (30 \text{ ml/kg} \times 3) = 36 \text{ kcal/kg}$$

Although glucosuria results in the loss of about 10–20% of these calories in the urine, parenteral dextrose administration remains a useful source of caloric support.

Management of Electrolyte Abnormalities. Polyuria is frequently associated with hypokalemia, particularly where dextrose diuresis is utilized. Serum potassium should be measured every 1–3 days. Potassium supplementation (2–6 mEq/kg/day unless hyperkalemic) can be achieved by several routes including 1) oral tablet (Urocit-K, Mission Pharmacal), elixir (Kaon, Adria Laboratories), or powder (Tumil-K, Daniels Pharmaceuticals) in animals that are not vomiting; 2) subcutaneously administered lactated Ringer's solution supplemented with 40–80 mEq K^+/L; or 3) intravenously administered lactated Ringer's solution supplemented with 10–30 mEq K^+/L. Intravenous potassium administration should not exceed 0.5 mEq/kg/hr.

Control of Vomiting. Uremic patients are usually vomiting. Cimetidine (Tagamet, SmithKline Beecham) at a dosage of 10 mg/kg given three times daily can be administered parenterally at first and orally once vomiting is controlled. Additional antiemetics, such as triethylperazine (Torecan, Sandoz) at a dosage of 0.125–0.250 mg/kg q8h, may be necessary to control vomiting initially.

Monitoring Therapy. Uremic animals should undergo daily assessment of serum electrolytes, degree of azotemia (SCr and BUN), caloric intake, and body weight. In polyuric animals, especially those receiving osmotic diuretic therapy, the BUN falls more rapidly than the SCr. In this case, BUN may serve as an index of the effectiveness of diuretic therapy (values of BUN below 100 mg/dl often coincide with the resolution of uremic signs), and SCr is a superior index of renal function (GFR). Therapy should be adjusted daily on the basis of results of diagnostic testing.

Prognosis for Recovery. Prognosis is generally guarded for uremic patients. The prognosis is better for animals with acute renal failure, as the compensatory response has not already been exhausted. However, the compensatory response is not necessarily rapid. For example, dogs with acute renal failure due to gentamicin toxicity often require 4–5 days of intensive therapy before the SCr begins to decline. Animals with chronic renal failure with acute exacerbations may also improve. In contrast, dogs or cats with a steady decline of renal function over several months should not be expected to improve dramatically.

Once a stable level of renal function is attained and the patient resumes food intake, fluid therapy should be discontinued gradually, over 2–3 days. The patient's level of azotemia and serum electrolyte and acid-base status should be assessed during this time. Unless the SCr can be maintained below 5 mg/dl, the prognosis is guarded. Further therapy for such patients is then handled in the same manner as that for a polyuric, azotemic animal.

Alternative Therapy. Because anorexia of more than 5 days' duration leads to a catabolic state that worsens uremia, there is likely to be a benefit to enteral or parenteral nutritional therapy in the uremic animal. Although this hypothesis remains to be evaluated, it has been established that intravenous administration of amino acid solutions enhances survival in experimental acute renal failure in dogs. Liquid diets for enteral support (e.g., RenalCare, Pet-Ag) may be administered by nasogastric, gastrostomy, or enterostomy tube .

Oliguric, Uremic Renal Failure

Oliguria is generally defined as urine production of less than 0.5 ml/kg/hr. Oliguria due to renal failure and reduced urine output due to prerenal factors, e.g., severe dehydration, may be confused. True oliguria carries a poor prognosis, particularly if standard therapy does not induce urine formation.

Standard Therapy. These patients usually require immediate care and have many metabolic derangements. Therapy should include 1) fluid administration, 2) attempts to induce urine production, and 3) correction of derangements in acid-base and electrolyte status.

Fluid Therapy. In oliguric patients it is imperative that an indwelling urinary catheter and an intravenous catheter be maintained. They should be aseptically placed, as uremic patients have reduced immune function. Lactated Ringer's solution should be administered intravenously to correct dehydration over 2–4 hours. Some patients, including those with an unrecognized prerenal insult, become polyuric at this time. Oliguric patients should be monitored carefully for signs of overhydration, which include pulmonary edema, serous exudate from eyes and nose, and an elevated central venous pressure (see Chapter 1). If fluid therapy alone does not lead to urine production, the following therapies can be attempted sequentially in an attempt to induce urine formation.

Induction of Urine Formation. Although the quantity of urine formed should not be confused with the amount of renal function (GFR), oliguria is a poor prognostic sign in part because urinary clearance of endogenous compounds is absent. Consequently, maneuvers that result in urine formation without further compromising the animal are generally beneficial. For some derangements present in uremia, e.g., hyperkalemia and metabolic acidosis, increasing urine flow rate in the absence of changes of GFR enhances urinary clearance of the offending metabolic compound (here, potassium and hydrogen ions). The excretion of some uremic toxins may similarly be enhanced in polyuric states. However, if urine formation is adequate (1 ml/kg/hr), the administration of pharmaceutical agents for the sole purpose of increasing urine production is not without risk.

The only way to adequately monitor urine output is with an indwelling urinary catheter. This catheter should be managed as are other indwelling urinary catheters (Table 11-1), with particular concern for asepsis in this immunocompromised patient.

The following methods may be successful for inducing urine formation in patients not responding to fluid therapy alone within the first 3–4 hours of treatment:

1. *Osmotic diuresis.* Osmotic diuresis can be accomplished with hypertonic dextrose (usually 10%) or mannitol. Because these hypertonic solutions may produce irritation and swelling if given into a peripheral vein (e.g., cephalic), they should be delivered through a central venous line (e.g., jugular catheter). An initial dosage of 0.5 ml of 10% dextrose/kg/min for 30 minutes should result in hyperglycemia and may induce an osmotic diuresis with glucosuria. If urine production is observed, a qualitative test for glucose (dipstick) should be performed to verify the presence of glucosuria, and the patient should be

TABLE 11-1. Appropriate Use of an Indwelling Urinary Catheter

1. A soft, sterile, lubricated catheter is preferred.

2. Aseptic technique during placement is required.

3. A closed-drainage system should be established immediately.

4. The drainage system should always remain below the level of the patient's bladder.

5. An antiseptic added to drainage bag (e.g., 60 ml of 1:500 chlorhexidine (Nolvasan, Fort Dodge) or 30 ml of 3% hydrogen peroxide) may reduce the incidence of iatrogenic urinary tract infections.

6. Hands should be washed prior to catheter manipulation.

7. Every effort should be made to *avoid the following:*

   a. Catheter manipulation and port contamination by clinician and by patient

   b. Catheter obstruction (even temporary)

   c. Retrograde flushing of the catheter

   d. Disconnection of the catheter

8. If possible, antibiotic therapy should be withheld until the catheter is removed.

9. A urine culture and sensitivity test should be obtained at time of catheter removal and 7 days later. If antibiotic therapy was employed during catheterization, a culture should be repeated 7–10 days after discontinuation of therapy. If a urinary tract infection is identified, it should be managed as outlined in the section of this chapter on treatment of simple, acute urinary tract infections.

---

further managed as a polyuric, uremic animal (see section in this chapter on treatment of polyuric, uremic renal failure). If little or no urine is produced (< 0.5 ml/kg in 1 hour), discontinue the hypertonic solution administration to avoid overhydration and proceed to an alternative method of therapy.

An alternative osmotic agent is mannitol (1.0 g/kg IV over 30 minutes). Mannitol, unlike dextrose, remains in the vascular space, which offers some advantage over dextrose in oliguric renal failure that is due to ischemia. However, this property of mannitol may lead to hyperosmolarity if urine is not formed in response to its use. Mannitol should not be repeated unless oliguria is resolved by the first administration.

2. *Loop diuresis.* Administer furosemide (Lasix, Hoechst-Roussel) at a dosage of 2–8 mg/kg IV. If a response to this medication is to occur, it should be expected within 30 minutes. Potential side effects include renal vasoconstriction. If used multiple times, hypokalemia or volume depletion (or both) may ensue. The clinician should not confuse enhanced polyuria with improvement of the GFR. That is, the goal of therapy with loop diuretics is to cause the animal to produce urine, not to enhance urine volume in a dog or cat already producing adequate quantities of urine. Although polyuria may enhance urinary clearance of some uremic toxins, urine volume is not proportional to renal function (GFR), and the two should not be confused.

3. *Loop diuresis plus vasodilator.* If furosemide (Lasix) is ineffective, there may be a response to the concurrent administration of furosemide (2–8 mg/kg IV) plus dopamine (Inotropin, Anar-Stone) at a dosage of 1–5 µg/kg/min diluted in 50–250 ml of an isotonic solution such as 5% dextrose, delivered at a steady, known drip rate. The most likely potential side effect of dopamine is tachyarrhythmia, particularly if dosage is too high. If an irregular heart rate occurs, or a tachyarrhythmia is diagnosed by electrocardiogram (ECG), the dopamine drip should be discontinued and can subsequently be reinstituted at a lower dose if the arrhythmia resolves.

4. *Conservative Management.* If the animal does not respond to therapy to induce urine formation, continued aggressive fluid administration may result in overhydration and death from pulmonary edema. One approach in the mildly uremic animal is to deliver daily fluid therapy at a volume calculated to correct dehydration and supply maintenance needs (see section on treatment of prerenal azotemia in this chapter). Occasionally, an animal converts from oliguric to polyuric spontaneously as the kidney undergoes the compensatory healing process. This situation is more likely in acute, than chronic, renal failure.

Electrolyte and Acid-Base Abnormalities. Patients with oliguric renal failure are often markedly hyperkalemic, which may be the first clue that oliguria is present. The degree of hyperkalemia is usually not high enough to necessitate specific therapy beyond the administration of solutions low in potassium concentration (e.g., lactated Ringer's solution). If the serum potassium concentration exceeds 8.0 mEq/L, appropriate measures should be taken, including the administration of either sodium bicarbonate *or* glucose-insulin solutions (see Chapter 1). If measures to induce urine formation are unsuccessful, an alternative therapy such as dialysis should be considered.

Although generally not necessary, metabolic acidosis should be corrected if TCO_2 falls below 15 mmol/L. The amount (mEq) of bicarbonate required to correct metabolic acidosis can be estimated from the following formula:

$$0.5 \times \text{body wt (kg)} \times [\text{normal } TCO_2 - \text{patient } TCO_2)$$

This quantity of bicarbonate or bicarbonate equivalent (e.g., lactate) should be administered in lactated Ringer's solution over 24–48 hours, and the acid-base status reassessed daily in any patient receiving base therapy.

Prognosis for Oliguric, Uremic Patients. If standard therapy does not induce urine formation, oliguria carries a poor prognosis. However, efforts should be made to eliminate the possibility that apparent oliguric renal failure is due to severe prerenal factors that resolve with standard therapy.

Alternative Therapies. Patients with oliguric renal failure have a poor prognosis. If fluid, diuretic, and vasodilator therapy does not induce polyuria, these patients rarely respond to further manipulations.

For nonresponding patients, renal transplantation (especially in cats) and dialysis (continuous ambulatory peritoneal dialysis or hemodialysis) remain potentially useful therapies. However, these techniques are not appropriate for all uremic patients, and they are best performed by, or with the guidance of, experienced clinicians. Both are costly and involve a great deal of nursing care. Dialysis, in particular, is labor intensive and is generally employed for less than 3 weeks, being reserved for animals with acute renal failure in which a compensatory response is anticipated. Appropriate patients for dialysis or transplantation (or both) are those with oliguria or uremia that do not respond to traditional medical therapy and do not have serious untreatable, concurrent diseases. Severely uremic patients are not good candidates for dialysis or transplantation.

Monitoring the Oliguric Patient. Urine output is the single most important parameter in the patient with oliguric renal failure, and a closed, aseptically maintained indwelling urinary catheter (Table 11-1) is essential. Other parameters that should be evaluated daily include degree of dehydration, body weight, caloric intake, serum potassium level, acidosis, and degree of azotemia. However, if the oliguria does not resolve, worsening in all of these parameters can be expected.

Proteinuric Patient

Azotemic patients with significant proteinuria should be managed similarly to other patients with renal disease, although they require special consideration because proteinuria may lead to hypoalbuminemia and peripheral edema.

Proteinuric patients may be edematous, azotemic, both, or neither. Supportive therapy for animals with proteinuric renal failure is similar to that for nonproteinuric ones; however, aggressive fluid therapy, including osmotic diuresis should be employed cautiously, if at all, in severely hypoalbuminemic patients. Otherwise, serious pulmonary edema may occur.

Specific therapeutic modalities might include corticosteroids, cyclosporin A (Sandimmune, Sandoz), cyclophosphamide (Cytoxan, Mead Johnson), and captopril (Capoten, Squibb). However, these treatments remain unevaluated in dogs and cats. More importantly, if an underlying etiology can be identified, the predisposing or contributory condition should be resolved if possible.

Similar to the situation for other azotemic patients, the diet should be low in phosphate, and dietary protein must be of high quality (e.g., Hill's Prescription Diet k/d). Reduction of dietary protein intake is appropriate in uremic patients and may slow renal injury in azotemic animals. However, any reduction in dietary protein intake in nonuremic animals should be followed for several months to determine the effects of this manipulation on the serum concentration of albumin and on lean body mass. A precipitous fall in serum albumin and muscle wasting are grounds for increasing the quality and quantity of protein in the diet.

If proteinuric patients develop edema, therapy should include sodium restriction (Prescription Diet k/d, h/d, or u/d, Hills Pet Products) and a diuretic such as furosemide (Lasix, Hoechst-Roussel) at a dosage of 1–4 mg/kg PO q8h.

Severely proteinuric patients may develop thrombotic disease secondary to antithrombin III deficiency or hypoalbuminemia-associated platelet hypersensitivity. If patients have severe hypoalbuminemia (serum albumin < 1.0 g/dl) or antithrombin III levels are less than 30% of normal, aspirin therapy (5–10 mg/kg every other day in dogs) should be considered. Because aspirin may depress renal function, especially in animals with preexisting renal disease on a low sodium diet, the SCr and BUN should be measured if aspirin or other nonsteroidal antiinflammatory agents are utilized. Signs of toxicity from these medications include polyuria, worsening azotemia, melena, blood loss anemia, vomiting, and anorexia.

The degree of proteinuria and azotemia should be evaluated at 2- to 4-month intervals by measuring the urine protein/creatinine ratio, serum albumin concentration, SCr, and BUN. The prognosis varies with the cause. Some glomerular diseases resolve spontaneously (e.g., glomerulonephritis associated with pyometra), whereas others carry a poor prognosis (e.g., amyloidosis).

Use of Medications in Animals with Compromised Renal Function

Many pharmaceutical agents are eliminated by the kidneys, and their administration to patients with renal failure may result in toxicity due to accumulation of the drug. To avoid this complication, dosage of medications eliminated by the kidneys can be adjusted on the basis of renal function. Some medications, including chloramphenicol, short-acting barbiturates, lincomycin, erythromycin, and phenothiazines, are metabolized predominantly by the liver, and no adjustment in dosing is generally necessary in animals with compromised renal function. Other generally safe medications can potentially accumulate to toxic levels in animals only with severe renal failure. This group includes penicillin, ampicillin, and cephalothin. Dose adjustment for these medications in animals with decreased renal clearance is not necessary until severe renal failure (SCr > 4.0 mg/dl) is present, in which case either the interdose interval should be increased or the dose reduced by multiplying the normal interval or dose by one of the following factors:

$$\text{Factor A} = (\text{normal GFR})/(\text{patient GFR})$$
$$\text{Factor B} = (\text{patient SCr})/(\text{normal SCr})$$

These correction factors are reliable only in animals in which renal function is stable. This point is especially true for factor B, as changes in SCr lag a day or more behind changes in GFR. Factor A is preferred, and creatinine clearance or other marker of filtration may be used to measure the GFR. In most patients, however, only factor B can be determined.

For comparatively nontoxic medications, if in doubt about how to dose a medication in an animal with renal failure, a pharmacology text or other reference should be consulted to determine the method of excretion and the appropriate method of adjustment if there is significant renal elimination.

The third group of medications includes those agents that should be avoided because of toxicity or the potential to worsen uremia. They include corticosteroids, tetracycline, nonsteroidal antiinflammatory agents, and nephrotoxic agents such as the aminoglycoside antibiotics. These agents should be utilized in animals with renal failure only if safer alternative medications have been eliminated from consideration. If used, the interdose interval or dosage should be adjusted. For some medications, lengthening the interdose interval may be preferred (e.g., aminoglycosides), whereas for others the dose reduction method is superior (e.g., bacteriostatic antibiotics).

For example, if it is absolutely necessary to administer gentamicin to a dog with a stable SCr of 2.0 mg/dl, the increased interdose interval should be employed. The dose of 2.2 mg/kg would remain the same. However, if the SCr is normal at 1.0 mg/dl, the interdose interval should be increased by factor B = (patient SCr)/(normal SCr) = (2.0 mg/dl)/(1.0 mg/dl) = 2.0. Because the interdose interval in normal animals is 8 hours, the interval would become 8.0 hours × 2.0 = 16 hours. Hence gentamicin would be administered at a dose of 2.2 mg/kg q16h in this dog. This toxic antibiotic has a narrow therapeutic index and can reach nephrotoxic levels despite this dose correction. Use of gentamicin in animals with renal failure should be monitored by measuring the trough serum gentamicin concentrations (the goal is a serum gentamicin concentration of < 2.0 µg/ml just prior to dosing).

Postrenal Azotemia

Azotemia due to obstruction to urine outflow or rupture of the lower urinary tract is referred to as postrenal azotemia. Such obstruction or rupture may occur at any point along the urinary tract, from the renal pelvis to the distal urethra. For ureteral or renal pelvic abnormalities to produce azotemia, bilateral obstruction or unilateral obstruction plus contralateral renal dysfunction must be present. By itself, unilateral ureteral obstruction does not produce azotemia. Isolated unilateral ureteral rupture is similarly unlikely to produce azotemia, unless the rupture allows leakage of urine produced by the contralateral kidney.

Standard Therapy: Obstructive Uropathy. *Relieve Obstruction.* Animals with an obstructed urinary tract should be treated as a medical emergency. In dogs and cats, the obstruction is almost always urethral, and immediate relief of obstruction should be attempted. The only prior consideration is therapy for hyperkalemia (see Chapter 1), which should be considered if sinoatrial standstill and bradycardia are present. Hyperkalemia and associated ECG abnormalities (peaked T waves and flattened or absent P waves) generally resolve rapidly once the urethral obstruction is relieved. The most appropriate treatment for all but the severest of ECG changes is to seek immediate relief of obstruction.

Anesthesia is generally not necessary for dogs. If needed, dogs may be anesthetized with ultra-short-acting barbiturates or a halothane-nitrous oxide mixture administered by face mask. Although some sedate or depressed cats tolerate attempts to catheterize the urethra, relief of urethral obstruction generally requires anesthesia in this species. Ketamine hydrochloride (Ketalar, Parke-Davis) at a dosage of 2–10 mg/kg IV or atropine 0.05 mg/kg IM plus thiamylal sodium (Surital, Parke-Davis) at a dosage of 10–18 mg/kg IV often suffices. An alternative anesthetic regimen in cats is halothane and nitrous oxide administered to effect by face mask or with the cat placed in an aquarium. Following induction of anesthesia the perineum or penis should be carefully cleansed, and attention must be paid to asepsis at each subsequent point of the procedure. At this time, digital compression of the bladder or cystocentesis may rupture the bladder, greatly worsening the prognosis for recovery. However, because some matrix-crystalline plugs occur in the distal penile urethra of the male cat, gentle manual massage should be attempted initially in these animals. Reverse flushing of the urethra, utilizing a feline olive tipped (Minnesota Olive Tipped Catheter, EJAY International Inc) or a 3.5 French open-ended (Tom Cat Catheter, Sherwood Medical) urethral catheter in cats or a 5–8 French feeding tube with the end removed in dogs (Feeding Tube and Urethral Catheter, Sherwood Medical) may unblock the urethra. Urethral catheters should be sterile and well lubricated. Copious amounts of physiologic saline or lactated Ringer's solution for flush and lots of patience are often beneficial. Asepsis is critical to avoid an iatrogenic urinary tract infection. When all else fails, cystocentesis may be attempted to decompress the bladder, followed by further attempts to establish urethral patency. However, it should be done only after other, safer methods fail and with the realization that the bladder may rupture as a result.

After urine flow has been reestablished, a soft French catheter (3.5 French in cats and 5–8 French in dogs) should be passed and urine removed from the bladder, if it can be accomplished with a combination of mild manual compression and gentle suction. If a great deal of debris is present in the urine (more common in cats), flushing the bladder with sterile lactated Ringer's solution, employing 10–25 ml at a time, is appropriate. The catheter should be maintained as a closed system (Table 11-1). The urinary bladder and urethral catheter should be evaluated hourly for 4–6 hours to ascertain that urethral patency remains. Although bladder manipulation should be minimized, gentle compression of the bladder may be employed to encourage bladder emptying.

Fluid Therapy. Following establishment of urethral patency, postobstructive diuresis occurs, lasting 1–5 days. It may result in excessive losses of water, sodium, and in particular potassium. Therefore proper fluid therapy is mandatory and ideally is designed so that fluid input equals output (urine flow plus insensible loss of 20 ml/kg/day). A closed catheter system should be employed and fluid output measured to determine the appropriate fluid therapy. Unless potassium supplementation is utilized, the patient usually makes the transition from hyperkalemia to hypokalemia within 1–5 days. Consequently, serum potassium should be measured daily for 3–5 days, and potassium should generally be supplemented at a dosage of 2–6 mEq/kg/day unless the patient is hyperkalemic. The potassium can be given by several routes including oral tablet (Urocit-K, Mission Pharmacal), elixir (Kaon, Adria Laboratories), and powder (Tumil-K, Daniels Pharmaceuticals) in cats that are not vomiting. Alternatively, subcutaneously administered lactated Ringer's solution supplemented with 40–80 mEq potassium per liter or intravenously administered lactated Ringer's solution supplemented with 10–30 mEq of potassium per liter may be employed. Intravenous potassium administration should not exceed 0.5 mEq/kg/hr.

Monitoring Therapy. When an indwelling catheter is removed, the residual bladder volume should be carefully monitored, as postobstructive bladder atony may develop. Therapy for animals with bladder atony is aimed at keeping the bladder empty for 3–5 days to allow healing. It is accomplished in dogs with an indwelling urethral catheter or frequent (every 6–8 hours) intermittent catheterizations. Compared to an indwelling urethral catheter, use of aseptic, intermittent catheterization poses somewhat less risk for the development of a urinary tract infection in dogs. However, an indwelling catheter may more effectively decompress the bladder, especially in polyuric dogs. The choice of which method to use in dogs depends on the degree of polyuria, the patient's tolerance of an indwelling catheter, and the availability of support personnel in the veterinary hospital. In cats, frequent catheterization is technically difficult, and an indwelling catheter is preferred. To achieve effective bladder "decompression," the bladder volume should be maintained below 10 ml/kg. In animals with bladder atony, bethanechol (Urecholine, Merck) at a dosage of 5–15 mg (1.25–5.00 mg in cats) PO q8h may be used to enhance detrusor tone. An excessive dose of this medication may cause gastrointestinal cramping leading to anorexia, salivation, or diarrhea.

In some cats, where excessive force or a stiff indwelling catheter is employed, urethral trauma may lead to outflow obstruction secondary to inflammation (edema and spasm) of the mucosa. Phenoxybenzamine (Dibenzyline, SmithKline) at a dosage of 0.25 mg/kg PO q12h may facilitate urination in these cases by reducing urethral spasm. Because bladder atony and urethral spasm are difficult to distinguish, bethanechol and phenoxybenzamine are often used in conjunction with each other. If urination is not accomplished within 12 hours, reinsertion of a soft urethral catheter, such as a feeding tube (3.5 French or smaller), may be necessary.

Daily assessment of the degree of azotemia, acid-base status, and serum potassium concentration should be maintained for 3–5 days after an obstructive episode. These abnormalities should rapidly and continuously improve during this time period. If it is not the case, reobstruction, superimposed renal azotemia, septicemia originating from an infected urinary tract, or other complicating factor should be suspected.

In an uncomplicated case of urethral obstruction, antibiotics should be withheld until catheterization is discontinued (Table 11-1). Antibiotics should not be used on a "prophylactic" basis. However, if a urinary tract infection is identified in an animal with bladder atony and urine stasis, antibiotic therapy may be necessary. Following any bout of urethral obstruction, a urine culture should be performed at discharge and repeated 7 days later to verify the sterility of the urinary tract. If infection is identified, it should be treated as outlined in the section in this chapter on urinary tract infections.

Prognosis. If obstruction is relieved, the prognosis for recovery from post-renal azotemia is good. However, the primary disease process (e.g., urethral neoplasia) may carry a poor prognosis, or repetitive bouts of obstruction may not always be relieved in time (e.g., urethral obstruction in male cats).

Standard Therapy: Rupture of the Urinary Tract. Standard therapy for animals with a rupture of the lower urinary tract includes 1) supportive fluids; 2) urinary catheterization, peritoneal lavage, or both; 3) antibiotics; 4) surgical correction of defect; and 5) postoperative care.

Fluid Therapy. Animals with a rupture of the urinary tract should receive intravenous lactated Ringer's solution to correct dehydration and supply maintenance needs (see Chapter 1 and section in this chapter on Prerenal Azotemia). Serum electrolyte concentrations should be determined, as hyper-kalemia or metabolic acidosis may be present. If the patient is nonuremic, immediate surgery to repair the rupture is appropriate. If possible, the cause of the rupture should be determined by radiographic studies prior to surgery.

Urinary Catheterization/Peritoneal Lavage. The decision on whether to attempt supportive therapy prior to surgery depends in part on the degree of azotemia and, in particular, on the degree of hyperkalemia and metabolic acidosis. The latter two metabolic derangements pose particular risks to animals under anesthesia. If uremic, animals with a lower urinary tract rupture can be treated with an indwelling urethral or peritoneal lavage cath-eter. In cases of bladder rupture, an indwelling urinary catheter often provides adequate clearance of urine to stabilize and improve the metabolic status of a uremic animal. If needed, additional benefit may be derived from sterile placement of an indwelling peritoneal catheter. Because this method of ther-apy is intended for short-term treatment only (12–36 hours), the type of peritoneal catheter utilized is less important than with chronic use, where fibrin and omentum necessitate the use of specialized, more expensive cath-eters, e.g., the column disc catheter (LifeCath, Quinton). Either a less expen-sive fenestrated catheter (Peritoneal Dialysis Catheter, Travenol) or a 16–20 French urethral catheter (Feeding Tube and Urethral Catheter, Sherwood Medical) may be employed. To improve drainage, the feeding tube may be fenestrated, although it is important to avoid weakening the catheter during the fenestration process as it may tear when it is removed, necessitating laparotomy for removal.

Antibiotic Therapy. In cases of uroperitoneum or uroretroperitoneum, where the sterility of the urinary tract is uncertain, antibiotic therapy is

TABLE 11-2. Antimicrobial Selection for Common Uropathogens (see Ling 1984, 1986)

Pathogen	Drug
Staphylococcus	Penicillins, trimethoprim-sulfas, nitrofurantoin, cephalexin, or chloramphenicol
Streptococcus	Penicillins or trimethoprim-sulfas
Escherichia coli	Trimethoprim, nitrofurantoin, or cephalexin
Proteus	Penicillins, trimethoprim-sulfas, or cephalexin
Pseudomonas	Tetracycline
Klebsiella	Cephalexin or trimethoprim-sulfas
Polymicrobic UTI	
Staph. plus Strep.	Penicillins
Staph./Strep. plus E. coli/Proteus	Trimethoprim-sulfas
Any combination of E. coli, Proteus, and Klebsiella	Trimethoprim-sulfas or cephalexin
Pseudomonas plus any other microbe	Treat other microbe first, then tetracycline

appropriate. Because renal clearance is reduced, it is necessary to use a nontoxic antibiotic. An antibiotic concentrated in the urine is desirable. Appropriate choices depend on previous urine culture; or for empiric therapy, ampicillin, a first generation cephalosporin such as cephalothin, or a trimethoprim-sulfa combination may be used (Tables 11-2 and 11-3). An oral route for administration of antibiotics is appropriate unless vomiting has occurred.

Surgical Correction of Defects. Resolution of a urinary tract rupture generally requires surgical correction. The appropriate definitive therapy depends on the defect present. Fluid therapy should be maintained prior to, during, and after anesthesia.

Postoperative Monitoring. To ensure adequate urine flow and to decompress the lower urinary tract, an indwelling catheter should be maintained postoperatively for a minimum of 3 days. Following removal of the catheter, the animal should be provided ample opportunity for urination (three to five times per day and more often if polyuric). Fluid therapy postoperatively should be directed toward correction of dehydration, supplying maintenance needs, and meeting output if postoperative diuresis is present (see Chapter 1 and section in this chapter on Prerenal Azotemia). However, diuresis should not be purposely induced by administration of increased quantities of fluid, as diuresis increases stress on the lower urinary tract while having little if any beneficial effect on the GFR. Although these patients often are initially hyperkalemic, the serum

TABLE 11-3. Recommended Therapy for Urinary Tract Infections[a] (see Ling 1984, 1986)

Generic Name	Dosage (mg/kg)	Route	Frequency	Mean Urine Conc. (µg/ml)
Antimicrobials				
Penicillin G	37,500 U/kg	PO	q8h	294
Penicillin V	25	PO	q8h	148
Ampicillin	25	PO	q8h	309
Amoxicillin	12	PO	q8h	202
Tetracycline	18	PO	q8h	138
Chloramphenicol	33	PO	q8h	124
Sulfisoxazole	22	PO	q8h	1466
Cephalexin	17	PO	q8h	805
Trimethoprim-sulfa	13.2	PO	q12h	55
Amikacin	5.5	SC	q8h	342
Gentamicin	2.2	SC	q8h	107
Kanamycin	3.8	SC	q8h	530
Tobramycin	1.1	SC	q8h	66
Ticarcillin	40	PO	q6h	ND
Antiseptics				
Enrofloxacin[b]	2.5–5.0	PO	q12h	ND
Norfloxacin[b,c]	10–20	PO	q12h	ND
Methenamine Mandelate	10	PO	q6h	ND
Nitrofurantoin	6	PO	q8h	100
Acidifiers				
D,L-Methionine	100	PO	q12h	ND
Ammonium chloride	100	PO	q12h	ND

[a]Prior to instituting therapy, clinicians should familiarize themselves with the side effects, drug interactions, and other important specifics of each agent used. Listed dosages are for normal dogs; some modifications for cats or animals with hepatic or renal disease may be necessary. ND = not determined.
[b]Should not be used in growing animals.
[c]Dose extrapolated from that for humans.

potassium concentration may fall below the normal range within 24 hours after correction of the rupture. Consequently, the fluid solution administered to correct dehydration and supply maintenance needs in normo- and hypo-kalemic animals should be lactated Ringer's solution supplemented with

KCl (10–30 mEq/L). The maximum advisable rate of intravenous potassium administration is 0 5 mEq/kg/hr.

A urine culture should be obtained at the time of surgery and 7–10 days after discharge. If identified, an infection should be treated as outlined in the section of this chapter on therapy of urinary tract infections.

URINARY TRACT INFECTIONS

Urinary tract infections (UTIs) should be managed on the basis of the results of urinalysis and urine culture. A urine sample obtained by cystocentesis provides the most reliable results for both of these tests. Therapy of UTIs requires adequate characterization of the location (lower or both upper and lower tract involvement), time course (acute or recurrent), and the presence or absence of predisposing factors (simple or complicated). Acute infections are defined as those not previously treated and are generally characterized by sudden onset of hematuria and dysuria coincident with significant bacteriuria. Complicated infections are present when identifiable abnormalities of host defense mechanisms are present, e.g., urolithiasis. Prostatic infection is presumed to occur in any male dog with a UTI; hence all UTIs in male dogs are considered complicated. Recurrent infections are also assumed to be complicated, unless thorough examination of the patient proves otherwise.

Standard Therapy and Monitoring

Standard treatment and monitoring of UTIs are based on classifying the UTI into one of several categories as outlined below.

Simple, Acute UTI. If clinical signs and urinalysis results are consistent with the existence of a simple, acute UTI (first time occurrence with no complicating factors apparent), a urine culture is recommended to identify the causative organism. The choice of antibiotics is based on the identity of the organism (Table 11-2) or minimum inhibitory concentration testing (Table 11-3). If no urine culture is obtained, a broad spectrum antibiotic such as ampicillin or trimethoprim-sulfa may be used (Table 11-3). Therapy should be employed for 14 days and urinalysis and urine culture repeated 1 week after discontinuation of therapy.

Complicated, Acute UTI. A complete urinalysis, including quantitative culture of a cystocentesis, is recommended. Complete evaluation and appropriate therapy of complicating factors are essential for the management of these infections. Therapy for UTI in all male dogs (assumed to be complicated owing to prostatic involvement) should be instituted, with careful follow-up and an antibiotic with prostatic penetrance such as chloramphenicol, carbenicillin, or macrolides (e.g., erythromycin) is recommended.

Therapy for other complicated UTIs depends on successful control of the complicating factors. Otherwise, it is unlikely the UTI can be successfully managed. If the complicating factor is temporary (e.g., urinary catheterization or transient bladder atony), antibiotic therapy should be withheld until it is resolved. Urinary antiseptics can be used during the intervening period. Methenamine (Mandelamine, Parke-Davis), given in conjunction with mandelic or hippuric acid to lower urine pH (goal < 6.0), can be used in this circumstance (Table 11-3). If used, urine pH should be monitored, and other urinary acidifiers (Table 11-3) can be added to effect (urine pH $\leqslant$ 6.0). Antibiotic therapy is again based on identifying the offending organism and the minimum inhibitory concentrations, if available (Tables 11-2 and 11-3). The appropriate time course for therapy is a minimum of 3 weeks and is often several times longer, depending on the complicating factor. Urinalysis and quantitative urine culture should be performed during therapy and 1 week and 1 month after discontinuation of therapy.

Recurrent UTI. A recurrent UTI is an infection that is detected after discontinuation of therapy. Such infections may be classified as relapsing, persistent (same microorganism) or as reinfections (different microorganisms).

Reinfections. Because reinfections represent recurrent bouts of simple acute UTIs, management is the same. Appropriate diagnostic tests should be performed to identify any possible complicating or predisposing factors. Trimethoprim-sulfa, cephalexin, or nitrofurantoin (Macrodantin, Norwich-Eaton) may be used for dogs with recurrent UTIs due to most gram-negative bacteria, and penicillin G or ampicillin may be used in dogs with Proteus spp. or gram-positive infections (Table 11-3). Length of therapy is generally 10–14 days. However, if recurrences are frequent (more than three per year), then low dose, continuous therapy should be considered. This method generally employs trimethoprim-sulfa combinations at one-half to two-thirds the normal dose (milligrams per kilogram), given once daily (at night). This lower dosage should be employed only after a 10- to 14-day regimen of full-dose therapy has been documented to eliminate bacteriuria. Monthly urine cultures should be performed while on the low-dose, suppressive therapy. If six consecutive cultures are negative, the low-dose therapy can be discontinued. Long-term side effects with trimethoprim-sulfa combinations include keratoconjunctivitis sicca or folate deficiency anemia. Patients should receive folate supplementation if this regimen is used for more than 6 weeks. Trimethoprim-sulfa combinations have the advantage of achieving high concentrations in the vagina and urethra, which reduce urinary tract colonization. However, other nontoxic antibiotics can be used in this regimen. Nitrofurantoin (Macrodantin, Norwich-Eaton) or a first generation cephalosporin such as cephalothin are suitable examples.

Relapsing or Persistent Infections. Relapsing infections are those that recur within a few weeks of discontinuation of therapy in which the original microorganism is again identified as the causative agent. These situations are generally therapeutic failures. Unidentified complicating factors, inadequate dose, inappropriate antibiotic, and development of microbial resistance are the most common reasons for these persistent infections. Appropriate diagnostic tests are essential to the management of this problem.

Antibiotic sensitivity testing, preferably determination of the minimum inhibitory concentration, is essential to the successful management of persistent infections. The bacterium is likely susceptible to the antimicrobial if the mean urine concentration is four times the minimum inhibitory concentration (see Table 11-3).

Involvement of the upper urinary tract generally results in a recurring urinary tract infection. With recurring UTIs, appropriate diagnostic tests (e.g., excretory urography) may suggest the possibility of upper tract involvement, and antibiotics with good medullary penetrance should be utilized. These drugs include trimethoprim-sulfa combinations, chloramphenicol, and the quinolones (norfloxacin, enrofloxacin, ciprofloxacin).

Antibiotic therapy should be continued for 6–8 weeks, with urinalysis and urine culture performed 1 week after initiation of therapy and immediately prior to discontinuation of therapy. Urinalysis and urine culture should be repeated 1 week and 1 month later. For highly resistant infections, urinary antiseptics may represent an alternative therapy, although only nitrofurantoin and the quinolones (norfloxacin, enrofloxacin, ciprofloxacin) are useful for upper tract (renal) involvement. Because recurrent infections generally require a minimum of 6 weeks of therapy, the toxicity of the aminoglycosides make them an unreasonable choice. Despite an exhaustive search for complicating factors and appropriate periods of antibiotic therapy, some reinfections can be controlled during therapy but recur as soon as therapy is discontinued. Continuous, nightly, low-dose suppressive therapy (as outlined in the section in this chapter on therapy for Reinfections) should be considered in these cases.

CANINE UROLITHIASIS

Diagnostic considerations are important in the management of urolithiasis. Predisposing factors should be resolved, if possible. A urinalysis, urine culture, and radiographic studies of the entire urinary tract are essential components of the diagnostic evaluation of affected dogs. Standard therapy is based on quantitative analysis of the mineral composition of the urolith.

Struvite (Magnesium Ammonium Phosphate) Urolithiasis

Surgical removal in conjunction with appropriate antibiotic therapy is an effective treatment for the struvite urolith and is generally preferred. However, in some patients, anesthesia and surgery may pose an undue risk, and some uroliths are difficult to remove surgically. For these reasons and others, medical dissolution of uroliths may be appropriate.

Medical therapy involves eradication of any UTI, induction of polyuria, use of calculolytic diets, and urinary acidification. Although some struvite uroliths are sterile, most are associated with infection (acute complicated or recurrent UTI). These cases should be managed as outlined above for UTIs. Although the urolith is present as a complicating factor, it may be possible only to control rather than to eradicate the UTI. A calculolytic diet (Prescription Diet Canine s/d, Hill's Pet Products) can reduce the concentration of urea, magnesium, and phosphate in the urine and is supplemented with salt to induce diuresis. This diet can generally be fed safely to dogs for 2–6 months, but reductions of serum albumin concentration preclude longer use. This low protein diet also reduces the BUN and increases serum alkaline phosphatase activity.

Urinalysis, urine culture, and radiographs to follow the size of the urolith should be repeated at monthly intervals. In addition, the BUN (as an index of dietary compliance), serum albumin, and hepatic alkaline phosphatase should be measured monthly. If the urolith is not reduced after 2 months of this therapy, surgical management should be reconsidered.

Potential side effects of medical therapy include an increased serum concentration of hepatic alkaline phosphatase and reduced serum albumin concentration. These effects are generally mild. Prescription Diet Canine s/d should not be used in patients predisposed to systemic hypertension, as it is sodium supplemented. As uroliths decrease in size, they may become lodged in the urethra or ureter. Calculi in the urethra can generally be managed by retrohydropropulsion of the offending urolith into the bladder, utilizing an open-ended catheter and a syringe to apply pressure with saline or a saline/K-Y lubricant mixture. The presence of calculi in the ureter(s) necessitates immediate surgical intervention.

Poor results from medical therapy can be anticipated if the identity of the stone is unknown. The recommended method of therapy (antibiotics and calculolytic diet) does not dissolve nonstruvite stones, and the delay in appropriate treatment of these uroliths is generally detrimental to the patient. For dogs with calcium-containing stones, the calculolytic diet is contraindicated, as it induces calciuresis. For dogs with urate stones, Canine s/d diet induces aciduria, in which urate is less soluble.

Efforts aimed at preventing recurrence include the management of any UTI present. In cases where a UTI is not involved in struvite urolithiasis, urinary acidification (see Table 11-3) may be beneficial.

Urate Urolithiasis

Urate calculi form in dalmatian dogs (incomplete hepatic conversion of uric acid to allantoin, producing hyperuricosuria) and in dogs with portosystemic shunts (hyperammonemia and hyperuricosuria). These calculi are usually treated surgically, although medical dissolution is possible in those cases in which location of the uroliths or patient factors preclude surgical intervention.

Medical dissolution is accomplished by a combination of calculolytic diets, xanthine oxidase inhibitors, alkalinization of urine, and eradication of any UTIs. The Prescription Diet u/d (Hill's Pet Products) is purine-restricted and does not acidify the urine. The Prescription Diet s/d (Hill's Pet Products) is also low in purine content, although it contains supplemental sodium and it generally acidifies urine. Consequently, if the latter diet is used, a non-sodium-containing alkalinizing agent should be employed (e.g., potassium citrate rather than sodium bicarbonate) to avoid excessive dietary sodium intake. Urinary alkalinization, which should be based on measurement of urine pH, can be accomplished with the addition of sodium bicarbonate (initial dose of 10 mg/kg given two or three times daily) or potassium citrate (Urocit-K, Mission Pharmacal) at an initial dose of 35 mg/kg PO three times daily. These alkalinizing agents should be increased to effect, although metabolic alkalosis should be avoided by routine measurement of the serum TCO_2 or bicarbonate concentration. The goal is a urine pH between 7.0 and 7.5. The calculolytic diet s/d should not be used as a long-term source of nutrition (>6 months); and if it is employed, serum hepatic alkaline phosphatase activity and serum albumin concentration should be measured monthly.

The size of the uroliths should be monitored monthly, utilizing contrast radiography if necessary. Urine pH should be checked at least once every 2 weeks at home and at monthly evaluations. Urate uroliths may become lodged in the urethra and usually can be returned to the bladder by retrohydropropulsion. If the stones remain unchanged 3 months after the initiation of therapy, surgical intervention should be considered.

After surgical removal or medical dissolution, preventive measures should be employed. In animals with portosystemic shunts, surgical correction of the shunt should preclude recurrence and assists in medical dissolution. Diets restricted in purine content (e.g., Prescription Diet u/d) can be utilized in dalmatian dogs with a history of recurrent urate uroliths. Dietary therapy should be supplemented with serial evaluations of urine pH to verify the presence of alkaline urine, employing appropriate dosages of alkalinizing agents as needed to maintain a urine pH between 7.0 and 7.5. Allopurinol (Zyloprim, Burroughs-Wellcome) at a daily dosage of 10–20 mg/kg/day PO may be used long term, although the formation of xanthine uroliths remains a possible side effect of long-term use of this medication.

Other Uroliths. Cystine, calcium oxalate, calcium phosphate, and silica uroliths together account for approximately 10–20% of canine uroliths. Surgical removal followed by preventive therapy is the method of choice. Cystine calculi may best be managed by the use of a low protein diet (Prescription Diet u/d), D-penicillamine (Cuprimine, Merck) at a dosage of

14 mg/kg PO twice daily to block the conversion of cysteine to cystine, and urinary alkalinization as needed. D-Penicillamine can produce side effects including vomiting, rash, fever, lymphadenopathy, and increased pyridoxine requirements (vitamin B supplementation recommended). Another medication, N-(2-mercaptopropionyl)-glycine, or MPG (14 mg/kg PO twice daily), is reportedly beneficial as a replacement therapy for D-penicillamine in this disease. MPG, however, is an investigational therapy at present and cannot yet be recommended as a standard therapeutic replacement for D-penicillamine. Potassium citrate (Urocit-K, Mission Pharmacal) at an initial dosage of 35 mg/kg PO three times daily is preferable to sodium bicarbonate as an alkalinizing agent.

Calcium oxalate uroliths are a diagnostic challenge, as there are many possible contributory mechanisms. A complete evaluation of affected patients, which precedes therapeutic trials, is a requirement. Some general guidelines of therapy include the avoidance of dietary calcium supplementation, restriction of dietary sodium intake, and potassium citrate supplementation (initial dose of 35 mg/kg PO three times daily to achieve urine pH > 7.0). The appropriate diet remains unknown, although general recommendations are for a diet restricted in sodium, calcium, oxalate, and phosphate content. Canine Prescription Diet k/d or u/d may be appropriate first choices for a diet. Although of unproved benefit in dogs, thiazide diuretics (e.g., chlorothiazide 15 mg/kg PO twice daily) to decrease urinary calcium excretion may be employed in normocalcemic dogs not responding to other therapy.

Silica uroliths are best treated by surgical removal followed by use of a meat-based (rather than vegetable protein) diet, induction of diuresis through the addition of sodium chloride (50–100 mg/kg/day; 1 teaspoon = 6000 mg; goal = urine specific gravity < 1.030) to the diet, and eradication of UTI.

In dogs, calcium phosphate uroliths are most commonly associated with hypercalcemia, and the appropriate therapy should be directed at treating the primary condition. Although preventive medical therapy remains unevaluated for this form of urolith in dogs, citrate supplementation (potassium citrate, initial dose 35 mg/kg PO three times daily), dietary sodium restriction, and urinary acidification are theoretically sound medical practices that can be employed in refractory cases, where they do not confound therapy for a primary condition. Urinary acidification is contraindicated in cases of calcium phosphate urolithiasis associated with renal tubular acidosis.

FELINE UROLITHIASIS

Lower urinary tract disease in the cat is similar to that in the dog in that UTIs, urolithiasis, and neoplasia occur in both species. However, an as yet unexplained high incidence of sterile urethrocystitis and struvite crystalluria, with or without the presence of an obstructive urethral plug, occurs in this species. This syndrome has been referred to as feline urologic syndrome (FUS).

Standard Therapy

Hematuria and dysuria in most nonobstructed cats with urethrocystitis spontaneously resolve in a few days, with or without therapy. However, more than one-third of cases recur despite therapy. Medical prevention of the recurrence may be attempted but remains unproved at this time. UTI, if present, should be appropriately treated. If uroliths are present in the bladder (usually documented by radiography or ultrasonography), specific therapy should be employed, generally including surgical removal. Other appropriate therapy includes the induction of polyuria by the use of canned cat food. Weight loss and exercise should be encouraged in obese, sedentary cats. Sodium chloride (50–100 mg/kg/day) may be added to the diet, unless a sodium-supplemented diet is utilized. Feline Prescription Diet s/d (Hill's Pet Products) is sodium supplemented and acidifying. DL-Methionine or ammonium chloride may be used to acidify the urine of cats (Table 11-3) but should be used only as needed to maintain the urine pH between 6.0 and 7.0. Urinary acidifiers and the s/d diet should not be used in young cats, as they may induce acidemia and anorexia. Other low mineral diets, such as Feline c/d, may be of benefit in the prevention of recurrence.

Alternative Therapy

If urethral obstruction recurs two or more times, some recommend a perineal urethrostomy. Before performing this operative procedure, a thorough diagnostic workup is appropriate. Many obstructive conditions or predisposing factors are best treated with alternative methods of therapy. For the sterile urethral plug (FUS) perineal urethrostomy may provide an effective therapy to reduce the prevalence of obstruction recurrence. However, it apparently has no effect on the incidence of urethrocystitis, and owners should be cautioned of this fact. In addition, a perineal urethrostomy is not appropriate therapy for other forms of feline urolithiasis in which grossly observable uroliths form in the bladder or upper urinary tract. Potential side effects of perineal urethrostomy include bacterial UTI (and associated struvite urolithiasis), urethral strictures, and urinary incontinence.

URINARY INCONTINENCE

Urinary incontinence is defined as a lack of voluntary control of urination. This complaint should be carefully evaluated to avoid confusion with dysuria, polyuria, and inappropriate urination, for which therapy is different.

Standard Therapy

The standard therapy for urinary incontinence includes the following: 1) identification of the abnormality by physical examination, careful observation of urination, measurement of the residual bladder urine volume, complete urinalysis, and other appropriate diagnostic tests (e.g., radiographic studies, urinary tract electrophysiology, and urodynamic studies); 2) treatment of identified primary diseases (e.g., UTI, neurologic lesions, and urolithiasis); 3) pharmacologic management of micturition; 4) reevaluation of response to therapy in 2–3 weeks; and 5) reevaluation of treatment failures, which may include repetition of appropriate diagnostic tests and consideration of increased drug dosage, change in drug agent, or other therapy.

Specific Therapy. For the purposes of therapy, incontinence may be divided into neurogenic and nonneurogenic causes on the basis of a thorough neurologic evaluation. For neurogenic incontinence, appropriate specific therapy should be directed at resolution of the underlying neurologic disease. Therapy for incontinence to assist the micturition process should be employed until the neurologic problem is resolved. Causes of incontinence in animals with neurologic disease include detrusor atonia, detrusor hyperreflexia, and reflex dyssynergia.

If the neurologic evaluation reveals no abnormalities, the incontinence is generally categorized as nonneurogenic. Nonneurogenic incontinence can be further subdivided into urethral incompetence, ectopic ureter, patent urachus, urge incontinence, and FeLV-associated incontinence in cats. Anatomic anomalies, such as ectopic ureters or patent urachus, should be identified and treated by appropriate surgical intervention. Urinary tract infections, if present, should be eradicated or controlled as outlined in another section of this chapter.

Therapy for Incontinence. Regardless of the cause of the incontinence (neurogenic or nonneurogenic), pharmacologic management of the incontinent patient, in combination with nursing care, may be used temporarily until continence is reestablished. This regimen is used for lifelong therapy in some patients.

The disorders of micturition may be divided into those affecting the storage phase and those affecting the voiding phase. Storage of urine requires bladder muscle (detrusor) relaxation and maintenance of adequate urethral tone. Consequently, disorders of the storage phase of micturition may include detrusor hyperreflexia (urge incontinence) or urethral incompetence. Bladder hypercontractility (hyperreflexia) may be treated by anticholinergic medications such as propantheline (Pro-Banthine, Searle) at a dosage of 7.5–15.0 mg PO q8h in dogs and 5.0–7.5 mg PO q4–8h in cats. Other medications, e.g., oxybutynin (Ditropan, Marion) at a dosage of 0.2 mg/kg PO q12h remain investigational at this time. Urethral hyporeflexia (urethral incompetence) is perhaps the most common cause of urinary incontinence in dogs. Hormone-responsive urinary incontinence may best be managed by the use of estrogen (diethylstilbestrol 0.1 mg PO for 3–5 days, subsequently repeated no more often than every 7 days) in females and testosterone at a dosage of 2.2 mg/kg IM every 3 days for testosterone propionate (Androlan) and every 30 days for testosterone cypionate (Depo-testosterone, Upjohn) in males. Side effects of hormonal therapy include aplastic anemia and signs of estrus (estrogenic compounds) and behavioral effect, perianal gland adenoma, and perineal hernia (testosterone). In dogs not responding to hormone therapy or in those in which hormonal therapy is not desired as a first-choice agent, urethral incompetence may be treated with α-adrenergic agents such as phenylpropanolamine (Ornade, Smith-Kline) at a dosage of 1.5 mg/kg PO q12h or sympathomimetic agents such as imipramine (Tofranil, Geigy) at a dosage of 5–15 mg PO q12h (2.5–5.0 mg PO q12h in cats). The use of surgical procedures to augment the urethral sphincter mechanism should be reserved for nonre sponding dogs and be performed only by experienced surgeons.

Voiding of urine requires a coordinated detrusor contraction and urethral relaxation. Disorders of the voiding phase of micturition include bladder hypotonia or atonia, urethral hyperreflexia, and reflex dyssynergia (a lack of synergism between bladder contraction and urethral relaxation during voiding). Bladder atony or hypotonia is best treated by a combination of bladder decompression (closed indwelling catheter or multiple intermittent catheterizations, with the latter being preferred if practical) plus cholinergic drugs such as bethanechol (Urecholine, Merck) at a dosage of 5–15 mg PO q8h in dogs and 1.25–5.00 mg PO q8h in cats to enhance bladder contractility. Urethral hyperreflexia and reflex dyssynergia may be managed in dogs with a combination of muscle relaxants, including those affecting smooth muscle [phenoxybenzamine (Dibenzyline, Smith-Kline) 0.25 mg/kg PO q12h] or skeletal muscle [baclofen (Lioresal, Geigy) 1–2 mg/kg PO q8h]; the feline doses are unknown. Diazepam (Valium, Roche), which affects skeletal muscle, may also be used at a dosage of 0.2 mg/kg PO q8h in dogs and 2.5 mg PO q8h in cats.

PROSTATIC DISEASES

Treatment of prostatic diseases should be based on a thorough diagnostic evaluation, including urinalysis, urine culture, prostatic palpation, and evaluation of a prostatic discharge sample (either ejaculate or prostatic massage sample). Other diagnostic tests that may be appropriate include prostatic imaging (radiographic or ultrasonic), prostatic aspiration, and prostatic biopsy. Prostatic diseases of importance in the dog include benign prostatic hyperplasia, paraprostatic cysts, bacterial prostatitis, and prostatic neoplasia. These conditions frequently coexist in the same organ, and some degree of benign hyperplasia should be expected in all older, intact male dogs. Prostatic neoplasia carries a poor prognosis, and surgical plus adjuvant therapy should be considered (see appropriate oncology textbooks).

Benign Prostatic Hyperplasia and Hypertrophy

Treatment for benign hyperplasia is necessary only if related clinical signs are present, which are most likely to include tenesmus and urethral obstruction. The most effective and appropriate therapy is castration, which results in prostatic involution within several days to, at most, a few weeks. If castration is not a viable option, low doses of estrogen (0.2 mg diethylstilbestrol daily for 5 days) may be effective. Higher doses are associated with aplastic anemia, and use of repeated doses may cause prostatic fibromuscular hyperplasia and induce squamous metaplasia. Other antiadrogenic drugs, such as megestrol acetate (Ovaban, Schering), ketoconazole (Nizoral, Janssen), and flutamide (5 mg/kg/day PO—not currently marketed in the United States) may prove clinically useful treatment for prostatic hyperplasia in dogs.

Paraprostatic Cysts

Large paraprostatic cysts may cause tenesmus or dysuria. The recommended therapy is surgical excision or marsupialization if excision is not possible, coupled with castration.

Bacterial Prostatitis

As outlined in the section on treatment of urinary tract infection, bacterial prostatitis is assumed in any male dog with a UTI. However, primary or secondary involvement of the prostate deserves special consideration. Acute bacterial prostatitis should be treated with 3–4 weeks of antibiotic based on urine culture and antibiotic sensitivity testing (preferably minimum inhibitory concentration determination). In acute bacterial prostatitis, the blood-prostatic fluid barrier is disrupted, and antibiotics should adequately penetrate this inflamed tissue.

Occasionally, clinical signs warrant fluid therapy and parenteral antibiotic administration, but generally oral antimicrobials are adequate. At 1–4 weeks after discontinuation of therapy, urinalysis, urine culture, and prostatic fluid (ejaculate or massage sample) evaluation should be repeated. If recurrence is documented, the prostate should be reevaluated by diagnostic testing, and antibiotics with good prostatic penetrance (see below) should be chosen on the basis of culture and sensitivity results and instituted for 8–12 weeks, with subsequent reevaluation at 1 and 4 weeks after discontinuation of therapy. Because the blood-prostatic fluid barrier is intact, chronic bacterial prostatitis is more difficult to manage. Antibiotics appropriate for therapy of chronic prostatic infection due to gram-positive bacteria include trimethoprim-sulfa combinations, chloramphenicol, carbenicillin (22–33 mg/kg PO q8h), erythromycin, clindamycin (3–10 mg/kg PO q8h in dogs; 12–25 mg/kg PO q12h in cats), and norfloxacin (Table 11-3). For gram-negative bacterial infection of the prostate, chloramphenicol, trimethoprim-sulfa, and carbenicillin are appropriate choices. Antibiotic therapy should be continued for a minimum of 6 weeks, with follow-up urinalysis, urine culture, and culture and cytology of prostatic fluid (ejaculate or massage sample) 7 days after discontinuation of therapy. The prognosis for cure is only fair, although chronic therapy may result in control of the condition. As with recurrent UTIs, chronic suppressive therapy with trimethoprim-sulfa combinations may be effective, although folate deficiency anemia and keratoconjunctivitis sicca may develop. The former can be avoided by folate supplementation. Castration is also generally recommended although as yet unproved for chronic canine bacterial prostatitis.

Prostatic abscessation, a severe form of bacterial prostatitis, must be managed surgically through drainage or prostatectomy. These therapies are expensive and difficult; and complications such as urinary incontinence, urethral fistula, and ascending UTI are frequent with both procedures. Antibiotic therapy with chloramphenicol, trimethoprim-sulfa, or carbenicillin should accompany the surgical procedure. Castration is also recommended.

The prognosis for recovery from acute prostatitis is fair. Chronic bacterial prostatitis is often difficult to resolve, although long-term therapy may prove capable of adequate control for a normal quality of life. Prostatic abscessation carries a poor prognosis for complete recovery.

PYOMETRA

Standard Therapy

Pyometra, the most common uterine disease in the bitch, is most appropriately managed by ovariohysterectomy. Rapid (1–2 hours) correction of dehydration with fluid therapy should be accompanied by antibiotics (e.g., ampicillin, cephalexin, trimethoprim-sulfa combinations). In severely debilitated animals, a combination of an aminoglycoside (amikacin or gentamicin) plus a penicillin or first generation cephalosporin (e.g., cephalexin) may be appropriate. If utilized, the aminoglycoside should be started after rehydration and employed only as long as necessary, generally 3–5 days. Other antibiotics, based on results of culture and sensitivity testing of the uterine wall, should be continued for 2–3 weeks postoperatively. Complications that may occur in association with the ovarariohysterectomy include peritonitis secondary to leakage of material into the abdominal cavity prior to or at the time of surgery and subsequent development of a uterine stump granuloma. The latter condition should be managed by surgical resection plus appropriate antibiotic therapy based on results of culture and sensitivity testing.

Although recovery from pyometra and its sequelae (including the associated renal disease) is generally rapid and complete, some animals develop hypothermia or cardiac arrhythmias (or both) postoperatively. These abnormalities may last for several days and are generally best treated by supportive care, including fluids and antibiotics.

Alternative Therapy

Medical therapy for pyrometra may be attempted in those cases where ovariohysterectomy is unacceptable to the owner. However, it should be emphasized that this therapy is associated with recurrence and therapeutic failures. Following correction of dehydration and initiation of antibiotic therapy, naturally occurring prostaglandin $F_{2\alpha}$ ($PGF_{2\alpha}$) (Lutalyse, Upjohn) is administered at a dose of 0.25 mg/kg in the bitch (0.1 mg/kg in the queen) subcutaneously once daily for 5 days; side effects include restlessness, vomiting, ataxia, muscle tremors, tenesmus, diarrhea, panting, and pupillary dilation/constriction. These side effects are common and are worse for 2–3 hours immediately following the injection. In addition, the uterus may rupture after administration of $PGF_{2\alpha}$.

The white blood cell count should be normal 10–14 days after treatment. The presence of a serous discharge for 10–14 days after therapy is normal. If clinical signs do not resolve and the uterus remains palpably enlarged, repeat treatments may be necessary during the subsequent 2 months. One-third of successfully treated dogs require a second 5-day regimen of $PGF_{2\alpha}$. About half of the bitches treated in this manner are subsequently able to deliver puppies.

METRITIS

Acute bacterial infection of the uterus almost always occurs postpartum and is managed similarly to pyrometra, with appropriate antibiotic and fluid therapy accompanying ovariohysterectomy. Medical management may be attempted if the cervix can be cannulated to allow flushing of the uterus with sterile isotonic solutions, with or without the addition of 2% povidone-iodine (Betadine) solution. An alternative adjunct therapy is the use of agents to enhance myometrial contractility. Such agents include $PGF_{2\alpha}$ (0.10–0.25 mg/kg SC for 3–5 days), oxytocin (0.25–0.50 unit/kg IM given once), or ergonovine (0.2 mg/kg IM given once). The latter drugs may lead to uterine rupture, and ovariohysterectomy is the preferred therapy instead of these drugs.

VAGINITIS

In prepuberal bitches, conservative medical therapy usually allows vaginal inflammation and discharge to resolve spontaneously at puberty. Conservative therapy includes the use of cleaning the perivulvar area to prevent moist dermatitis. In some cases, a urinary antiseptic such as methenamine mandelate (Table 11-3) reduces clinical signs. It has been recommended that affected bitches be allowed to cycle prior to neutering. In affected adults, predisposing causes should be considered and a 2- to 3-week trial of antibiotics tried (e.g., trimethoprim-sulfa combinations or ampicillin). Results of bacterial culture and sensitivity tests of the vaginal mucosa are difficult to interpret, as this area is normally inhabited by a microflora. Medicated douches and antibiotic instillation might prove useful in individual cases, although these therapies have not been systematically evaluated. It should be remembered that absorbance across an inflamed mucosal surface may occur, and toxic medications should not be instilled vaginally without consideration of this possibility.

SUGGESTED READINGS

Azotemia

Allen TA: Specialized nutritional support. In: Ettinger SJ, ed. Textbook of Veterinary Internal Medicine. Philadelphia: WB Saunders, 1989; 450.

Allen TA, Jaenke RS, Fettman, MJ: A technique for estimating progression of chronic renal failure in the dog. J Am Vet Med Assoc 1987;190:866.

Barsanti JA, Finco DR, Vaden S: Medical management of canine glomerulonephropathies. In: Kirk RW, ed. Current Veterinary Therapy X. Philadelphia: WB Saunders, 1989;1170.

Chew DC: Proceedings. Washington, DC: American College of Veterinary Internal Medicine Scientific Meeting, 1990.

Cowgill L: Proceedings. Washington, DC: American College of Veterinary Internal Medicine Scientific Meeting, 1990.

Cowgill L, Kallet AJ: Recognition and management of hypertension in the dog. In: Kirk RW, ed. Current Veterinary Therapy VIII. Philadelphia: WB Saunders, 1983;1205.

Cowgill LD, Kallet AJ: Systemic hypertension. In: Kirk RW, ed. Current Veterinary Therapy IX. Philadelphia: WB Saunders, 1986; 360.

Crowe DT: Clinical use of an indwelling nasogastric tube for enteral nutrition and fluid therapy in the dog and cat. J Am Anim Hosp Assoc 1986;22:675.

Grauer GF, Thrall MA: Ethylene glycol poisoning. In: Kirk RW, ed. Current Veterinary Therapy IX. Philadelphia: WB Saunders, 1986; 206.

Krawiec DR, Gelberg HB: Chronic renal disease in cats. In: Kirk RW, ed. Current Veterinary Therapy X. Philadelphia: WB Saunders, 1989; 1170.

Polzin DJ: Diseases of the kidneys and ureters. In: Ettinger SJ, ed. Textbook of Veterinary Internal Medicine. Philadelphia: WB Saunders, 1989;1962.

Ross LA, Labato MA: Use of drugs to control hypertension in renal failure. In: Kirk RW, ed. Current Veterinary Therapy X. Philadelphia: WB Saunders, 1989;1201.

White JV: Diagnostic approach to proteinuria. In: Kirk RW, ed. Current Veterinary Therapy X. Philadelphia: WB Saunders, 1989;1139.

Urinary Tract Infections

Brown SA, Barsanti JA: Diseases of the bladder and urethra. In: Ettinger SJ, ed. Textbook of Veterinary Internal Medicine. Philadelphia: WB Saunders, 1989;2108.

Ling GV: Management of urinary tract infections. In: Kirk RW, ed. Current Veterinary Therapy IX. Philadelphia: WB Saunders, 1986;1174.

Ling GV: Therapeutic strategies involving antimicrobial treatment of the canine urinary tract. J Am Vet Med Assoc 1984;185:1162.

Urolithiasis

Lees GE, Moreau PM: Management of hypotonic and atonic urinary bladders in cats. Vet Clin North Am 1984;14:641.

Osborne CA, Kruger JM, Johnston GR, Polzin DJ: Feline lower urinary tract disorders. In: Ettinger SJ, ed. Textbook of Veterinary Internal Medicine. Philadelphia: WB Saunders, 1989;2057.

Osborne CA, Polzin DJ, Johnston GR, O'Brien TD: Canine urolithiasis. In: Ettinger SJ, ed. Textbook of Veterinary Internal Medicine. Philadelphia: WB Saunders, 1989;2083.

Urinary Incontinence

Chew DJ, DiBartola SP, Fenner WR: Pharmacologic manipulation of urination. In: Kirk RW, ed. Current Veterinary Therapy IX. Philadelphia: WB Saunders, 1986;1207.

Lappin MR, Barsanti JA: Urinary incontinence secondary to idiopathic detrusor instability. J Am Vet Med Assoc. 1987;191:1439.

Moreau PM, Lappin MR: Pharmacologic management of urinary incontinence. In: Kirk RW, ed. Current Veterinary Therapy X. Philadelphia: WB Saunders, 1989;1214.

Reproductive Tract Diseases

Barsanti JA, Finco DR: Canine prostatic diseases. In: Ettinger SJ, ed. Textbook of Veterinary Internal Medicine. Philadelphia: WB Saunders, 1989; 1859.

Mosier JE: Parturient and periparturient diseases. In: Ettinger SJ, ed. Textbook of Veterinary Internal Medicine. Philadelphia: WB Saunders, 1989; 1826.

Olson PN, Wrigley RH, Husted PW, et al: Persistent estrus in the bitch. In: Ettinger SJ, ed. Textbook of Veterinary Internal Medicine. Philadelphia: WB Saunders, 1989;1792.

Turrel JM: Management of prostatic neoplasia. In: Kirk RW, ed. Current Veterinary Therapy X. Philadelphia: WB Saunders, 1989; 1193.

CHAPTER TWELVE

Musculoskeletal Diseases

Steven C. Budsberg

The goal of this chapter is to present concise therapeutic management schemes for selected common problems that may be faced by the practitioner. For ease of understanding, the chapter is divided into disorders that primarily affect joints, bones, and muscles.

JOINT DISEASES

In a practical approach to treating joint disease, establishing whether the joint's response to the condition is noninflammatory or inflammatory is paramount. It is easily accomplished through joint taps and cytologic evaluation of the synovial fluid. Once this differentiation is made, therapeutic avenues can be addressed.

Noninflammatory Joint Disease

Noninflammatory joint disorders are defined as having synovial fluid with normal or minimal increases in cellularity (mainly mononuclear) and all other fluid parameters within normal limits. In practice, the most common noninflammatory joint disorders seen are degenerative joint disease (primary or secondary), traumatic joint disease, and developmental arthropathies.

Degenerative Joint Disease. Degenerative joint disease (DJD) is the most common noninflammatory joint disorder in companion animals. This disorder is characterized grossly by fragmentation and loss of articular cartilage and radiographically by sclerosis of subchondral bone and osteophyte production. Primary DJD is a specific syndrome in which no underlying cause can be found for the above described changes seen in the joint. This form of DJD is *extremely rare* in small animals. Secondary DJD is far more common in dogs and cats and follows a known disturbance of the affected joint or supporting tissues. As stated, in the clinical setting, one is most likely faced with DJD that is secondary in nature. Therefore, it is essential to establish the predisposing cause of the DJD and treat that problem (i.e., stifle DJD commonly caused by cruciate instability requires reestablishment of joint stability through surgery). Yet once the DJD is present (regardless of the cause) and it begins to manifest as a clinical problem, it must be managed. Management can be broken down into medical and limited surgical options and again varies with each patient.

Standard Therapy. The treatment of DJD is symptomatic and nonspecific in nature; it is directed toward relieving pain and decreasing the inflammatory response in the joint. The objective is to return the animal to acceptable activity levels without pain or lameness. One must examine each case differently, assessing the age, normal activity levels, and most importantly the owner's expectant demands for performance for the animal. Success largely depends on this accurate assessment of client expectations and demands for the pet's performance.

The medical therapeutic regimen is divided into a three-pronged strategy in which all components are equally important for clinical improvement: 1) rest and exercise modification; 2) weight loss; and 3) anti-inflammatory and analgesic medical management.

Enforced rest and exercise modification are different for each animal, but their importance must be stressed to the owner. Jumping for balls or frisbees or jogging with the owner must be discouraged in favor of leash walks, swimming, and controlled off-leash exercise. In general, activities that cause acute lameness regardless of time or intensity levels, should be used as measures of excess and must be avoided. Complete removal of exercise should also be avoided if possible, as exercise is important for maintaining muscle mass and tone, joint mobility, and the health of the remaining cartilage in the joint. However, in some cases complete rest must be used initially, although with time some exercise should be encouraged. Swimming is an excellent exercise for patients with DJD and should always be strongly encouraged.

Weight control is a must when dealing with DJD. The vast majority of animals seen with clinical manifestations of DJD are obese. Owner education and proper dietary management must be used in every case (see Chapter 2). In many cases, the implementation of rest and exercise modification along with weight reduction diminishes or completely alleviates the clinical signs of DJD.

Anti-inflammatory and analgesic agents are useful for the management of DJD in combination with rest and weight reduction. Buffered aspirin (i.e., Ascriptin, Rorer) at a dose of 20–25 mg/kg three times a day in dogs provides the most consistent and reproducible results for difficult cases. This dosage regimen should be given for at least 2 weeks or until positive effects are noted—whichever comes first. Then the dosage should be titrated down to as low a level as possible to maintain clinical improvement. An example is a 27 kg dog started at 650 mg of Ascriptin (two tablets) every 8 hours for 2 weeks, then 650 mg every 12 hours for a week. If no relapse is seen clinically, the dosage is further decreased to 325 mg every 12 hours for a week, then to 325 mg every 24 hours, then to every 48 hours, and so on. Drug therapy of 1 or 2 days without success is not a sufficient time frame to accurately assess if aspirin will be successful in a case. Side effects commonly seen are vomiting, diarrhea, and melena. It must be stressed that gastrointestinal hemorrhage, especially gastric ulceration, is not uncommon in dogs. Once signs of side effects are observed, immediate discontinuance with no further aspirin usage is strongly recommended. If there is evidence of excessive blood loss or dehydration due to gastrointestinal bleeding or profuse diarrhea on physical examination, measurement of packed cell volume and total solids is advisable. Implementation of intravenous fluid therapy to replace calculated fluid volume losses, or occasionally blood transfusion may be indicated. Dogs on protracted regimens of aspirin (several months to years) who present acutely ill should be carefully examined for any evidence of gastric perforation and peritonitis.

The variability in individual tolerance to aspirin has led some individuals to recommend lower dosages followed by increasing amounts if desired effects are not achieved. This mode of management, although acceptable, in inexperienced hands has a tendency to underestimate the effectiveness of aspirin and often results in premature discontinuance of the drug for lack of clinical response.

For cats, the need for treatment of DJD is rare. Considering the long half-life of aspirin in the cat (52 hours) and the possibility of toxic side effects, the use of aspirin is not as widely recommended as in the dog. These side effects include pulmonary edema, gastrointestinal bleeding and ulceration, and in gross overdosage cases severe acid-base disturbances, hyperthermia, electrolyte imbalances, renal damage, and convulsions or coma. Feline aspirin dosages vary widely, with 25 mg/kg once a day as a high end dosage and 10–15 mg/kg *every other day* as a more conservative dosage. The author has little experience with aspirin therapy in treating DJD in cats, yet I believe that one should first do no harm to the patient, and thus recommend using the lower dosage. If aspirin is used and found to be effective, every effort should be made to decrease to the lowest effective level for long-term usage. The goal should be to discontinue aspirin and administer the drug again only during acute exacerbations.

Alternative Therapies. If aspirin is unsuccessful after a sufficiently long trial or if the dog cannot tolerate it, *phenylbutazone* can be tried. It should be remembered, however, that many clinicians believe that phenylbutazone will not be effective if aspirin was not, and that risk of serious toxicity may be greater with phenylbutazone. The dosage is 13 mg/kg given three times a day. After 2 or 3 days, the dosage should be decreased to the lowest possible levels that maintain a clinical response. The maximum dosage is 800 mg/day regardless of the dog's body size or weight. Bone marrow suppression with accompanying anemia is the most common side effect seen with chronic usage of the drug. Chronic usage should be accompanied with a complete blood count (CBC) every 2–3 months.

Corticosteroid therapy should be limited to those dogs in which no other treatment has worked. There is much evidence that steroid therapy speeds up progression of DJD, and thus any positive short-term results are negated by long-term loss of the remaining cartilage. Whenever steroids are used, owners must be made aware of the probable detrimental side effects. Prednisone or prednisolone dosage levels should start at 0.5–1.0 mg/kg once a day (or divided into two equal doses every 12 hours) and be reduced to as low a dosage as possible as soon as possible, with a goal of every other day or every third day attempted. Chronic maintenance dosage should not exceed 1 mg/kg every other day. Repeated intraarticular injections of steroids should be avoided. Especially detrimental is the use of long-acting steroids such as methylprednisolone acetate (Depo-Medrol, Upjohn). These drugs can dramatically expedite the damage to the cartilage and the progression of DJD. The major side effects of chronic steroid usage are associated with iatrogenic induction of Cushing's syndrome. Other side effects, of which the owner must be made aware, are increased appetite and water consumption, with compensatory urination.

The use of corticosteroids may be preferential in the cat for treatment of DJD. Prednisone or prednisolone should be administered initially at a dosage of 0.5–2.0 mg/kg once a day for 5–7 days. The drug should then be tapered to as low a dosage as possible with every second or third day chronic therapy as a goal. As for the dog, chronic maintenance dosage should not exceed 1 mg/kg every other day. The side effects and monitoring are similar to those described for the dog.

There are a large number of *nonsteroidal anti-inflammatory and analgesic agents* that have been developed for treatment of DJD in humans. In fact, many are sold over the counter and are readily available to clients. Various dosage regimens have been advocated for some of these drugs. Unfortunately, many have been used in dogs and cats with severe side effects including severe gastrointestinal hemorrhage. Propionic acid derivatives (including naproxen and ibuprofen), indomethacin, and piroxicam (Feldene, Pfizer) have been reported to cause severe gastrointestinal hemorrhage and are much more gastrotoxic than aspirin in the dog. Many veterinarians report successfully using ibuprofen when aspirin fails. I have seen an increasing number of such cases in which ibuprofen was prescribed for DJD (at a variety of dosage regimens), associated with serious gastrointestinal bleeding with documentation of severe gastric ulcerations. Thus because of the lack of adequate toxicity studies, controlled research, and clinical trials on each of these drugs, they cannot yet be recommended for the dog and cat.

The goals of *surgery* should be to treat the primary cause of the joint abnormality (i.e., ruptured cranial cruciate ligament) and to relieve pain in the affected joint during normal activity. In many instances, treatment of the primary cause does not effectively accomplish these goals, and thus orthopedic salvage procedures are needed to relieve the pain and provide some function to the joint.

The options most widely used are excision arthroplasty, arthrodesis, and joint replacement. Table 12-1 briefly outlines the possible options for surgical intervention; however, one should consult a qualified surgeon if any of these procedures are to be used for therapy because each can have serious complications.

TABLE 12-1. Surgical Options for Degenerative Joint Disease in Dogs and Cats

| | Procedure | | |
Joint	Arthrodesis	Excision Arthroplasty	Joint Replacement
Fore limb			
Shoulder	X	X	
Elbow	X		
Carpus	X		
Rear limb			
Hip		X	X
Stifle	X		
Tarsus	X		

Investigational Therapy. Presently, in dogs, there is work being done with intraarticular products including hyaluronic acid and polysulfated glycosaminoglycans. This work is primarily in research models but will be making its way into clinical usage within a few years. Also, there is at least one nonsteroidal anti-inflammatory drug (e.g., Carprofen, Hoffman-LaRoche) presently under investigation that has fewer gastrointestinal side effects and is still effective. None of these drugs has been cleared by the U.S. Food and Drug Administration (FDA) for clinical use in the dog or cat.

Osteochondrosis. Osteochondrosis is characterized by a disruption in normal endochondral ossification involving the deeper layers of chondrocytes within growth plates. Specifically, the germinal zone of cartilage is irregularly arranged, and the progression of cartilage growth to calcification is abnormal. Osteochondrosis can be clinically silent, apparent only histologically, or evident upon gross or radiographic examination of the joint. Although technically a disease of the bone, clinical signs of the disease including lameness and joint effusion are associated with exposure of the joint fluid to the subchondral bone through fissures in the cartilage overlying the lesion. Osteochondritis dissecans (OCD) refers to a specific disease entity when the overlying cartilage forms a flap that may still be attached or may be free-floating in the joint. OCD is the process that is commonly referred to in clinical medicine. Other diseases that are thought to be defects in endochondral ossification include nonunited anconeal processes and fragmented (or nonunited) coronoid processes of the ulna.

Standard Therapy. Surgical intervention prior to the development of degenerative changes offers superior results that are the most predictable in terms of both long-term outcome and immediately reducing clinical signs. The only exception to this statement *may be* OCD of the hock, which is discussed below. Remember, the keys to success are diagnosis and surgical intervention prior to development of degenerative changes in the joint.

The objectives of surgery involve three goals: 1) removing the cartilage flap and/or free joint mice; 2) hastening healing of the defect; and 3) slowing the development and progression of the degenerative joint disease. The cartilage flap or the free-floating joint mouse is first removed. The defect in the cartilage is then examined to ensure that there is no undermining of the remaining cartilage. The edges of the cartilage should be made as perpendicular as possible around the lesion. Curettage of the lesion is recommended to remove any areas of subchondral eburnation, stimulate granulation tissue to form, and hasten the formation of replacement fibrocartilage. As an alternative to, or in combination with curettage, small holes may be drilled with a k-wire (also known as forage).

Success of surgery depends on the amount and severity of degenerative joint disease, which is present in the joint prior to surgery and to some degree on the specific joint involved. Remember, no surgical procedure removes preexisting DJD or completely prevents its insidious progression.

Scapulohumeral OCD responds well to surgical treatment and carries a good to excellent prognosis. Expectations for OCD in the elbow (medial humeral condyle) are more dependent on preexisting DJD in the joint than would be the case for the shoulder, but the prognosis is still generally favorable. The prognosis for OCD of the stifle again depends on the amount of DJD present. The stifle seems to respond less favorably than the elbow to surgical intervention, and the prognosis is guarded. The tarsocural joint is the only joint in which early surgical management of OCD may not provide consistent results. However, surgery is still recommended, especially in cases in which appreciable DJD has not already formed or free floating joint mice are present.

Alternative Therapy. The conservative modes of therapy—rest and analgesics—can be attempted in a *very* few selected cases. One example is a dog in which early stages of osteochondrosis are found radiographically without a visible cartilage flap (osteochondritis dissecans) or free-floating joint mouse, and there are no clinical signs. In this instance, rest and a balanced nonsupplemented commercial diet can be recommended. Also, if the dog is under the age of 6 months and has had mild lameness for 2–4 weeks, exercise restricted to leash walks and performance of passive flexion and extension for 2–3 weeks may alleviate clinical signs. However, if lameness is still present after attempts with conservative management, if the dog is older than 6 months, or if there is radiographic evidence of a cartilage flap or a free-floating cartilage piece, surgery is indicated. Finally, medical management is necessary in DJD cases that are severe and where the DJD is causing clinical signs. In these cases, surgical intervention will likely not improve the clinical outcome.

Fragmented Coronoid Process of the Ulna. Surgical removal of the loose osteochondral fragment is the standard approach to treatment. Conservative therapy is *not* recommended unless there is severe DJD already present in the patient, and even then one may still consider removing the fragmented coronoid.

The prognosis is good if surgical intervention is accomplished prior to the development of considerable DJD. In cases where there is severe DJD prior to therapy, one must treat for DJD with previously described medical therapy.

Nonunited Anconeal Process. Surgical removal is the only option. The prognosis is favorable if performed prior to the development of severe DJD.

Canine Hip Dysplasia. Hip dysplasia in dogs is a developmental disorder of the coxofemoral joint. The exact pathogenesis is unclear, with multiple factors probably involved to varying degrees in its development in each dog. Formation of a normal hip joint requires close conformity between the femoral head and the acetabular cup; but, for whatever reasons in an individual patient, hip dysplasia develops when this conformity fails to occur. Treatment options are varied and numerous, with sometimes confusing overlap in usage. Remember that many dogs with hip dysplasia show no signs of pain or show intermittent signs usually requiring minimal or no treatment. In an attempt to simplify the decision-making process for this disorder, one can subdivide patients into groups based on skeletal maturity (i.e., immature and mature).

Immature Dogs (5–11 Months). When dealing with this disease process, there is no single correct way to treat an individual dog. First, physical and radiographic findings can differentiate these young dogs into three groups by examining the parameters of pain, amount of locomotion dysfunction, degree of joint subluxation (or luxation), and degree of bony changes to the femoral head, femoral neck, and acetabulum. Next, one should consider the dog's size and activity levels in an effort to determine the expectations for development of signs.

1. *Group I.* Dogs with minimal bony changes and mild subluxation but who are showing signs of pain are the first group to discuss. In these dogs, medical management as outlined for treatment of DJD may be tried initially. This therapy includes weight reduction and control, exercise restriction and modification, and anti-inflammatory agents (aspirin). Reassessment should occur every 2–3 weeks to document clinical response to the therapy. Smaller or relatively inactive dogs are much more likely to benefit from this therapy and thus require no further treatment.

In the dog who is going to be large or used in active pursuits during its life, one should consider performing one of the surgical corrective osteotomies (triple pelvic osteotomy), which attempt to provide more stability to the hip joint by improving the congruity of the coxofemoral joint. However, the question of whether, in these mild cases, corrective osteotomies are a necessity for improvement of each dog is still strongly debated.

2. *Group II.* Dogs that have moderate to severe subluxation, have minimal bony changes, and are showing signs of pain form the next group.

These dogs may be far better served by undergoing one of the corrective osteotomies to improve the coverage of the femoral head and increase the articular surface contact of the head and acetabulum. These osteotomies can be divided into two groups: those that osteotomize the pelvis, rotating the acetabulum over the femoral head, and those that osteotomize the femur, thus placing the femoral head deeper into the acetabulum. Long-term follow-up on the clinical responses to these procedures is limited but encouraging. One drawback to such procedures is that they do not uniformly stop the progression of degenerative changes already present in the hip; and at some later time, the dog may need further medical management for DJD or additional surgery.

A second viable option in the larger and the more active dog is to consider medical management of these cases until the dog is skeletally mature and the affected joint can be replaced with a prosthetic hip replacement. The latter provides a more final, definitive, successful mode of therapy in the long run.

Medical therapy for group II dogs is the same as previously described; however, the likelihood of success of medical management alone is unpredictable and may be closely correlated with the size of the dog and its activity levels. Remember that this treatment is palliative and does not address the disease process. However, medical management combined with surgical intervention after the animal is skeletally mature can be used with much success. Likewise, in the small dog, excision arthroplasty may be considered, either after medical management or immediately.

3. *Group III.* Dogs with marked bony changes (degenerative changes) on the acetabulum or femoral head and neck, with any amount of subluxation, and who are in pain comprise the final group.

In this group, the benefits of corrective osteotomies are questionable. Results are highly variable owing to the fact that DJD is established. Also, there is a misshapened femoral head or acetabulum, and they never remodel to normal again. Thus surgical options are limited to excision arthroplasty immediately or total hip replacement at skeletal maturity.

Medical therapy is the same as previously described.

Skeletally Mature (> 12 Months). In these patients, one should treat DJD conservatively, as previously described. Medical management is sufficient to reduce the pain and allow normal modified activity for many dogs for several years. However, some dogs are refractory to this conservative therapy or need to be more active than medical management allows. For these dogs surgery is the best option.

The best option for dogs over 45–50 pounds (lean body weight) in this disease is total hip replacement. If costs are prohibitive, femoral head and neck excision is an alternative. However, excision arthroplasty is a nonreversible procedure and must be considered a salvage procedure. The goal of excision arthroplasty is to relieve pain. There is no doubt the operation does relieve pain in large dogs, but gait changes are usually evident, although highly variable. In dogs smaller than 45–50 pounds, femoral head and neck excision seems to afford sufficient pain relief, with minimal gait aberration, to make hip replacement unnecessary. Finally, there are a number of myotomy procedures for which the sole purpose is to relieve pain. The techniques are so limited in their application that they cannot be uniformly recommended.

Aseptic Necrosis of the Femoral Head. Aseptic necrosis of the femoral head is a noninflammatory disease process that is thought to be caused by disruption of the blood supply to the femoral head. The overlying cartilage, which is initially intact, often begins to form fissures owing to the collapse of the subchondral bone causing the development of noninflammatory joint disease. Also, collapse of the head and neck causes joint incongruity and instability, further predisposing the joint to DJD. The condition is seen in toy and small breed dogs usually during their first year of life.

Standard Therapy. Femoral head and neck excision arthroplasty provides the most predictable results for the treatment of this disease when there is any deformity in the femoral head. A good prognosis for return to normal function can be expected in these cases, with only a rare instance in which the animal has a mild limp following properly performed surgery.

Alternative Therapy. Conservative management may be attempted initially when there is no deformity of the femoral head, if the signs are mild, or if the owner is hesitant to allow surgery. Rest, analgesics, and placing the leg in a non-weight-bearing sling for 2–3 weeks can be attempted. If this therapy does not improve the clinical signs, surgery is indicated.

Inflammatory Joint Disease

Inflammatory joint disorders are characterized by inflammatory changes in the synovial membrane and fluid. Systemic signs are variable and may include lethargy, fever, and leukocytosis. Joint taps are diagnostic. Within the general category of inflammatory joint disease, the next differentiation is infectious versus noninfectious. This distinction is made from joint fluid cytologic examination and culture. Once this subdivision has been made, treatment can then progress.

Infectious Inflammatory Arthritis. Infectious inflammatory arthritis can be caused by bacteria, mycoplasmae, rickettsiae, spirochetes, fungi, and viral agents. Bacterial arthritis, spread hematogenously (usually in neonates or debilitated patients), is usually the result of direct contamination from a penetrating wound or surgical incision and is the most common cause of infectious arthritis. Regardless of the cause, infectious arthritis warrants aggressive early treatment. The overall goals of treatment of infectious arthritis are eradication of the causative agent and preservation of as much of the articular cartilage of the joint as possible.

Bacterial Inflammatory Arthritis. *Single Joint.* In cases with single joint involvement, regardless of cause, one must provide early aggressive therapy. It should include adequate drainage of suppurative material, débridement of accessible necrotic tissue, and decompression of the joint to avoid further vascular embarrassment of the epiphysis in the immature patient. Parenteral bactericidal antibiotics are also indicated.

Specifically, adequate drainage and débridement of the joint is best accomplished by arthrotomy. In acute cases, primary closure of the joint following copious lavage is usually adequate. In more advanced cases, partial closure or application of a drainage system may be considered. Both of these methods require intensive postsurgical management. Multiple aspirations are difficult and do not provide for adequate débridement, drainage, or decompression of the joint. This technique may be the only alternative for multiple joint involvement due to hematogenous spread (see multiple joint treatment).

Choice for antimicrobial therapy should be based on culture and sensitivity test results. However, during the initial time period prior to obtaining these results, or in cases in which cultures are negative, antimicrobial therapy should be based on the following criteria. The drug should be bactericidal, active against penicillinase-producing staphylococcal species, parenteral, and broad-spectrum (see Chapter 15). Some examples are the first-generation cephalosporins, e.g., cefazolin (Ancef, SmithKline & French; Kefzol, Lilly) at 22 mg/kg q6–8h, or one of the semisynthetic penicillins such as oxacillin (Bactocil, Beecham) at 22 mg/kg q6–8h. Antibiotics should be initially administered intravenously for 24–48 hours and then switched to the oral route for at least 14 days. For more advanced cases, the antibiotic should be administered for 4–6 weeks. Posttreatment joint aspiration for cytology and culture should be considered in all cases.

In all cases, passive flexion and extension of the affected joint is advisable as soon as the patient can tolerate the procedure. Exercise should be restricted to leash walks during the antimicrobial treatment period. For an additional 6–10 weeks, exercise should be increased gradually, but the dog should always be on a leash. Alternatively or in addition, swimming is an excellent mode of physical therapy and can be encouraged as soon as all skin incisions or wounds are healed.

The prognosis, primarily determined by the amount of destruction of the articular cartilage, is difficult to estimate. Clinical evaluation over the next 1–2 months with radiographs on the second visit may begin to define the amount and severity of changes that have occurred; however, DJD development may take months to progress to the point where the patient is showing clinical signs.

Multiple Joints. Treatment of polyarthropathies due to bacterial agents that have spread hematogenously is far more difficult. In these cases, diagnosis of the cause of the septic event must be addressed simultaneously with management of the joint infection. As stated previously, multiple arthrotomies are not feasible in most cases, and needle aspiration may be the only viable option for removing the suppurative material Antibiotic therapy is the mainstay of treatment and should be aggressive, as described above. Follow-up evaluations, physical therapy, and prognosis are similar to those described for single joint treatment.

Rickettsial and Spirochetal Inflammatory Arthritis. Polyarthropathies of infectious nature other than bacterial are being recognized more frequently with improvement of diagnostic abilities. Diseases such as ehrlichiosis, Rocky mountain spotted fever, and more recently Lyme disease have been associated with polyarthropathies. Fungal and protozoal arthritis (leishmaniasis) are rare and are usually signs of systemic disorders. See Chapter 16 for details of the treatment of these diseases.

Noninfectious Inflammatory Arthritis. Noninfectious inflammatory arthritis in small animal practice can be primarily considered to be caused by immunologic mechanisms. Within this classification, there are two major subgroups: erosive (deforming) and nonerosive (nondeforming) arthritides.

Erosive Arthritides. Treatment goals with canine rheumatoid arthritis center around reducing the destructive inflammatory activity occurring within the joint, relieving patient discomfort, and preserving joint function. Realizing that it is a progressive chronic disease for which there is no known cure, extensive client education is vital. Initially, the owner must realize that medical therapy may take 2 weeks or more before a decrease in severity of clinical signs is seen, and possibly up to 8–10 weeks for remission to occur. Furthermore, the owner must be made aware that even if therapy is successful in abating the clinical signs and slowing the progression of the disease, exacerbations are likely, and the medications themselves often have side effects. Although systemic medical management is a mainstay of treatment of this disease, one must not forget the aspects of complete patient management for chronic generalized joint disease, which include weight loss and modification of exercise (including the addition of swimming whenever feasible).

The *standard therapy* in humans with this disease is aspirin as the initial treatment. Its effectiveness is far less in our patients, however. A possible explanation for this variation is that, as veterinarians, we rarely are able to document and institute treatment in the early, mild stages of the disease as is done in human medicine. Thus patients presented to us are usually in the severe phases of the disease and require much more aggressive initial treatment. Glucocorticoids in combination with cyclophosphamide seem to have the best chance of inducing remission in the dog.

Dogs weighing more than 15 kg should be started on prednisone or prednisolone at a dosage of 0.75–1.50 mg/kg PO q12h for 14 days. One should then reevaluate the patient and begin to reduce the steroid dosage at 2-week intervals to a level of no more than 1 mg/kg once every other day. Dogs weighing less than 15 kg should be started on prednisone or prednisolone at a dosage of 1.0–2.0 mg/kg PO q12h for 14 days and follow the same decreasing dosage regimen to a level of no more than 1.0 mg/kg given every other day. This therapy should be maintained for at least 2–3 months after clinical signs and synovial fluids values return to normal. If remission occurs, prednisone can be reduced to every third day and then every fourth day prior to complete removal of the drug.

Dogs weighing more than 25 kg require a cyclophosphamide (Cytoxan, Mead Johnson) dosage of 1.75 mg/kg, and dogs 10–25 kg require a dosage of 2 mg/kg. Dogs less than 10 kg require 2.5 mg/kg. Treatment consists of oral administration of cyclophosphamide once a day for 4 days, followed by 3 days of no therapy, then back on therapy for 4 days, and so on. This therapy should be discontinued 1 month after remission of synovial inflammation (joint tap evaluation), if hemorrhagic cystitis occurs, or after 2–3 months of treatment.

If prolonged cytotoxic therapy is required to attain or maintain remission (2–3 months), cyclophosphamide is discontinued and replaced with either azathioprine (Imuran, Burroughs Wellcome) or 6-mercaptopurine (Purinethol, Burroughs Wellcome). The dosage of each drug is 2.0 mg/kg PO once a day for 14 days and then every other day, usually on alternating days with the glucocorticoids.

If animals on glucocorticoids and cyclophosphamide do not improve or do not make sufficient progress, one may replace the cyclophosphamide with azathioprine, as some dogs seem to have a better response on this protocol. Thus these dogs would stay on the steroid treatment described earlier and begin on azathioprine at 2.0 mg/kg PO once a day for 14 days and then every other day.

Weekly CBCs are done on all animals receiving cytotoxic drugs beginning 2 weeks after initiation of therapy. If the white blood cell (WBC) count falls to 6000 cells/mm^3 or less, and the platelet count is below 125,000/mm^3, the cytotoxic drug dosage should be reduced by 25%. If the WBC count falls below 4000 cells/mm^3 and the platelet count below 100,000/mm^3, the cytotoxic drugs should be discontinued for 1 week and another WBC count and platelet count should be done. If the WBC count is more than 6000–7000 cells/mm^3 and the platelet count is more than 100,000/mm^3, cytotoxic drug treatment is reinstituted at half the previous dosage. When cyclophosphamide is used, owners must monitor urine color carefully; and if blood is noted the drug is stopped and urinalysis performed to determine the cause of the blood. If sterile hemorrhagic cystitis is present, the drug should be discontinued and azathioprine substituted.

The *alternative therapy* for canine rheumatoid arthritis is palliative; aspirin at a dosage of 25 mg/kg three times a day has been recommended, although it does not slow the progression of the disease. Also, remember that it may take 2–3 weeks for this treatment to produce any effect. One should then try to decrease the dosage as much as possible.

Surgical therapy consists of arthrodesis of the affected joint(s) if after remission the joint is nonfunctional due to pain. Synovectomy is a routine procedure for treatment of human rheumatoid arthritis but has not been reported in veterinary medicine.

The prognosis for canine rheumatoid arthritis is guarded at best, with relapse occurring commonly.

Nonerosive Arthritides. *Idiopathic nondeforming inflammatory arthritis* is by far the most common disorder of dogs manifesting immune-mediated arthritis. As the name indicates, radiographic abnormalities are usually absent from this disease, and no primary cause can be identified such as systemic lupus erythematosus. Diagnosis is suspected by the clinical signs including generalized stiffness, cyclic fever, lameness, and anorexia. The syndrome is usually seen in multiple joints including and distal to the elbow and stifle. Joint taps reveal synovial fluid that produces increased cell counts, with the predominant cells being nontoxic neutrophils. The fluid is sterile for all infectious agents.

Glucocorticoids are most often used to begin *standard therapy* for this disease. However, some authors believe that these agents are inferior to a combination of glucocorticoids with a cytotoxic drug such as cyclophosphamide or azathioprine. Initially, prednisone or prednisolone is used at a dosage of 1.5 mg/kg for dogs weighing more than 15 kg and 2.0 mg/kg for dogs less than 15 kg every 12 hours for 2 weeks. The clinical response and a single joint tap are then reevaluated. If the synovial fluid cell count has dropped to the range of 1000 cells/mm^3 and most of the cells are now mononuclear, the glucocorticoid therapy is likely to be effective by itself. It is then a matter of decreasing the steroid dosage down to a maximum of 1.0 mg/kg every other day while maintaining remission. If this dosage decrease is not possible or if no substantial improvement is seen at the 2-week recheck, the addition of azathioprine or 6-mercaptopurine is advisable. The dosage regimen and patient monitoring are the same as described for rheumatoid arthritis.

Physical therapy should include passive flexion and extension of the affected joint three or four times a day for 30–40 repetitions, swimming if possible, and controlled exercise, which should be limited to short leash walks until remission is obtained.

The prognosis for remission is good, although many (about 25–50%) of the patients have recurrences after drug therapy is stopped.

The standard treatment for *systemic lupus erythematosus* is identical to that mentioned for idiopathic polyarthritis. See Chapter 5 for further details. The prognosis is guarded to fair for initial remission of the polyarthropathy; however, the disease process itself carries a guarded to poor prognosis, as there is no known cure and most animals eventually succumb to one of the many complications.

Drug-induced arthritides have been well documented to occasionally cause many signs including polyarthropathies. Trimethoprim-sulfa therapy in Doberman pinschers is the best known of these reactions. Golden retrievers are also reported to have the same reaction on occasion.

Discontinue the offending agent and restrict exercise for 2–3 weeks. The prognosis is excellent following removal of the offending drug.

BONE DISEASES

Metabolic Bone Diseases

Hypertrophic Osteodystrophy. Hypertrophic osteodystrophy is a developmental skeletal disease of unknown etiology. It primarily affects young, rapidly growing large and giant breed dogs. It involves most commonly the metaphyseal regions of the long bones distal to the elbow and stifle, causing warm and often painful swellings of the affected metaphyseal regions. The clinical presentation of this disease can vary tremendously from intermittent lameness to recumbency, anorexia, and dehydration.

Standard Therapy. The treatment of this syndrome is not uniform owing to the lack of knowledge about the inciting cause. In many cases, especially the milder ones, the disease is self-limiting, and treatment probably does not affect the outcome at all. In more severely affected patients, supportive therapy is essential. Treatment varies with the severity of the case but should be centered around three areas.

1. Nutritional imbalances (i.e., eliminate overfeeding, high protein diets, vitamin or mineral supplements)
2. Analgesics (buffered aspirin at 15–20 mg/kg given two to three times a day) to moderate the pain and prevent constant recumbency and its associated problems
3. Supportive care, which may include parenteral fluids (lactated Ringer's at 2.2 ml/kg/hr IV over a 24-hour period), forced feeding (total daily caloric needs divided into three or four meals), and extensive nursing care to prevent decubital ulcers

This disease is episodic in nature and usually bilaterally symmetric in affliction. The signs usually recede within a week, but multiple reccurrences at 1- to 6-week intervals are not uncommon. Those dogs experiencing multiple bouts of clinical signs are usually the ones that have prolonged recumbency, anorexia, and fever. It is these patients for which close careful monitoring of calorie intake, hydration status, and secondary decubital problems is mandatory. Furthermore, all cases in which there is involvement of the radius and ulna there should be follow-up radiographs along with careful, frequent physical examination of the legs to detect any bony bridging of growth plates and premature closure of the limb with subsequent angular limb deformity (i.e., radius curvus). In these severe cases, steroids (prednisone at 0.5–1.0 mg/kg divided into two daily doses) may be beneficial.

Although hypertrophic osteodystrophy is usually a self-limiting disease, the prognosis varies with the severity of each case. Although uncommon, death has been reported with this disease. When hypertrophic osteodystrophy affects the bones of the antebrachium (radius and ulna), another sequela that can affect the prognosis is secondary bridging or trauma to the growth plates with subsequent angular limb deformities.

Panosteitis. Panosteitis is a common cause of lameness in the young, fast growing dog. It is a spontaneously occurring disease of the long bones, usually seen in large breed dogs, especially the German shepherd. The most prominent clinical sign is lameness in a limb that may occur acutely and persist for 4–6 weeks. The dog may show a shifting leg-lameness due to multiple limb involvement. The cause is unknown. The diagnostic hallmarks are pain on palpation directly over the affected long bone and radiographic changes within the medullary canal that vary with the stage of the disease. These radiographic abnormalities most commonly involve an increased intramedullary opacity of the diaphyseal region of the bone.

Standard Therapy. The treatment for panosteitis is nonspecific and symptomatic in nature. The disease is a self-limiting process that may last up to 6–10 weeks for each affected long bone. However, the dog can be lame for several months if the other long bones of the limb are affected at different times and each elicits separate clinical signs.

Restricted exercise and buffered aspirin at 15–20 mg/kg two to three times a day as necessary to help alleviate pain are recommended. Complete resolution of signs with aspirin therapy cannot always be expected. Mineral and vitamin supplements are contraindicated.

Panosteitis is a self-limiting disease that may take 2–10 months to resolve depending on the number of bones that become clinically affected. There is no residual lameness from the disease. Occasionally, a dog may continue with clinical signs for more than a year.

Secondary Hyperparathyroidism. Secondary hyperparathyroidism is a complication of either chronic renal failure or a disturbance of mineral homeostasis induced by nutritional imbalances (diets low in calcium and excessive in phosphorus). For different reasons both syndromes cause excessive or increased secretion of parathyroid hormone. The common sequelae of both diseases are increased osteoclastic resorption and bone remodeling resulting in release of stored calcium from bone. As a result clinical signs vary from lameness due to pain to pathologic fractures of the skeleton.

Renal Hyperparathyroidism. The treatment aim is to manage the renal disease (see Chapter 11). Specific supportive care and exercise restrictions vary greatly depending on the skeletal components affected in each case.

Nutritional Hyperparathyroidism. Occasionally, an animal is presented with multiple pathologic fractures secondary to an exclusively meat diet. In such cases the diet must be replaced with a balanced commercial diet. Supplementation with calcium gluconate (or lactate or carbonate) to achieve a 2:1 calcium/phosphorous ratio only during the healing phase in severely affected animals may be advisable but is *not mandatory*. Do not continue the supplementation beyond the time of healing of the fractures. The calcium/phosphorous ratio should then be decreased to 1.2:1.0, which is the ratio found in most good quality commercial foods. The exercise and physical therapy prescribed are highly variable and depend on the clinical condition of each patient. Moderate controlled loading to the skeleton through limited exercise supplies positive physiologic stimulus to bone formation and remodeling.

Diet-Induced Hypercalcemia. Many breeders and owners of large breed dogs do not heed warnings regarding supplementation of calcium and phosphorus above and beyond what is in a good balanced diet and thus create skeletal problems in their animals. Although this practice has long been attributed to several problems, scientific data have been limited. One study produced skeletal changes that included osteochondrosis, retained cartilage cores, radius curvus syndrome, and stunted growth by inducing hypercalcemia with the diet.

Standard Therapy. The oversupplemented diet should be replaced by a balanced diet at levels that do not push the dog but allow growth at a slower rate. Just as important is client education regarding the possible detrimental effects of nutritionally pushing the dog to be as large as possible as fast as possible. The bottom line to emphasize to the client is that no supplementation is necessary if the dog is on a good quality national commercial diet produced by a reputable manufacturer. In some cases fractures are present and must be reduced and stabilized at the same time medical management is instituted.

Infections of Bone

Osteomyelitis, although correctly defined as an inflammatory event of bone, can be due to numerous causes including infectious agents, radiation, implants, and a variety of other irritants. In clinical practice, osteomyelitis is usually caused by bacterial infection. Even though bacteria are involved, osteomyelitis can be more correctly thought of as primarily a disease of ischemia with subsequent bacterial colonization. For practical purposes, infections of osseous tissue can be placed in two categories: diskospondylitis and primary osteomyelitis.

Diskospondylitis. Diskospondylitis is defined as a concurrent intervertebral disk infection and vertebral osteomyelitis of contiguous vertebrae. Although clinical signs are somewhat dependent on the location of the lesion, back pain with an abnormal gait and reluctance to ambulate are common presenting signs. Neurologic abnormalities may or may not be present depending on lesion location and severity. The diagnosis is made from the patient history, physical examination, and radiographic findings of a lesion.

Standard Therapy. When discussing treatment in the individual patient, there are a number of clinical aspects that need to be considered. Most important is the neurologic status of the animal. If the dog has minimal to no neurologic dysfunction, treatment with the appropriate antimicrobial agent is usually sufficient to treat the infection. If, however, the dog shows moderate dysfunction including ataxia, paresis, and some motor dysfunction, initial treatment consideration should center around aggressive parenteral antibiotic therapy, with the owner aware that treatment, in rare instances, may include relieving the extradural cord compression with surgical decompression.

If the dog has complete paralysis, the owner must be strongly advised that if intensive parenteral antibiotic therapy is not dramatically successful within 24–48 hours decompression of the cord and stabilization of the vertebral column may be necessary. As stated previously, surgical intervention regardless of presenting clinical signs, is rarely necessary so long as medical management is immediate and aggressive. When considering surgery, it is necessary to consider the number and accessibility of the vertebral lesions. If there are multiple lesions, one may still recommend surgery but only if a myelogram is performed first to identify compressed areas. If one disk space and associated vertebral bodies are causing all compression, and the neurologic signs from physical examination support the myelographic findings, surgery can be recommended. However, if multiple lesions are causing compression, surgical intervention, including decompression, may not be feasible or advisable *unless* the goal of surgery is only to obtain a direct bone biopsy for microbiologic culture and sensitivity.

Other major considerations when treating diskospondylitis are the best antibiotic for systemic treatment and the most appropriate route of administration. Ideally, treatment is based on culture results from blood, urine, or optimally bone; however, during the initial phase when cultures are still pending, one must empirically choose an antimicrobial agent and route of administration. It should be initially assumed that the offending bacteria are a staphylococcal species that produces penicillinase, rendering penicillin, amoxicillin, and ampicillin useless. Use of a bactericidal, penicillinase-resistant agent that is primarily effective against gram-positive organisms is preferred. Several drugs fit these criteria (Table 12-2):

1. Semisynthetic penicillins (parenteral and oral):
   Oxacillin (Bactocil, Beecham) 22 mg/kg q6–8h
   Cloxacillin (Cloxapen, Beecham) 11 mg/kg q8–12h
2. First-generation cephalosporins
   Parenteral: Cefazolin (Kefzol, Lilly; Ancef, Smith Kline & French), cephalothin (Keflin, Lilly), or cefazolin 22 mg/kg q6–8h
   Oral: cephradine (Velosef, Squibb) or cephalexin (Keflex, Dista) 22 mg/kg q8h
3. Clindamycin (Cleocin, Upjohn; Antirobe, Upjohn) 11 mg/kg q8h IV or q12h PO

The next decision is route of administration. The clinical presentation and progression of the disease should dictate the route. For instance, an acute and rapidly progressive case or a case of severe neurologic dysfunction regardless of length of onset, requires intravenous administration of antibiotics for 2–5 days, followed by oral administration. In a more slowly progressive situation, a single loading dose of antibiotics administered intravenously, intramuscularly,

TABLE 12-2. Select Groups of Antimicrobial Agents Commonly Used for Orthopedic Infections in Dogs and Cats.

Generic Drug	Trade Name	Dose (mg/kg)	Route	Interval (hr)
Amoxicillin-clavulanate	Clavamox	22	PO	8
Cefadroxil	Cefa Tabs	22	PO	8–12
Cefazolin	Ancef, Kefzol	22	IV, IM, SC	6–8
Cephalexin	Keflex	22–30	PO	8
Cephalothin	Keflin	22–30	IV, IM, SC	6–8
Cephapirin	Cefadyl	22	IV, IM, SC	6–8
Cephradine	Velosef	22	IV, IM, SC, PO	6–8
Ciprofloxacin	Cipro	11	PO	12
Clindamycin	Cleocin, Antirobe	11	IV, IM, PO	8 12
Cloxacillin	Cloxapen	10–15	IV, IM, PO	6–8
Enrofloxacin	Baytril	5–11	SC, PO	12
Oxacillin	Bactocil	22	IV, IM, SC, PO	6–8

or subcutaneously may be followed by oral treatment. Length of treatment is a minimum of 4–6 weeks regardless of a favorable patient response during the first week or so. If *Brucella canis* titers come back positive, switching to tetracycline therapy is advisable (see Chapter 15). If the *Brucella*-positive dog is an intact male, castration is a must.

One should begin to see improvement within 5–7 days after initiation of therapy. Cultures should be back within this initial time frame; if no response has been achieved and cultures of blood and urine are negative, one may consider surgical curettage of the lesion to obtain a direct bone culture. The patient should be closely monitored over the first few days and then be evaluated at 2-week intervals once the therapy begins to show signs of success. Radiographs have been recommended for every 2 weeks, but they are often difficult to interpret. Therefore, I recommend radiographic evaluation 3 weeks after initiation of treatment and following cessation of therapy. However, remember that the clinical signs usually resolve well before radiographic improvement. Thus radiographs may be of more benefit to document cases of aggressive infections that are not responsive to treatment. Finally, confinement and exercise restriction are necessary in all cases for the length of antibiotic treatment.

The prognosis is largely dependent on the degree of pretreatment neurologic involvement in each animal. Dogs with minimal to no neurologic dysfunction have a good prognosis, whereas cases with severe neurologic dysfunction have a fair to guarded prognosis.

Osteomyelitis. Osteomyelitis, as stated previously, is a disease of ischemia with concurrent bacterial colonization. In terms of treatment, it is important to consider osteomyelitis in two distinct forms, hematogenous and posttraumatic. Acute hematogenous osteomyelitis is rare in the dog and cat; and it is usually seen in the neonate with septicemia, causing emboli to be lodged in the blood vessels of the metaphyseal region and infection in the physis. Occasionally, this infection progresses to a septic arthritis.

Posttraumatic osteomyelitis, the form most commonly encountered in veterinary surgery, is caused by ischemia (i.e., fracture and/or a surgical event), and direct contamination. Posttraumatic osteomyelitis can be further subdivided into acute and chronic cases.

Standard Therapy. Animals with *acute hematogenous osteomyelitis* are usually septic and have systemic involvement. After evaluation of the systemic problems, it is paramount to detect any joint involvement via joint taps and radiographs. If joints are affected, aggressive management should be undertaken as described previously for infectious arthritis. If no joint involvement can be demonstrated, any fluctuant, warm, or painful area around the affected bone can be used to obtain an aspirate aseptically for culture and sensitivity. If there is an obvious fluctuant area, one should attempt to open and copiously lavage the region with a sterile isotonic solution and then perform any débridement necessary. Systemic intravenous antibiotics should be given for 2–3 days before switching to the oral route. Bactericidal agents that are active against penicillinase-producing staphylococci should be used (Table 12-2). If the infection is severe, the combination of oxacillin or cefazolin at 22 mg/kg and gentamicin at 2.2 mg/kg, both given intravenously every 8 hours, provides broad-spectrum activity until culture results are obtained. Remember, monitoring of urine sediment for casts is recommended during gentamicin administration.

Systemic considerations of sepsis and any joint involvement demand the most amount of time when managing these patients. Radiographs following treatment at 2 weeks can help evaluate progression and response to therapy. Systemic and joint involvement are the best indicators of prognosis. There are few reported studies from which to assess success rates because it is such an uncommon process.

Acute posttraumatic osteomyelitis occurs within a few (2–5) days after the insult and may be difficult to differentiate from soft tissue wound infections. In fact, most wound complications are not osteomyelitis but infections of the soft tissues. Regardless, treatment is similar, and absolute differentiation is not always necessary. It is good to remind all clients of the possibility of the development of osteomyelitis in every case. Treatment should be aggressive and prompt in an effort to prevent these infections from developing into chronic processes. Treatment includes drainage and débridement, use of systemic antimicrobial agents, rigid stabilization, direct bone culture, and a delayed closure of some type.

Drainage and débridement of both soft tissue and bone (e.g., all necrotic tissue or bone, hematoma), should be done. In many cases decompression of the medullary cavity with a drill or trephine should also be performed. Culture and biopsy samples are obtained at this time followed by copious lavage of the area with lactated Ringer's or saline. Additions to the flush, which may include various antibiotics, dilute chlorhexidine (Nolvasan, Fort Dodge), or dilute povidone-iodine (Betadine, Purdue Frederick), is a topic of much controversy, research, and individual bias. A good rule to remember is that these agents are all irritants to some degree and can be cytotoxic. When in doubt, do not use anything in the lavage solution except large amounts of fluids such as lactated Ringer's. Use of closed suction units or simply using open wound management with daily flushing are options to be considered depending on the case and the clinician. Choice of antibiotics is the same as described previously under diskospondylitis, given intravenously or intramuscularly for the first 2–3 days followed by oral therapy for a minimum of 4 weeks with most cases needing 8 weeks.

Patient monitoring must be intense and regular. If patients show a response within 24–72 hours of beginning antimicrobial therapy, they may not require surgical intervention. In all cases radiographs should be obtained 2–3 weeks after intervention and then sequentially as needed. Remember, many of these dogs have fractures that need to be concurrently monitored for healing.

In most cases that respond to therapy, the prognosis is fair to good. Unfortunately, some of these cases progress to chronic osteomyelitis regardless of the therapy instituted.

Unfortunately, *chronic posttraumatic osteomyelitis* is the type of bone infection the veterinary surgeon sees most commonly in practice. Remembering that osteomyelitis is more of a disease of ischemia than anything else, it is obvious that therapy with antibiotics alone is usually not successful. It is because the drugs do not enter the tissue in which they are most needed. Thus without attempting to improve the ischemic, necrotic environment, success with bacterial eradication is minimal. Treatment is based on the fundamental objectives of débridement and removal of bony sequestra, necrotic tissue, and all foreign material, including old implants, if possible. Isolation of the causative organism, removal of deadspace, establishing drainage, and finally rigid stabilization of the bone should be accomplished. It is important to remember that bone heals in the face of infection if it is stable.

Débridement and sequestra removal are vital. All scar tissue, devitalized or necrotic soft tissues (including fat, fascia, muscle), all sinus tracts, and necrotic skin must be removed. It is within this avascular tissue that organisms are harbored away from the antibiotics given to eradicate them. Removing places for bacteria to hide and removing all implants (if the fracture is healed) or implants that are not adding to the stabilization are mandatory. Meticulous eradication of deadspace and removal of unnecessary foreign material (including suture material) and hematomas are key steps in treatment. Drainage can be established by a number of techniques. Closed suction units, saucerization (suturing the skin directly to the soft tissues around the bone), or treating an open wound without suturing the skin to the soft tissues are all viable methods. When using either saucerization or simple open wound management, following the formation of granulation tissue in the defect, one should consider performing a secondary closure. Another option that has been used is the placement of vascularized muscle flaps over the defect after the infection has been controlled.

The particular type of drainage used varies depending on the type, site, and severity of the wound and the temperament of the patient. Copious lavage is performed during and after the débridement phase. Again, as stressed earlier, it is far more important to use large amounts of fluid (liters) than to place additional solutions into the isotonic, sterile lavage fluid (lactated Ringer's).

Fracture stability should then be evaluated. If implants are loose, they must be removed. Intramedullary implants should be removed in favor of plates and screws or external skeletal fixators. It is imperative to have rigid fixation for the fracture to heal and to achieve eradication of the infection. In some cases, implants may have to be removed after clinical union of the bone before the infection is eradicated.

Finally, antibiotic therapy is the last point to consider in treatment. Once again, the choice of antibiotic must be based on culture and sensitivity results. Remember, however, that there is a lack of correlation of clinical response and in vitro sensitivity of some microorganisms. These failures can in part be attributed to the inability of the antibiotic to achieve sufficient concentrations in the affected tissue. With these limitations in mind, the best chance to reach and maintain levels at consistent concentrations would be intravenous infusions over the treatment period of a minimum of 4–6 weeks. Unfortunately, in practice we are usually limited to initial short parenteral regimens followed by administration of oral preparations, which may decrease the chance for success. Antibiotics that fit the criteria previously discussed for penicillinase-producing staphylococci that can be used successfully in this oral long-term mode include oxacillin (Bactocil, Beecham) 22 mg/kg q8h, clindamycin (Antirobe, Upjohn) 11 mg/kg q12h, cephalexin (Keflex, Astra) 22 mg/kg q8h, cephradine (Velosef) 22 mg/kg q8h, and ciprofloxacin (Cipro, Miles) 10 mg/kg q12h (Table 12-2).

It must also be noted that culturing for anaerobic infections is important. The difficulty in obtaining proper samples and growth is being eliminated with better understanding and laboratory techniques. Remember that clindamycin, penicillins, and second and third generation cephalosporins have activity against many anaerobic bacteria.

Management of the open wound or the suction system is the initial problem to work with in every case. Open wound management and possible secondary delayed closure may take 1–3 weeks or longer. Suction units are usually maintained for 1–2 weeks. Once this early phase is finished, rechecks weekly and radiographs at 3-week intervals are advised but may vary. Antibiotics must be continued for the 4- to 6-week period regardless of any early positive response.

Successful management is reasonably common in these cases, but multiple surgeries may be required. Also, wound management and close observation are vital in each animal. The owners must be reminded that chronic osteomyelitis can remain quiescent for weeks, months, or years; and one must be careful about using the word "cure" in these cases.

Investigational Therapy. Chronic osteomyelitis is a much more severe problem in human medicine and has sparked a number of ideas for the treatment of refractory cases of this disease. Presently, a large amount of effort has been placed on attempting to improve the ischemic environment with hyperbaric oxygen and to increase the direct application of the antibiotics to the affected region. Antibiotic-impregnated bone cement, beads, and direct infusion into the bone with implantable pumps are being tried. Presently, however, many of these procedures are not applicable to animals primarily because of expense.

DISEASES OF MUSCLE

Primary skeletal muscle disorders, once differentiated from primary neurologic or neuromuscular disorders, can be categorized as either inflammatory or noninflammatory.

Inflammatory Myopathies (Myositis)

The inflammatory myopathies are characterized by weakness, muscle pain, intermittent pyrexia, high serum muscle enzyme values, and muscle biopsy evidence of inflammation. Inflammatory myopathies can be categorized as infectious and noninfectious.

Infectious Myopathies. Inflammatory infectious myositis can be caused by bacteria, protozoa, and some parasites. The presenting myositis can be localized or generalized. The vast majority of these infections are polysystemic, with muscular complications as a part of the entire disease process.

Toxoplasmosis. Toxoplasmosis is a systemic infection that shows muscular signs of a progressive, nonpainful weakness with muscle atrophy. Concurrent central nervous signs often occur.

Standard therapy is as follows (see also Chapter 16). When approaching a case of infectious myositis caused by *Toxoplasma*, the owner must be fully informed of the protracted treatment and supportive care that will be necessary to allow for any improvement. It is not a disease process that improves dramatically within the first few days of treatment in general. Therapy begins with clindamycin 25 mg/kg divided into three equal doses per day. Initially, treatment should be parenteral and then switched to oral. Therapy should be continued for a minimum of 6–8 weeks.

Supportive nursing care is equally important in these cases because of the protracted time frame for the resolution of clinical signs. With severe cases the patient may need constant nursing care, which may include feeding either through a pharyngostomy or gastrostomy tube, intravenous fluid therapy, and so on. One of the biggest problems that needs to be addressed is basic patient management in relation to daily needs. Procedures such as turning a recumbent animal every 2–4 hours, supplying proper bedding support to prevent or diminish decubital ulcer formation, and some system to prevent fecal and urine scalding and contamination is required. This patient cannot be managed unattended in a standard cage all day waiting for its next clindamycin treatment. For further information on toxoplasmosis treatment, see Chapter 16.

The prognosis is guarded to grave. It depends more on the presence of other systemic complications, such as central nervous system involvement or immunosuppression, than on the muscle disease itself.

Non-infectious Myopathies. *Idiopathic Inflammatory Polymyositis.* Idiopathic polymyositis has been recognized, and various clinical syndromes have been described. Affected dogs usually have stiffness and gait abnormalities. They may also have some component of masticatory muscle involvement, but the immunologic mechanism is different than for dogs with masticatory muscle myositis. Dogs with idiopathic inflammatory polymyositis do not have difficulty opening or closing their mouths.

Standard Therapy. When treating these animals, one must remember that the disease is immune-mediated. The owner must be aware that these patients require long-term therapy, and recurrences are possible. Glucocorticoids, specifically prednisone or prednisolone at a dosage of 1.0–1.5 mg/kg q12h, are the cornerstone of the initial treatment. This therapy should be maintained for 3–4 weeks as one monitors for improvement in the dog's clinical condition. Creatine phosphokinase (CPK) levels should be monitored during the initial treatment, which can help in revising the steroid regimen. The goal of treatment is to reduce the frequency of steroid treatment to every other day or every third day. In some dogs it is possible to stop glucocorticoid treatment after a long initial therapy period. If treatment is unsuccessful, the addition of azathioprine and a compensatory decrease in steroid therapy can be implemented (for dosages and monitoring see the section on rheumatoid arthritis in this chapter).

The objective of treatment should be to control rather than to cure the disease. Recurrence of signs periodically is not unexpected, at which point steroid treatment should be reinstituted. The glucocorticoids should again start at 1.0–1.5 mg/kg q12h, but the dose usually can be decreased at a faster pace than during the initial treatment. The response to appropriate therapy is usually favorable, and a fair to good prognosis for remission is warranted.

Masticatory Muscle Myositis. Disorders of the muscles involved in mastication are far more common than idiopathic polymyositis. This process is an inflammatory myopathy that selectively involves the muscles of mastication. Clinically, the dogs present with either swelling or atrophy of the masticatory muscles, which can be manifested as difficulty opening or closing the mouth, respectively.

In early stages of the disease, aggressive immunosuppressive therapy with prednisone at 1.0–1.5 mg/kg PO q12h is usually effective. Response to treatment is seen clinically as improvement in jaw mobility and chemically with decreases in CPK levels. Both of these parameters should be monitored throughout treatment; and if the animal is responding after 3 weeks or so, an effort should be made to begin to decrease the steroid dose. The goal, as for all the immune-mediated diseases, is to administer steroids, at most, every other day. In some dogs, complete removal from the drugs may be possible. However, remember that recurrences of the disease are common. Clinical improvement can be expected in more chronic cases, yet there may be some residual dysfunction of the jaw. If steroid therapy is not successful, addition of azathioprine may be considered as described in the section on rheumatoid arthritis.

Although some have recommended anesthesia and manually opening the mouth as part of the therapy, these procedures are not without risk; and with proper steroid therapy they have been found not to be necessary. These dogs have a fair to good prognosis if the owner understands that the above treatment will not result in a cure but rather control of the disease.

Familial Canine Dermatomyositis. This syndrome has been identified in collies and shetland sheepdogs. The cause of canine dermatomyositis is unknown. Signs of muscle disease follow the onset of skin lesions; and although generalized muscle involvement can occur, the temporalis muscle seems to be the most affected. Thus clinical signs are characterized by prehension difficulties and dysphagia.

The variation of severity of the disease among different dogs and the cyclic progression of the disease and its self-limiting nature make assessment of therapy difficult. Affected young dogs may improve without any therapy. Dermatitis may be in part caused by any cutaneous trauma, so every effort should be made to prevent injury to the skin. Affected dogs should be housed away from littermates and not on hard surfaces. Baths with hypoallergenic shampoos have been found to be beneficial (see Chapter 3). When therapy is initiated, prednisone at a dosage of 1–2 mg/kg PO q12h should be used for induction. This dosage should then be tapered slowly, with a goal of every other day treatment. Just as important is to treat the secondary staphylococcal skin infection often present in these patients. Systemic antibiotics and antimicrobial baths should be used to treat the staphylococcal pyodermas (see Chapter 3). These dogs have a fair prognosis.

Noninflammatory Myopathies

The noninflammatory myopathies primarily cause degenerative muscle disease, which can present with weakness, muscle atrophy, high serum muscle enzyme values, and biopsy evidence of degeneration.

Muscular Dystrophies. Muscular dystrophy is defined as a group of primary myopathies that are genetically determined (inherited) and characterized by progressive degeneration of skeletal muscle. Unfortunately, little is known about any of these disorders in animals, and consequently little advice regarding treatment can be offered for these patients. The following represent some of the identified disorders in dogs.

Muscular Dystrophy in Golden Retrievers. There is no known effective therapy, and prognosis is poor for these dogs.

Hereditary Myopathy of Labrador Retrievers. Diazepam (Valium, Roche) 10 mg q12h has been reported to help in some cases. To reduce the likelihood of exacerbations, do not expose affected dogs to cold weather. Clinical signs seem to stabilize between 6 months and 1 year of age. Owners should avoid stressing these animals. The life-span does not appear to be directly affected by the condition; but if megaesophagus is present, the prognosis is far more guarded.

Congenital Myotonia in the Chow Chow. There is no known effective therapy. Efforts have been made to use drugs that stabilize muscle cell membranes, e.g., procainamide, quinidine, and phenytoin. Dogs should not have extended periods of exercise. The prognosis is poor for recovery; however, it is usually not a progressive disorder.

Sex-Linked Myopathy of Irish Terriers. There is no known treatment, and the prognosis is poor because the disease is progressive.

Metabolic Myopathies. *Hypokalemic Polymyopathy in Cats.* An idiopathic polymyopathy has been documented in cats. The disorder has been linked to severe hypokalemia and potassium depletion. This syndrome is now thought to be a relatively common cause of generalized muscle weakness in cats. The most common clinical sign is ventroflexion of the neck. Other signs include reluctance to walk, sudden fatigue, and a stiff and stilted gait.

Treatment (also see Chapter 1) consists of parenteral administration of potassium either as potassium chloride diluted in a balanced electrolyte solution or orally as potassium-containing elixirs. In severely affected cats, KCl at a dosage of 0.4 mEq/kg/hr in lactated Ringer's solution has been successful. However, infusions of highly concentrated potassium solutions may induce lethal cardiac arrhythmias, and so they should always be administered via a constant-rate infusion pump. Serum potassium concentrations should be monitored every 3–6 hours and the infusion rate slowed once serum potassium concentrations reach 3.5 mEq/L.

Infusion of dopamine at 0.5 μg/kg/min can induce a transient elevation in serum potassium concentration that may be life-saving and avoid some of the inherent risks of concentrated potassium infusion. However, concurrent oral potassium supplementation *must be* started immediately with the dopamine infusion. Oral administration of potassium gluconate elixir (Kaon, Adria Laboratories) can be used and is well tolerated by most cats. For long-term dietary potassium supplementation, a palatable potassium gluconate powder (Tumil-K, Daniels Pharmaceuticals) is available. Oral dosage is empiric; cats with severe hypokalemia (serum potassium < 3.0 mEq/L) are given 5–8 mEq of potassium every day divided into two equal doses. Oral potassium treatment rarely causes hyperkalemia. Instead, rather persistent hypokalemia is the most common problem. Serum potassium concentration should be measured until the concentration has increased to the normal range. Normal concentrations are usually reached within 1–3 days following the initiation of therapy. Response to treatment may be seen within 24 hours of starting therapy. Most cats are significantly improved within 3–4 days, but complete resolution may take weeks.

Once in the normal range, the serum potassium concentration should be monitored weekly and the dose of potassium increased or decreased to maintain serum concentration in the normal range. Most cats require 2–4 mEq of potassium per day to maintain normal serum concentration.

The prognosis for these cats is excellent; however, polymyopathy may recur if diet is not continuously supplemented with potassium. Periodic monitoring of serum potassium concentration is indicated.

Endocrine Myopathies. *Polymyopathy Associated with Canine Hyperadrenocorticism.* A degenerative noninflammatory myopathy, clinically characterized by muscle stiffness, weakness, and concomitant gait abnormalities, has been documented with hyperadrenocorticism. See Chapter 4 for a discussion of the treatment of hyperadrenocorticism. The reversibility of the myopathy is variable. Some animals reach near-normal gaits, whereas others improve somewhat but then plateau.

Myopathies Associated with Canine Hypothyroidism. Myopathies associated with hypothyroidism have been recognized in clinical practice. The cause of such musculoskeletal dysfunction is unclear. Treatment of hypothyroidism is described in Chapter 4.

Prognosis is uncertain. There is little documented information regarding the resolution of muscular signs. The clinical impression is that if improvement is going to occur it will be gradual and seen within 4–6 weeks after the initiation of therapy.

SUGGESTED READINGS

Degenerative Joint Disease

Alexander JW: Aging and the joints. Compend Contin Educ Pract Vet 1984;12: 1074.
Booth NH: Non-narcotic analgesics. In: Jones LM, et al, eds. Veterinary Pharmacology

and Therapeutics, 5th ed. Ames: Iowa State University Press, 1982;297.

Conlon PD: Nonsteroidal drugs used in the treatment of inflammation. Vet Clin North Am (Small Anim) 1988;18:1115.

Davis LE: Clinical pharmacology of salicylates. J Am Vet Med Assoc 1980;176:65.

Osteochondrosis

Egger EL: Development and etiologics of the osteochondrosis-itis syndrome. In: Proceedings 16th Annual Meeting Veterinary Orthopedic Society 1989;18.

Lenehan TM, VanSickel DC: Osteochondrosis. In: Newton CD, Nunamaker DM, eds. Textbook of Small Animal Orthopaedics. Philadelphia: JB Lippincott, 1985:981.

Pedersen NC, Wind A, Morgan JP, et al: Joint diseases of dogs and cats. In: Ettinger SJ, ed. Textbook of Veterinary Internal Medicine, 2nd ed. Philadelphia: WB Saunders, 1989;2348.

Smith MM, Vassuer PB, Morgan JP: Clinical evaluation of dogs after surgical and nonsurgical management of osteochondritis dissecans of the talus. J Am Vet Met Assoc 1985;187:31.

Hip Dysplasia

Braden TD, Prieur WD, Kaneene JB: Clinical evaluation of intertrochanteric osteotomy for treatment of dogs with early-stage hip dysplasia: 37 cases (1980–1987). J Am Vet Med Assoc 1990;196:337.

Lust G, Rendano VT, Summer BA: Canine hip dysplasia: concepts and diagnosis. J Am Vet Med Assoc 1985;6:638.

Olmstead ML: Total hip replacement. Vet Clin North Am (Small Anim) 1987; 4:943.

Riser WH: A half century of canine hip dysplasia. Semin Vet Med Surg (Small Anim) 1987;2:87.

Schrader SC: Triple osteotomy of the pelvis and trochanteric osteotomy as a treatment for hip dysplasia in immature dogs: the surgical technique and results in 77 consecutive operations. J Am Vet Med Assoc 1986;187:659.

Walker TL, Prieur WD: Intertrochanteric femoral osteotomy. Semin Vet Med Surg (Small Anim) 1987;2:117.

Wallace LJ: Canine hip dysplasia: past and present. Semin Vet Med Surg (Small Anim) 1987;2:92.

Infectious Arthritis

Brown SG, Newton CD: Infectious arthritis and wounds of joints. In: Newton CD, Nunamaker DM, eds. Textbook of Small Animal Orthopaedics. Philadelphia: JB Lippincott, 1985:1047.

Noninfectious Inflammatory Arthritis

Giger U, Werner LL, Miiichamp NJ, Gorman NT: Sulfadiazine-induced allergy in six doberman pinschers. J Am Vet Med Assoc 1985;186:479.

Pedersen NC, Wind A. Morgan JP, Pool RR: Joint disease of dogs and cats. In: Ettinger SJ, ed. Textbook of Veterinary Internal Medicine, 2nd ed. Philadelphia: WB Saunders, 1989;2366.

Romatowski J: Comparative therapeutics of canine and human rheumatoid arthritis. J Am Vet Med Assoc 1984;185:558.

Stanton ME, Legendre AM: Effects of cyclophosphamide in dogs and cats. J Am Med Assoc 1986;188:1319.

Hypertrophic Osteodystrophy

Woodward JC: Canine hypertrophic osteodystrophy: a study of the spontaneous disease in littermates. Vet Pathol 1982;199:337.

Secondary Hyperparathyroidism

Hazewinkel HAW, Goedegebuure SA, Poulos PW, Wolvekamp WThC: Influences of chronic calcium excess on the skeletal development of growing Great Danes. J Am Anim Hosp Assoc 1985;21:377.

Kornfield DS: Nutrition in orthopaedics. In: Newton CD, Nunamaker DM, eds. Textbook of Small Animal Orthopedics. Philadelphia: JB Lippincott, 1985;655.

Diskospondylitis

Betts CW: Osteomyelitis of the vertebral body and the intervertebral disk: diskospondylitis. In: Newton CD, Nunamaker DM, eds. Textbook of Small Animal Orthopaedics, 1st ed. Philadelphia: JB Lippincott, 1985:725.

Kornegay JN: Diskospondylitis. In: Kirk R, ed. Current Therapy IX. Philadelphia: WB Saunders, 1988;810.

Turnwald GH, Shires PK, Turk MA et al: Diskospondylitis in a kennel of dogs: clinicopathologic findings. J Am Vet Med Assoc 1986;2:178.

Osteomyelitis

Braden TD, Johnson CA, Wakenell P, et al: Efficacy of clindamycin in the treatment of Staphylococcus aureus osteomyelitis in dogs. J Am Vet Med Assoc 1988;12:1721.

Caywood DD: Osteomyelitis. Vet Clin North Am 1983;1:47.

Daly WR: Orthopedic infections. In: Slatter DH, ed. Textbook of Small Animal Surgery, 1st ed. Philadelphia: WB Saunders, 1985;2020.

Nunamaker DM: Osteomyelitis. In: Newton CD, Nunamaker DM, eds. Textbook of Small Animal Orthopedics, 1st ed. Philadelphia: JB Lippincott, 1985;499.

Parker RB: Treatment of post-traumatic osteomyelitis. Vet Clin North Am (Small Anim) 1987;17:841.

Waldvogel FA, Vasy H. Osteomyelitis: the past decade. N Engl J Med 1980;303:360.

Walker RD, Richardson DC, Bryant MJ, et al: Anaerobic bacteria associated with osteomyelitis in domestic animals. J Am Vet Med Assoc 1983;182:814.

Inflammatory Myopathies

Greene CE, Cook JR, Mahaffey EA: Clindamycin for treatment of Toxoplasma polymyositis in a dog. J Am Vet Med Assoc 1985;187:631.

Haupt KH, Hargis AM: Familial dermatomyositis. In: Kirk RW, ed. Current Veterinary Therapy X. Philadelphia: WB Saunders, 1989;606.

Kornegay JN, Gorgacz EJ, Dawe DL, et al: Polymyositis in dogs. J Am Vet Assoc 1980; 176:431.

Shelton GD, Cardinet GH: Pathophysiologic basis of canine muscle disorders. J Vet Intern Med 1987;1:36.

Shelton GD, Cardinet GH: Canine masticatory muscle disorders. In: Kirk RW, ed. Current Veterinary Therapy X. Philadelphia: WB Saunders, 1989:816.

Muscular Dystrophies

Kornegay JN, Tuler SM, Miller DM, Levesque DC: Muscular dystrophy in a litter of golden retriever dogs. Muscle Nerve 1988;11:1056.

McKerrell RE, Braund KG: Hereditary myopathy of Labrador retrievers. In: Kirk RW, ed. Current Veterinary Therapy X. Philadelphia: WB Saunders, 1989;820.

Shelton GD, Cardinet GH. Pathophysiologic basis of canine muscle disorders. J Vet Intern Med 1987;1:36.

Hypokalemic Polymyopathy in Cats

Dow SW, LeCouteur RA: Hypokalemic polymyopathy of cats. In: Kirk RW, ed. Current Veterinary Therapy X. Philadelphia: WB Saunders, 1989;812.

Dow SW, LeCouteur RA, Fettman MJ, Spurgeon TL: Potassium depletion in cats: hypokalemic polymyopathy. J Am Vet Med Assoc 1987;191:1563.

Metabolic Myopathies

Feldman EC: Adrenal gland disease. In: Ettinger SJ, ed. Textbook of Veterinary Internal Medicine. Philadelphia: WB Saunders, 1989;1721.

Greene CE, Lorenz MD, Munnell JF, et al: Myopathy associated with hyperadrenocorticism in the dog. JAMA 1979;174:1310.

Peterson ME, Ferguson DC: Thyroid diseases. In: Ettinger SJ, ed. Textbook of Veterinary Internal Medicine. Philadelphia: WB Saunders, 1989;1642.

CHAPTER THIRTEEN

Neurologic Disorders

John E. Oliver

Primary neurologic disorders that require medical treatment include trauma, infections, and seizures. The nervous system is affected in many systemic disorders including infectious diseases, endocrine abnormalities, immune-mediated reactions, and neoplasia. Most of these conditions are discussed in other chapters.

CENTRAL NERVOUS SYSTEM TRAUMA

Traumatic injury to the central nervous system (CNS) is often life-threatening, especially in the case of brain or cervical spinal cord trauma. Even if the animal survives, consequences of injury may be incompatible with normal function. Assessment of the location and severity of injury is discussed in several sources. Surgery may be indicated for some injuries, especially compressive spinal cord injury. This discussion is limited to management of the early effects of trauma to the nervous system.

Trauma to nervous tissue causes hemorrhage and edema. If hemorrhage is sufficient to cause a space-occupying mass, surgical decompression is indicated; otherwise there is no specific treatment for hemorrhage. Edema is the most common reaction of the CNS to any injury. It is increased if hypoxia or hypercarbia occurs. Brain injury is often accompanied by decreased respiration, enhancing the probability of severe edema. The brain is in an enclosed compartment, so any increase of the intracranial contents causes severe compression and distortion of the brain. If the mass effect is sufficient, the brain herniates through the tentorium cerebelli and foramen magnum. It is imperative that herniations are prevented. Once they occur, treatment is often ineffective, and the animal frequently dies. The spinal cord reacts like the brain. Considerable research on medical treatment of spinal cord injury probably applies to brain injury as well.

Standard Therapy

Brain Injury. An animal with severe head injury causing stupor or coma is a medical emergency. The priorities for management on presentation of the animal to the veterinary clinic are 1) maintenance of adequate ventilation by endotracheal catheter or tracheostomy if necessary and 2) treatment of shock (see Chapter 17). An intravenous catheter should be established, and lactated Ringer's solution should be administered to maintain a route for other medications. The rate of administration and amount of fluid are dictated by the condition of the animal. The objective is to maintain normal fluid balance without overhydrating the animal. Intravenous corticosteroids (methylprednisolone sodium succinate, Solu-Medrol, Upjohn, 30 mg/kg) usually are given for shock and are probably beneficial in the reduction and prevention of traumatic cerebral edema. The efficacy of corticosteroids in trauma-induced edema has been questioned. Other studies, however, have provided objective evidence of reduced intracranial pressure with high doses. Studies on spinal cord trauma indicate that high dose corticosteroid therapy during the first day of injury have significant benefit. The two key factors appear to be adequate dose and early administration. The soluble steroids, such as methylprednisolone sodium succinate, are essential to the early therapy. They must be given as early as possible, preferably during the first hour after injury. Within 6 hours of injury there is neuronal and axonal loss that is irreversible. Mannitol (0.25–1.00 g/kg) should be given intravenously if the patient is comatose but not if the patient is hypovolemic.

The extent of the injury must be determined quickly. Cardiopulmonary function, internal hemorrhage, and fractures of the limbs or the spinal column should be evaluated. The nervous system is then examined as has been described elsewhere. Evaluations of the level of consciousness, pupillary function and eye movements, dysfunction of other cranial nerves, and motor function are adequate for assessing the level and extent of the damage to the CNS.

After the patient is stabilized, frequent monitoring of the severity of signs is imperative. A coma scale is useful for comparison between examinations. Radiography should be performed on the patient with minimal deficits (alert or depressed) in order to detect skull fractures, and the animal should be observed closely for 24–48 hours for signs of progression. Depressed skull fractures in conscious patients are elevated surgically when the animal is stable. Animals with linear fractures do not need surgery unless progressive signs indicate continuing intracranial hemorrhage. Open fractures are débrided and closed as early as possible.

Stuporous or comatose patients require more critical assessment and care and have a poorer prognosis. Brain stem hemorrhage usually can be differentiated from tentorial herniation from the time course of the neurologic signs. Intramedullary brain stem hemorrhage, which usually occurs in the midbrain or the pons, produces coma immediately after the trauma, and there is little or no improvement in this case. Tentorial herniation may develop from cerebral edema (usually bilateral) or from rostrotentorial hemorrhage (epidural or subdural). The progression of signs is usually characteristic. Animals with brain stem hemorrhage rarely recover, and those that do usually have severe neurologic deficits. Tentorial herniation must be managed early in order for the treatment to be successful. Severe tentorial herniation with compression and distortion of the brain stem produces secondary brain hemorrhages that are irreversible. In addition, increased pressure transmitted to the caudotentorial compartment produces cerebellar herniation through the foramen magnum, causing death by interference with the medullary respiratory centers and their descending pathways.

Brain stem hemorrhage is treated as was outlined previously: corticosteroids, mannitol, ventilation, and nursing care. The initial management of tentorial herniation involves the same procedures. If the signs do not improve or if progression is observed during the first few hours, craniotomy for evacuation of the hematoma and relief of intracranial pressure is indicated.

Management of the comatose patient must include maintaining hydration and nutrition; regulating body temperature; providing adequate ventilation (including hyperventilation in the early stages, see Chapter 17); preventing decubital ulcers by frequent turning, meticulous cleaning of the skin, and cushioning with sponge rubber or fleece pads; and maintaining urinary and fecal elimination. Management of the comatose patient can be time-consuming and expensive but is rewarding when successful.

Spinal Cord Injury. Medical management of spinal cord injury is the same as that for brain injury, except that consciousness is not a problem. Respiration is usually normal unless the cervical spinal cord is severely involved. Compression of the spinal cord or instability of the vertebral column are indications for decompressive or stabilizing surgery. The earlier decompression is accomplished, the better are the chances for recovery. The only reason for delay is if other injuries make anesthesia too hazardous. Early administration of methylprednisolone sodium succinate at a dosage of 30 mg/kg is indicated. Continued infusion of methylprednisolone sodium succinate at a rate of 5 mg/kg/hr for the first 24 hours is recommended in humans. Studies in experimental animals generally support this approach. Longer periods of corticosteroid administration may have benefit, but side effects are more likely and significant benefits have not been proved.

After surgical correction of spinal cord injury, physical therapy is initiated as soon as the patient's condition permits. Turning of paralyzed animals every 2–4 hours helps prevent pressure necrosis of the skin. Slings for supporting the animal are useful. Hydrotherapy twice a day, either whirlpool or just a tub of warm water, increases circulation, keeps the skin clean, and promotes movement of the limbs. Passive exercise of the limbs is useful for maintaining muscle function and can be done by the owner once or twice a day.

Side Effects. High dose corticosteroid therapy for spinal injury may have adverse effects on the digestive tract, causing bleeding and ulceration. Based on large studies in humans, using corticosteroids in large doses for only 24 hours avoids these effects. Corticosteroids should not be continued for days, nor is a tapering withdrawal necessary. If corticosteroids are used for longer intervals, cimetidine or sucralfate may be protective (see Chapter 8).

Administration of mannitol causes an osmotic diuresis that can seriously dehydrate the animal and cause electrolyte abnormalities. Replacement fluid therapy is indicated based on an assessment of the serum electrolytes and an estimate of dehydration. Mannitol should not be given if the animal is hypovolemic, as it is potentially lethal.

CNS INFECTIONS

Infectious diseases are discussed in Chapter 16. The CNS is involved in many of the diseases reviewed there. The most common treatable bacterial infection of the CNS is meningitis caused by *Staphylococcus* sp. The primary concerns when treating any CNS infection are 1) using an antimicrobial effective for the agent and 2) providing an adequate level of the drug to the site of infection. Culture and sensitivity tests of cerebrospinal fluid (CSF) are important diagnostic tools for establishing the agent and its sensitivity to drugs. The blood-brain barrier selectively excludes many chemicals from reaching adequate concentrations in the CNS. Choosing an antibiotic that penetrates the CNS is critical for successful treatment.

Standard Therapy

When a diagnosis of bacterial meningitis is made based on positive culture from the CSF, the choice of appropriate antibiotic may be made. Table 13-1 lists the antibiotics with their ability to penetrate the CNS in concentrations adequate for effective treatment. Most of the synthetic penicillin derivatives (e.g., ampicillin, oxacillin) are good choices. Combinations of one of the synthetic penicillins with clavulinic acid may also be effective. Resistant organisms do occur, but they have not been frequent. If the animal is severely affected or the organism is not known, the third generation cephalosporins (moxalactam, cefotaxime) are a better choice because of a broader spectrum of activity and less-resistant organisms. Chloramphenicol has been the antibiotic most frequently used for treating CNS infections in the past, as it penetrates the CNS better than any other antibiotic. However, most of the bacterial infections of the CNS in our hospital have been resistant to chloramphenicol. Moreover, it is bacteriostatic, rather than being bactericidal, another disadvantage. The aminoglycosides are poor choices for CNS infections because of poor penetration, even in inflammation. They may be used in combination with another antibiotic if there is a focus of infection elsewhere.

Diskospondylitis (vertebral osteomyelitis) may cause spinal cord compression and pain. The most frequent causative organism is *Staphylococcus* sp. Blood and urine cultures are frequently useful for identifying the organism. One of

TABLE 13-1. Antimicrobial Drugs: Ability to Penetrate the Blood-Brain Barrier

Good	Intermediate	Poor
Bactericidal		
Trimethoprim	Penicillin G[a]	Penicillin G benzathine
Moxalactam	Ampicillin[a]	Cephalosporins[b]
Cefotaxime	Methicillin[a]	Aminoglycosides
Ceftazidime	Nafcillin[a]	
Metronidazole	Carbenicillin[a]	
	Oxacillin	
Bacteriostatic		
Chloramphenicol	Tetracycline	Amphotericin B[c]
Sulfonamides	Flucytosine	Erythromycin[d]
Isoniazid		
Minocycline[e]		
Doxycycline[e]		
Rifampin		

[a]High intravenous doses are needed to achieve the maximal effect.
[b]First and second generation; may be effective early in bacterial meningitis; concentrations dramatically decrease with repair of the blood-brain barrier.
[c]May be effective in cryptococcal meningitis.
[d]Penetration in the face of inflammation is unpredictable.
[e]Lipid-soluble tetracyclines that achieve higher concentrations in CSF than do other tetracyclines.

the cephalosporins, such as cephalexin or cephradine 20–40 mg/kg q8h, is the first choice for most cases. Treatment should be continued for 6 weeks. If there is no response in 5 days, or if significant neurologic deficits other than pain develop despite treatment, decompressive surgery, curettage of the lesion, and direct culture are indicated. Prognosis is good if pain is the only sign and there is response to therapy. Extensive lysis of the vertebra and poor response to initial therapy indicate a poor prognosis. Pathologic fractures with severe spinal cord compression may result. *Brucella canis* is the causative organism in a small group of these patients. Because of the potential public health implication and the difference in treatment, *Brucella* titers should be obtained in all cases. Treatment of *B. canis* is with tetracycline (22 mg/kg q8h for 4 weeks) and dihydrostreptomycin (5 mg/kg q12h, weeks 1 and 4 of therapy). Minocycline may be more effective but is expensive in large dogs.

OTITIS MEDIA AND OTITIS INTERNA

Infections of the middle and inner ear cause signs of a peripheral vestibular dysfunction. Common findings are head tilt, nystagmus, positional ventral strabismus, and asymmetric ataxia. Postural reactions and other signs of central disease are absent. Noninfectious peripheral vestibular syndromes are common, so therapy should not be used unless there is evidence of infection.

Standard Therapy

The diagnosis is confirmed by otoscopic examination and radiographs of the bulla ossea. When the diagnosis is made during otoscopic examination, the tympanic membrane should be punctured or incised (if it is intact) and a sample of material obtained for culture and sensitivity. A 22 gauge spinal needle can be inserted through the otoscope for sampling. Aspiration may obtain fluid for culture. If not, 0.5 ml of sterile saline is injected and then aspirated. After the sample is obtained, the membrane is incised and the bulla flushed with sterile saline. Low pressure suction is useful for removing the fluid.

Systemic and topical antibiotics are administered based on culture results. Aminoglycoside antibiotics are avoided, especially in the ear canal because of ototoxicity. Therapy is continued for at least 2 weeks. The tympanic membrane usually heals within 7–14 days if the infection is controlled.

Alternative Therapy

Many animals with otitis media and interna have severely infected ear canals. Granulomatous changes may preclude otoscopic examination, and topical therapy is useless. Surgical ablation of the ear canal and ventral or lateral bulla osteotomy are indicated in these cases.

SEIZURES

Epilepsy is a disorder of the brain that is characterized by recurring seizures. Seizures, fits, and convulsions are synonymous terms used to describe the manifestations of abnormal brain function that are characterized by paroxysmal stereotyped alterations in behavior. Seizures can be caused by numerous abnormalities that affect neuronal function of the brain. Seizures with no demonstrable cause require anticonvulsant therapy.

Treatment of seizures is a client decision. If the seizures are frequent or severe, treatment is strongly recommended. The more seizures an animal has, the more likely it is that more will occur. Therefore treatment of infrequent seizures has merit, but the daily administration of medication is difficult for some owners. The client must understand some basic principles of treatment of seizures. Every animal is different in terms of their response to medication, and the dose must be adjusted to the response. One or more drugs may be tried to find the most effective regimen. Medication must be given as scheduled. Severe seizures can result from missed doses. Efficacy may not be judged for

TABLE 13-2. Anticonvulsant Drugs for Dogs and Cats

Drug	Dosage (mg/kg)	Serum Conc. (μg/ml)	Half-life (hours ± SE)	Time to Steady State (days)
Phenobarbital	1.5–5.0 q12h	15–45	70 ± 16	10–18
Potassium bromide	20–60 q24h or divided	1000–1500	25 days	4 months
Diazepam (cats)	0.5–1.0 q12h	200–500 ng/ml	1.5–2.0	
Clonazepam	0.02–0.50 q12h	0.02–0.08	1.4 ± 0.3	
Valproic acid	60 q8h	40–100	1.7 ± 0.4	6–10
Primidone	10–15 q8h	5–15	9–12	6–8
Metabolites				
PEMA		4–20	10–16	
Phenobarbital		15–45	70 ± 16	10–18
Anticonvulsants not recommended				
Phenytoin	35 q8h	10	4.4 ± 0.78	0.5–1.0
Carbamazepine		5–12 (human)	1.1–1.9	4–12 hours

some time, usually several weeks, depending on the frequency of seizures and the drug being used. Sudden changes in medication must be avoided. Usually medication must be given for the life of the animal. Finally, the owner must agree that success is reducing the frequency and severity of seizures, as complete control of seizures is unusual.

Standard Therapy

Phenobarbital is the drug of choice for control of seizures in dogs and cats (see Table 13-2 for dosages and serum levels for all anticonvulsants). It should be used first in all cases. The usual starting dose is 1.5–5.0 mg/kg PO twice daily. The lower dose is used if seizures are infrequent and occur as single episodes; the higher dose is used if seizures are frequent or tend to cluster. Dosage is adjusted as needed to prevent seizures and as dictated by side effects, e.g., sedation. Blood levels should be measured when seizure control is inadequate before arbitrarily raising the dose. A level of 15–45 μg/ml is in the therapeutic range. Many dogs need levels near the high end to achieve control. Doses as high as 10–20 mg/kg/day are needed in some dogs to maintain therapeutic blood levels.

Diazepam (Valium, Roche) is also a good choice for control of seizures in cats. It may be used at a dose of 0.2–0.5 mg/kg three times daily.

Primidone is metabolized to phenobarbital and phenylethylmalonic acid (PEMA), and a small amount remains as primidone. It has been estimated that more than 80% of the activity is from the phenobarbital. Primidone is more expensive and potentially more hepatotoxic than phenobarbital; therefore its use is not recommended unless phenobarbital is ineffective. It should not be used in cats.

Phenytoin is an effective drug in humans but has not been effective in dogs and cannot be used in cats.

Alternative Therapy

Animals that cannot be controlled with phenobarbital when serum levels are in the therapeutic range are candidates for combination therapy. Phenobarbital is continued while other drugs are added to the regimen. The choice of alternative drugs is limited, and guidelines are not clearly documented by controlled trials in most cases.

Currently, my first choice for an additional drug is potassium bromide (KBr). KBr was used at the turn of the century for treating seizures in humans but was discontinued because of the efficacy of other drugs and some problems with side effects, especially skin disorders. Chemical grade KBr can be obtained and put into capsules or dissolved in sucrose or water (250 mg/ml), which can be mixed with food. KBr is slow to reach steady state and has a long half-life (Table 13-2). Two to three months are needed for therapeutic effect. It has been recommended that a loading dose of 400–600 mg/kg can be given to achieve adequate therapeutic levels more quickly. It takes up to 4 months to achieve a steady state in the dog. Therapeutic levels are 1.0–1.5 mg/ml. KBr has not been used in cats.

Animals that have frequent or severe seizures and are not controlled with phenobarbital alone are a special problem. Because of the long time required to achieve efficacy with KBr, it may be necessary to do something in the interim. Currently, we give clonazepam (Klonopin, Roche) at a dosage of 0.02 mg/kg twice daily. Clonazepam has a longer half-life than diazepam and may help achieve seizure control. However, it is not recommended for long-term use, as most animals develop seizures, despite medication, within several months. Its use during the time until KBr becomes effective is still being evaluated, but it appears promising.

Valproic acid (Depakene, Abbott) in combination with phenobarbital has been useful in a limited number of cases. The half-life is short, and therapeutic levels are difficult to achieve. Tissue levels in the CNS are reportedly higher than might be expected from the serum levels.

Side Effects

Most of the anticonvulsants produce some sedation, especially when medication is first started. Generally, normal activity returns within a week. Animals that are not having severe or frequent seizures may be started at lower doses and gradually brought into the therapeutic range. Polydipsia and polyphagia may be seen with phenobarbital and primidone. Some animals may have to be monitored for weight gain. Some young animals have a paradoxical hyperactive reaction to phenobarbital. Hepatotoxicity, resulting in chronic hepatic insufficiency, is seen most frequently with primidone. It can occur with phenobarbital but is rare. Liver enzymes are frequently elevated with both drugs. We have had several dogs with hepatotoxicity after several months on clonazepam. Currently we recommend limiting the use of clonazepam to 2 months, primarily while achieving efficacy with KBr.

SUGGESTED READINGS

Central Nervous System Trauma

Bracken MB, Shepard MJ, Collins WF, et al: A randomized, controlled trial of methylprednisolone or naloxone in the treatment of acute spinal-cord injury. N Engl J Med 1990;322:1405.

Griffiths IR: Central nervous system trauma. In: Oliver JE, Hoerlein BF, Mayhew IG, eds. Veterinary Neurology. Philadelphia: WB Saunders, 1987;303.

Hall ED, Braughler IM, McCall JM: Glucocorticoid and nonglucocorticoid steroids: experimental studies on head and spinal cord injuries. In: Capildeo R, ed. Steroids in Diseases of the Central Nervous System. New York: John Wiley & Sons, 1989;125.

Hoerlein BF, Redding RW, Hoff EJ Jr, McGuire JA: Evaluation of naloxone, crocetin, thyrotropin releasing hormone, methylprednisolone, partial myelotomy, and hemilaminectomy in the treatment of acute spinal cord trauma. J Am Anim Hosp Assoc 1985;21:67.

Kornegay JN, Oliver JE Jr, Gorgacz EJ: Clinicopathologic features of brain herniation in animals. J Am Vet Med Assoc 1983;182:1111.

Oliver J: Neurologic examination and the diagnostic plan. In: Oliver JE, Hoerlein BF, Mayhew IG, eds. Veterinary Neurology. Philadelphia: WB Saunders, 1987;7.

Oliver J, Hoerlein B: Cranial surgery. In: Oliver JE, Hoerlein BF, Mayhew IG, eds. Veterinary Neurology. Philadelphia: WB Saunders, 1987;470.

Oliver JE: Coma. In: Lorenz MD, Cornelius LM, eds. Small Animal Medical Diagnosis. Philadelphia: JB Lippincott, 1987:458.

Shores A: Craniocerebral trauma. In: Kirk RW, ed. Current Veterinary Therapy. Philadelphia: WB Saunders, 1989;847.

Toombs J, Collins L, Graves G, et al: Colonic perforation in corticosteroid-treated dogs. JAVMA 1986;188:145.

Central Nervous System Infections

Carmichael LE, Greene CE: Canine brucellosis. In: Greene CE, ed. Infectious Diseases of the Dog and Cat. Philadelphia: WB Saunders, 1990;573.

Greene CE: Principles of medical therapy. In: Oliver JE, Hoerlein BF, Mayhew IG, eds. Veterinary Neurology. Philadelphia: WB Saunders, 1987;393.

Oliver JE: Head tilt. In: Lorenz MD, Cornelius LM, eds. Small Animal Medical Diagnosis. Philadelphia: JB Lippincott, 1987;443.

Oliver JE Jr, Lorenz M: Ataxia of the head and limbs. In: Oliver JE Jr, Lorenz M, eds. Handbook of Veterinary Neurologic Diagnosis. Philadelphia: WB Saunders, 1983;223.

Oliver JE Jr, Lorenz M: Principles of medical treatment of the nervous system. In: Oliver JE Jr, Lorenz M, eds. Handbook of Veterinary Neurologic Diagnosis. Philadelphia: WB Saunders, 1983;122.

Sharp NJH: Chronic otitis externa and otitis media treated by total ear canal ablation and ventral bulla osteotomy in thirteen dogs. Vet Surg 1990;19:162.

Seizures

Bunch SE, Castleman WL, Baldwin BH, et al: Effects of long-term primidone and phenytoin administration on canine hepatic function and morphology. Am J Vet Res 1985;46:105.

Frey H-H: Use of anticonvulsants in small animals. Vet Rec 1986;118:484.

Lane SB, Bunch SE: Medical management of recurrent seizures in dogs and cats. J Vet Intern Med 1990;4:26.

Oliver JE: Collapse (seizures, syncope, and narcolepsy). In: Lorenz MD, Cornelius LM, eds. Small Animal Medical Diagnosis. Philadelphia: JB Lippincott, 1987;448.

Oliver JE Jr: Seizure disorders and narcolepsy. In: Oliver JE Jr, Hoerlein BF, Mayhew IG, eds. Veterinary Neurology. Philadelphia: WB Saunders, 1987;285.

Schwartz-Porsche D: Epidemiological, clinical, and pharmacokinetic studies in spontaneously epileptic dogs and cats. In: Proceedings ACVIM Forum, Washington DC 1986;11:61.

CHAPTER FOURTEEN

External Ophthalmic Diseases and Glaucoma

Victoria W. Pentlarge

THERAPEUTIC FORMULATIONS

Ophthalmic drugs for topical therapy are manufactured in four vehicles: solutions (aqueous, oily, and suspension), ointments, gels, and inserts. The veterinarian's choice of vehicle is based on commercial availability, characteristics of the ophthalmic disease, and capabilities of the owner. At this time, drug-impregnated insoluble inserts and membrane-controlled diffusional systems are not practical because of expense and poor retention by animals. However, drug-soaked hydrophilic soft contact lenses and collagen shields may offer approaches to providing prolonged and high concentrations of the drug in the tear film, cornea, and anterior chamber (see Ulcerative Keratitis). Solutions and ointments are by far the most common vehicles used.

The design of the vehicle considers drug solubility, pH, stability, tonicity, and electrolyte composition. The pH range tolerated by the ocular surface is 3.5–10.5. The tonicity of the formulation needs to be near isotonicity for patient comfort.

Vehicles that increase viscosity or decrease surface tension prolong the drug's corneal contact time, which enhances drug absorption. Liquid and solid oils increase the viscosity of formulations. Oily vehicles include lanolin and liquid fats, whereas ointments are primarily composed of bland petrolatum and lanolin. Wetting agents, such as methylcellulose, polyvinyl alcohol, and other polymeric systems, are liquid vehicles that decrease surface tension. The respective half-lives for corneal contact time are 4, 24, and 50 minutes, respectively, for pure water, solution, and ointment vehicles in the non-inflamed eye. The prolonged corneal contact of ointments may be slightly offset by the ointments' slow release of the drug. To compensate for slow drug release, ointments can be formulated with a higher drug concentration.

Ointment formulations have the following advantages: 1) more stable than other vehicles; 2) longer corneal contact time than solutions; 3) less loss through the nasolacrimal system; 4) less frequent applications required; 5) moisten the ocular surface; 6) soften crusts and discharges; and 7) do not interfere with corneal healing. The disadvantages of using an ointment include: 1) trapping debris in conjunctival fornices; 2) blurred vision (primarily a concern for human patients); 3) difficulty of administration by some owners; 4) higher incidence of contact dermatitis; and 5) intraocular injury if the petrolatum gets inside the eye through a corneal perforation. Oil-based solutions are also toxic to intraocular structures.

Benzalkonium chloride, chlorobutanol, phenols, thimerosal, edetate disodium, and substituted alcohols are additives used to maintain the sterility of preparations. Occasionally, preservatives cause ocular irritation, inflammation, or allergy, and these reactions can be confused as a worsening of the ocular ailment. Benzalkonium chloride is toxic to the corneal epithelium at concentrations higher than those used in commercial formulations. However, toxic concentrations of benzalkonium chloride could develop with frequent applications or in dry eye states. Allergic conjunctivitis in humans has been associated with thimerosal.

ROUTES OF ADMINISTRATION

Diseases of the eyelids, conjunctiva, and cornea are managed by topical and occasionally subconjunctival and systemic routes.

Topical Route

The topical route is the main therapeutic route for external ocular diseases. An advantage of this route is that higher ocular and lower systemic drug concentrations can be attained. Commercial eyedroppers deliver between 50 and 75 µl of medication, a volume two to three times more than can be retained in the cul-de-sac compartment. The extra volume overflows onto the skin or leaves by way of lacrimal drainage. More than one drop at a time is excessive and increases systemic absorption. A minimum of 5 minutes should elapse between drops to minimize drug washout and loss of effect. The recommended ointment dose is a 5 mm strip; excessive ointment coats and matts periocular hair.

Topical drugs leave the ocular surface by overflow, corneal penetration, conjunctival vessels, and the lacrimal duct. Drug loss is accentuated with epiphora, blinking, and conjunctival inflammation. Compared to solutions, less ointment is lost by absorption into conjunctival vessels and passage through the lacrimal system. Drugs that pass through the lacrimal duct empty into the oral and nasal cavities and are swallowed or absorbed across mucous membranes. Systemic absorption of ophthalmic drugs can be significant and in some cases causes side effects. Side effects are more likely to be observed in tiny patients or when high dosages are used.

In human patients the drug is instilled into the lower conjunctival sac, and the eyelids are closed for 2 minutes to immobilize the lacrimal pump system and thereby prolong corneal contact time. This method of topical

TABLE 14-1. Guidelines for the Use of Liquid and Ointment Ophthalmic Vehicles

Liquid vehicles (solutions, suspensions)

1. Remove ocular discharges before administration.
2. Shake suspensions vigorously.
3. Direct head and eye upward, hold container above and away from eye, allow drop to fall onto the eye.
4. Administer only one drop per dose.
5. Space sequential or additional doses apart by at least 5 minutes.
6. Give solutions before ointments.
7. Contact time is approximately 24 minutes.
8. Allergic or irritative drug and preservative reactions occasionally develop.

Ointments

1. Remove ocular discharges before administration.
2. Use approximately a 5 mm strip.
3. Warm tube in hand to liquefy the ointment and ease administration.
4. Minimize nozzle contact with eye or eyelids.
5. Contact time is approximately 50 minutes.
6. They are contraindicated in corneal perforations.
7. Passage through nasolacrimal system is less than solutions.
8. Allergic or irritative drug and preservative reactions occasionally develop.

administration is not practical in most animal patients. To prevent contamination of the medication, bottles should be held above and away from the eye and the drop allowed to fall to the eye. Ointments are more difficult to administer without contamination because the ribbon of ointment does not easily separate from the nozzle without contacting the eye or eyelids. Holding the ointment tube in the hand for a minute warms and liquefies the ointment making it easier to deliver. Table 14-1 lists guidelines for selection and use of liquid and ointment ophthalmic vehicles.

Subconjunctival Route

The bulbar subconjunctival route supplies drug to the eye by leakage through the conjunctival puncture and tissue diffusion. This route is most useful when drug combinations or increased local drug concentration are needed. However, the subconjunctival route does not replace topical therapy. The co-administration of similar or different drugs by the subconjunctival and topical routes can provide additive or synergistic therapeutic effects. Corneal concentrations for poorly adsorbed drugs (i.e., antibiotics) may be higher than with

TABLE 14-2.   Subconjuctival Antibiotic Dosages

Antibiotic [a]	Dosage [b] (mg)
Ampicillin	40–100
Amoxicillin	40–50
Carbenicillin	100–250
Cefazolin	100
Cephalothin	25–100
Chloramphenicol[c]	40–100
Gentamicin[d]	10–20
Lincomycin	50–150
Methicillin	20–100
Penicillin G	300,000–1,000,000 units
Tobramycin	10–20

[a]Use only the soluble aqueous form of the antibiotic.
[b]Dosage varies with different references and can be repeated once daily if necessary.
[c]Sodium succinate suspension.
[d]Subconjunctival administration is painful.

traditional topical therapy. However, aggressive topical therapy (e.g., fortified eyedrops or high frequency of administration) can achieve comparable drug concentrations within the cornea especially if there is a loss of the epithelial barrier. Subconjunctivally administered drugs are systemically absorbed and can reach blood levels that are comparable to those achieved by intramuscular injection. Care must be taken to prevent overdosage, especially when using drugs with a small safety margin (e.g., aminoglycosides). Drugs given subconjunctivally should be near physiologic tonicity, be water soluble, and have a pH between 3.5 to 10.5. Tables 14-2 and 14-3 list drugs and their dosages for subconjunctival administration.

Parenteral Route

Parenteral therapy may complement but not replace the other routes of drug administration for managing external ocular diseases. The parenteral route is most important for eyelid diseases.

GENERAL GOALS OF OPHTHALMIC THERAPEUTICS

The delicate and transparent tissues of the eye can be rapidly and irreversibly damaged, threatening normal visual function and causing pain. To minimize

TABLE 14-3. Subconjunctival Corticosteroid Dosages

Corticosteroid*	Dosage (mg)
Dexamethasone	1–2
Methylprednisolone	10–20
Triamcinolone	10–20

*Use the soluble aqueous form of the corticosteroid.

damage, external ocular problems should be diagnosed early so appropriate therapy can be immediately implemented. The goals of managing diseases of the eyelids, conjunctiva, and cornea include the following: 1) promote good hygiene; 2) prevent or treat existing infection; 3) minimize inflammation; 4) decrease pain; and 5) prohibit self-trauma.

Promote Good Hygiene

Ocular hygiene is essential yet frequently overlooked. Discharges hold bacteria, inflammatory cells, toxins, proteolytic enzymes, and inflammatory mediators that can cause ocular irritation and enhance tissue damage. Accumulated debris also inhibits antibiotic activity. Therefore, ocular and periocular discharges should be removed by compresses, tissues, and/or irrigating solutions before each application of an ophthalmic medication. Eyewash solutions should be sterile and isotonic. Most of the solutions listed in Table 14-4 are over-the-counter products, and all can be used repeatedly and indefinitely to irrigate the external ocular and periocular surfaces. The patient's comfort and cooperation may be improved if the solution is first warmed to body temperature by placing the container in a warm water bath. Inadvertent contamination of irrigating solutions by nozzle contact to the eyelids or eyes should be avoided, especially if the solution does not contain preservatives.

Antimicrobial Therapy

Antimicrobial therapy is always indicated for suspected or confirmed bacterial infections of the eye. Mycotic infections are rare, except for dermatomycoses of the eyelids, and viral infections are usually self-limiting. Bacterial infection should be suspected for the following: 1) foreign body trauma; 2) animal inflicted wounds; 3) mucopurulent ocular discharge; 4) deep or progressive corneal ulceration; 5) stromal infiltrates around an ulcer; and 6) immunocompromised patients. Cytologic evaluations, Gram stain, cultures, and sensitivity studies can help identify bacteria and facilitate selection of appropriate antibiotics. However, therapy should not be delayed for culture results. Even in the absence of infection, antibiotic therapy is justified for certain ocular diseases (e.g., noninfected corneal ulcers) to inhibit the development of secondary

TABLE 14-4. Sterile Ophthalmic Irrigating Solutions

Trade Name	Components	Preservative	Company
Ak/Rinse*	Sodium, potassium, calcium, and magnesium chlorides; sodium acetate and citrate	Benzalkonium chloride	Akorn
Collyrium*	Antipyrine; boric acid; borax	Thimerosal	Wyeth-Ayerst
Dacriose*	Sodium and potassium chloride; sodium phosphate	Benzalkonium chloride Edetate disodium	IOLAB
Eye-Stream*	Sodium, potassium, magnesium, and calcium chloride; sodium acetate and citrate	Benzalkonium chloride	Alcon
Lactated Ringer's Injection USP	Sodium, potassium, and calcium chloride; sodium lactate	None	Travenol
Sensitive Eyes* saline solution for soft lenses	Boric acid; sodium borate; sodium chloride	Sorbic acid Edetate disodium	Bausch & Lomb
0.9% Sodium Chloride Injection USP	Sodium chloride	None	Travenol

*Over the counter preparations.

bacterial infections which might result in significant tissue damage and loss of function. Concern about the increased risk of developing resistant bacterial infections is outweighed by the need to protect susceptible ocular tissues from damage that can cause blindness. The stroma of the cornea, in contrast to the epithelium, is susceptible to infection by bacteria of low pathogenicity. However, the indiscriminate use of antibiotic therapy for ocular diseases is not warranted.

Anti-inflammatory Therapy

Anti-inflammatory therapy tempers the host's inflammatory processes, which although beneficial can become excessive and damage the fragile ocular tissues. Anti-inflammatory therapy includes compresses, corticosteroids, nonsteroidal anti-inflammatory drugs (NSAIDs), and immunosuppressive agents (Tables 14-5 and 14-6).

TABLE 14-5. Nonsteroidal Anti-inflammatory Therapy

Therapy	Mechanism of Action	Dosage	Side Effects and Recommendations	Contraindications
Compresses				
Cold	Vasocon-striction	q8–12h × 5–15 min first 24–48 hrs.	Keep eyelids closed to prevent corneal trauma. Avoid extreme temperatures.	Deep corneal ulcers or pending ocular perforations. Extreme patient resistance.
Warm	Vasodi-lation	q8–12h × 5–15 min	*See* Cold Compresses, above.	*See* Cold Compresses, above.
Aspirin (acetyl salicylic acid)	Inhibits synthesis of prosta-glandins	Dog: 10 mg/kg PO q12h following a meal Cat: 10 mg/kg PO every 3rd day following a meal	Vomiting, diarrhea, gastrointestinal bleeding, melena, decreased appetite, decreased platelet function, displaces other albumin-bound medications.	Coagulopathies, thrombocytopathias, gastrointestinal diseases, hyphema, renal insufficiency.
Flunixin meglumine[a] (Banamine, Schering)	Inhibits synthesis of prosta-glandins	Dog: 0.55 mg/kg IV daily × 1–2 days. Cat: Not recommended	Gastrointestinal ulceration and erosion, acute renal necrosis.	Renal insufficiency, gastrointestinal disease, coagulopathies, dehydration.
Cyclosporine[a,b] (2% solution)	Immuno-suppression (T cell suppression)	Dog and cat: 1 drop topically q6–12h	Pustular blepharitis, stinging.	Blood dyscrasias, immunosuppressed patients, infectious ocular diseases.
Megestrol acetate (Ovaban, Schering)	Synthetic progestogen with anti-inflammatory activity	2.5–5 mg/cat/day for 5–7 days then 2.5–5 mg/cat once weekly until recovered	Diabetes mellitus, weight gain, lethargy, pyometra, adrenocortical suppression, mammary gland hyperplasia.	Unspayed, diabetes mellitus.

[a]Not FDA approved for use in small animals.
[b]A 2% solution can be made by mixing 2ml of cyclosporine oral solution, 100 mg/ml, (Sandimmune, Sandoz) with 8 mls of corn oil.

TABLE 14-6. Ophthalmic Corticosteroid Preparations[a,b]

Generic Name	Concentration (%)	Trade Name	Company
Hydrocortisone			
acetate suspension, ointment	2.5, 1.5	Hydrocortisone acetate	Merck Sharp & Dohme
ointment, solution	1.0	Cortisporin[c]	Burroughs Wellcome
	1.0	Vetropolycin-HC[c]	Pitman-Moore
ointment	0.5	Ophthocort[c]	Parke-Davis
Prednisolone			
acetate suspension	1.0	Pred Forte	Allergan
	1.0	Econopred Plus	Alcon
Dexamethasone			
phosphate suspension ointment	0.1, 0.5	Maxidex	Alcon
	0.1	Maxitrol[c]	Alcon
	0.1	Dexacidin[c]	CooperVision
	0.1	Dexasporin[c]	Pharmafair
	0.1	Decadron	Akorn
Betamethasone			
acetate solution	0.1	Gentocin Durafilm[c]	Schering
Isoflupredone			
ointment	0.1	Neopredef[c]	Upjohn
Fluorometholone			
suspension, ointment	0.1, 0.25	FML FML Forte	Allergan

[a]Relative glucocorticoid activity: hydrocortisone < prednisolone < dexamethasone, betamethasone, isoflupredone, and fluorometholone. The activity is also influenced by drug concentration, formulation, and drug derivative.
[b]List is not complete.
[c]Contains antibiotics.

Corticosteroids inhibit cellular infiltration, epithelial and fibroblastic proliferation, and neovascularization. Corticosteroids stabilize cell membranes, are lymphocytotoxic, and decrease the synthesis of prostaglandins, leukotrienes, and free oxygen radicals from arachidonic acid. Corticosteroids are used to treat ocular and periocular allergy, immune-mediated diseases, trauma, and inflammation. Because corticosteroids suppress the humoral and cell-mediated aspects of immune defense, concomitant bactericidal antimicrobial therapy is required when there is a risk of infection. Ophthalmic corticosteroids are contraindicated in ulcerative keratitis unless immune mechanisms are responsible for the pathology, and that is rarely recognized in animal patients. Ophthalmic corticosteroids accentuate collagenase activity, delay initial corneal wound healing, and predispose the eye to infections. Topically administered corticosteroids are systemically absorbed, result in adrenocortical suppression, and can cause an elevation of serum alkaline phosphatase. Furthermore, the side effects of polyuria, polydipsia, and polyphagia are rarely noted.

NSAIDs irreversibly bind to enzymes involved in the arachidonic acid cyclooxygenase pathway to inhibit the formation of prostaglandins, thromboxane, and prostacycline. In contrast to corticosteroids, NSAIDs do not block the production of leukotrienes and superoxide radicals from arachidonic acid by the lipoxygenase pathway. It has been suggested that inhibition of the cyclooxygenase pathway in certain circumstances potentiates the lipoxygenase pathway, causing a more severe leukocyte response. Anti-inflammatory synergism may be attained by concomitant use of an NSAID and a corticosteroid, but great care should be used if both are administered systemically at the same time as side effects overlap (Table 14-5). The concurrent use of more than one NSAID is not recommended because it may enhance the development of systemic adverse reactions, including gastroenteritis, gastrointestinal ulceration and erosion, bleeding disorders, acute renal insufficiency, and acute renal papillary necrosis.

Management of Pain and Self-Trauma

Ocular pain due to external diseases results from painful sensory stimulation of the ophthalmic branch of the trigeminal nerve terminating in conjunctiva, sclera, and cornea. Trigeminal stimulation can also elicit reflex ciliary muscle spasms, which add to the patient's discomfort. The signs of pain, which may be obvious or subtle, include head tilt, depression, lethargy, anorexia, epiphora, blepharospasm, elevation of the nictitating membrane, enophthalmos, and pawing or rubbing at the eye. Pain can be lessened by systemic NSAIDs (e.g., aspirin), systemic opioids, and topical cycloplegics (if ciliary muscle spasms are present).

Painful and irritative ocular diseases may result in the animal rubbing or pawing the eye. Self-trauma can cause, perpetuate, or exaggerate ocular damage. Restraint collars that extend beyond the animal's nose may be indicated to prevent self-trauma. Tranquilization is occasionally required to calm a patient that refuses topical care.

BLEPHARITIS

The eyelid is composed of an outer layer of skin, a middle layer of muscle, connective tissue, adnexal glands, and an inner layer of mucous membrane (palpebral conjunctiva). In blepharitis, the outer or middle layers (or both) are inflamed; the conjunctiva frequently becomes secondarily involved. The cutaneous surface of the eyelid is susceptible to the same diseases as the skin covering the rest of the body. However, the clinical responses of the eyelids to diseases are frequently exaggerated because of the high number of mast cells within the conjunctival submucosa and the eyelids' rich vascular supply.

The clinical signs of blepharitis depend on the cause and include blepharospasm, ocular discharge, pruritus, pain, eyelid hyperemia, edema, thickening, crusts, papules, abscesses, erosions, ulcers, alopecia, and depigmentation. Concurrent keratitis and conjunctivitis may be observed. Chronic blepharitis can lead to cicatrization and abnormal eyelid function, which can compromise the health of the cornea and conjunctiva.

Identifying the cause of blepharitis is based on the findings from the history, a careful examination, skin scrapings, cultures and cytology of exudate, and occasionally a skin biopsy. Common treatment principles for all causes of blepharitis include good hygiene and warm compresses. Ophthalmic ointment vehicles may be preferred over solutions because ointments maintain longer upper eyelid contact and moisten crusts, conjunctiva, and cornea.

Hordeolum

A hordeolum is a localized inflammation of the lid adenoidal adnexa. Staphylococcal infection is believed to be an important factor in the pathogenesis. As normal inhabitants of canine and feline skin and conjunctiva, *Staphylococcus* species rarely invade healthy tissue. Trauma, irritation, and altered or impaired sebaceous gland secretion may be inciting causes for a staphylococcal infection and hordeolum development. Hordeolums can usually be differentiated from eyelid neoplasms by their smooth surface. Uncharacteristic eyelid masses should be biopsied. The occurrence of hordeolums in cats appears to be rare.

External Hordeolums. An external hordeolum is called a sty and is a focal suppurative inflammatory reaction of the glands of Moll and Zeis. External hordeolums occur primarily in young animals and may be recurrent until maturity. Solitary or multiple erythematous swellings (abscesses) are observed on or near the external eyelid margin. Pain, ocular discharge, and eyelid crusting may be concurrent signs. Resistant, recurrent, or severe cases may require bacterial culture and sensitivity studies, fungal culture, skin scrapings, biopsy, systemic antibiotic therapy, and rarely systemic corticosteroid therapy.

Standard Therapy. The goals of therapy are to resolve the infection and control inflammation. A combination broad spectrum antibiotic and corticosteroid ointment should be applied four to six times a day for 10–21 days onto the eye and hordeolum but only if there is an absence of corneal ulceration (negative fluorescein corneal staining), eyelid demodicosis, and eyelid dermatophytosis. Topical antibiotics with an anticipated spectrum of activity against *Staphylococcus* species include bacitracin, chloramphenicol, erythromycin, polymyxin B, neomycin, gentamicin, and occasionally sulfonamides. Initial ophthalmic ointment selections include the following: 1) neomycin, polymyxin B, and bacitracin with hydrocortisone (e.g., Cortisporin, Burroughs Wellcome); 2) neomycin, polymyxin B, and dexamethasone (e.g., Dexacidin, CooperVision Pharmaceuticals); and 3) chloramphenicol, polymyxin B, and hydrocortisone (e.g., Ophthocort, Parke-Davis).

Warm compresses should be applied for 5–15 minutes three times a day to help resolve inflammation and to soften crusts. The eyelids and ocular area must be kept clean with tissues and sterile irrigating solutions (Table 14-4).

Systemic antibiotics and corticosteroids or lancing and drainage are usually not necessary unless the condition is severe (see Bacterial Blepharitis). When bacterial culture is indicated, the contents of the hordeolum should be cultured after puncture with a sterile 20 gauge hypodermic needle.

Meibomianitis. The meibomian glands number 20–40 per eyelid and exit along the furrow of the lid margin. When meibomian glands become inflamed, yellowish swollen bands oriented perpendicular to the lid margin can be observed underneath the palpebral conjunctiva. The yellowish bands are due to the accumulation of sebaceous secretions within the meibomian glands. The tarsal conjunctiva may become inflamed and contain superficial yellow calcareous deposits from the meibomian secretions.

Standard Therapy. Meibomianitis is treated similarly to external hordeolum with the addition of gentle manual expression of the meibomian glands with cotton swabs following topical anesthesia. Topical anesthesia is achieved by administering several drops of 0.5% proparacaine hydrochloride (e.g., Ophthetic, Allergan Pharmaceuticals). After warm compresses, the owner may be able to gently massage the eyelids with warm moistened cotton balls to stimulate expression of meibomian secretions. Any conjunctival calcareous deposits require surgical removal to eliminate secondary corneal irritation.

Chalazion. A chalazion is an internal hordeolum that develops because of obstruction of a meibomian gland duct with retention of the oily glandular secretions. Escape of the secretions into surrounding tissue elicits a foreign body reaction with formation of a granuloma, the chalazion. Chalazia are observed on the conjunctival side of the palpebrae near the margin as firm, yellowish, smooth, roundish masses. They occur most frequently in middle-aged dogs and may be single or multiple. Except in the acute stage, chalazia appear to be nonpainful and are usually an incidental finding.

Standard Therapy. One to several small, smooth, nonirritating chalazia may require no therapy. For acute chalazia, the conservative medical treatment described for external hordeolum is appropriate. Gentle expression of the contents of a chalazion is usually not possible but can be carefully attempted. Rupture of contents elicits inflammation of the surrounding tissue.

Chronic, multiple, or resistant chalazia that are symptomatic are managed by incision and drainage. Following topical, local, or general anesthesia, an incision is made through the palpebral conjunctiva over the mass and perpendicular to the lid margin with a small scalpel. Another surgical approach is to make a cruciate incision with excision of the four corners to produce a circular opening. A chalazion clamp placed on the eyelid decreases intraoperative bleeding and makes it easier to incise the tissue. The accumulated secretions and surrounding inflammatory tissue are removed with small scissors or a curette. The incision is allowed to heal by secondary intention. The ocular area is kept clean with an irrigating solution (Table 14-4), and warm compresses should be applied three to four times a day. A combination broad spectrum antibiotic and corticosteroid ointment, (e.g., bacitracin, neomycin, and polymyxin B with hydrocortisone (e.g., Cortisporin, Burroughs Wellcome Co.) is used four to six times a day for 1–2 weeks. Chalazion recurrence is common and may necessitate biopsy to rule out neoplasia.

Investigational Therapy. Recurrent or chronic chalazia in human patients who have not responded to conservative medical management (warm compresses, lid scrubs, and topical antibiotic-corticosteroid combination) have been successfully managed by an intralesional corticosteroid injection with or without incision and drainage. Triamcinolone acetate or acetonide was used in these patients. Without surgery, the triamcinolone acetate (20 mg/ml) was diluted with normal saline to 4–5 mg/ml and then a volume of 0.05–0.50 ml was injected intralesionally depending on the size of the chalazion and ease of injection. If the chalazion was not reduced in size by 50% within 1 week, another injection was performed. Persistence of the chalazion after 6 weeks warranted surgical excision.

Other investigators combine incision and drainage with a postoperative perilesional corticosteroid injection of 8 mg of triamcinolone acetonide (40 mg/ml). Conservative medical management was continued after surgery. For human patients, the use of a corticosteroid injection with or without surgery may be more effective than conservative management alone. Information regarding these methods in animals is not available.

Bacterial Blepharitis

Bacterial blepharitis is characterized by inflammation of the conjunctiva, eyelid margins, meibomian glands, and eyelids. The inflammation is therefore more diffuse than with hordeolums. Clinical signs include pain, mucopurulent ocular discharge, conjunctivitis, eyelid crusting, erythema, swelling, erosions, abscesses, and hordeolums. With chronicity, keratitis and eyelid alopecia, ulceration, and fibrosis may develop. Bacterial dermatitis may be evident on other parts of the body. Purulent blepharitis can be the first sign of juvenile pyoderma in puppies.

The diagnosis is based on the findings from physical examination and diagnostic tests, which include skin scrapings, cytology, and cultures. Deep skin scrapings should be evaluated for parasites (see Parasitic Blepharitis). Dermatophyte cultures should also be considered (see Mycotic Blepharitis). Gram and Giemsa (or Wright-Giemsa) stained cytology of exudate or scrapings usually demonstrates abundant degenerate neutrophils and bacteria, some of which may be intracellular. A skin biopsy may be necessary to rule out immune-mediated skin diseases (see Chapter 3).

Standard Therapy. The goals of therapy are to eradicate the infection, control inflammation, and identify and eliminate predisposing factors. Mild cases are managed with good hygiene, warm compresses, and topical and systemic antibiotics. Moderate to severe cases may require careful antiinflammatory therapy to minimize eyelid scarring.

Warm compresses are applied for 5–15 minutes three or four times a day. Crusts and discharges are gently removed with tissues and sterile irrigating solutions (Table 14-4) before each treatment. Promoting good hygiene in long-haired animals is easier if the periocular hair is clipped. A restraint collar may be required to prevent self-trauma. Eyelid abscesses should be lanced with a sterile 20 gauge hypodermic needle from the conjunctival or cutaneous surface. The expressed exudate should be cultured and cytologically examined, especially in severe or chronic cases. Lid margins, conjunctiva, or meibomian gland contents may also be cultured. *Staphylococcus* species and *Streptococcus* species are the most common organisms isolated. Staphylococci can enhance tissue damage by elaborating dermonecrotizing toxins and stimulating allergic reactions.

The initial antibiotic selection should have an anticipated spectrum of activity against *Staphylococcus* and *Streptococcus* species. Ophthalmic antibiotic choices include chloramphenicol (e.g., Chloroptic, Allergan Pharmaceuticals), erythromycin (e.g., Pharmafair), and the combination of bacitracin (or gramicidin), neomycin, and polymyxin B (e.g., Neosporin, Burroughs Wellcome). Topical gentamicin should be reserved for resistant cases. The topical antibiotic ointment should be applied on the eye and eyelids four to six times daily. Systemic antibiotics hasten recovery and are especially indicated if the blepharitis is severe or chronic. Initial systemic antibiotic selections and dosages are listed in Table 14-7. Systemic and topical therapy should be given for at least 3 weeks. Improvement should be noted within 3–7 days.

The most common causes for treatment failure are using subinhibitory antibiotic concentrations, stopping antibiotic therapy too soon, and not correcting any predisposing factors. Immune incompetence, hypothyroidism, seborrhea, demodicosis, dermatophytosis, atopy, food allergies, immune-mediated skin disorders, and staphylococcal hypersensitivity may be responsible for a poor clinical response. Further testing (e.g., skin scrapings, cultures,

TABLE 14-7. Recommended Initial Oral Antibiotic Selections for Treating Bacterial Blepharitis

Antibiotic	Dosage[a] (mg/kg)	Company
Cefadroxil	D: 22 q12h	Fort Dodge
Cephalexin	D & C: 22–66 q8h	Dista, Barr
Cephradine	D & C: 22–66 q8h	Barr, Zenith
Chloramphenicol	D & C: 22–55 q6–8h	Parke-Davis, Vedco
Clavulanic acid-amoxicillin	D & C: 22 q8h	Beecham
Erythromycin	D & C: 22 q8h	Abbott
Oxacillin	D & C: 22 q8h	Biocraft
Trimethoprim-sulfadiazine[b]	D & C: 15–22 q12h	Coopers

[a]D = dog; C = cat.
[b] Trimethoprim-sulfadiazine can cause keratoconjunctivitis sicca in the dog.

skin biopsy, allergy testing, and blood tests) should be considered in nonresponsive or recurrent cases (see Chapter 3).

In moderate to severe or poorly responsive cases of confirmed bacterial blepharitis, concomitant topical and systemic corticosteroid therapy is indicated to temper inflammation in the absence of corneal ulceration, demodicosis, diffuse pyoderma, and fungal infection. Topical antibiotic corticosteroid preparations include Cortisporin (Burroughs Wellcome), Dexacidin (CooperVision Pharmaceutical), Maxitrol (Alcon Laboratories), and Blephamide (Allergan Pharmaceuticals). Furthermore, an oral corticosteroid is combined with a 14- to 21-day course of systemic antibiotic therapy based on antimicrobial sensitivity testing. Oral prednisolone or prednisone is given for a minimum of 4 weeks on a decreasing dosage regimen (i.e., 1 mg/kg body weight twice daily for 1 week, 0.5 mg/kg twice daily for the second week, 0.5 mg/kg once a day for the third week, and 0.25–0.5 mg/kg once every other day) until eyelid inflammation resolves.

Alternative Therapy. Recurrent or nonresponsive bacterial blepharitis in dogs is suggestive of staphylococcal hypersensitivity, especially if a pathogenic *Staphylococcus* species has been cultured. However, staphylococcal hypersensitivity remains an unproved clinical entity. If systemic and topical corticosteroid and antibiotic therapy have been ineffective, injections of homologous *Staphylococcus aureus* bacterin in combination with appropriate systemic antibiotic therapy may be helpful for reducing inflammation and preventing recurrence of staphylococcal blepharitis in dogs. The bacterin is used to stimulate host antibody production against the bacterial cell wall and some exotoxins. The bacterin must be carefully prepared from a canine strain of *S. aureus* isolated from active ocular lesions as described by Chambers and Severin (see suggested reading list). Weekly 1 ml subcutaneous injections are given until eyelid inflammation resolves, and then the injection interval is *slowly* extended to 3 weeks. At that time, the bacterin may be stopped if there are no clinical signs of inflammation. The prognosis is fair to good, although some dogs require long-term therapy. Autogenous staphylococcal bacterin has been reported to be successful in cats with resistant staphylococcal dermatitis.

Commercial staphylococcal bacterins may be an alternative to homologous bacterin. Staphage Lysate (Delmont Laboratories) is a whole-culture staphylococcal bacterin used to treat canine pyodermas. Staphage Lysate is initially administered subcutaneously once or twice weekly at 0.2 ml increments until a maintenance dose of 1 ml is reached. This dose is continued once or twice weekly for approximately 4–18 weeks and then as needed. Alternatively, 0.5 ml of the staphage can be given twice weekly at 3–4 day intervals.

Investigational Therapy. *Propionibacterium acnes* immunotherapy as an adjunct to antibiotic therapy has been shown to be helpful in dogs with chronic recurrent canine pyoderma. A poor clinical response may be from acquired immunodeficiency due to staphylococcal pyoderma and/or host inherent immunodeficiency. *P. acnes* is a nonspecific immunostimulant. Nonviable *P. acnes* is suspended in a 12.5% ethanol in saline solution at a concentration of 0.4 mg/ml and administered intravenously at dosages ranging from 0.25 ml for dogs weighing less than 7 kg to 2 ml for those weighing more than 34 kg.

Long-term, low dose clindamycin therapy has been helpful in human patients with recurrent staphylococcal infections.

There is no available information about specifically using these therapies for chronic or recurrent bacterial blepharitis.

Mycotic Blepharitis

Mycotic blepharitis is rarely due to any fungi other than dermatophytes, with *Microsporum* and *Trichophyton* being the most common isolates. The eyelids may be the only site of infection, but usually there are lesions elsewhere. Eyelid dermatophytosis is characterized by circular areas of alopecia, scaling, and sometimes hyperemia, crusting, and edema. Pruritus is uncommon. The diagnosis is confirmed by culture of hairs and scale removed from the periphery of active lesions and placed on Sabouraud dextrose agar or Dermatophyte Test Medium (Fungassay, Pitman-Moore). Other diagnostic tests include ultraviolet illumination with a Wood's light, KOH preparations, and biopsy. The lesion should also be scraped for *Demodex* mites.

Standard Therapy. Most *Microsporum canis* infections are self-limiting. However, topical therapy may hasten resolution, control secondary bacterial infections, decrease environmental contamination, and prevent transmission to man and other animals. Whether topical preparations are effective is controversial because of the difficulty distinguishing between spontaneous resolution and cure.

Affected areas of the skin should be clipped to prevent reinfestation from infected hairs. Topical preparations reported effective against dermatophytes for periocular use include 2% miconazole cream (Conofite, Pitman-Moore), 1% clotrimazole cream (Lotrimin, Schering Animal Health), and diluted povidone-iodine solution (Betadine Solution, Purdue Frederick). Care must be taken to *not* use any dermatologic lotions around the eyes because they contain alcohols. Diluted povidone-iodine solution is made by mixing 1 part povidone-iodine with 300 parts sterile water; the final mixture is yellow. These topical preparations are applied once or twice daily. Alternatively, 2% chlorhexidine diacetate (Nolvasan, Fort Dodge Laboratories) once every 5 days has been recommended.

Applications of antidermatophyte medications should extend well beyond the edges of the visible lesion where dermatophytes may be residing. A bland ophthalmic ointment can be used to protect the cornea, and attempts should be made to keep antidermatophyte preparations out of the eye. If there is ocular contamination, flush the eye with a sterile irrigating solution (Table 14-4) or water. The owner should be instructed to wear protective clothing and rubber gloves when applying antidermatophyte medications and when handling the animal to reduce the risk of human infection. Therapy is continued 2 weeks after clinical cure or negative fungal cultures. The duration of treatment should be at least 6 weeks. Severe ringworm infection that is caused by dermatophytes other than *Microsporum canis* may be resistant to treatment or recrudesce after withdrawal of treatment. Recurrence is believed to be due to latent infection rather than reinfection. Systemic therapy with griseofulvin or an imidazole is probably best reserved for generalized or poorly responsive cases and is discussed in Chapter 3.

Because dermatophytes are contagious to humans and other animals, animal and human exposure must be minimized and the environment treated. Care should be taken that the animal handler does not act as a fomite. Carpets should be frequently vaccum-cleaned; and hard surfaces, cages, baskets, and runs should be washed with one of the following solutions: 1) 1 part 5.25% sodium hypochlorite (Clorox, The Clorox Company) with 10 parts water; 2) undiluted Lysol (Lehn and Fink Products); or 3) 0.5% chlorhexidine (diluted Novalsan, Fort Dodge Laboratories). Otherwise, under favorable conditions the spores of *Microsporum canis* can survive in the environment for many months. Other household pets (especially cats) should be evaluated for infection (see Chapter 3).

Parasitic Blepharitis

Parasitic blepharitis from mite infestation is caused by *Demodex* and Sarcoptic mange.

Demodectic Blepharitis. Demodicosis is rare in cats and older dogs but is fairly common in young dogs. Immunodeficiency should be suspected in all cases of demodicosis in that this normal inhabitant of the skin is allowed to

proliferate and incite inflammation. Endogenous and exogenous immunosuppressive factors include corticosteroid administration, hyperadrenocorticism,
neoplasia, hereditary immunodeficiencies, feline leukemia virus infection, and
feline immunodeficiency virus infection.

Demodicosis has two clinical forms: localized and generalized. Localized
demodicosis is characterized by one to five small, well circumscribed, erythematous, scaly areas of alopecia. Pruritus is uncommon. The most common site
of infection in the dog is the face, especially the periocular area and commis-
sures of the mouth. In cats, localized demodicosis also has a predilection for
the face with lesions that appear similar to the dog. Generalized demodicosis affects large areas of the body. The diagnosis is made by finding large
numbers of mites by microscopic examination of deep and extensive skin
scrapings. The presence of an occasional adult mite may be reflective of
normal inhabitation.

Standard Therapy. Localized demodicosis is considered a mild disease that
may spontaneously resolve within 4–8 weeks without miticide treatment or
with the amelioration of any immunosuppressive disorders. In young dogs,
approximately 10% of localized cases become the generalized form. Treatment
appears not to prevent generalization of the infection, nor does it hasten
recovery. If topical therapy is thought to be indicated, 0.025% isoflurophate
ophthalmic ointment (Floropryl, Merck Sharp & Dohme), undiluted benzyl
benzoate solution, or diluted amitraz (Mitaban, Liquid concentrate, Upjohn)
are considered to be fairly safe around the eyes. Rotenone ointment (Goodwinol Ointment, Goodwin Products) and benzoyl peroxide gel should be
avoided for periocular use. Isoflurophate is a cholinesterase inhibitor with
sustained activity that causes miosis and can result in systemic toxicity.
Isoflurophate should be avoided in the cat, in tiny patients, and in the presence
of other organophosphates. Benzyl benzoate should also not be used in the cat.
Diluted amitraz is formulated by mixing 1 part amitraz with 9 parts of mineral
oil. The cornea can be protected with a bland ophthalmic ointment, but if the
eye becomes contaminated it should be irrigated with water or a sterile
irrigating solution (Table 14-4). The miticide is gently rubbed into the skin
lesions with a rubber-gloved hand or cotton-tipped swab once or twice daily
except for the diluted amitraz, which is applied once every 3 days in the dog
and once weekly in the cat. Hair loss from parasitized follicles is accentuated
by the required rubbing for application of the miticide, and therefore the
lesions initially appear to enlarge. In rare cases, the diluted amitraz can cause
marked eyelid irritation requiring discontinuation of the drug. Otherwise,
topical treatment is continued until hair regrowth is observed, which usually
takes 4–8 weeks. Topical or systemic corticosteroid administration is contraindicated. The overall health status and care of the patient should be critically
evaluated.

Skin scrapings and examination are repeated in 4 weeks to evaluate for
generalization. As localized demodicosis resolves, there are fewer or no mites

and fewer immature forms. Spread of the lesions, increased mite count, and lymphadenopathy are suggestive of generalization of the infection. Therapy for generalized demodicosis is discussed in Chapter 3.

Sarcoptic Blepharitis. Sarcoptic mange, a transmissible mite infestation, is caused by *Sarcoptes scabiei canis* in the dog and *Notoedres cati* in the cat. Eyelid involvement is usually only a small part of a larger, intensely pruritic dermatitis. Therapy is discussed in Chapter 3.

CONJUNCTIVITIS

Conjunctiva lines the underside of the eyelids (palpebral conjunctiva), reflecting over at the superior and inferior conjunctival fornices to cover the sclera to the limbus (bulbar conjunctiva). A fold of conjutiva also covers the anterior and posterior surface of the third eyelid. Inflammation of the conjunctiva occurs commonly in the dog and cat with the acute signs of chemosis, hyperemia, and ocular discharge. The ocular discharge can be serous, mucoid, or mucopurulent. Some degree of discomfort is usually manifested by variable degrees of blepharospasm, enophthalmos, elevation of the third eyelid, and occasionally lethargy and spastic entropion. In severe or chronic cases, the conjunctiva becomes thickened and may develop follicles or papillae. Furthermore, the inflammation can spread to the cornea, eyelids, and sclera.

It is of utmost importance to rule out other causes for a "red eye" (e.g., glaucoma, anterior uveitis, keratoconjunctivitis sicca, scleritis, hyphema, and enophthalmitis). A thorough ophthalmic examination is necessary to identify underlying or predisposing problems, such as entropion, distichiasis, low tear production, dacryocystitis, skin diseases, and corneal ulcers. The conjunctival fornices, eyelids, cornea, and underside of the third eyelid should be examined, preferably with magnification and a good light source, for foreign bodies, follicles, distended meibomian glands, and aberrant hairs. Eyelid conformation is assessed without and with topical anesthesia. Furthermore, conjunctival cytologic examination may be helpful in determining the type of conjunctivitis and is most informative when performed early in the disease.

Mucoid ocular discharges trap medications, bacteria, debris, toxins, proteolytic enzymes, and inflammatory cells that can enhance the inflammation and interfere with the activity of drugs. Ocular discharges should be removed with tissues and irrigating solutions (Table 14-4) before each treatment. Clipping long periocular hair makes it easier to keep the area clean. Warm compresses applied for 5–15 minutes two to four times daily can be helpful in softening eyelid crusts and decreasing inflammation. A restraint collar is indicated to prevent self-mutilation in animals rubbing or pawing at their eyes. Systemic NSAIDs (e.g., aspirin) are occasionally needed (Table 14-5).

Infectious Conjunctivitis in Cats

Viruses, *Chlamydia psittaci,* and perhaps *Mycoplasma* are the major etiologic agents of infectious conjunctivitis in cats. Bacteria other than *Mycoplasma* and *Chlamydia,* are an uncommon cause of conjunctivitis in cats. Because the clinical syndromes share many similarities, distinguishing among infectious causes is frequently difficult. Furthermore, more than one infectious agent may be contributing to the conjunctivitis.

Infectious conjunctivitis tends to be bilateral but frequently begins in one eye. Multiple cats in a household may become infected, but asymptomatic carriers are possible. Even immunized cats can develop mild disease and shed the organism. Young or immunosuppressed cats tend to have the worst clinical manifestations.

Viral Conjunctivitis in Cats. Conjunctivitis has been associated with reovirus, feline calicivirus, feline herpesvirus type 1, and feline immunodeficiency virus infections in cats. Viral conjunctivitis usually starts with a serous discharge that frequently becomes mucopurulent as secondary bacterial infections develop. Upper respiratory and, uncommonly, lower respiratory signs may accompany the conjunctivitis. Clinically differentiating which virus is responsible may be difficult without viral cultures, serologic tests, and fluorescent antibody techniques. Except when dealing with a cattery or multiple-cat household, identification of the virus is not necessary with acute conjunctivitis because it does not alter patient management.

Standard Therapy. Acute and benign viral conjunctivitis does not require specific therapy (i.e., antiviral drugs) because the condition ordinarily is transient. Symptomatic care provides good hygiene and nutrition, minimizes stress, and manages secondary bacterial infections and corneal ulcers (see Ulcerative Keratitis). Sterile irrigating solution (Table 14-4) and tissues are used to remove ocular discharges and crusts. Occasionally, warm soaks are needed to loosen eyelid crusts. Secondary bacterial infections are suspected when mucopurulent discharge is observed or when numerous bacteria or neutrophils are present in conjunctival cytology. Corneal ulcers are identified by corneal uptake of fluorescein dye. Bacterial infections and corneal ulcers are treated with a broad spectrum topical antibiotic four to six times a day. Because concurrent infection with *Chlamydia* or *Mycoplasma* is possible, ophthalmic tetracycline (e.g., Achromycin, Lederle Laboratories) or chloramphenicol (e.g., Chlorofair, Pharmafair) are good initial choices. Chloramphenicol may be preferred in young cats when there is a concern about the systemic absorption of tetracycline causing dental staining. The owner should be instructed to wash hands after handling chloramphenicol to minimize exposure to this drug. Topical antibiotic therapy is continued a few days beyond ulcer healing or resolution of the conjunctivitis. The clinical course usually ranges from 10 days to 4 weeks. Concurrent herpesvirus corneal ulcers may require topical antiviral therapy, which is discussed below under Herpesvirus Ulcerative Keratitis in Cats.

Depressed tear production necessitates tear replacement (see Keratoconjunctivitis Sicca). Parenteral fluids and systemic antibiotics are indicated when systemic disease warrants. A cat with chronic or recurrent viral conjunctivitis should be evaluated for an immunosuppressive disorder, e.g., feline leukemia virus infection, feline immunodeficiency virus infection, or systemic disease. Chronic herpesvirus conjunctivitis may respond to antiviral therapy (see Herpesvirus Ulcerative Keratitis).

Infected cats should be isolated from other cats during active disease to prevent viral transmission. Herpesvirus-infected cats that have recovered can be asymptomatic carriers. Rhinotracheitis and calicivirus immunoprophylaxis may protect against severe systemic signs. However, vaccinated cats can still develop symptomatic ocular infection or become chronic carriers without evidence of clinical disease.

Chlamydial Conjunctivitis in Cats. *Chlamydia psittaci* is responsible for causing conjunctivitis and occasionally rhinitis and neonatal conjunctivitis in cats. The disease frequently starts in one eye and progresses to the other eye within 1 week. In the early stages, there is chemosis and a serous ocular discharge. Subsequently, the conjunctiva becomes hyperemic and thickened, and a mucopurulent discharge develops. Conjunctival follicles may be observed.

The diagnosis is based on Giemsa-stained conjunctival cytology, fluorescent antibody microscopy, serologic tests, tissue culture, or a dramatic response to therapy.

Standard Therapy. Without treatment, chlamydial conjunctivitis may persist for several months. Therapy is most effective in the early stages of the disease. Topical tetracycline (e.g., Achromycin, Lederle Laboratories) or chloramphenicol (e.g., Chlorofair, Pharmafair) should be applied six times a day until 2 weeks after clinical signs have resolved. The frequent applications are necessary because tetracycline and chloramphenicol are bacteriostatic. Topical chloramphenicol may be preferred in young cats if the systemic absorption of topical tetracycline causes dental staining. In unilateral cases, both eyes are treated to prevent the development of conjunctivitis in the asymptomatic eye. An occasional cat experiences ocular irritation due to topical tetracycline or chloramphenicol. Ocular irritation requires switching therapy to the alternate drug. In chronic or severe cases, topical therapy should be supplemented with oral tetracycline or chloramphenicol at 22–55 mg/kg PO three times daily on an empty stomach for 2 weeks. Tetracycline should not be given when the animal's adult teeth are developing. All cats in the household should be treated because asymptomatic carriers may exist. Carrier queens should receive topical and systemic therapy, as *Chlamydia* in the birth canal can be transmitted to the neonate. Persons handling chloramphenicol or the infected cat should be instructed to wash hands after each contact because of the remote possibility of chloramphenicol absorption and aplastic anemia and because chlamydial conjunctivitis is a zoonotic disease.

Subcutaneous chlamydial immunization may temper the severity and duration of clinical signs depending on the type of vaccination and field strain. Immunization may be beneficial in catteries with an endemic problem but is probably not indicated for the private cat owner.

Mycoplasmal Conjunctivitis in Cats. *Mycoplasma* species have been isolated from normal and diseased conjunctiva in cats. The development of mycoplasmal conjunctivitis may require the presence of stress, immunosuppression, or other disease because experimental attempts to induce conjunctivitis have not been successful. The conjunctivitis may involve only one eye the first week. The conjunctiva can be pale or hyperemic, and a pseudodiphtheritic membrane may cover the third eyelid. Other agents that cause conjunctivitis have also been isolated from cats with mycoplasmal conjunctivitis. The diagnosis may be confirmed by conjunctival cytology and culture or by inference from a positive response to therapy.

Standard Therapy. The natural course of the disease is usually 4 or 5 days to 1 month, but therapy can shorten this interval. Topical tetracycline, chloramphenicol, or erythromycin (Pharmafair) is applied four to six times a day for 2 weeks (see Chlamydial Conjunctivitis).

Bacterial Conjunctivitis

Under poorly understood circumstances, normal conjunctival bacterial flora can become pathogenic. Factors that may predispose the ocular surface to infection include abnormal eyelid conformation, local trauma, impaired host immune status, stress, increased virulence and number of organisms, tear film deficiency, and concurrent diseases. Primary bacterial conjunctivitis, excluding the mycoplasmal and chlamydial forms, is uncommon in the cat.

Acute bacterial conjunctivitis presents as a sudden onset of severe mucopurulent ocular discharge, marked diffuse conjunctival hyperemia, moderate chemosis, and occasional blepharitis. It is frequently unilateral and often has a predisposing factor of recent grooming, foreign body, or trauma. Conjunctival fornices and the underside of the third eyelid must be carefully inspected for a foreign body. Pain and blepharospasm may result in secondary spastic entropion. Care must be taken to differentiate anatomic entropion from spastic eyelid inversion.

Chronic bacterial conjunctivitis is usually bilateral and associated with poor lid conformation or other diseases. Chronic bacterial conjunctivitis results in thickening of the conjunctiva with mild follicular hyperplasia. Secondary blepharitis with marginal depigmentation and erosion can develop. The superficial peripheral cornea may become inflamed and ulcerated. Inflammatory occlusion and scarring of tear ductules may cause secondary keratoconjunctivitis sicca.

The diagnosis is based on findings from the examination and conjunctival cytology. Bacterial cultures and sensitivity testing are usually reserved for severe, relapsing, or chronic cases because of expense, delay in results, and the

TABLE 14-8. Initial Antibiotic Choice for External Ocular Infections Based on Gram Stain and Clinical Impressions

Organism and Clinical Findings	Therapy		
	Topical	Subconjunctival*	Systemic
No organism identified and not a deep or progressive corneal ulcer	Chloramphenicol Erythromycin Neomycin, polymyxin, and bacitracin		Ampicillin Amoxicillin Cephalosporin Chloramphenicol Dicloxacillin
Gram-positive	Bacitracin Carbenicillin Cefazolin Chloramphenicol Erythromycin Gentamicin Gramicidin	Amoxicillin Ampicillin Carbenicillin Cephalosporin Chloramphenicol Gentamicin Methicillin	Amoxicillin Ampicillin Cephalosporin Dicloxacillin Methicillin
Gram-negative	Carbenicillin Chloramphenicol Gentamicin Polymyxin Tobramycin	Carbenicillin Gentamicin	Amoxicillin Ampicillin Carbenicillin Cephalosporin
Pseudomonas spp., progressive corneal ulcer, or deep ulcer	Carbenicillin Gentamicin Tobramycin	Carbenicillin Gentamicin	Amoxicillin Carbenicillin Cephalosporin
Mycoplasma or *Chlamydia*	Chloramphenicol Erythromycin Tetracycline		Chloramphenicol Tetracycline

*See Table 14-2.

usual dramatic response to therapy. Samples for culture must be taken before any drugs are instilled in the eye.

Standard Therapy. Sterile irrigating solutions (Table 14-4) and tissues are used to clean the eye, conjunctiva, and eyelids. Ocular discharges must be removed before each treatment. If the animal tolerates warm compresses, apply for 5–15 minutes two to four times daily. Warm compresses help resolve the inflammation and soften and remove crusted discharges. A topical antibiotic may be initially selected based on the findings from cytologic studies or Gram staining (Table 14-8). Otherwise, the antibiotic should have an anticipated spectrum of activity against *Staphylococcus* and *Streptococcus* species, e.g., bacitracin, chloramphenicol, neomycin, and gentamicin. The combination of bacitracin, neomycin, and polymyxin B (or gramicidin) (e.g., Neosporin, Burroughs Wellcome) is usually a good initial choice. The topical antibiotic is applied four or more times daily depending on the severity of the disease. Improvement should be noted within 2–5 days. Therapy is continued for at least 7 days beyond resolution of clinical signs. Complementing topical antibiotic therapy with systemic antibiotic administration is considered when there is chronicity, when the conjunctivitis is deep-seated, or when the eyelids are involved. Initial systemic antibiotic selections and dosages are listed in Table 14-7. The systemic antibiotic should be used for at least 2 weeks. Concurrent or exacerbating problems, such as ectropion, entropion, keratoconjunctivitis sicca, dermatitis, seborrhea, and otitis externa, may have to be corrected or controlled in order to achieve complete resolution of the conjunctivitis. Eyelid surgery should be postponed until the inflammation has resolved. Depressed tear production warrants tear supplementation (see Keratoconjunctivitis Sicca).

Chronic or recurrent cases may reflect an undiscovered nidus of infection in the meibomian glands or nasolacrimal drainage system. Meibomianitis and dacryocystitis can be a primary or secondary problem with bacterial conjunctivitis. The meibomian glands are examined for abnormal retention of sebaceous material, which should be gently expressed (see Meibomianitis). The nasolacrimal drainage system is mechanically flushed with sterile saline. Purulent material exiting from the opposite puncta or obstruction of the nasolacrimal duct indicates nasolacrimal drainage system disease (e.g., foreign body or dacryocystitis). General anesthesia may be necessary either to flush out all purulent material or to unobstruct the system.

Culture and sensitivity studies are required in poorly responsive, chronic, or recurrent cases. *Staphylococcus* and *Streptococcus* species are the most frequently isolated bacteria from eyes of normal dogs and dogs with external ocular disease. Furthermore, *Pseudomonas* species were isolated in 14% of 150 clinically normal dogs in one study. This overlap of similar conjunctival flora under diseased and normal conditions makes the interpretation of bacterial cultures difficult. At these stages of the disease, it may be best to wait on the sensitivity profile for topical and systemic antibiotic selections. Some chronic cases require indefinite or intermittent therapy. Occasionally patients develop drug-induced allergic or toxic conjunctivitis with chronic topical therapy; this must not be misinterpreted as a worsening of the bacterial conjunctivitis. Neomycin is a common culprit for toxic conjunctivitis in human patients. In the absence of ulcerative keratitis or other diseases, and with appropriate bactericidal antibiotic therapy, chronic cases may benefit from the concurrent use of a topical corticosteroid (i.e., 1.0% hydrocortisone, 0.1% dexamethasone, or 0.1% isoflupredone) (Table 14-6), as immune responses to staphylococcal toxins and antigens may be responsible for chronic corneal and conjunctival inflammation. The topical corticosteroid should be applied four times a day until at least 7 days beyond resolution of the conjunctivitis.

Alternative Therapy. Perhaps chronic unresponsive staphylococcal conjunctivitis would respond to *Staphylococcus aureus* bacterin administration, as do some cases of chronic staphylococcal blepharitis (see Bacterial Blepharitis).

Allergic Conjunctivitis

Allergic conjunctivitis involves different degrees of hypersensitivity reactions I and IV with resultant degranulation of sensitized mast cells. Mast cell degranulation releases numerous chemical mediators which elicit inflammation and attract eosinophils. With allergic disease, the protective processes of the conjunctival mast cells become excessive and result in tissue damage.

The conjunctiva initially is hyperemic and chemotic. Blepharospasm and ocular discharge are usually present. The discharge may be serous, mucoid, or mucopurulent. Over time, the conjunctiva becomes thickened and may develop a granular or cobblestone texture. A superficial keratitis may also be observed. Tear production can become depressed by inflammatory occlusion of tear ductules. Interestingly, the conjunctivitis may be only unilateral.

Ocular pruritus, seasonality, and concurrent systemic signs (sneezing, serous nasal discharge, and regional pruritus) are variably observed. Allergic conjunctivitis in the dog may be a component of atopy.

Conjunctival cytology can be helpful in making a diagnosis. The finding of mast cells, free eosinophilic granules, or a single eosinophil is supportive of allergic disease. In cats, extreme numbers of mast cells are sometimes observed. A predominance of plasma cells, Russell body cells, lymphocytes, and neutrophils may also reflect allergic disease. If a hemogram is performed, some cases have a peripheral eosinophilia.

Standard Therapy. The goal of therapy is to minimize the clinical signs, as there is no cure. The treatment modalities employed in human patients with ocular allergies include cold packs, a change in climate, systemic antihistamines, hygiene, protective goggles, irrigation of the eye, avoidance of the antigen, immunotherapy, and topical corticosteroids, vasoconstrictors, antihistamines, cromolyn sodium, and cyclosporine. Many of these therapies are impractical or of undetermined benefit in canine and feline patients. Human patients have a great variation in their response to therapy, and frequently treatments must be changed or combined for the best response.

At this time, topical corticosteroids are the mainstay of therapy in animals. Topical corticosteroids are usually effective in decreasing the inflammation that follows mast cell degranulation. Corticosteroids with more potency than hydrocortisone are recommended (Table 14-6). Initially, four to six applications are administered daily. Mild cases may respond to fewer doses. The applications do not have to be spaced apart by regular intervals throughout the day. Once the conjunctivitis is in remission, the frequency of administration is *slowly* tapered over 2–4 weeks to the lowest level that controls the inflammation. Intermittent, chronic, or lifelong therapy may be needed. Topical corticosteroids should not be used when there is a break in the corneal epithelium or a surface infection. Owners are instructed to discontinue therapy and seek assistance should the animal develop blepharospasm or ocular discharge. The adverse effects from the topical administration of corticosteroids include adrenocortical suppression, increased susceptibility to local infection, delayed ocular healing, and increased collagenase activity. These adverse effects are usually not observed as a problem in animal patients unless the cornea becomes ulcerated.

Topical corticosteroid therapy is complemented with good hygiene, tear replacement, tear supplementation, and ocular irrigation. Ocular discharges that trap medication and hold pollens and dust should be removed before each treatment (Table 14-4). The amount of discharge decreases with resolution of the inflammation. Tear replacement is indicated in animals with low Schirmer tear test values (see Keratoconjunctivitis Sicca). The values usually return to normal as the inflammation resolves. Tear supplementation and ocular irrigation are employed theoretically to decrease the antigen load solubilized within the tear film.

Some cats with "eosinophilic conjunctivitis" have tested positive for feline herpesvirus type 1 infection and have improved following topical antiviral therapy. The relation between these two diseases is not known, but cats with eosinophilic conjunctivitis should be tested for feline herpesvirus infection. If infected, treatment with an antiviral agent can be tried (see Feline Ulcerative Herpesvirus Keratitis). There have also been reports that some cats with eosinophilic conjunctivitis respond to a hypoallergenic diet.

The effectiveness of therapy can be monitored by clinical signs, sequential conjunctival cytologic examinations, and perhaps peripheral eosinophil counts.

Alternative and Investigational Therapies. Adjunctive, alternative, or investigational therapies for managing refractory cases of allergic conjunctivitis in animals include immunotherapy, topical cromolyn sodium, topical cyclosporine, systemic corticosteroids, and in the cat, megestrol acetate.

If offending allergens are identified by cutaneous allergy testing, desensitization or avoidance can be tried. Allergy testing and desensitization have been beneficial in animals with cutaneous allergies and in cats with eosinophilic granuloma complex, but to my knowledge these procedures have not been employed in animals with ocular allergies. Immunotherapy or avoidance would be especially important if the conjunctivitis was part of a systemic allergic disease, such as atopy or food allergy.

Cromolyn sodium inhibits the degranulation of immunologically sensitized mast cells in rats, primates, and humans, but not in guinea pigs. Cromolyn sodium has been shown to be effective in human patients with ocular allergy. The disadvantages of cromolyn sodium are that it may cause transient stinging upon instillation, its applications must be spaced apart at regular intervals throughout the day, and it may take up to 6 weeks before improvement is noted. Cromolyn sodium is applied five or six times daily; a lower dosage may be effective when used concurrently with a topical corticosteroid. The drug is not U.S. Food and Drug Administration (FDA) approved for use in domestic animals and its effectiveness in dogs and cats needs investigation.

Cyclosporine is an immunosuppressive drug with anti-inflammatory prop-erties. Its efficacy for allergic conjunctivitis may depend on the degree that hypersensitivity reaction IV is causing the inflammation and on the subtype of mast cell involved in the hypersensitivity reaction. Topical 2% cyclosporine in olive oil used four times daily for 2 weeks and slowly tapered thereafter has been helpful in human patients with allergic conjunctivitis. See Table 14-5, footnote b, for instructions on mixing cyclosporine.

Megestrol acetate (Ovaban, Schering Animal Health) is an oral progestogen with anti-inflammatory properties that has been used in cats with eosinophilic keratitis and eosinophilic granuloma complex, both of which may have an allergic component. The potential for serious side effects (i.e., pyometra, lethal adrenocortical suppression, diabetes mellitus, and mammary gland hyperpla-sia) warrants careful patient monitoring and using the lowest effective meg-estrol acetate dosage. The dosage and contraindications are listed in Table 14-5. Megesterol acetate is not approved for feline use and in my opinion should be used only when all other therapies are unsuccessful.

Follicular Conjunctivitis

Follicular conjunctivitis is characterized as conjunctival inflammation with numerous nodules on the inner (bulbar) surface of the third eyelid and occasionally all conjunctival surfaces. The proliferation of nodules on the posterior surface of the third eyelid causes a cobblestone or granular texture that is hyperemic and thickened. Topical anesthesia and Adson forceps or a cotton-tipped swab are used to evert the third eyelid for examination. These nodules have been thought to develop from chronic irritation or stimulation due to pollens, allergens, or infective agents. Follicular conjunctivitis is usually associated with an abundant grayish to yellow mucoid discharge and mild diffuse conjunctival hyperemia. In my experience, the disease is most common in adult working dogs. Follicular conjunctivitis is uncommon in cats.

Standard Therapy. Without therapy, the conjunctivitis may persist for months. If the condition is mild, the corneal epithelium intact, and the ocular discharge not discolored green, ocular irrigation and applications of a topical corticosteroid ointment with potency greater than hydrocortisone (Table 14-6) may be effective. After cleaning the eyes, the corticosteroid is applied four to six times a day for 2–3 weeks. If a mucopurulent discharge is present, an antibiotic and corticosteroid combination (e.g., Maxitrol, Alcon; Neopredef, Upjohn; Dexasporin, Pharmafair) is used. Mucoid ocular discharges must be removed before each treatment, as discharges trap medications, irritants, and allergens. Even in the absence of excessive ocular discharge, ocular irrigation theoretically removes irritants and antigens that have solubilized in the tear film. Twice-daily irrigation with a sterile ophthalmic irrigating solution (Table 14-4) is recom-mended, and may be used indefinitely.

Recurrent cases or cases with marked nodular proliferation usually benefit from mechanical débridement or rupture of the nodules with gauze or a blunt instrument. Five to seven drops of 0.5% proparacaine hydrochloride (e.g., Ophthetic, Allergan Pharmaceuticals) are administered over 1–2 minutes to provide maximal topical anesthesia for débridement. A topical corticosteroid and broad spectrum antibiotic (e.g., Maxitrol, Alcon; Dexasporin, Pharmafair; Neopredef, Upjohn) is employed four to six times a day for 2–3 weeks after débridement.

Intermittent topical therapy is needed in some cases; recurrence may be seasonal. Long-term ocular irrigation may be helpful in those cases that accumulate excessive ocular discharge in their lower conjunctival fornix (Table 14-4).

KERATOCONJUNCTIVITIS SICCA (DRY EYE SYNDROME)

Keratoconjunctivitis sicca (KCS) refers to a qualitative or quantitative deficiency of any layer of the precorneal tear film that produces disease of the ocular surface. Deficiency of the aqueous layer of the tear film is the most common form of KCS in dogs and cats, but rarely mucin deficiency KCS has been recognized. Decreased tear production causes drying and metaplasia of corneal and conjunctival epithelial cells, increased eyelid friction, excessive surface mucus due to increased production by conjunctival goblet cells and decreased removal, enhanced tear film evaporation, increased tear film osmolarity, and increased susceptibility to surface infections.

Clinical signs of KCS are variable depending on the severity of deficiency, rapidity of development, and chronicity. The hallmark sign of the dry eye syndrome is excessive mucoid or mucopurulent ocular discharge. Other signs include conjunctivitis (i.e., a "red eye"), lusterless cornea, blepharospasm, elevation of the nictitating membrane, eyelid crusts, pawing or rubbing at the eye, keratitis, drying of the ipsilateral nostril, and corneal ulcers. Chronic changes include conjunctival thickening and impaired vision due to corneal pigmentation, neovascularization, granulation tissue, and cloudiness. In the cat, clinical signs are usually subtle.

KCS is common in the dog but less so in the cat. Despite the disease usually being easy to diagnose by an abnormal Schirmer tear test (STT), the condition is frequently overlooked. It is important to suspect tear deficiencies in any patient displaying one or more of the listed clinical signs. KCS is a painful disease with serious sequelae that can be stopped or dampened with rapid diagnosis and therapy.

Because the gland of the third eyelid contributes significantly to the aqueous tear film, the gland should never be excised unless neoplasia is suspected because removal may predispose the animal to the development of KCS. In my opinion, the treatment of choice for "cherry eye" (prolapsed gland of the third eyelid) is surgical replacement of the gland of the third eyelid.

TABLE 14-9. Lacrimotoxic and Tear Depressant Drugs

Lacrimotoxic Drugs	Tear Depressant Drugs
Dapsone (Jacobus Pharmaceutical)	Antihistamines
Phenazopyridine hydrochloride (e.g., Azo Gantrisin, Roche Dermatologics)	General anesthetics
Sulfadiazine (e.g., Tribrissen, Coopers Animal Health; Di-Trim, Syntex)	Systemic and topical atropine
Sulfamethoxazole (Bactrim, Roche Laboratories)	
Sulfasalazine (e.g., Asulfidine, Pharmacia)	
Other sulfonamides	

Standard Therapy. The goals of therapy for KCS are to: 1) determine the cause; 2) stop lacrimotoxic drugs; 3) provide good hygiene; 4) treat surface infections; 5) treat corneal ulcers; 6) provide tear replacement; 7) promote tear secretion; 8) provide antiinflammatory therapy; and 9) enhance tear preservation. Medical management of dry eye should continue a minimum of 3 months before it is deemed ineffective.

Determine the Cause. Causes of KCS in animals include congenital hypoplasia or agenesis of lacrimal tissue, infections (e.g., canine distemper virus and feline herpesvirus type 1 ocular infections), trauma, drug toxemia, drug-induced tear depression, megavoltage x-irradiation, neoplasia, senile atrophy, neurologic deficits (e.g., feline dysautonomia), anesthesia, and abnormal hormonal regulation. Hypoestrogenemia, hypovitaminosis A, and Sjögren's syndrome can also result in a deficiency of tears in humans. In most animals a cause for KCS is usually not obvious. However, there is evidence to support immune-mediated gland destruction or abnormal hormonal or neurologic regulation of tear secretion in idiopathic cases. Biopsy of lacrimal tissue is not a routine diagnostic or prognostic procedure.

Diseases that cause KCS-like signs must be differentiated from primary KCS. Facial nerve paresis, lagophthalmos, and eyelid deformities do not depress tear production; but without normal eyelid activity to distribute the tear film over the surface of the eye, a horizontal paracentral band of keratitis develops (exposure keratitis). Dysfunction of the ophthalmic branch of the trigeminal nerve causes decreased reflex lacrimation. Inflammatory and cicatricial closure of lacrimal ductules due to chronic conjunctivitis can secondarily depress tear production, which usually resolves once the inflammation subsides.

Stop Lacrimotoxic and Tear Depressant Drugs. Drugs reported to decrease tear production are listed in Table 14-9. Owners of animals treated with a lacrimotoxic or tear depressant drug should be instructed to seek evaluation if conjunctivitis or mucoid ocular discharge develops. Furthermore, STT values should be monitored when using lacrimotoxic drugs at high dosages or for a prolonged therapeutic course. If the STT value becomes depressed (< 15 mm and 10 mm in 60 seconds for the dog and cat, respectively) and clinical signs are observed, the drug should be immediately discontinued, if possible, and dry eye therapy implemented. A return of normal lacrimation may take several days to 8 weeks after withdrawal of a lacrimotoxic drug. In some cases, tear production never returns to normal. With the sulfonamides, the prognosis for a return of normal lacrimation is worse with therapy longer than 6 months. The reduction of tear production from tear depressant drugs (e.g., atropine, general anesthetics, and antihistamines) is transient and usually resolves within several hours to days after drug withdrawal.

Provide Good Hygiene. Keep the eye and eyelids clean with tissues, cotton-tipped swabs, and sterile irrigating solutions (Table 14-4). Clipping long periocular hair makes ocular hygiene easier. Most cases of KCS have copious amounts of tenacious mucus that especially accumulates in the conjunctival fornices. Stagnant mucin can be irritating, and it traps medications, microorganisms, and irritants. The amount of ocular discharge decreases with therapy, but initially the eye may need cleaning three to four times daily. If tear insufficiency persists, the affected eye has chronically excessive mucoid to mucopurulent discharge.

The patient's nose may also become dry and crusted ipsilaterally. The nose should be kept clean in order to enable the animal to breath easily. Applications of white petrolatum (e.g., Vasoline, Chesebrough-Ponds) protect the nose from drying and cracking.

Treat Surface Infections. Mucopurulent ocular discharges are suggestive of a secondary bacterial infection. The tear film's antimicrobial activities are greatly impaired in dry eye syndromes. A broad spectrum antibiotic ointment (e.g., Neosporin, Burroughs Wellcome) is applied topically four to six times a day for 5–7 days beyond resolution of the infection. Ointments are preferable because they provide longer surface contact time than solutions. Intermittent therapy may be required so long as tear insufficiency persists. Chronic topical neomycin therapy results in toxic or allergic conjunctivitis in an occasional patient, and it must not be misinterpreted as a worsening of the disease.

Treat Corneal Ulcers. KCS-associated corneal ulcers must be aggressively managed and closely monitored because they can rapidly progress to perforation and enophthalmitis. Effective antimicrobial therapy is important because the normal surface defenses are significantly impaired with tear insufficiency. The reader is referred to the Ulcerative Keratitis section for an in-depth discussion of ulcer management.

Superficial ulcers should be treated topically with a broad spectrum bactericidal antibiotic ointment six times a day until several days after complete healing. The combination of neomycin, bacitracin, and polymyxin B (or gramicidin) (e.g., Neosporin, Burroughs Wellcome) is a good initial selection. Animals with lagophthalmos, conformational exophthalmos, corneal anesthesia, or facial nerve paresis require more frequent applications or a protective surgical flap (e.g., third eyelid flap, conjunctival flap, or temporary tarsorrhaphy). Because it depresses lacrimation, topical atropine is avoided unless there are spasms of the ciliary and iridal muscles. Superficial ulcers should be monitored daily.

Deep ulcers require frequent applications (i.e., 6–24 times daily) of a topical bactericidal antibiotic. Gentamicin ophthalmic ointment or solution (Schering) is a good initial selection. The one drawback to frequent doses of commercial antibiotic preparations with preservatives is that the preservatives can become concentrated on the ocular surface because of the lack of tears, which may cause irritation or delayed epithelial healing in an occasional patient. Gram stain and bacterial culture and sensitivity studies are diagnostically helpful in the management of deeper ulcers (Table 14-8). If the edges of the ulcer are soft (melting), a topical anticollagenase is indicated (see Deep Corneal Ulcers). Slow healing and deep ulcers require a surgical graft or flap to aid with the healing process, provide structural support, and improve the patient's comfort. Topical atropine is usually necessary for deep ulcers and is definitely indicated if there is an accompanying secondary anterior uveitis or miosis. Atropine sulfate ointment or solution (1%) is used two to six times a day until the pupil is widely dilated and the patient is more comfortable. Subsequently, the atropine doses are slowly decreased to the lowest frequency needed to maintain mydriasis until the ulcer has healed. Atropine's depression of tear production should subside within several days after discontinuation. Patients with KCS and deep ulcers must be monitored several times daily during early case management.

Provide Tear Replacement. Tear replacement is the primary treatment of the dry eye and should complement all other forms of therapy. Artificial tears are used 2–24 times a day depending on the severity of the disease, the patient's discomfort, and the artificial tear formulation. Tear substitutes are available as solutions, ointments, and inserts. Solutions have the shortest contact time, thereby requiring the most frequent instillations. Viscous, absorptive polymers (e.g., methylcellulose, polyvinyl alcohol, hydroxypropyl methylcellulose) are added to liquid tear substitutes to thicken and stabilize the tear film. Polymers prolong the contact time of the artificial tears to 30–40 minutes. However, the polymer polyvinyl alcohol can cause ocular irritation in some dogs. Liquid tear substitutes that have the synthetic mucin polyvinylpyrrolidone (e.g., Adsorbotear, Alcon Laboratories; Adapt, Burton Parsons) have a longer contact time of up to 1.5 hours with perhaps better clinical efficacy in severe KCS. Tear substitutes with an artificial mucin are also the preferred choice for mucin deficiency KCS.

Ointment tear substitutes (e.g., AKWA Tears, Akorn; Duratears, Alcon Laboratories; Duolube, Muro Pharmaceutical; Tears Renewed, Akorn) are petrolatum based and have a longer contact time than solutions. The blurring of vision that bothers human patients is not observed as a problem in animal patients. Important advantages of artificial tear ointments over solutions are fewer required daily applications and lower cost. Artificial tear as an ointment is my choice for tear replacement in most cases. Furthermore, substitute tear ointments and solutions can be used concurrently in the same patient. If an artificial tear solution is desired, Adsorbotear and Adapt are excellent initial selections.

Artificial tear inserts (e.g., Lacrisert, Merck Sharp & Dohme) are made of solid hydroxypropylcellulose, which stabilizes the tear film and lubricates the eye. The insert is placed in the lower conjunctival sac one to three times daily. Expense, extrusion, and difficulty with insertion are distractors for veterinary use.

The preservatives in artificial tear formulations (benzalkonium chloride, thimerosol, edetate disodium, and chlorobutanol) can cause ocular irritation and discomfort. Preservatives can be toxic to the corneal epithelium, especially when there is an absence of tears to dilute the preservative. Thimerosol and chlorobutanol can be especially irritating. Preservative reactions are more common with frequent instillations or long-term therapy and require discontinued use of all products containing that preservative or perhaps any preservative. Alternatively, the concentration of the preservative in the product can be decreased by mixing the artificial tear substitute with methylcellulose or 1% sodium hyaluronate. A total of 15 ml of unpreserved 1% methylcellulose can be mixed with 6 ml of an artificial tear substitute. Commercial 1% sodium hyaluronate (Healon, Pharmacia Ophthalmics) is a glycosaminoglycan with viscoelastic and lubricating properties that can be added to tear solutions to achieve a sodium hyaluronate concentration of 0.10–0.04%. A 0.04% hyaluronic acid solution can be formulated by diluting 0.4 ml of sodium hyaluronate with 3 ml of Adapt. Clinical trials have shown diluted sodium hyaluronate solutions to be beneficial but not better than commercial artificial tears for the treatment of KCS. A relatively new product (Tears Naturale II, Alcon Laboratories) is marketed as containing a nonsensitizing preservative (quarternary ammonium). Unpreserved artificial tear products are commercially available but are expensive and can become contaminated. Artificial tear ointments do not contain preservatives, except Lacri-Lube, Allergan Pharmaceuticals, which has chlorobutanol.

Promote Tear Secretion. A new breakthrough for the management of KCS in animals and perhaps humans is topical cyclosporine, a third generation noncytotoxic immunosuppressant. Topical 2% cyclosporine has been reported to increase lacrimation in approximately 80% of idiopathic cases of canine KCS. The efficacy of 2% cyclosporine eyedrops on feline patients has not been very successful in the few cases I have treated. Even if tear production does not increase, corneal pathology (superficial granulation tissue, neovascularization, and pigmentation) may regress. Cyclosporine's mechanism of action is unknown, but it may alter the inflammatory processes or the hormonal or neurologic regulation of lacrimal tissue. For cyclosporine to be effective, some functional lacrimal tissue must remain. Furthermore, efficacy may be improved when therapy is started early in the disease or when the STT value is more than 4 mm/60 seconds. A 2% solution of cyclosporine is applied to the affected eye as a 1 drop dose two times a day. A 2% solution can be made by mixing 2 mls of cyclosporine oral solution, 100 mg/ml (Sandimmune, Sandoz), with 8 mls of corn oil. The drop is followed in 30 minutes by a dose of an artificial tear ointment (e.g., AKWA Tears, Akorn), antibiotic ointment (e.g., Neosporin, Burroughs Wellcome), or an antibiotic corticosteroid combination ointment (e.g., Cortisporin, Burroughs Wellcome). With unilateral KCS, both eyes may require treatment with topical cyclosporine to achieve the greatest efficacy. However, the normal eye may develop epiphora. In severe or chronic cases of KCS, the cyclosporine eyedrops should initially be administered into both eyes three times daily. Most patients respond to the cyclosporine eyedrops in 1–3 weeks, though some cases may take 1–3 months before tear production increases. Cessation of cyclosporine eyedrops usually results in regression of STT values within 1–3 days. Therefore, cyclosporine therapy is usually chronic and perhaps lifelong; however, once the patient is stabilized, a less frequent administration can be tried. Tear supplementation, good hygiene, antibiotic therapy, and anti-inflammatory therapy are continued as needed. Topical 2% cyclosporine can be carefully used in conjunction with topical antibiotic therapy in the presence of sterile corneal ulceration, as cyclosporine does not appear to delay corneal healing or accentuate collagenase activity. As an immunosuppressive drug, perhaps topical cyclosporine should not be used when corneal infection is suspected. The cyclosporine or its oil vehicle has rarely been associated with ocular or eyelid irritation requiring withdrawal of the drug.

The most frequently used lacrimomimetic for years was pilocarpine, a parasympathomimetic drug, until its replacement with cyclosporine eyedrops. Some functional lacrimal tissue is a prerequisite for pilocarpine effectiveness. Pilocarpine can be used topically or orally, but topical administration can cause conjunctival injection, chemosis, and blepharospasm. Furthermore, the induced miosis from topical pilocarpine can impair vision, especially if there are any axial ocular opacities. Topical pilocarpine is contraindicated with iridocyclitis. To minimize the side effects of topical pilocarpine, concentrations of 1% or less are recommended. Topical pilocarpine is used as a 1 drop dose two or three times a day depending on the patient's response and concentration of the solution.

Oral pilocarpine also has disadvantages. In addition to being a bitter tasting solution, systemic signs of intoxication, in order of increasing severity, include hypersalivation, vomiting, diarrhea, urinary incontinence, tachycardia, hypertension, and bronchiolar spasms. Oral pilocarpine is contraindicated with cardiovascular and gastrointestinal disorders. Human patients receiving oral or topical pilocarpine occasionally report the additional side effects of intestinal discomfort, headaches, and myopia that would be difficult to identify in animal patients. The oral pilocarpine dosage must be slowly titrated for each patient by starting at a low dosage and increasing the dosage by only 1 drop per day. The development of salivation 30–60 minutes after pilocarpine administration is a good indicator of a dose adequate to stimulate tear production, but it also indicates a dose in the toxic range. I recommend the use of a dosage slightly lower than the one that stimulates excessive salivation. As a basic guideline, administer 1–2 drops of pilocarpine (e.g., Pilocar, CooperVision) two to three times daily in a ball of food. The concentration of the solution varies with the weight of the patient, e.g., 0.5% for 2–4 kg; 1–2% for 5–10 kg; and 2–4% for 11–20 kg. The medication bottle should be kept tightly closed when not in use and completely out of reach of children. Hands should be washed after each application. The effect of pilocarpine lasts 6–8 hours. It has been suggested that a 4- to 6-week trial period might be necessary to detect a drug response. Clinical experience suggests that pilocarpine is effective in only 15–20% of canine KCS cases. If tear production returns to normal, an attempt should be made eventually to slowly discontinue the pilocarpine, though long-term therapy may be required. Perhaps pilocarpine and cyclosporine can be tried concurrently in cases resistant to cyclosporine.

KCS has been recognized in cats with feline herpesvirus type 1 ocular infection. The role of topical antiviral therapy for improving tear production in infected cats is not known. Whether cyclosporine eyedrops would complicate ocular herpesvirus infection is also not known.

Treat Inflammation. Mild corneal and conjunctival inflammation usually regress with improved tear production, topical cyclosporine therapy, adequate tear replacement, and resolution of secondary surface infections. However, persistent corneal inflammation impairs vision owing to corneal pigmentation, vascularization, and cloudiness. If there is moderate to severe corneal or conjunctival inflammation, then mild topical corticosteroid therapy in conjunction with cyclosporine therapy will improve the patient's response to treatment; however, the corneal epithelium must be intact as determined by fluorescein staining, and herpesvirus ocular infection must not be present. My preference is a 1% hydrocortisone-antibiotic combination ointment (e.g., Cortisporin, Burroughs Wellcome) used two to four times a day, instilled 30 minutes after cyclosporine instillation, until the inflammation has resolved. In the presence of a mucopurulent discharge or confirmed bacterial infection, steroid therapy should be delayed for several days while an appropriate topical antibiotic is used. Patients on both cyclosporine and a corticosteroid must be carefully monitored for external infections, as both drugs are immunosuppressants. If the external inflammation is judged to be a result of a toxic or allergic drug reaction, use of the suspected agent must be stopped.

Enhance Tear Preservation. Preservation of existing tears can be accomplished by lacrimal punctal occlusion or tarsorrhaphy. The efficacy of these procedures in dogs and cats is not known, as they are rarely employed. Temporary punctual occlusion with plugs (Freeman Punctal Plug, Eagle) or with an intracanalicular collagen insert allows assessment of the effectiveness of punctual closure. Diathermy, laser, and cyanoacrylate tissue adhesive have been used for permanent punctal occlusion in human patients.

By decreasing the size of the palpebral fissure, a partial tarsorrhaphy reduces the exposed ocular surface area and decreases tear evaporation. Lateral tarsorrhaphies are used in some human patients with KCS. In animals, a partial tarsorrhaphy may be beneficial when there is lagophthalmos, facial nerve paresis, or conformational exophthalmos.

Alternative Therapy. If medical therapy is impossible for the owner or ineffective after at least 3 months, parotid duct transposition should be considered in patients without xerostomia. Because the procedure can be associated with several complications (e.g., loss of duct patency, crystalline deposits on the eyelid margins and cornea, saliva overflow, and blepharoconjunctivitis), it is reserved as an alternative therapy for KCS.

Investigational Therapy. As KCS is a common, painful, often devastating ocular disease in humans and animals, numerous studies about several aspects of the disease continue. Investigational therapies include Gel tears, autologous serum tears, primrose oil, and topical retinoid (vitamin A).

Gel tears is a clear, semisolid formulation of synthetic, high molecular weight, cross-linked polymers of acrylic acid that has been investigated as a tear substitute. Patients with severe dry eye syndromes have subjective and objective clinical improvements with doses of Gel tears no more often than four times daily. However, Gel tears is not commercially available at the time. Autologous serum as another tear substitute has been shown to benefit some human patients with KCS who were refractory to commercially available artificial tear preparations.

Some female human patients with systemic signs of estrogen deficiency have demonstrated improvement of their dry eye syndrome after systemic estrogen therapy. Vasoactive intestinal peptide and porcine histidine isoleucine-containing peptide are being investigated as tear stimulants. Another study has explored the benefits of primrose oil, which consists primarily of *cis*-linoleic and γ-linolenic acid, in patients with Sjögren syndrome.

Topical retinoid therapy was once thought to be helpful in managing human patients with dry eye syndromes. However, another study has shown that topical tretinoin is not effective in alleviating the symptoms and clinical signs of noncicatricial dry eyes.

Investigations continue to explore the role of neurotransmitters and other immunosuppressants, anti-inflammatory drugs, and hormones in managing KCS.

KERATITIS

Keratitis refers to inflammation of the cornea that can result in cellular infiltrates, neovascularization, edema, pigmentation, ulceration, and scarring of this normally transparent structure. The ophthalmic examination should be thorough, and attempts should be made to identify etiologic factors to help determine therapy and prognosis. Lid margins, conjunctival fornices, and the bulbar side of the third eyelid should be carefully inspected, preferably with magnification and a bright light source, for foreign bodies and ectopic hairs. Eyelid conformation and function are assessed for entropion, ectropion, lagophthalmos, and facial nerve dysfunction. Gross corneal sensation should be determined with a cotton wisp, as lesions of the fifth cranial nerve can cause neurotrophic keratitis. Unless there is concern about perforation of a deep ulcer, a Schirmer tear test is necessary to rule out keratoconjunctivitis sicca. Corneal staining with fluorescein, a nonvital stain, or perhaps rose bengal, a vital dye, followed by examination with a Wood's lamp or cobalt blue light determines the integrity and health of the corneal epithelium. Finally, corneal edema or vascularization can be associated with blepharoconjunctivitis, scleritis, anterior segment inflammation, and glaucoma.

To facilitate a discussion about the treatment of keratitis, it is easiest to categorize corneal inflammation as ulcerative or nonulcerative.

Nonulcerative Keratitis

Nonulcerative keratitis is corneal inflammation without a break in the integrity of the corneal epithelium. Fluorescein is a water-soluble dye that requires an interruption in the hydrophobic epithelium to stain the hydrophilic corneal stroma. However, diseased epithelium can faintly retain fluorescein or allow passage of a small quantity of dye through intercellular epithelial spaces to stain stroma in the absence of ulceration. Corneal granulation tissue may also retain fluorescein dye. Pooling of fluorescein within an epithelialized corneal depression, called a facet or crater, should not be misinterpreted as an ulcer. While holding the eyelids apart, irrigation of the cornea removes fluorescein that pools within depressions.

Pannus (Chronic Superficial Keratitis). Pannus is a nonpainful, nonulcerative, bilateral, progressive, inflammatory disease of the cornea that can lead to blindness. This specific keratitis has also been called German shepherd pannus, chronic superficial keratitis, pigmentary keratitis, and Uberreiter's syndrome. Although it occurs predominantly in the German shepherd with a much lesser frequency in the German shepherd crossbreeds, Siberian husky, Scotch collie, greyhound, and border collie, the disease is not restricted to these breeds. Pannus is characterized by variable proportions of corneal vascularization, pigmentation, granulation tissue, and whitish opacities, which usually begin at the inferior temporal limbus. In some cases neovascularization and granulation tissue dominate the corneal changes, whereas in others, corneal pigmentation may be pronounced with little vascular response. The anterior face of the nictitating membrane occasionally becomes thickened and hyperemic, and the border may depigment. Nictitating membrane involvement can occur with or without corneal disease. Patients are usually presented for impaired vision, blindness, corneal opacification, or redness of the third eyelid.

Diagnosis is based on the clinical presentation in the absence of irritative ocular diseases, such as entropion, distichiasis, and keratoconjunctivitis sicca. Corneal fluorescein staining should always be done to rule out ulcerative keratitis; anticipate a speckled pattern of dye retention over the lesion. Cytology and histopathology are almost never needed because of the classic presentation of pannus. However, if cytology is performed, it will demonstrate many lymphocytes and plasma cells.

Standard Therapy. The goal of treatment is to control the disease sufficiently to preserve functional vision. There is no known cure for pannus. The pathogenesis is unknown, but an immune-mediated or hypersensitivity disease is suspected. The initial treatment of choice is a topical corticosteroid. The potency, concentration, and derivative of the corticosteroid and the severity of the corneal lesion influence the dosage. A corticosteroid either in an ointment or solution vehicle with a potency greater than hydrocortisone is selected, such as 1% prednisolone acetate, 0.1% isoflupredone, or 0.1% dexamethasone (Table 14-6). If a corticosteroid suspension is chosen, the owner should be instructed to vigorously shake the container in order to evenly disperse the drug particles for an accurate dose. The topical corticosteroid is initially administered 6–8 times a day (less often for mild conditions). In contrast to the administration of antibiotics, the doses do not have to be administered at regular intervals throughout the day, which helps with client compliance when frequent applications are necessary. Clearing of corneal neovascularization and granulation tissue (i.e., remission) usually takes 2–6 weeks. Magnification is helpful for evaluating corneal changes. Regression of corneal pigmentation is slow and frequently incomplete. An occasional large diameter corneal blood vessel persists. Evaluations are scheduled about every 2 weeks until the disease is in remission. Once in remission, the frequency of topical corticosteroid administration is *slowly* tapered over 4–6 weeks to the least number of daily administrations necessary for control of corneal revascularization. Tapering the dosage slowly allows time for reversal of adrenocortical suppression and prevents recurrence or rebound of the inflammation. Maintenance lifelong therapy is individually adjusted and usually ranges from one dose twice daily to twice weekly. Twice-yearly examinations are then scheduled. The owner should be told to look for corneal revascularization, which would require reevaluation and an adjustment of maintenance therapy. Furthermore, the owner is instructed to discontinue the topical corticosteroid and seek help should the dog develop blepharospasm or an abnormal ocular discharge. Topical corticosteroids are contraindicated when there is a break in the corneal epithelium. The side effects of topical corticosteroids (adrenocortical suppression, elevation of serum alkaline phosphatase, enhanced collagenase activity, and increased susceptibility to local infection) are usually not observed as a problem in canine patients treated for pannus unless the cornea becomes damaged. A rare dog develops polyuria and polydipsia due to systemic absorption of the corticosteroid. The lifelong therapy must be stressed to the owner. Flare-ups require a significant increase in the corticosteroid dosage, a change in the type of corticosteroid, or additional therapy. Some patients seem to respond better to one corticosteroid than to another.

Subconjunctivally administered corticosteroids may be necessary under the following circumstances: 1) more than 50% of the cornea is diseased; 2) the patient's vision is significantly impaired; 3) there is abundant corneal granulation tissue; 4) there has been a relapse or poor response to topical corticosteroid therapy; and 5) the owner is unable to give frequent topical applications. Subconjunctival therapy does not replace topical therapy but may allow fewer daily topical applications to achieve remission. Repositol preparations provide prolonged drug release; however, it is difficult to discontinue therapy, and therefore the diagnosis must be correct. Some repositol corticosteroids (e.g., Depo-Medrol, Upjohn) leave a residual white plaque that can become inflamed. The injection site is usually adjacent to the most severely affected region of the cornea. When the disease is diffuse, it is easiest to perform the injection dorsally (i.e., around 12 O'clock). Subconjunctivally administered drugs are systemically absorbed and can reach blood levels that are comparable to those levels achieved by intramuscular injection. Subconjunctival injection always requires topical anesthesia and firm restraint to prevent penetration of the globe. Occasionally, sedation is necessary. To provide maximal topical anesthesia, 5–7 drops of 0.5% proparacaine hydrochloride (e.g., Ophthetic, Allergan Pharmaceuticals) are administered, spacing the doses over 1–2 minutes. For additional anesthesia, a cotton pledget soaked in 2% lidocaine (e.g., Elkins-Sinn) is pressed onto the site of injection for 1 minute. Inflamed eyes are difficult to anesthetize topically because the anesthetic is rapidly carried away from the eye and the acidic pH of inflamed tissue decreases the membrane penetration of the anesthetic. A 25 or 26 gauge needle on a tuberculin or 3 ml syringe is used. One hand immobilizes the eyelids or uses small forceps to grasp bulbar conjunctiva while the hand holding the syringe is stabilized against the animal's head. The needle is directed parallel to the globe and is inserted through the bulbar conjunctiva about 2–5 mm from the limbus with the bevel up. The tip of the needle should be visible, and a bleb should form when a small quantity of the drug is given. Hyperemia or hemorrhage may develop around the site of injection and resolves in a few days. Recommended drug formulations and dosages are listed in Table 14-3. Subconjunctival injections can be repeated at time intervals influenced by the patient's response to therapy. Topical corticosteroid therapy should complement the subconjunctival injection.

The prognosis for control is usually good except in severe cases with a lot of pigment or when there is exacerbation during topical corticosteroid therapy. Relocation to an environment with less ultraviolet radiation exposure may be helpful for disease control and response to therapy.

Alternative Therapy. Other therapeutic modalities for the management of pannus include cryosurgery, beta radiation, and superficial keratectomy. These alternatives are usually reserved for those cases that did not respond to medical therapy and have significant visual impairment. Concurrent lifelong topical corticosteroid therapy is required to deter corneal revascularization. These procedures may best be reserved for a specialist.

Cryosurgery has been effectively employed in a small number of cases with heavily pigmented corneas and blindness. Cryotechniques have only recently been used for pannus, and a standardized procedure has not been determined. Cryosurgery damages tissue by causing cellular and vascular injuries. The cornea is fairly resistant to damage by freezing, whereas melanocytes are cold-sensitive. Cryogens that have been used include nitrous oxide, liquid nitrogen, and carbon dioxide. Nitrous oxide does not lower tissue temperatures as much as liquid nitrogen; therefore the use of a nitrous oxide cryosurgical system may decrease the likelihood of permanently damaging the corneal endothelium and causing secondary corneal edema.

Before surgery, patients are started on topical 1% atropine twice daily and a topical corticosteroid and broad-spectrum antibiotic combination (e.g., Maxitrol, Alcon Laboratories) two to four times a day. One group of investigators used the following procedure. Patients were placed under general anesthesia, and a nitrous oxide cryosurgical system was used with the temperature of the probe tip adjusted to $-70°C$. Areas of abnormal cornea and adjacent conjunctiva were frozen for 7–20 seconds depending on the severity of the lesion. Freezing did not go beyond 3 mm behind the limbus because of the concern about thermal damage to the ciliary body. The frozen site was allowed to completely thaw before probe removal to prevent stripping off of the corneal epithelium. Another group of investigators used liquid nitrogen spray. Treated areas were frozen for 15 seconds, allowed to thaw completely, and then refrozen for 15 seconds.

The postoperative management for cryosurgery includes a continuation of the topically administered atropine, antibiotic, and corticosteroid. Variable amounts of corneal edema and ocular pain are observed after cryotherapy. Restraint collars may be needed to prevent self-mutilation. Systemic aspirin 10 mg/kg PO q12h that is given following a small meal may help decrease discomfort and inflammation. The patient should be monitored closely for adverse gastrointestinal reactions due to aspirin. The eyes should be kept clean with tissues and sterile irrigating solutions (Table 14-4). The corneas initially appear worse owing to corneal edema. Fluorescein may be retained by the cornea because of epithelial loss and damage, yet topically administered corticosteroids must be carefully continued to impair corneal revascularization and pigmentation unless ulceration progresses or infection develops. The topical antibiotic and atropine can usually be stopped after 2 weeks. Cryosurgery can be repeated months later if deemed necessary. Lifelong topical corticosteroid therapy is required.

Beta radiation is administered by a strontium 90 probe. Up to six circular areas of the cornea are irradiated with 4500 to 7500 Rads. The irradiated region should extend 2–3 mm beyond the limbus. Topical or subconjunctival corticosteroids are also used. Improvement may take 2–4 weeks.

Superficial lamellar keratectomy is employed to remove all abnormal corneal tissue. A 2 mm wide strip of perilimbal episcleral and conjunctival tissue may also be excised. Postsurgical management requires careful use of a topical corticosteroid during the healing phase to inhibit revascularization of the cornea. If there is minimal corneal inflammation, the topical corticosteroid should be started after reepithelialization of the cornea. Topical 1% atropine (one dose administered two to four times a day) and a broad spectrum topical antibiotic (one dose administered four to six times daily) are also used until the cornea is healed. Topical corticosteroid therapy is continued indefinitely. A maximum of three keratectomies can be performed in severe cases. Corneal thinning and scarring, which can be severe, are the sequelae of this procedure.

Investigational Therapy. The topical use of the T cell immunosuppressant cyclosporine has been tried in only a few cases of pannus with variable results. The dosage was 1 drop of 2% cyclosporine four times daily (see Table 14-5 for cyclosporine formulation). The combination of topical corticosteroid therapy with cyclosporine eyedrops has not yet been investigated. Homoplastic lamellar corneal-penetrating scleral grafting for advanced pannus has been reported in four German shepherds with beneficial results in three. Graft rejection would hinder the success of this procedure.

Ulcerative Keratitis

Ulcerative keratitis is probably the most common corneal disease in dogs and cats. The clinical signs of ulcerative keratitis include blepharospasm, pawing or rubbing at the eye, head tilt, lethargy, enophthalmos, elevation of the third eyelid, ocular discharge, photophobia, loss of the smooth corneal surface contour, secondary anterior uveitis, and corneal edema, vascularization, pigmentation, and cellular infiltrates.

The diagnosis is made by visible inspection of the cornea with or without the aid of fluorescein stain. However, if stain is not used, small ulcers, superficial ulcers, and sealed microperforations may be easily overlooked. In certain animals, topical anesthesia or tranquilization is necessary to examine a painful eye. Regions of the cornea obscured by the third eyelid or chemotic conjunctiva must also be inspected.

Most ulcers in animals are probably a result of trauma. Other causes include aberrant hairs, entropion, infections (viral, bacterial, and mycotic), foreign bodies, corneal endotheliopathies with bulla formation, exposure (lagophthalmos, exophthalmos, abnormal eyelid structure, and corneal anethesia), burns, tear deficiencies, neurologic (neurotrophic keratitis), and immune mechanisms. The eye must be carefully scrutinized for local causes that can be corrected or managed.

A systematic approach to ulcer management is as follows: 1) classify the ulcer; 2) determine the etiology; 3) correct the cause; and 4) promote ulcer healing. The classification of an ulcer considers depth, presence or absence of sepsis, and healing rate. The depth of an ulcer can be broadly categorized as either superficial or deep. Descemetoceles and corneal perforations are the deepest corneal defects and require immediate attention. The presence of corneal infection is suggested by purulent discharge, stromal infiltrates, animal-inflicted injury, and progressive corneal ulceration. Ulcers caused by plant material or a cat scratch are likely to be inoculated with a microorganism. Furthermore, the normal ocular flora can contain pathogenic and opportunistic microorganisms that may be able to damage the cornea once the epithelial barrier has been disrupted. The amount of tissue damage depends on the pathogenicity of the microorganism and the host's defense mechanisms. Immunocompromised patients are at increased risk of developing infection. Cytologic evaluations, Gram stain, and cultures and sensitivity studies can help identify bacteria and facilitate selection of appropriate antibiotics. These tests are usually reserved for deep, progressive, or unusual ulcers. Samples for culture should be collected before any drugs or anesthetics are instilled in the eye. Antibiotics, carrier agents, and preservatives may interfere with bacterial growth. With uncooperative patients, a single drop of 0.5% proparacaine hydrochloride (e.g., Ophthetic, Allergan Pharmaceuticals) or 2% lidocaine (e.g., Elkins-Sinn) may have to be used before collecting samples. A moistened swab may improve bacterial isolation; thioglycollate broth or sterile physiologic saline can be used. The sample should be immediately plated onto blood agar, and the swab then broken off into a tube of thioglycollate broth. Antibacterial therapy must not be delayed for the culture and sensitivity results. In contrast, cytology can provide rapid information about the cell population and presence of infectious agents. However, the information from the Gram stain does not always correlate with culture results, and the absence of bacteria is not a guarantee that the ulcer is sterile. Furthermore, sensitivity studies using the Kirby-Bauer system do not consider the high antibiotic levels that can be obtained with topically and subconjunctivally administered antibiotics. Because of these drawbacks, laboratory testing is not always used, and antimicrobial therapy becomes based on the type of corneal ulcer and the response to therapy.

The rate of healing is classified as normal, progressive when the ulcer is worsening, or delayed when it is resistant to healing. Progressive and resistant ulcers indicate that there is a problem that was initially overlooked, poor epithelial adherence (see Superficial Epithelial Ulcers), or excessive enzymatic destruction of corneal tissue (see Deep Ulcers).

The promotion of ulcer healing requires good hygiene, antimicrobial, analgesic, and anticollagenase therapy, and ulcer protection and support. Furthermore, mydriatic, cycloplegic, and nonsteroidal anti-inflammatory therapy are important when anterior uveitis accompanies an ulcer. Good hygiene is of paramount importance in the treatment of ulcerative diseases. Ocular mucoid secretions trap medications, debris, bacteria, toxins, proteolytic enzymes, and inflammatory cells, which can further tissue destruction. Ulcers with necrotic or infected tissue may require mechanical or surgical débridement. These principles are discussed for each type of ulcer.

Superficial (Epithelial) Ulcers. A superficial ulcer refers to a loss of the epithelium with or without concurrent loss of the epithelium's basement membrane. These ulcers usually have a clean edge, unless they become indolent, and minimal corneal edema. Superficial ulcers frequently are painful and may elicit reflex spasms of the ciliary and iridal muscles.

Standard Therapy. The goals of therapy are to correct a local cause if identified and promote ulcer healing. The examination should include assessment of eyelid function, corneal sensation, and tear production. The eyelid surfaces and the underside of the third eyelid should be examined for foreign bodies and aberrant hairs, preferably with the aid of magnification and bright lighting. Uncomplicated superficial corneal ulcers do not warrant the expense of cytology and cultures. Ulcer healing is promoted by good hygiene, antimicrobial therapy, analgesic therapy, and ulcer protection.

Antibiotic therapy is indicated to prevent bacterial infection or to eradicate existing infection. A broad spectrum topical antibiotic ointment or solution should be used four times daily. Chloramphenicol (e.g., Chlorofair, Pharmafair) or the combination of neomycin, polymyxin, and bacitracin or gramicidin (e.g., Neosporin, Burroughs Wellcome) are good selections. Gentamicin is usually reserved for deeper or complicated ulcers. The antibiotic is continued until 2–3 days after healing.

Ocular pain may be decreased by the cycloplegic action of atropine. Atropine 1% is used one to four times a day as needed. Mydriasis and improved comfort suggest an effective dosage. However, mydriasis may elicit photophobia with resultant blepharospasm, and excessive eyelid motion may interfere with ulcer healing. Atropine solution passes through the nasolacrimal system and is bitter tasting. Cats that do not tolerate the taste of atropine can be treated with 1% tropicamide (e.g., Mydriacyl, Alcon Laboratories) or atropine ointment. Topical atropine decreases tear production, but artificial tear supplementation is rarely necessary unless the patient has tear deficiency, lagophthalmos, corneal anesthesia, or eyelid dysfunction. Normal lacrimation returns shortly after cessation of the atropine. Once atropine therapy is stopped, it may take up to 14 days for the pupil to return to its normal size and responsiveness. Owners should be instructed to wash hands after handling the atropine container to prevent inadvertent introduction into their own eyes. Topical anesthetics (e.g., 0.5% proparacaine hydrochloride) are toxic to the corneal epithelium and therefore cannot be used for pain relief except for ophthalmic examinations. Systemic analgesics (e.g., aspirin) are rarely necessary.

The eye should be kept clean of discharges with tissues and sterile ocular irrigating solutions (Table 14-4). Removal of discharges is especially important before the instillation of medications. Restraint collars are necessary in patients that paw or rub at the eye. Patients with exophthalmos, lagophthalmos, corneal anesthesia, or facial nerve paralysis may benefit from the protective effects of artificial tear administration, a third eyelid flap, or a temporary tarsorrhaphy. Surgical flaps and bandage contact lenses or collagen shields are usually reserved for nonhealing or deeper ulcers.

Uncomplicated superficial corneal ulcers should reepithelialize within 4–10 days if the cause has been removed and the animal is prevented from rubbing at the eye. Once epithelialized, the ulcer no longer retains fluorescein dye. Cornea experimentally denuded of all of its epithelium can be reepithelialized within 4–7 days by cells multiplying and sliding from the limbus. The ulcer is reevaluated every 2–3 days until healed and the owner is instructed to monitor for changes in the size of the ulcer and the character of the ocular discharge. The owner should seek attention if any problems develop. Complications and delays in healing warrant careful reevaluation to identify infection or causes for continued corneal irritation (e.g., tear deficiency, foreign body, abnormal eyelid conformation, conformational exophthalmos, or ectopic hairs). Otherwise, delayed healing of a superficial noninfected ulcer suggests a problem with epithelial adherence and is discussed next.

Refractory Superficial Ulcers (Indolent Corneal Ulcers). Refractory superficial corneal ulcers are common in the dog, less so in the cat. Refractory superficial ulcers are also called Boxer ulcers, refractory or recurrent corneal erosions, persistent corneal erosions, and refractory epithelial ulcers. These ulcers can occur in any breed. Refractory or indolent ulcers are characterized by the following: 1) loss of corneal epithelium with the epithelial basement membrane usually remaining intact, although the basement membrane may be damaged, lost, or abnormal; 2) delayed epithelial healing (i.e., > 1–2 weeks); 3) the presence of poorly adherent corneal epithelium; and 4) an absence of underlying ocular problems that would delay ulcer healing (i.e., infection or irritation).

Refractory ulcers are usually painful. Corneal edema can be mild to moderate. The edges of the ulcer are usually jagged because of a collarette of loose epithelium. Variable amounts of superficial vascularization and pigmentation may develop over time. Corneal vascularization seems to promote healing. The pathogenesis of delayed healing is incompletely understood. Considerations include a primary corneal epithelial (or basement membrane) dystrophy or an acquired corneal dysfunction that results in an inability of new epithelium to adhere to the underlying anterior stroma.

Standard Therapy. The primary goal of therapy is to promote adherence of the advancing epithelial cells to the underlying anterior stroma. Otherwise, refractory erosions may persist for up to 6 months despite the conventional use of topical atropine, hyperosmotic agents (discussed below), and numerous antibiotics. Therapeutic modalities include débridement, multiple superficial keratectomies, soft contact lens or collagen corneal shield wear, and surgical procedures. Unfortunately, no one therapy is always successful. Furthermore, recurrence may occasionally occur because the new epithelial covering is not tightly secured until the hemidesmosomal attachments between epithelial basal cells and their basement membrane are completely reformed. Even under normal conditions, this may take up to 6 weeks. During this time, excessive eyelid motion may sheer off any weakly attached epithelium.

Débridement of loose epithelium has traditionally been the initial therapy. Topical anesthesia is achieved by applying several drops of 0.5% proparacaine hydrochloride (e.g., Ophthetic, Allergan Pharmaceuticals) onto the cornea, spacing the applications over 1–2 minutes. Fine forceps or sterile dry cotton-tipped swabs are used to remove all loose epithelium. Because dry cotton-tipped swabs adhere to the epithelium better than moistened swabs, tear-soaked swabs should be replaced. Move the swab circumferentially around the edge of the ulcer rather than parallel to the ulcer's margin. Débridement removes variable amounts of epithelium with sometimes alarming amounts lifting off the cornea. Normally adhered epithelium does not lift off with gentle circumferential débridement. The corneal surface is flushed clean after dé-bridement with a sterile irrigating solution (Table 14-4). Aggressive epithelial and basement membrane débridement using magnification and a scalpel blade with the patient under general anesthesia has also been recommended. Chemical cautery may enhance removal of loose epithelium, but its use is not required and clinically it does not improve the final results. Chemical cauterizers include povidone-iodine solution, tincture of iodine, and ether. If chemical cautery is elected, my preference is 10% povidone-iodine solution (Betadine, Purdue Frederick). Débridement with a cotton-tipped swab dipped in 10% povidone-iodine solution is followed by copious lavage with a sterile irrigating solution (Table 14-4) to prevent iodophor irritation.

To further enhance ulcer healing, I prefer to follow corneal débridement by another procedure (multiple superficial keratotomies, placement of a bandage soft contact lens or collagen corneal shield, or a third eyelid flap). These procedures are discussed below.

After débridement, therapy is similar to that for superficial ulcer management (see previous section). A topical broad spectrum antibiotic solution or ointment (e.g., chloramphenicol or the combination of neosporin, polymyxin, and bacitracin or gramicidin) is used prophylactically three or four times daily. Refractory ulcers tend to be resistant to bacterial infection. If there is miosis or severe pain, ophthalmic 1% atropine should be used sparingly. Atropine therapy is minimized because the resultant mydriasis increases incident light stimulation of the retina, which may worsen photophobia and blepharospasm, and the increased eyelid activity may shear off any weakly attached advancing epithelium. The analgesic activity of aspirin may be helpful for decreasing ocular pain (Table 14-5). Animals that rub at the eye require a restraint collar. The owner is instructed to seek help if the ulcer progresses or a mucopurulent ocular discharge develops. The patient is reevaluated every 5–7 days, and any loose epithelium is gently removed. If loose epithelium is not observed with magnification, débridement is not necessary. In many patients, the ulcer's size gradually decreases and the ulcer heals over the next 2–6 weeks. If the ulcer continues to be refractory to healing, another therapeutic approach is warranted to improve the patient's comfort and relieve the owner's concerns. The options include (in order of my preference) multiple superficial keratotomies, a bandage soft contact lens, a collagen corneal shield, a surgical flap, investigational drugs, superficial keratectomy, and a topical hyperosmotic drug.

Multiple superficial keratotomies is a procedure that has been employed in humans and dogs, and it may offer better results than débridement alone. Investigators theorize that the procedure enhances epithelial adherence. Following topical anesthesia, loose epithelium is débrided as previously described. The corneal surface is flushed clean with a sterile ophthalmic irrigating solution (Table 14-4). Uncooperative patients require tranquilization or general anesthesia. A 25 gauge needle is used to make superficial scrapes in a cross-hatch pattern over the ulcer bed. The scrapes should extend 1–2 mm beyond the edge of the ulcer and be spaced apart by about 1.0 mm. An alternative technique makes perpendicular superficial corneal punctures rather than cross-hatch scrapes. This technique would probably be best performed with the patient completely immobilized by general anesthesia. Under low magnification, the depth of the puncture is determined by advancing a 20 gauge needle only until the cornea slightly indents. The punctures are spaced apart by 0.5–1.0 mm over the base of the ulcer and should extend 1–2 mm beyond the edge of the ulcer. Prophylactic antibiotic solution or ointment is applied four times daily until healing is complete. Topical atropine, a restraint collar, and aspirin are used if needed. The average time of healing is about 15 days. Multiple superficial keratotomies can be repeated in 2 weeks if there is minimal to no improvement. Multiple superficial keratotomies can also be combined with placement of soft contact lens, corneal collagen shield, or surgical flap, which may further improve epithelial healing.

Bandage soft contact lenses apply pressure to stabilize loosely adherent epithelium, protect weakly adherent epithelium from the shearing forces of the eyelids, and provide relief from corneal pain. The advantages of using soft contact lenses over surgical flaps include unobscured vision, ability to monitor the healing process, less expense, and no need for general anesthesia. The primary disadvantage with the use of soft contact lenses is poor retention by some patients. Soft contact lenses are usually contraindicated in active microbial infections, blepharitis, and dry eye syndromes. Most therapeutic soft contact lens are composed of hydrogels, which renders them hydrophilic. Hydrophilic soft contact lenses can absorb large quantities of water, which increases their oxygen and fluid transmissibility. Hard lenses and lenses with low oxygen permeability should not be used.

Contact lenses made for humans or animals[*] can be employed. Accurate fit is important for retention and successful therapy. The selection and proper fitting of bandage soft contact lenses should consider the following: 1) the lens should completely cover the cornea or extend 1–2 mm beyond the limbus; 2) the lens should undergo only a 1- to 2-mm excursion with blinking because

---

[*]Equine Specialty Products, Inc., Denton TX 76202, (1-800-874-6773) and The Cutting Edge Ltd., Santa Clara, CA 95054, (1-408-970-0200) manufacture large, medium, and small animal lenses.

excessive movement increases the shearing force between the lens and the corneal epithelium; 3) the curvature of the lens should approximate the curvature of the cornea or fit on the steeper side (i.e., the lens having a greater curvature than the cornea), as steeper fitting improves lens centration, especially with an irregular corneal surface; and 4) thicker lenses are easier to place and seem to have a better retention rate in animals than the ultrathin membrane lenses, which do not possess sufficient rigidity to center on an irregular surface. The normal range of corneal curvature in the dog is 7–9 mm and in the cat 8.4–8.9 mm. The smaller the radius of curvature, the steeper is the lens. The normal corneal horizontal diameter in the dog varies between 13 and 17 mm. In the cat, the horizontal diameter is about 17 mm. Manufactured lenses for humans have a maximal diameter of 16.0 mm. Therefore, human lenses are on the small side for many animals. Despite this less than ideal fit, human lenses with diameters of 14.0–16.0 mm can work well. Investigators report the best fit by Soflens (Bausch & Lomb) and Softcon lens (CIBA Vision) in the dog and cat, respectively.

The contact lens is placed after débridement of loose corneal epithelium with or without making multiple superficial keratotomies. Topical anesthesia is necessary, but tranquilization is rarely required. The ocular surface must first be irrigated to remove mucus, hair, and pieces of epithelium. Consider clipping periocular hair in long-hair breeds. The lens can be placed with fingers that have been washed with a disinfectant, rinsed, and dried. Alternatively, thumb forceps with the tongs covered by a small section of sterile intravenous tubing can be used to aseptically and gently manipulate the lens. Frequently, a hook or forceps must be used after lens placement to position the third eyelid on top of the lens rather than underneath it. Small air bubbles trapped between the cornea and lens resorb and do not require replacement of the lens if the fit is judged to be good. If the edges of the lens roll up after fitting, the lens is too flat and a lower radius of curvature should be tried. If the lens wrinkles or there is a central dome, the lens is too steep and a higher radius of curvature is selected. A topical broad spectrum antibiotic solution or ointment applied three or four times daily should be considered to prevent infection. Because preservatives in ophthalmic drugs can be absorbed and concentrated by the lens, applications more frequent than six to eight times daily are usually avoided to prevent the development of toxic keratitis. Complications of poor lens-to-cornea contact include discomfort, corneal edema, corneal neovascularization, sterile corneal infiltrates, secondary infections, and loss of the lens. Some animals display mild blepharospasm for the first 1–2 days after lens placement. This may reflect discomfort due to a foreign body sensation or from corneal débridement. Slight blepharospasm does not warrant lens removal. Severe lens reactions, such as keratitis, anterior uveitis, and surface infections, require immediate removal of the lens. Otherwise, the lens is left in place for 2–3 weeks or until the ulcer is healed. If the lens is well tolerated, it is best to refrain from early removal, as the bandage lens stabilizes and protects the regenerating epithelium to allow for hemidesmosome reformation. A restraint collar prevents the animal from rubbing at the eye, which improves retention of the lens. Owners are instructed to seek help if the animal develops mucopurulent ocular discharge or severe blepharospasm. Owners can also be asked to try to find lost lenses for resterilization and reuse. The owner should not replace a lost lens but, instead, store it in water or a saline solution until returned.

Soft contact lenses can be sterilized by boiling, dry heat, autoclaving, or hydrogen peroxide. The preservatives in cold disinfectants can be irritating or toxic and therefore should not be used. The lens is first cleaned with a commercial lens cleaner or baking soda. When using baking soda, place ¾ teaspoon in the palm of the hand. Add sterile 0.9% saline or an irrigating solution other than lactated Ringer's (Table 14-4) to make a watery consistency with no lumps or dry grains of soda. The lens is coated with the mixture and gently rubbed for 30 seconds per side. The lens is then thoroughly rinsed in sterile 0.9% saline or an irrigating solution. The lens can then be replaced in the same patient or sterilized for future use. When using hydrogen peroxide for sterilization, the lens is soaked in a 3% solution for 10 minutes. After the soak, the hydrogen peroxide is removed by rinsing the lens four times for several minutes each time in buffered normal saline with no preservatives. It is *important* to remove all of the hydrogen peroxide from the lens since as little concentration as 30 ppm can damage the cornea. The lens is then stored in sterile 0.9% saline solution.

A collagen corneal shield (Opti-Cor, Pitman-Moore) can be used to promote healing of the corneal epithelium. The shield dissolves completely within approximately 48–72 hours after application. The manufacturer recommends rehydrating the shield with methylcellulose to provide less curling and folding of the lens. The shield can also be rehydrated with an electrolyte solution or an antibiotic preparation. Concomitant use of ophthalmic ointments or solutions does not appear to cause any problems. Retention of shields may be improved by the use of a restraint collar.

Surgical flaps can also be used to protect the refractory superficial ulcer, relieve pain, and facilitate healing. Before the flap is placed, all loose epithelium is débrided as previously described. Multiple superficial keratotomies can also be performed. A third eyelid or 360-degree conjunctival flap can be employed; I prefer the third eyelid flap. However, there is some controversy regarding the efficacy of the third eyelid flap, as motion exists between the flap and the cornea when the third eyelid is sutured to the upper eyelid. Yet if the third eyelid flap is maintained for 5–6 weeks, most refractory ulcers heal. Topical antibiotic ointment or solution is applied on top of the flap four times daily for the first 1–2 weeks. The ocular environment should be kept clean with tissues and collyrium. Some animals need a restraint collar.

A superficial keratectomy is usually reserved for refractory cases. This procedure requires general anesthesia and magnification. Epithelium and basement membrane are scraped off with a scalpel blade. The theory is that the postoperative healing results in secure epithelial adhesion to the stroma by scar formation. The scarring also decreases recurrences. A surgical flap or bandage contact lens should be placed after the keratectomy, and topical antibiotic, cycloplegic therapy, aspirin, and a restraint collar are recommended as previously described.

Topical hyperosmotics (e.g., 5% NaCl and 10% boric acid) have been advocated for the treatment of refractory superficial ulcers. It has been theorized that decreases in corneal edema might improve epithelial adherence. NaCl (5%) ointment (Muro-128, Muro Pharmaceutical) can be tried once or twice daily. However, clinical experience suggests that hyperosmolar agents may not improve the clinical course of refractory superficial ulcers and can actually be irritating. If irritating, increased eyelid activity may pull off any loosely attached epithelium and actually delay healing.

Investigational Therapy. Research is active in this field because refractory corneal erosions are a common and frustrating ocular problem in humans and animals.

Epidermal growth factor is a polypeptide that stimulates the incorporation of RNA, DNA, and protein synthesis precursors, thereby increasing the rate of cell proliferation. Epidermal growth factor has no effect on cell attachment. In animal studies, topically administered epidermal growth factor enhances the rate of reepithelialization for various corneal wounds, but the regenerating cells may be loosely attached. Combining epidermal growth factor with an attachment factor (see below) or a bandage soft contact lens may improve epithelial adherence to the underlying stroma. In a clinical trial of dogs with refractory or recurrent superficial ulcers, topically administered human epidermal growth factor (Creative Biomolecules) demonstrated improvement in healing. The patients were treated with 1 drop four times a day, with many of the corneas being healed in 2 weeks.

Fibronectin is a glycoprotein found in plasma and in corneal wounds. Fibronectin is a cellular attachment factor that is thought to bridge the epithelial basal cell wall to the basement membrane. Topical fibronectin is being investigated for its ability to enhance reepithelialization by providing a temporary substratum for epithelial adhesion and migration. Other attachment factors might be laminin and chondroitin sulfate.

Topically administered aprotinin, a polypeptide that inhibits proteolytic enzymes, is being researched in Europe for use in refractory ulcers where endogenous or exogenous fibronectin is degraded inappropriately by the proteolytic enzyme plasmin. Topically administered aprotinin inhibits plasmin at the corneal surface. Tissue plasminogen activator, thought to be secreted by epithelial cells adjacent to the corneal defect, generates plasmin that degrades fibronectin in the normal regulation system of healing. This enzyme system may have increased activity in persistent epithelial defects.

Tissue adhesives (see Deep or Progressive Ulcers) applied as a thin layer over the ulcer may be successful in promoting epithelial healing in refractory superficial ulcers.

Deep or Progressive Ulcers. Ulcers that are progressive or that extend into the corneal stroma are regarded as a potential threat to the integrity of the globe and are considered an ocular emergency. Ulcers deeper than half the corneal thickness are especially vision threatening and require aggressive therapy. When the destructive enzymatic processes of the host or microorganisms become excessive, superficial ulcers can rapidly deepen and perforate within 48 hours. Cytology, Gram stain, and cultures may be informative, particularly if there is a purulent corneal stromal infiltrate, mucopurulent ocular discharge, or evidence of progression. Therapy should not, however, wait for culture and sensitivity results. Secondary anterior uveitis and perforations are complications of deep ulcers.

Standard Therapy. The goals of therapy are as follows: 1) identify and remove the cause; 2) débride necrotic tissue; 3) use appropriate medical therapy; 4) provide protection or support (or both); 5) use supplemental care; 6) closely monitor the eye; and 7) decrease scar formation. Also review the Ulcerative Keratitis section.

1. *Identify and remove the cause.* As with all ulcers, a thorough ophthalmic examination is performed to search for a local cause. If any is identified, it should be corrected.

2. *Débridement.* Necrotic or infected tissue should be gently débrided following topical anesthesia and proper patient restraint. Routine débridement of all deep ulcers is not recommended. If samples for culture are desired, it is best to collect them before instilling a topical anesthetic, which may interfere with the growth of microorganisms (see Ulcerative Keratitis). Topical anesthesia is achieved by applying several drops of 0.5% proparacaine hydrochloride (e.g., Ophthetic, Allergan Pharmaceuticals) spaced over 1–2 minutes. Sterile cotton-tipped swabs, a spatula, the blunt end of a scalpel with the sharp border protectively covered by the blade's foil wrapper, corneal forceps, and small scissors are effective tools for débridement. Unless there is a descemetocele, it is unlikely that gentle débridement will rupture the ulcer. The base of a descemetocele should not be débrided. Cytologic evaluation of the débrided material by Wright stain and Gram stain is recommended. After débridement, the ocular surface is flushed with copious amounts of diluted 10% povidone-iodine solution or sterile irrigating solution (Table 14-4) to assist with the removal of debris, bacteria, and inflammatory products. The diluted povidone-iodine solution is made by mixing 1 part of 10% povidone-iodine (Betadine, Purdue Frederick) with 50 parts of sterile 0.9% NaCl or lactated Ringer's solution. Infected tissue can also be swabbed with a sterile cotton-tipped swab that has been soaked in undiluted (10%) povidone-iodine solution. The cornea is then copiously flushed with a sterile irrigating solution (Table 14-4) to prevent iodophor irritation. Débridement does not usually need to be repeated during the course of ulcer management.

3. *Medical therapy.* The emphasis of medical therapy is to control infection, deter ulcer progression, improve the patient's comfort, and manage secondary anterior uveitis. Medical therapy involves the use of antimicrobics, a

TABLE 14-10. Formulas for Making Concentrated Antibiotic Eyedrops

Antibiotic	Available Form	Quantity of Antibiotic	Quantity of Artificial Tears (ml)	Final Volume (ml)	Final Concentration (mg/ml)
Bacitracin (Bacitracin, Upjohn)	50,000 IU/vial (3 vials)	150,000 IU Use artificial tears to reconstitute	15	15.6	9,600 IU/ml
Carbenicillin	1 g vial	1 ml (100 mg)	15	16	6.2
Cefazolin (Kefzol, Eli Lilly)	1 g vial	3 ml (1 vial)	15	18	50
Gentamicin (Gentocin, Schering)	100 mg/ml	2.5 ml	15	17	14
Gentamicin ophthalmic solution (Gentacidin, CooperVision)	3 mg/ml	1.7 ml of parenteral gentamicin (50 mg/ml)	0	6.7	15
Ticarcillin	1 g vial	1 ml (100 mg)	15	16	6.2
Tobramycin (Nebcin, Dista Products)	40 mg/ml	5.5 ml	15	20.5	11
Tobramycin ophthalmic solution (Tobrex, Alcon)	3 mg/ml	2 ml of parenteral tobramycin (40 mg/ml)	0	7	13.6

Adapted with permission from Nasisse MP. Canine ulcerative keratitis. *Compend Contin Educ Pract Vet* 1985;7:685.

cycloplegic-mydriatic, and perhaps an anticollagenase or systemic nonsteroidal anti-inflammatory agent. The topical route of administration is the principle route for acquiring high concentrations of the drug within the cornea, and fortified topical antibiotic solutions can be formulated with concentrations greater than commercial strength (Table 14-10). Topical therapy can be complemented with subconjunctival or parenteral routes (Tables 14-2 and 14-8), however, these routes do *not* replace topical therapy. Gram staining of corneal scrapings may assist with the initial antibiotic(s) selection (Table 14-8).

Ulcers that are progressive (melting), necrotic, deep, or associated with a gram-negative organism require the topical use of an antibiotic with an anticipated spectrum against *Pseudomonas*. Gentamicin (e.g., Schering) is a good first choice. Tobramycin (Tobrex, Alcon Laboratories) and carbenicillin are usually effective against gentamicin-resistant *Pseudomonas* strains. Carbenicillin (Geopen, Roerig) for topical ophthalmic use is reconstituted for intravenous administration and stored in the refrigerator, where the shelf life is 72 hours. Various drug and route combinations can be employed to improve drug concentration, broaden the antimicrobial coverage, or produce synergistic or additive effects. For example, gentamicin acts synergistically with carbenicillin, but they must be administered at different times topically. Topical aminoglyoside therapy can also be combined with a penicillinase-resistant penicillin applied subconjunctivally, parenterally, or at different times topically. Gentamicin can also be used concurrently with the triple antibiotic combination neomycin, polymyxin, and bacitracin or gramicidin. Whenever different drugs are given at the same or different times by the same or different routes, drug incompatibility must be considered.

The antibiotic should initially be administered topically at least every 1–2 hours and sometimes more often for rapidly progressive or infected ulcers. Subconjunctivally administered aqueous antibiotics can be repeated daily if needed (Table 14-2). As the ulcer heals, topical doses can be *slowly* tapered over several days to 1 week to four to eight treatments daily. Ointment or solution vehicles may be selected, but it may be best to use the same vehicle for all of the topical therapy. Ointments and oily vehicles are contraindicated with perforations or impending perforations, as the oils and petrolatum are toxic to intraocular structures. The preservatives in commercial antibiotic preparations can delay epithelial wound healing; however, dispensing topical medications without preservatives may be dangerous because of contamination and secondary corneal infection. Fortification of commercial antibiotics decreases the concentration of perservatives (Table 14-10). Antimicrobial therapy is continued for 5–7 days beyond ulcer healing.

Atropine 1% is topically applied two to six times a day as needed to promote mydriasis. Atropine therapy is especially important for secondary anterior uveitis because it decreases painful spasms of the ciliary muscle, synechia formation in the axial visual pathway, and uveal protein exudation into the aqueous humor. Atropine rarely has to be administered more than six times daily to produce mydriasis. However, severe miosis may require that atropine be used once hourly for 4–6 hours to dilate the pupil. Occasionally, the addition of a topical sympathomimetic helps induce mydriasis. One drop of 10% phenylephrine (e.g., Pharmafair) can be used two to four times a day until the pupil is dilated. Topical 10% phenylephrine frequently causes transient stinging upon instillation and is contraindicated in patients with hypertension; it should be used cautiously in patients with hyperthyroidism, cardiac disease, and pulmonary disease. Phenylephrine causes little or no cycloplegia. Some cats do not tolerate the taste of ophthalmic atropine, and 1% tropicamide (e.g., Mydriacyl, Alcon Laboratories) or atropine ointment can be substituted. Ointment formulations do not readily pass through the nasolacrimal system. Systemic atropine toxicity can develop in small patients receiving frequent doses, and the signs include dryness of mouth, fever, irritability, delirium, tachycardia, pacing, and dysuria. Owners should be instructed to wash hands after handling the atropine container to prevent inadvertent introduction into their own eyes.

A topical anticollagenase should be used in rapidly progressive or melting ulcers. Melting or collagenase ulcers have soft, ill-defined margins (keratomalacia). Collagenase is one of many enzymes that can be elaborated by the host (damaged corneal epithelial cells and fibroblasts) and certain bacteria in ulcerative conditions. Collagenase causes stromal destruction, as the corneal stroma is primarily composed of collagen. Tissue destruction is also due to exogenously and endogenously liberated toxins and other enzymes. Strains of *Pseudomonas, Staphylococcus,* and *Streptococcus* can produce many extracellular toxins and enzymes (e.g., hemolysins, proteases, lipases, hyaluronidase, and *Pseudomonas* exotoxins A, B, and C). Endotoxin release due to cell wall destruction of microorganisms can also cause local tissue damage. Antibiotics such as β-lactams destroy the cell wall. Furthermore, inflammatory cells have numerous lytic enzymes in their lysosomes that participate in stromal degradation. Tissue damage is further enhanced in patients with tear deficiencies, lagophthalmos (exophthalmic breeds), corneal anesthesia, abnormal eyelid function, and perhaps hyperadrenocorticism. Continued corneal destruction can quickly lead to perforation, iris prolapse, and secondary enophthalmitis. The efficacy of anticollagenase therapy is controversial, yet I recommend its use. Perhaps the beneficial effect I have observed is not due to the anticollagenase activity but, rather, to the mechanical flushing away of bacteria, toxins, enzymes, debris, and inflammatory cells by the addition of another solution onto the cornea. Serum, heparin, cysteine, ethylenediaminetetraacetate (EDTA), and acetylcysteine inhibit collagenase and protease activity. My preference is 5-10% acetylcysteine. Higher concentrations of acetylcysteine are irritating. Acetylcysteine 20% (Mucomyst, Bristol Laboratories) is diluted with artificial tears to a ratio of 1:1 or 1:2 and kept in a dark or opaque container. One drop is topically applied hourly until the edges of the ulcer appear firm. The dosage is then *slowly* tapered over several days to 1 drop six times a day. Acetylcysteine degradation starts within 48–72 hours, and refrigeration may not delay the degradation as was once thought. Despite the short shelf life, I have not observed any problems with using the diluted acetylcysteine for 1 week. Another recommended protocol is to apply the diluted acetylcysteine every 15 minutes for 2 hours, then every hour for 6–8 hours, followed by every 2 hours thereafter. There is some evidence that acetylcysteine antagonizes gentamicin and tobramycin in vitro. With this concern, these drugs should be given at different times. If acetylcysteine is not available, autologous serum can be used at the same frequency of administration. Serum may also supply other substances that promote healing. The serum should be aseptically harvested from the patient and allowed to clot for 15 minutes. The blood is then centrifuged for 15–20 minutes. Red-tinged serum should be discarded. Harvested serum is kept refrigerated in a sterile container and can be used for several days.

Oral aspirin or parenteral flunixin meglumine may be used to decrease ocular pain and anterior segment inflammation (Table 14-5).

4. *Protection and support.* Protection of corneal ulcers is achieved by surgical flaps (i.e., conjunctival, third eyelid, or a temporary tarsorrhaphy) and lubrication. Ulcers that are no deeper than half their corneal thickness do not require a surgical flap unless medical therapy cannot be intensive or the ulcer is progressing. Ulcer protection is especially beneficial when there is lagophthalmos, conformational exophthalmos, corneal anesthesia, or eyelid dysfunction.

Surgical flaps protect the ulcer, decrease the patient's pain, provide support, and improve ulcer healing. Pedical, advancement, bridge, or 360-degree conjunctival flaps are preferred because they also supply antimicrobial and anticollagenolytic products, eliminate motion between the cornea and flap, and can serve as a tissue graft. Furthermore, once a conjunctival flap is placed, topical therapy usually need not be as frequent. A third eyelid flap or tarsorrhaphy should not be placed if infection is suspected. Surgical flaps for ulcer protection are left in place for 2–4 weeks.

If the ulcer is deeper than three-fourths of the corneal thickness, corneal support is required. If the edges of the ulcer are firm, the defect is no larger than 5 mm in diameter, and infection is not suspected, the edges can be sutured with simple interrupted 7–0 absorbable sutures. The sutured cornea may still need to be covered by a tissue flap (third eyelid or conjunctival) depending on the strength of closure and the need for protection. Defects larger than 5 mm require a surgical grafting procedure, such as lamellar corneal-scleral transposition, conjunctival pedical grafts, tarsoconjunctival pedicle flaps, and free corneal or conjunctival grafts. An alternative would be to place a 360-degree conjunctival flap. It is beyond the scope of this chapter to describe these surgical procedures. Surgical grafts and flaps for corneal support are left in place for 2–6 weeks depending on the severity of the corneal disease.

Lubricants are not usually necessary during the early stages of therapy because so many other moisteners are placed on the cornea. However, lubrication or tear supplementation (see KCS) is an important prophylactic measure for recovered or unaffected eyes with lagophthalmos, keratoconjunctivitis sicca, conformational exophthalmos, corneal anesthesia, or eyelid dysfunction.

5. *Supplemental care.* Good ocular hygiene is absolutely essential in the management of corneal ulcers. Ocular irrigation removes bacteria, enzymes, toxins, debris, and inflammatory cells that can accentuate corneal destruction. One of the irrigating solutions in Table 14-4 can be used. It may be helpful to clip short periocular hair. During the acute stages of ulcer management, hospitalization should be considered. Restraint collars are recommended for all patients with deep ulcers. Patients should be allowed only minimal activity.

6. *Monitoring.* Patients should be monitored daily and therapy adjusted accordingly during the acute stages of the ulcer. Progressive ulcers require evaluations more often until the condition has stabilized. Ulcers less than half the corneal depth usually have a good prognosis with intensive therapy and

close monitoring. Ulcers deeper than three-fourths the corneal thickness, but without corneal perforation and enophthalmitis, also have a fair to good prognosis if aggressive medical therapy is complemented by surgical repair, a conjunctival flap, or a surgical graft. Rapidly progressive (melting) corneal ulcers warrant a guarded prognosis and require intensive management and monitoring. Topical antibiotic therapy is usually continued for 5–7 days after complete ulcer reepithelialization. Negative fluorescein retention by the ulcer indicates complete reepithclialization. A thinning or focal depression (facet or crater) of the cornea may be a result of deep ulceration, as major losses of stroma cannot be completely replenished.

7. *Decrease scar formation.* A corneal opacity (scar) usually remains after a deep ulcer heals. Disorganization of corneal stromal collagen fibrils and transplantation of grafted tissue are responsible for the loss of corneal transparency. Anterior synechiae and corneal endothelial dysfunction also interfere with corneal transparency. Corneal scarring tends to be less in young animals and cats. The density of the scar usually decreases over the subsequent months as the collagen fibrils approach a more regular arrangement. If the endothelium is damaged, an area of permanent corneal edema may persist. Corneal vascularization and pigmentation also impair corneal clarity, but these changes lessen over time.

Once the ulcer has completely healed and there is no evidence of infection, careful use of a topical corticosteroid can be employed to decrease scar formation and corneal vascularization. However, corticosteroid therapy should be reserved for those patients in which it is absolutely necessary to improve the animal's vision, as scarring and vascularization normally lessen over time. Abundant corneal vascularization and granulation tissue resolve more rapidly with the use of a topical corticosteroid. Topical corticosteroid therapy is contraindicated in cats with a history or a suspicion of ocular herpesvirus infection because of possible reactivation of latent virus. Furthermore, caution should be used whenever a topical corticosteroid is employed after the healing of a melting or infected corneal ulcer. A corticosteroid with more potency than hydrocortisone (i.e., dexamethasone, isoflupredone) is used two to four times a day for 1–2 weeks (Table 14-6). The use of a topical corticosteroid to temper corneal inflammation during the ulcerative process is controversial at this time and *cannot* be recommended for canine and feline patients because of possible serious complications.

Alternative Therapy. Hydrogel bandage contact lenses have been used to protect and support deep ulcers and microperforations. Furthermore, the lens may facilitate healing by limiting neutrophil access to the stroma and stimulating vascularization. However, necrotic or infected material and ocular discharges may build up underneath the lens and may enhance corneal damage. Therefore, bandage lenses are usually contraindicated in the presence of corneal infection unless they are first loaded with an antibiotic (see Investigational Therapy, below). The management of ulcers by bandage soft lenses is described under Refractory Superficial Ulcers.

Collagen corneal shields (Opti-Cor, Pitman-Moore) have been used to treat deep corneal ulcers, descemetoceles, infected corneal ulcers, and melting ulcers. As the shield slowly dissolves, it conforms to the cornea and offers ulcer protection and support. Rehydrating the shield with an antibiotic can deliver high and sustained levels of the drug to the infected cornea. In contrast to soft contact lens, collagen shields do not become colonized by bacteria. Ophthalmic ointments and solutions can be used after placement of the shield.

Tissue adhesives (e.g., Nexaband, Bionexas) have been successfully used as a temporizing procedure or as the definitive treatment for sterile melting ulcers, corneal perforation, and descemetocele in human patients since 1968. Their use in veterinary ophthalmology developed thereafter but has not gained wide use because the commercially available adhesives can be difficult to work with. Low viscosity and rapid polymerization cause "running" of the adhesive down the corneal surface, and one is unable to mold the glue to the exact shape of the defect. Furthermore, cyanoacrylate on the cornea elicits a marked foreign body reaction, causing edema, vascularization, and discomfort. Tissue adhesives should probably be reserved for corneal defects smaller than 5 mm. Furthermore, the smallest possible quantity of the glue should be used. The high alkyl derivatives of cyanoacrylate (isobutyl and *n*-butyl) that are free from impurities are the best tolerated.

Tissue adhesives work by tectonic support, and they may inhibit further tissue destruction by excluding tear film inflammatory cells from exposed stroma. Complications in human patients are uncommon but include septic and nonseptic corneal infiltrates, increased intraocular pressure, and repeat perforation.

The application of tissue adhesives in animal patients usually requires tranquilization or anesthesia. An eyelid speculum is placed to hold the eyelids apart. While using magnification, epithelium and necrotic tissue are débrided with a spatula or sterile cotton-tipped swab from the perforation, descemetocele, or deep ulcer and from the adjacent cornea. The base of a descemetocele, Descemet's membrane, should not be débrided for fear of rupturing the membrane with resultant leakage of aqueous humor. The adhesive must be applied to a clean, dry surface as a smooth, thin layer. Building up layers of adhesive or using a large quantity of adhesive to cover large defects gives poor results. The formation of a large, elevated, jagged seal causes discomfort and is likely to become dislodged by eyelid activity. Dislodgement of the adhesive seal may cause corneal perforation. The deepithelialized area must be well dried with sterile cellulose sponges (Weck-cel, Edward Weck & Co.) or cotton-tipped swabs, as the adhesive rapidly polymerizes on contact with water and results in poor adherence. The tissue adhesive can be sparingly applied by a 25- to 27-gauge needle on a tuberculin syringe, by a microapplicator that accompanies the adhesive, or by a small polyurethane disk (or soft contact lens). If a needle is used, the tip can be filed smooth or bent back to make it easier to spread glue over the ulcer. The use of a polyurethane disk helps create a smooth outer surface to the adhesive seal The size of the disk is cut slightly larger than the corneal defect, and the disk is picked up with the end of a cotton-tipped swab covered with ointment. A small drop of adhesive is placed on the other side of the disk and then the adhesive and disk are applied to the corneal defect with gentle pressure. After any technique for applying the adhesive, wait 90 seconds and then irrigate the eye with sterile 0.9% saline solution to finish polymerization. If a polyurethane disk is used, it is removed with small forceps after adhesive polymerization is complete. In human patients, a bandage soft contact lens is usually placed to provide comfort and to protect the adhesive seal from dislodgement. Retention of the lens is lessened by an irregular and elevated surface to the adhesive seal. To improve lens retention, the adhesive can be used to focally weld the lens onto the cornea. In animal patients, a nictitating membrane flap or temporary tarsorrhaphy are alternatives to placement of a bandage soft lens. Prophylactic topical antibiotics should be employed after application of the tissue adhesive at four applications daily for 2 weeks or longer. Topical 1% atropine, one dose two to four times daily, is also required if there is miosis or anterior uveitis. The tissue adhesive can be left in place until it is sloughed or it can be removed after 5–8 weeks. Earlier removal becomes necessary when there is leakage of aqueous humor at the perforation site or when corneal infiltrates develop around or under the adhesive. Anticipate a marked corneal reaction consisting of vascularization and edema in response to the glue. However, periadhesive corneal infiltrates may reflect a septic keratitis. When the adhesive stays in place longer than 3–5 weeks, the patient should be closely monitored for signs of corneal infection.

Investigational Therapy. Soft contact lenses can also be used for antibiotic delivery to an infected cornea. By loading the lens with a water-soluble antibiotic, high and prolonged concentrations can be delivered to the tissue. Unpreserved antibiotic solutions must be used for soaking because preservative uptake and subsequent release by the lens may damage the cornea. The high water content and large intermolecular pore size of hydrogel lenses allows diffusion, absorption, and release of most water-soluble drugs, all of which are influenced by the drug's molecular weight. Hydrogel lenses soaked in 1 ml of 0.5% gentamicin solution overnight provide bactericidal tear film concentrations against many *Pseudomonas* strains for 72 hours in normal human volunteers. Ocular inflammation and infection would probably reduce the duration of bactericidal concentrations. There are other published reports of loading hydrophilic contact lenses with carbenicillin, chloramphenicol, and tetracycline. A lens can be loaded with a water-soluble antibiotic by presoaking for as little as 30 minutes or perhaps for even just 2 minutes. Sustaining the high concentration of the water-soluble antibiotic can be achieved by superinstillation of drops at 2- to 4-hour intervals with the lens left in place or reapplication of a drug soaked lens. Similar corneal antibiotic concentrations can be attained by frequent topical applications of fortified concentrations at 1 drop four times an hour. Retention of the lens is decreased when the corneal surface is irregular. Furthermore, necrotic or infected material and ocular discharges can accumulate underneath the lens, which may enhance corneal damage. Soft contact lenses are not recommended in patients with low tear production. See Refractory Ulcers for more information about soft contact lenses.

Frozen corneal allografts and heterografts and lamellar to penetrating autografts and allografts of corneal or corneoscleral tissue have been reported in veterinary medicine for surgical repair of corneal perforation and descemetocele. Modern nonsteroidal anti-inflammatory drugs may be beneficial in limiting corneal inflammation without impairing healing or protective immune processes. Topical cyclosporine eyedrops may have a role in decreasing corneal inflammation and scarring due to nonseptic ulcerative conditions without the risk of enhanced collagenase activity and delayed healing. Finally, other antibiotic preparations for ophthalmic use are also being explored (e.g., fusidic acid, imipenem, and enoxacin).

Herpesvirus Ulcerative Keratitis in Cats. Herpesvirus keratitis is the most serious consequence of feline ocular herpesvirus type 1 infection. Although cats of all ages can develop keratitis, it occurs more commonly in older cats. Conjunctivitis and previous or concurrent upper respiratory signs are frequently (but not always) associated with the corneal disease. Slight blepharospasm, tearing, or low tear production are sometimes the only signs. Unilateral corneal involvement is possible.

Ulcerative corneal disease can be superficial or deep. Superficial or epithelial ulcers usually present as one of several patterns: 1) numerous small and punctate; 2) linear and branching (dendritic ulcers); and 3) geographic. Deep corneal ulceration can lead to descemetocele formation, perforation, and secondary bacterial enophthalmitis. The ulcerative disease can be associated with variable amounts of corneal vascularization and cloudiness.

The diagnosis of feline herpesvirus ulcerative keratitis may be suspected after completion of the clinical history and ophthalmic and physical examinations. All cats suspected for herpesvirus infection should have their corneal sensation ascertained and tear production measured. Both corneas should be stained with fluorescein dye; otherwise, small and superficial ulcers will not be identified in affected or asymptomatic eyes. Diagnostic tests include conjunctival scrapings for fluorescent antibody testing, serum neutralization or hemagglutination inhibition tests for anti-FHV (feline herpesvirus) antibody, and viral culture.

Standard Therapy. Except for ulcer management and antiviral therapy, the general goals of therapy for herpesvirus ulcerative keratitis are the same as for other types of corneal ulcers (see Ulcerative Keratitis). Anticipate recurrences, as latent virus may survive within corneal or nervous tissues. Good health care, minimizing stress, and good nutrition may deter recurrences. Cats with chronic, severe, or recurrent herpesvirus disease should be scrutinized for an immunosuppressive factor, such as feline leukemia virus infection, feline immunodeficiency virus infection, and systemic disease. The infected cat should be isolated from other cats during an outbreak because this disease is contagious. Recovered, vaccinated, and unvaccinated cats can be symptomatic or asymptomatic carriers.

1. *Ulcer management.* Superficial corneal ulceration with loose epithelium requires débridement as described in the Standard Therapy section of Refractory Superficial Ulcers. The rationale for débridement is to remove virus-infected tissue and loose epithelium that could delay healing. Chemical cautery of the ulcer margins has been recommended after débridement. Undiluted (10%) povidone-iodine solution (Betadine, Purdue Frederick) is a good choice, but ether has been suggested because it inactivates herpesvirus. After débridement and cauterization, the cornea should be copiously irrigated with a sterile irrigating solution (Table 14-4) to remove debris and prevent iodophor irritation. A protective third eyelid flap can be placed to provide comfort, but it may impair access of antiviral drugs to the cornea. Corneal ulcers that are deep require surgical flaps or grafts for ulcer protection and support (see Deep Ulcers).

2. *Antiviral therapy.* Several topical antiviral agents are available for the treatment of ulcerative herpetic keratitis, and more may become available as research continues. These agents are usually used singly, but when treatment is unsuccessful the antiviral agents can be tried in combinations or consecutively. The various strains of feline herpesvirus can have differences in their susceptibility to antiviral drugs. The presently available antiviral drugs are virustatic, requiring treatments at frequent intervals for a sufficient length of time. Treatment is usually continued for 2 weeks or longer. Early withdrawal of an antiviral drug in human patients can result in a rebound of viral particles to above pretreatment levels. Virustatic drugs also require a competent immune system. Unfortunately, antiviral therapy is not always effective. An in vitro study of the antiviral effectiveness of available antiviral drugs against six strains of feline herpesvirus 1 demonstrated a potency of most to least as trifluridine, idoxuridine, and vidarabine.

Trifluridine (trifluorothymidine) (Viroptic, Burroughs Wellcome) works by becoming incorporated into viral DNA and causing synthesis of defective proteins. Trifluridine affects only virus-infected cells. I recommend trifluridine as the first drug of choice. Trifluridine is considered more soluble, less toxic, and more effective than idoxuridine and vidarabine. However, trifluridine is more expensive than the other drugs. The rare drug reactions of pain and severe chemosis necessitate withdrawal of the drug. One drop of 1% trifluridine is administered every 2 hours during waking hours until reepithelialization is complete and then every 4 hours during the day for 2 weeks more.

Idoxuridine (IDU)(Stoxil, Smith Kline & French) was the first approved topical antiviral drug for human ocular herpesvirus infection. IDU inhibits viral DNA synthesis by competing with the nucleotide thymidine for incorporation into the viral DNA, rendering it nonfunctional. Reepithelialization of the cornea appears not to be delayed or only minimally delayed by IDU. IDU is poorly soluble and does not easily penetrate intact corneal epithelium. The 0.1% solution is recommended every 2 hours around the clock until the ulcer is healed and then five times daily thereafter. The 0.5% ointment may be effective when administered five times daily. Severe local allergic or toxic reactions consisting of chemosis, keratitis, and conjunctivitis require immediate withdrawal of IDU. Regenerating corneal epithelial cells of experimentally treated rabbit's eyes can show signs of toxicity, which include intraepithelial edema and roughening of the epithelium. Human patients can develop superficial punctate erosions during IDU therapy.

Vidarabine (adenine arabinoside) is a purine nucleoside that inhibits viral protein synthesis. Compared to IDU, vidarabine is more soluble and less likely to cause conjunctival irritation and corneal epithelial toxicity. Vidarabine is available as a 3% ointment (VIRA-A, Parke-Davis) that should be applied five times daily at 3-hour intervals for 14–21 days. After reepithelialization, the dosage can be decreased to twice daily for 7 days to prevent recurrence.

Investigational Therapy. Acycloguanosine (Acyclovir, Burroughs Wellcome) is an antiviral agent being effectively used for the management of herpes simplex virus infections in man. Systemic and topical administration have been shown to be beneficial in human patients. Acyclovir is a purine nucleoside analogue with a wide safety margin between toxicity for host cells and herpesvirus. Activation of Acyclovir depends primarily on virus-induced thymidine kinase. Acyclovir's role for feline herpesvirus infection requires investigation. In vitro susceptibility testing found Acyclovir to be less effective than IDU, vidarabine, and trifluridine against feline herpesvirus 1.

Research for effective antiviral agents is active because herpes simplex virus infection is one of the leading causes of visual impairment in humans. Other agents that have been investigated for the treatment of herpes simplex virus infections in human cell cultures, patients, and rabbits include topical polyinosinic acid: polycytidylic acid, intravenous foscarnet (trisodium phosphonoformate), and the co-administration of topical Acyclovir and interferon. These drugs cannot be recommended in feline patients without further investigations. However, co-administration of an antiviral drug and topical or systemic interferon may offer a new therapeutic approach to resistant cases.

GLAUCOMA

Glaucoma is an elevation of intraocular pressure (IOP) that is detrimental to the maintenance of vision. As one of the most common causes of blindness in animals, glaucoma must not be overlooked when evaluating a patient presented for ocular pain, conjunctivitis (a "red eye"), corneal cloudiness, decreased vision, blindness, buphthalmos, mydriasis, or lens dislocations. Unfortunately, early glaucoma is frequently misdiagnosed as conjunctivitis or anterior uveitis, as these diseases share similar signs. Suspicion of glaucoma should be

TABLE 14-11. Canine Breeds Predisposed to Primary Glaucoma

American cocker spaniel	English springer spaniel
Basset hound	Malamute
Beagle	Norwegian elkhound
Boston terrier	Poodle (miniature and toy)
Brittany spaniel	Samoyed
Chihuahua	Shar pei
Chow chow	Siberian husky
Dalmation	Welsh springer spaniel
Dachshund	Wirehaired fox terrier
English cocker spaniel	

especially high in predisposed breeds (Table 14-11), though it can occur in any breed. Education of clients who own predisposed breeds may promote periodic evaluations and encourage them to seek immediate veterinary assistance when ocular problems arise. Glaucoma is less common in the cat and is more difficult to recognize as ocular signs are frequently subtle. The most common signs in the cat are squinting, mydriasis, decreased vision, and buphthalmos.

The observation of any sign compatible with glaucoma warrants determination of IOP by tonometry. Tonometry is also essential for the prognosis and management of glaucoma. The Schiotz tonometer is the least expensive of tonometers (less than $250) but more difficult to use and perhaps less reliable than applanation tonometers. Both eyes must be evaluated, as the uninvolved eye may have a high normal or mildly elevated IOP with no outward signs. Specialists also perform bilateral gonioscopy to elevate the drainage angles.

Glaucoma can be divided into primary and secondary types. Either type can have an open, narrow, or closed drainage angle. The primary glaucomas are believed to be due to drainage angle abnormalities in the absence of any other ocular disease. Primary glaucoma is considered a hereditary condition with a high incidence of bilateral involvement. Patients may initially present with only one eye affected, but the other eye frequently becomes involved within several weeks, months, or sometimes years. Causes of secondary glaucoma include intraocular neoplasia, inflammation, and hemorrhage, as well as trauma, pigment proliferation, lens displacements, lens intumescence, chronic lens resorption (e.g., resorbing cataract), and orbital diseases.

Standard Therapy. Glaucoma therapy includes medical management and a variety of ocular surgeries. This section focuses on medical management. The goals of therapy are to restore or preserve vision and alleviate or decrease pain. To achieve these goals, aqueous humor flow must be decreased to maintain the IOP within the normal range of 15–27 mm Hg for the dog and 15–29 mm Hg for the cat. Aqueous flow can be decreased by suppressing aqueous production or increasing aqueous outflow (or both).

The type and cause of glaucoma, prognosis for vision, patient's overall health status, veterinarian's resources, and desires of the owner influence therapy. With secondary glaucomas the emphasis of therapy is directed at the underlying disease while controlling the IOP medically. Glaucoma due to intraocular neoplasia warrants enucleation and histopathology following complete patient evaluation. Unresponsive or severe enophthalmitis mayalso require enucleation and histopathology after patient evaluation. Pupillary block glaucoma due to anterior lens luxation requires emergency medical glaucoma therapy to decrease the IOP followed by intracapsular lens extraction. Glaucoma secondary to anterior uveitis warrants a complete patient workup in search of an etiology for the anterior uveitis, medical control of the IOP, and specific therapy directed at the anterior uveitis.

Emergency and Maintenance Medical Management. All recently (e.g., within 2 weeks) visual eyes should receive emergency medical therapy. The survivability of the retina is influenced by the age of the animal, species, elasticity of the globe, rate of increase in IOP, and the length of time the IOP has been elevated. The survivability of the retina may be only hours when pressures are higher than 60 mm Hg—hence the importance of early diagnosis and treatment.

The therapeutic response of animals to medical therapy may be less encouraging than that experienced with human patients. The reasons for this difference are not known, but considerations include species differences in the drainage angle and response to drugs and the presentation of animals at an advanced stage of the disease. The response to medical therapy is better with an IOP of less than 55 mm Hg, an open drainage angle, or an acute episode. Unfortunately, medical therapy may be ineffective or partially effective in some patients. In other patients, medical therapy is effective only for an indefinite period of time.

Emergency and maintenance glaucoma therapy are discussed together because all of the drugs (except hyperosmotics) can be used for either therapy; moreover, maintenance therapy is usually started with emergency therapy. Emergency and maintenance medical management uses drugs from the following classes: hyperosmotics, carbonic anhydrase inhibitors, parasympathomimetics, sympathomimetics, and β-blockers. One drug from each class can be used concurrently for additive effects on lowering IOP in the absence of contraindications and side effects.

Hyperosmotics. Systemic hyperosmotic therapy is the most important aspect of emergency glaucoma management. The pressure-lowering effect is observed within 30 minutes of administration with a maximum effect within 1 hour. By increasing serum osmolality, hyperosmotics dehydrate the vitreous and perhaps decrease aqueous production. Decreasing vitreous volume also opens the drainage angle, which may improve aqueous outflow. Finally, the reduction of IOP may increase the eye's response to other antiglaucoma drugs and surgeries.

The two most commonly used hyperosmotics are intravenous mannitol and oral glycerol. Mannitol is more consistent in its pressure-lowering effect and is usually the preferred drug for emergency treatment of acute glaucoma. Mannitol is also the preferred hyperosmotic when there is intraocular inflammation because it does not enter the inflamed eye in sufficient amounts to offset the blood-ocular osmotic gradient. However, the degree of pressure reduction may be less with intraocular inflammation.

Contraindications for the use of hyperosmotics include preexisting cardiac disease, renal insufficiency, hypertension, and dehydration. Glycerol should not be used in diabetic patients because its metabolism elevates blood glucose levels. Mannitol is contraindicated during methoxyflurane anesthesia, as there may be an increased risk of death.

The side effects of hyperosmotics include vomiting, diuresis, dehydration, potassium deficiency, confusion, disorientation, congestive heart failure with concomitant pulmonary edema, hypertension, subdural hematoma, and death. Cerebral dehydration results in disorientation. These side effects, except vomiting, are more likely to occur with mannitol. Congestive heart failure and pulmonary edema may be precipitated in patients with borderline cardiac function by expanding the extracellular fluid volume and overloading the cardiovascular system. With impaired renal function, mannitol accumulates and increases blood volume. Prior to the administration of a hyperosmotic, patients should have a complete physical examination and measurements of packed cell volume, total plasma protein, blood urea nitrogen, urine specific gravity, and blood or urine glucose concentration.

The dosage of mannitol is 1.4–1.6 g/kg in dogs and cats given slowly intravenously over 15 minutes to 2.5 hours. Before withdrawing the dosage, the bottle of mannitol should first be slowly warmed to dissolve any mannitol crystals. If the patient is stable and healthy, water is usually restricted for several hours following administration to maintain the increased serum osmolality. Care should be taken when restricting water in older patients, and signs of dehydration and disorientation warrant fluid therapy. Sometimes I do not restrict water in older patients and still observe adequate ocular pressure reduction. Mannitol's maximal effect lasts for about 6–8 hours.

The dosage of glycerol and glycerine is 1.4–1.6 g/kg slowly per os in dogs and cats. Glycerol may induce emesis, especially at higher dosages. The pressure reduction effect lasts about 10 hours and is more variable than that seen with mannitol.

Both mannitol and glycerol can be repeated two or three times at 6- to 12-hour intervals, if indicated. However, the pressure-lowering effect may not be as marked. These patients must be carefully monitored for dehydration and cardiovascular stress (acquired heart murmurs, respiratory distress, abnormal lung sounds). Mannitol and glycerol are not recommended for maintenance glaucoma therapy.

Oral Carbonic Anhydrase Inhibitors. Carbonic anhydrase inhibitors (CAIs) lower IOP in a dose-dependent manner by decreasing aqueous humor production. CAI therapy can be implemented during hyperosmotic therapy for

TABLE 14-12. Dosages for Oral Carbonic Anhydrase Inhibitors Used for Glaucoma in Dogs and Cats

Drug	Dosage
Acetazolamide 　(Diamox, Lederle Laboratories)	5–15 mg/kg q8–12h (only for short-term therapy)
Dichlorphenamide 　(Daranide, Merck Sharp & Dohme)	2.2 mg/kg q8–12h
Ethoxzolamide 　(Cardrase, Upjohn)	5 mg/kg q12h
Methazolamide 　(Neptazane, Lederle Laboratories)	2.2 mg/kg q8–12h

emergency glaucoma management. The pressure-lowering effect is observed within 1 hour, with the duration of action approximating 6–8 hours. CAI are especially useful for maintenance therapy. Concurrent therapy with a miotic, sympathomimetic, or β-blocker may further decrease the IOP.

Contraindications for the use of CAIs include renal and hepatic insufficiency, dehydration, electrolyte abnormalities (hypokalemia, hyponatremia), and hyperchloremic acidosis. The side effects of CAIs include lethargy, anorexia, vomiting, diarrhea, panting, weight loss, depression, irritability, polyuria, and paresthesia. Patients receiving chronic CAI therapy should have their serum electrolytes and acid-base status evaluated before undergoing general anesthesia.

Dichlorphenamide (Daranide, Merck Sharp & Dohme) and methazolamide (Neptazane, Lederle Laboratories) are usually the best tolerated CAIs, but they may have to be ordered by a local pharmacist. On the other hand, acetazolamide (Diamox, Lederle Laboratories) is usually readily available at pharmacies, though it is the poorest tolerated CAI in animals. Acetazolamide is more likely to induce hypokalemia and an acidotic state than other CAIs. Therefore acetazolamide should only be used for several days until another CAI can be obtained. The CAI dosages are listed in Table 14-12 and should be tailored individually. A patient may tolerate one CAI better than another. The lower dosages are usually used for long-term management to minimize side effects. For long-term therapy, I use dichlorphenamide at 2.2 mg/kg q12–8h PO. Potassium supplementation appears to be unnecessary in healthy patients that are eating a balanced diet. For small patients, a dichlorphenamide 10 mg/ml suspension can be formulated by mixing five crushed 50 mg tablets into 10 ml of water, then adding 15 ml of corn syrup (CPC International). The dichlorphenamide suspension shelf life may be only about 1 month.

Topical Miotics (Parasympathomimetics). Direct-acting parasympathomimetics and indirect-acting cholinergic stimulating drugs (cholinesterase inhibitors) lower the IOP by causing contraction of the longitudinal ciliary muscle, which then opens the ciliary cleft and increases the facility of aqueous outflow. Miotic therapy may be most effective for open angle glaucomas. Miotic therapy can be considered for emergency or maintenance treatment if there are no contraindications. A topical miotic can be used with hyperosmotic, CAI, sympathomimetic, and β-blocker therapy.

The induced miosis is not responsible for the reduction in IOP. However, the alteration of the pupil size changes the iris–lens relation, which may impede aqueous flow through the posterior chamber. This point is especially important with anterior lens displacements and intumescent lenses where pupillary block glaucoma may develop. The patient's IOP should be monitored 1–2 hours after the initial dose. A paradoxical increase in IOP can be alleviated by a topical dose of a sympathomimetic, e.g., 10% phenylephrine (AK-Dilate, Akorn).

Contraindications for the use of topical miotics are anterior lens dislocations, anterior uveitis, and lens-induced uveitis (i.e., hypermature cataract). If there is any suspicion of intraocular inflammation, miotic therapy should be avoided because it may enhance active uveitis or reactivate latent uveitis. Adverse side effects include ciliary muscle spasms, conjunctival vascular congestion, stinging upon instillation, eyelid muscle twitching, and lacrimation. The constriction of the pupil may produce blindness in animals with axial corneal or lenticular opacities. Furthermore, the miosis may cause difficulty in dark adaptation. Miotic therapy in human patients has been associated with iris cysts, retinal detachments, and anterior subcapsular cataracts (with prolonged use). Adverse systemic reactions following systemic absorption from topical administration include salivation, nausea, vomiting, diarrhea, urinary incontinence, hypertension, tachycardia, and bronchiolar spasm. Therefore, the owner should be instructed to instill only *one* drop at each dose to minimize systemic absorption. The medication bottle should be kept tightly closed when not in use and completely out of reach of children. Hands should be washed after each application.

The most commonly used direct-acting miotic is pilocarpine. Concentrations from 0.5% to 8.0% appear to be equally effective in decreasing IOP in dogs, but the higher concentrations are more likely to cause local and systemic adverse reactions. Therefore, the 1% concentration (e.g., Pilocar, CooperVision Pharmaceuticals) is recommended as a single drop topically two to four times daily. The pressure-lowering effect is observed within 15 minutes and lasts longer than 6 hours. Pilocarpine is also available as a gel (Pilopine HS 4% Gel, Alcon Laboratories) with a duration of action approximating 24 hours. The pilocarpine gel has been demonstrated to lower the IOP by 25–35% in normotensive and glaucomatous beagles. The dosage is 0.25 inch in the lower conjunctival sac at bedtime. Twice-daily administration does not improve the pressure-lowering effect. The side effects of conjunctival irritation and blepharospasm with pilocarpine therapy may decrease after the first few days of treatment. Corneal haze and keratitis have been reported in human patients using pilocarpine gel. Pilocarpine 1% is also available as a combination antiglaucoma drug with 1% epinephrine (E-Pilo-l, CooperVision Pharmaceutical). The epinephrine-pilocarpine solution dosage is 1 drop topically two or three times daily. (See the next section for a discussion of topical sympathomimetics.)

The indirect-acting miotics are long-acting cholinesterase inhibitors that enhance the effect of endogenously liberated acetylcholine in the eye. These drugs are usually reserved for human patients who are not satisfactorily controlled with pilocarpine. In veterinary ophthalmology, the long-acting miotics are sometimes used to keep the pupil small to prevent movement of a displaced lens into the anterior chamber. Topical cholinesterase inhibitors are contraindicated in the cat. Ophthalmic cholinesterase inhibitors are also contraindicated in dogs exposed to carbamate or organophosphate insecticides or in dogs being treated with a systemic anticholinesterase for myasthenia gravis. In human patients, plasma and erythrocyte cholinesterase levels can become depressed after a few weeks of eyedrop therapy. Ophthalmic cholinesterase inhibitors enhance intraocular inflammation and hemorrhage during ocular surgery for up to 2 weeks after discontinuation. The indirect-acting miotics include echothiophate iodide (Phospholine Iodide, Ayerst Laboratories) and demecarium bromide (Humorsol, Merck Sharp & Dohme). Echothiophate iodide is usually prescribed at 0.03% strength. Higher strengths (0.06% and 0.125%) are available but are more likely to induce adverse effects. The reconstituted powder of echothiophate iodide remains stable for 1 month at room temperatures and 6 months if refrigerated. The 0.125% strength of the demecarium bromide is usually used. The dosage is 1 drop topically once or twice daily. Because they are long-acting drugs, the two daily doses should not be exceeded.

Topical Sympathomimetics. The direct adrenergics lower IOP by decreasing aqueous production and increasing outflow. They demonstrate an additive pressure-lowering effect when used with a hyperosmotic, CAI, pilocarpine, or β-blocker. Topical sympathomimetic therapy can be used for emergency and chronic glaucoma management if there are no adverse side effects. The onset of action occurs in about 30 minutes with a maximum effect about 1 hour after treatment. The topical sympathomimetics include epinephrine (e.g., Epifrin, Allergan Pharmaceuticals; Glaucon, Alcon Laboratories; E-Pilo-1, CooperVision Pharmaceutical) and dipivefrin hydrochloride (Propine, Allergan Pharmaceuticals).

Topical sympathomimetics are usually contraindicated in narrow, shallow, or angle closure glaucomas, as they may precipitate a rise in IOP. Therefore, the IOP should be reevaluated 1–2 hours after administration of the first dose. Ophthalmic adverse reactions with prolonged use of topical epinephrine include allergic lid and conjunctival reactions and conjunctival or corneal pigmentation due to adrenochrome deposits. Tears can become discolored pink, but this change does not require withdrawal of the drug. In rabbit studies, topical administration can cause meibomian gland retention cysts. Systemic side effects reported in human patients treated with topical epinephrine include headache, palpitation, faintness, tachycardia, extrasystoles, hypertension, and cardiac arrhythmia. Sympathomimetics should be used cautiously in patients with hyperthyroidism, hypertension, cardiac disease, and pulmonary disease.

The dosage of epinephrine is 1 drop topically two or three times daily. The 1% concentration is recommended as higher concentrations are more likely to induce mydriasis, a burning sensation upon instillation, and local irritation consisting of epiphora, conjunctival hyperemia, and chemosis. The owner should be instructed to instill only one drop at each dose to minimize systemic absorption. The medication bottle should be kept tightly closed when not in use, away from light and excessive heat, and completely out of reach of children. A discolored solution should be discarded. Hands should be washed after each application.

Dipivefrin hydrochloride is a newer product that is a prodrug of epinephrine with enhanced intraocular penetration. Once inside the eye, the prodrug is enzymatically hydrolyzed to liberate epinephrine. It causes less of a burning sensation upon instillation and less systemic absorption than epinephrine. Dipivefrin hydrochloride is available in 0.1% and 0.5% concentrations, and the dosage is 1 drop topically twice daily. The most frequent side effects reported in human patients are conjunctival hyperemia and stinging.

Topical β-Blockers. The topical β-blockers lower IOP by decreasing aqueous production and perhaps by increasing outflow. The IOP reduction is enhanced when β-blockers are combined with a miotic, CAI, or sympathomimetic agent. β-Blocker therapy can be part of emergency or long-term glaucoma management. The available products include timolol maleate (Timoptic, Merck Sharp & Dohme), betaxolol hydrochloride (Betopic, Alcon Laboratories) and levobunolol (Betagan, Allergan Pharmaceuticals). My preference is timolol maleate.

Timolol maleate is a β_1 and β_2 (nonselective) adrenergic receptor blocking agent. Timolol has dominated glaucoma therapy in human patients since 1978. However, its effectiveness in animal patients is unclear. In pentobarbital anesthetized normal dogs, ocularly applied timolol lowered IOP and demonstrated systemic β-adrenergic antagonism with a decrease in heart rate and blood pressure. However, another study showed that topically applied timolol and betaxolol in normal unanesthetized dogs did not reduce IOP, heart rate, or blood pressure. In normal cats, topically applied timolol lowers IOP. My clinical impression is that timolol is effective in many animal patients.

Timolol is contraindicated in patients with hypotension, bradycardia, congestive heart failure, and pulmonary disease, as transocular systemic absorption can result in systemic β-blockade. I have observed one canine and one feline patient that developed respiratory distress during timolol therapy. The reported human side effects include depression, fatigue, weakness, disorientation, bradycardia, hypotension, syncope, congestive heart failure, asthmatic attacks, aggravation of myasthenia gravis, impotence, superficial punctate keratitis, allergic blepharoconjunctivitis, pain upon instillation, corneal anesthesia, visual disturbances, and rare dry eye problems. Stinging upon instillation and eyelid inflammation have been rare complications in animals. Patients should undergo a thorough physical examination prior to the institution of a β-blocker. Furthermore, the owner should be instructed to administer only one drop per dose to minimize systemic absorption.

Timolol maleate is available as 0.25% and 0.5% solutions. In human patients, the 0.5% solution demonstrates the maximum IOP lowering effect. However, in small animal patients (<10 lb) the 0.25% may be less likely to induce systemic side effects.

Betaxolol hydrochloride is a selective β_1-blocker. The absence of β_2 antagonism allows this drug to be used in glaucoma patients with pulmonary disease. Reported human side effects include mild ocular discomfort, erythema, corneal punctate staining, keratitis, anisocoria, photophobia, and ocular pruritis. Betaxolol is available only as a 0.5% solution, and the dosage is 1 drop on the affected eye twice daily.

Levobunolol is a nonselective β-blocker with no information on its use in animals.

Follow-up Examinations. Follow-up evaluations are important in the glaucoma patient. During acute management, the IOP should be measured several times daily until it is stabilized. Anticipate small to moderate fluctuations in IOP readings throughout the day. Some patients have an initial IOP drop into the normal range only to have the IOP increase within one to several days despite continued medical therapy. In part, this reaction may be due to the pressure-lowering effect of hyperosmotic therapy wearing off. If the IOP does not descend into and remain within the normal range, a surgical decision is required (see below). If the IOP stabilizes within the normal range, the frequency of evaluations depends on the level of IOP, the type of glaucoma and drainage angle, the health of the nonglaucomatous eye, and the desires of the owner. Evaluations may range from weekly to monthly intervals. Both eyes should be carefully examined at each follow-up evaluation. Furthermore, the owner should be carefully instructed to seek immediate help should either eye develop any changes.

Prophylactic Therapy. Prophylactic treatment of the nonglaucomatous second eye in a patient with primary glaucoma may delay the onset of glaucoma in the second eye. A study in dogs demonstrated that prophylactic medical treatment significantly lengthened the time that the second eye remained normal. Prophylactic treatment includes the use of one or more of the antiglaucoma drugs previously described. Surgical prophylaxis is less commonly used. The second eye should be frequently monitored (e.g., monthly or every other month), depending on its IOP, the type of glaucoma, the characteristics of the drainage angle, and the wishes of the owner. The owner should be carefully counseled about the early signs of glaucoma. Any ocular changes warrant immediate evaluation.

Surgical Therapy for Potentially Visual Eyes with Primary Glaucoma. Surgery should be considered in potentially visual eyes when the IOP cannot be controlled medically. In this situation, a surgical decision must not be delayed beyond several hours to several days depending on the IOP. Surgical procedures that have been developed to increase aqueous humor outflow include iridencleisis, cyclodialysis, trabeculectomy, and shunts. Modern drainage tubes and pharmacologic manipulation of inflammation and fibrosis may offer improved results with filtering surgeries. Surgical procedures used to decrease aqueous production by destroying the secretory epithelium of the ciliary body include transscleral cyclocryotherapy and neodymium-YAG laser cyclocoagulation. Focused transscleral ultrasonography has been used experimentally to destroy the ciliary body and create scleral flow holes.

Surgical Therapy for Blind Eyes with Primary Glaucoma. Permanently blind eyes with primary glaucoma can be maintained on medical therapy indefinitely if it is successful in controlling IOP. However, drug side effects and cost may be drawbacks. Furthermore, buphthalmic blind globes frequently develop corneal problems due to lagophthalmos or trauma. My clinical impression is that eyes with an IOP of more than 40 mm Hg are painful. However, most animals outwardly compensate for the ocular discomfort and display no obvious signs of pain to the owner. The surgical procedures for permanently blind glaucomatous eyes include enucleation, ocular evisceration with silicone sphere implantation, and pharmacologic ablation of the ciliary body. All enucleated eyes should be submitted for histopathology. Pharmacologic ablation of the ciliary epithelium and a silicone sphere prosthesis are contraindicated when there is intraocular infection or suspicion of intraocular neoplasia. Idiopathic intraocular hemorrhage or inflammation may reflect intraocular neoplasia. Evisceration with silicone sphere implantation provides an excellent cosmetic result, eliminates antiglaucoma drug therapy, and terminates ocular pain after surgical recovery.

Investigational Medical Therapy. The emphasis of research in humans is geared at controlling IOP medically, and therefore the search for more effective drugs with minimal side effects continues. Apraclonidine (Iopidine, Alcon) is a selective α_2-agonist that lowers IOP in human patients. N-Demethylated carbachol is an experimental cholinergic agent that has been shown to lower IOP in glaucomatous dogs. The use of topical carbonic anhydrase inhibitors and prostaglandins is being explored. Determining the location and roles of α- and β-receptors in the ciliary body and trabecular meshwork may improve the medical management of patients with glaucoma. Drugs that directly affect the trabecular meshwork to decrease aqueous humor outflow resistance are also being investigated.

SUGGESTED READINGS

Blepharitis

Chambers ED, Severin GA: Staphylococcal bacterin for treatment of chronic staphylococcal blepharitis in the dog. JAVMA 1984;185:422.

Peiffer RL, Gelatt KN, Karpinski LG: The canine eyelids. In: Gelatt KN, ed. Textbook of Veterinary Ophthalmology. Philadelphia: Lea & Febiger, 1981;277.

Conjunctivitis

Martin CL: Conjunctivitis. Vet Clin North Am 1973;3:367.
Peiffer RL: Feline ophthalmology. In: Gelatt KN, ed. Textbook of Veterinary Ophthalmology. Philadelphia: Lea & Febiger, 1981;530.

Keratoconjunctivitis Sicca (Dry Eye Syndrome)

Salisbury MA, Kaswan RL, Ward DA, et al: Topical application of cyclosporine in the management of keratoconjunctivitis sicca in dogs. J Am Anim Hosp Assoc 1990;26:269.

Keratitis

Bistner SL: Clinical diagnosis and treatment of infectious keratitis. Comp Contin Educ Prac Vet 1981;3:1056.
Busin M, Spitznas M: Sustained gentamicin release by presoaked medicated bandage contact lenses. Ophthalmology 1988;95:796.
Dice PF: The canine cornea. In: Gelatt KN, ed. Textbook of Veterinary Ophthalmology. Philadelphia: Lea & Febiger, 1981;355.
Dice PF, Cooley PL: Use of contact lenses to treat corneal diseases in small animals. Semin Vet Med Surg (Small Anim) 1988;3:46.
Gelatt KN, Samuelson DA: Recurrent corneal erosions and epithelial dystrophy in the boxer dog. J Am Anim Hosp Assn 1982;18:453.
Holmberg DL, Scheifer HB, Parent J: The cryosurgical treatment of pigmentary keratitis in dogs an experimental and clinical study. Vet Surg 1986;15:1.
Kirschner SE, Cooley P, Kern T, et al. Epidermal growth factor for treatment of persistent corneal erosions. Proc Am Col Vet Ophthalmol 1988;59.
Kirschner SE, Niyo Y, Betts DM: Idiopathic persistent corneal erosions: clinical and pathological findings in 18 dogs. J Am Anim Hosp Assoc 1989;25:84–90.
McLean EN, MacRae SM, Rich LF. Recurrent erosion treatment by anterior stromal puncture. Ophthalmology 1986;93:784.
Munger RJ, Champagne ES: Multiple superficial punctate keratotomies for the treatment of recurrent erosions in dogs. Proc Am Col Vet Ophthalmol 1987;103.
Nasisse MP: Canine ulcerative keratitis. Comp Contin Educ Prac Vet 1985;7:686.
Nasisse MP: Manifestations, diagnosis, and treatment of ocular herpesvirus infection in the cat. Comp Contin Educ Prac Vet 1982;4:962.
Nasisse MP, Guy JS, Davidson MG, et al: In vitro susceptibility of feline herpesvirus-1 to vidarbine, idoxuridine, trifluridine, acyclovir, or bromovinyl deoxyuridine. Am J Vet Res 1989;50:158.
Weiss JL, Williams P, Lindstrom RL, Doughman DJ: The use of tissue adhesive in corneal perforations. Am Acad Ophthalmol 1983;90:610.

Glaucoma

Brooks DE, Dziezyc J: The canine glaucomas: pathogenesis, diagnosis, and treatment. Comp Contin Educ Prac Vet 1983;5:292.
Dugan SJ, Roberts SM, Severin A: Systemic osmotherapy for ophthalmic disease in dogs and cats. JAVMA 1989;194:115.
Gelatt KN: The canine glaucomas. In: Textbook of Veterinary Ophthalmology. Philadelphia: Lea & Febiger, 1981;390.
Slater MR, Erb HN: Effects of risk factors and prophylactic treatment on primary glaucoma in the dog. JAVMA 1986;188:1030.

CHAPTER FIFTEEN

Antimicrobial Therapy

Duncan C. Ferguson and Michael R. Lappin

ANTIBACTERIAL DRUGS

For clinical application, it is most useful to classify the antimicrobial drugs according to their spectrum of activity, their mechanism of action, and their toxicity. When choosing antimicrobials without the benefit of a culture and sensitivity result, the clinician should attempt to evaluate a Gram stain of appropriate infected material. Knowledge of the nature of the organism(s) together with a knowledge of common organisms involved with infections at that organ site constitutes rational decision-making about antimicrobial agents. Because detailed information on the treatment of specific bacterial infections is covered in the organ system related chapters, the following discussion focuses on the basic characteristics of antimicrobial drugs (Table 15-1), their metabolism, and their toxicity; and it applies this information to the empiric choice of an antimicrobial for key organ site infections.

Classification by Spectrum of Activity

Broad Spectrum Activity. Broad spectrum antimicrobials are those that control gram-negative, gram-positive, and possibly other organisms such as rickettsia and protozoa. Examples of broad spectrum agents include chloramphenicol, tetracycline, cephalosporins, and some penicillins, e.g., ampicillin and amoxicillin.

Narrow Spectrum Activity. The narrow spectrum agents can be divided into those that control predominantly gram-positive organisms such as the older penicillins (e.g., penicillin G), the macrolides (e.g., erythromycin), and the lincosamides. Agents that control predominantly gram-negative organisms include the aminoglycosides.

Bactericidal or Bacteriostatic Drugs

Another clinically useful way to classify antimicrobial drugs is according to their capability to kill a microorganism (i.e., bactericidal) or simply inhibit its growth and replication (i.e., bacteriostatic). It is a common misconception that

TABLE 15-1.   Antibiotics in Small Animal Practice

Drug	Acid/ Base	Binding in Serum	Serum Half-life (hours)	Primary Elim. Route(s)	Suggested Dosage (mg/kg), Interval, Routes
Penicillins	Acids	Mod		R or H	
Ampicillin	Neutral	Mod	1.4	R,H	D: 10–50 q6–8h IM,SC, PO, IV C: 10–20 q8–12h PO
Hetacillin		Mod	1.4	R,H	As for Ampicillin
Penicillin G		Mod	0.5	R,H	D,C: 22,000–88,000 units/kg q12h
Amoxicillin		Mod	1.4	R,H	D,C: 11–22 q8–12h
Amoxicillin/clavulanate		Mod	—	R,H	D,C: 13.8–22 q8–12h
Carbenicillin		Mod	1.3	R	D,C: 15–50 q6–8h IM,PO,IV (UTI); D,C: 100–150 q6–8h (systemic)
Cloxacillin		High	0.5	H	D,C: 10 q6h IM
Oxacillin		High	0.5	H	D,C: 7–15 q8h IM,PO
Dicloxacillin		High	0.7	H	D,C: 10–25 q8h PO
Piperacillin		Mod	—	H	D,C: 50–70 q4–8h IV, IM
Nafcillin		Mod	—	H	D,C: 10 q6h IV
Methicillin		Mod	—	H	D,C: 20–40 q4–6h IV,IM
Ticarcillin		Mod	—	R,H	D,C: 25–33 q6–8h IV,SC
Cephalosporins	Acids	Low		R or R,H	
Cephalothin		Mod	0.5-1.0	R,H	D,C: 15–35 q6–8h IM,IV,SC
Cephalexin		Low	1.3–2.8	R	D,C: 8–30 q6–8h PO
Cephazolin		High	0.8–1.5	R	D,C: 15–25 q6–8h IM
Cephradine		Low	1.5	R,H	D,C: 12–25 q6h IM,IV,PO
Cefamandole		—	0.5–1.0	R,H	D,C: 15 q4–6h IM,IV
Cefadroxil		Low	2–3	R,H	D,C: 20–30 q12h PO
Cephapirin		—	0.4	R	D,C: 30 q4–6h IM,IV
Cefoxitin		—	0.7	R,H	D,C: 6–40 q4–6h
Ceftazidime		—	—	R,H	D,C: 35 q8–12h IM,SC
Cefotaxime		—	—	R	D: 20–80 q8h IV,IM,SC
Ceftriaxone		—	—	R	Man: 20 q12h IV,SC
Moxalactam			—	H	Man: 50 q6–8h IV,IM
Tetracyclines	Bases			R	
Oxytetracycline		Mod	6	R	D,C: 10 q12h IV
Tetracycline		Mod	5.5	R	D,C: 25 q6–8h PO; 4.4–11 q8–12h IV

continued

TABLE 15-1. Antibiotics in Small Animal Practice *(continued)*

Drug	Acid/ Base	Binding in Serum	Serum Half-life (hours)	Primary Elim. Route(s)	Suggested Dosage (mg/kg), Interval, Routes
Chlortetracycline		Mod	5.5 (humans)	R	D,C: 20 q8h PO
Minocycline		High	6.9	R	D,C: 5–15 q12h PO
Doxycycline		High	—	G	D,C: 5–20 q12h PO
Macrolides and lincosamides	Bases			H or H,R	
Erythromycin		Low	1.5	H,R	D,C. 5–20 q8h PO
Lincomycin		High	5	H,R	D,C: 15–25 q12h PO: 10 q12h IM
Tylosin		—	1	H,R	D,C: 6.6–11 q12–24h IM
Clindamycin		—	14.5	H	D,C: 5–20 q8–12h IV,IM,SC,PO
Aminoglycosides	Bases	Low		R	
Gentamicin		Low	2.5	R	D,C: 2–4 q6–8h IM,IV,SC
Streptomycin		Low	2.4	R	D,C: 11 q6–12 h IM,SC
Kanamycin		Low	0.7–1.0	R	D,C: 5–15 q6–12h IV,IM,SC
Tobramycin		Low	1.5–2.2	R	D: 1 q8h SC
Amikacin		Low	0.8	R	D,C: 5 q8h IV,IM,SC
Sulfas/potent. sulfas	Acids				
Sulfadiazine		Mod	3.9	R,H	D,C: 110 q12h PO
Trimethoprim/sulfadiazine		Mod	TMP 2.5/ SDZ 9.8	R,H	D,C: 5 TMP/25 SDZ q12h PO,SC
Fluoroquinolones					
Ciprofloxacin		Low	—	R, H	D: 5–11 q12h PO (UTI) 11–22 q12h PO (tissue)
Norfloxacin		Low	6	R,H	D,C: 5–11 q12h PO
Enrofloxacin		Low	—	R,H	D,C: 2.5–5.0 q12h PO,SC (UTI) D: 5–15 q12h PO (tissue)
Miscellaneous					
Chloramphenicol	Neutral	Mod	4–5	R,H	D: 40–50 q6–8h IV,IM,PO C: 40–50 q8–12h IV,IM,PO
Rifampin	Base	High	2–3	H	D: 10–20 q12h PO
Nitrofurantoin	Acid	Low	—	R	D: 4.4 q8h PO
Metronidazole	Neutral	Low	—	H,R	D,C: 7.5–15.0 q8–12h IV,PO

R = renal; H = hepatic, G = gastrointestinal mucosa; metabolic and excretory pathways are listed in order of increasing to decreasing importance; UTI = urinary tract infection.
Low serum binding < 30%; moderate binding 30–70%; high binding > 70%.

a drug fits into one category or the other. It is more useful to think that the tendency to be bacteriostatic is dose-dependent. At low concentrations even "bactericidal" agents may only inhibit growth, and at high concentrations "bacteriostatic" agents may become bactericidal. Bacteriostatic agents may reduce the efficacy of a simultaneously administered dose of bactericidal drug. The choice between a bacteriostatic and bactericidal drug becomes important when there is a question about the competence of the animal's immune system. A bactericidal drug is clearly preferable when the immune system is not capable of destroying the organism. Such situations occur when immunosuppressant drugs such as glucocorticoids, azathioprine, or cyclophosphamide are used. Examples of bacteriostatic agents include tetracyclines, chloramphenicol, macrolides, lincosamides (lincomycin), sulfonamides, and nitrofurans. Examples of bactericidal drugs include penicillins, cephalosporins, aminoglycosides, polymyxins, and trimethoprim-sulfonamide combinations. Bactericidal agents generally require active multiplication of organisms to be effective. These agents are also more likely to destroy the normal flora of the body, particularly that in the gut.

Mechanism of Antibacterial Drug Action

The antimicrobial agents are best classified according to their mechanisms of action, which can be divided into four general categories.

Inhibitors of Bacterial Cell Wall Synthesis. Cell wall synthesis inhibitors, characterized by the penicillins, cephalosporins, and bacitracin, are usually bactericidal and require active multiplication to be effective. The efficacy of these agents may therefore be impaired by the simultaneous use of bacteriostatic agents. Resistance may develop as microorganisms produce β-lactamase enzymes (penicillinase and cephalosporinase). Given their efficacy with *Escherichia coli* and anaerobes, these agents may result in superinfection in the gut.

Disruptors of Bacterial Cell Membrane. Bacterial membrane inhibitors are generally bactericidal but are not dependent on rate of bacterial growth. These agents may be combined with bacteriostatic drugs with no loss of efficacy. Examples of this class include polymyxin B, colistin, novobiocin, and the antifungal drugs nystatin and amphotericin.

Inhibitors of Protein Synthesis. Drugs in this category inhibit one or more steps in the pathway from ribosomal transcription to protein synthesis. Bacteriostatic examples of this class include the tetracyclines, chloramphenicol, the macrolides (erythyromycin), and the lincosamides (lincomycin, clindamycin). The primary bactericidal examples of this class are the aminoglycosides (streptomycin, neomycin, kanamycin, gentamicin, amikacin, tobramycin).

Inhibitors of Nucleic Acid and Intermediary Metabolism. Bacterial growth may be inhibited by disruption in the replicative machinery of the microorganism. Bacteriostatic examples of this category include the sulfonamides, griseofulvin (antifungal), nalidixic acid, and the nitrofurans. Bactericidal examples include trimethoprim-sulfonamide combinations and the quinolones.

Toxicity of Antibacterial Drugs

At the time of a therapeutic decision involving antimicrobials, it is important to consider the negative effects of the drug and to consider if the animal's medical condition precludes the use of the drug because of its toxicity or the route of metabolism. Several key forms of toxicity produced by antimicrobials are as follows.

1. **Neurotoxicity**
   a. Ototoxicity (damage to eighth cranial nerve), e.g., aminoglycosides
   b. Neuromuscular blockade, e.g., aminoglycosides, polymyxin
2. **Nephrotoxicity**
   a. Tubular toxins, e.g., aminoglycosides, polymyxins, tetracyclines
   b. Collecting ducts and beyond, e.g., crystalluria with sulfonamides
3. **Hepatotoxicity** (parenchymal degeneration), e.g., tetracyclines, erythromycin
4. **Enterocolotoxicity** (damage to mucous lining of gastrointestinal tract, e.g., pseudomembranous colitis), e.g., ampicillin, lincomycin, clindamycin
5. **Marrow toxicity.** Antibacterials may depress bone marrow resulting in aplastic anemia. Chloramphenicol causes irreversible aplastic anemia in humans and cats. The bone marrow suppression in dogs is dose- and time-dependent and reversible. Trimethoprim also may cause a reversible anemia in dogs with long-term usage.
6. **Other drug toxicity.** Inhibitors of drug metabolism, e.g., chloramphenicol and tetracyclines, reduce the activity of microsomal drug metabolizing enzymes, resulting in slowing of the clearance of other drugs handled by these mechanisms, e.g., barbiturates.

Combination Antimicrobial Therapy

In vitro sensitivity tests should be used, when possible and available, to provide the agents that might be successful and to rule out those that show in vitro resistance. Intermediate in vitro responses may translate to a positive clinical outcome if high concentrations of the drug can be achieved. The best example of this phenomenon is in the empiric choice of ampicillin for urinary tract infections because of renal secretion and concentration of this drug in the urine.

However, it is not uncommon that antimicrobial therapy must be chosen without a culture and sensitivity result. The choice of a single drug is always preferable because side effects are minimized. However, empiric selection requires at least an 80% historical efficacy rate. When a multiple organism infection is known to exist, such as with intraabdominal sepsis due to a perforated colon or when an undiagnosed infection is life-threatening, it is necessary to choose two or more antimicrobial agents that cover a broad spectrum with bactericidal results. Such a choice may also discourage the development of drug resistance if an initial single agent is chosen. However, the reduced specificity increases the possibility for adverse side effects and the possibility of superinfection.

The rational combination of antimicrobial drugs generally takes advantage of synergistic or additive drug interactions of certain drugs and avoids the antagonistic combination of others.

Synergistic combinations include those that result in an antimicrobial effect greater than the sum of the individual effects of the drugs and may result in a bactericidal effect when each drug alone produces only a bacterio-static effect.

1. Penicillins or cephalosporins with aminoglycosides
2. Sulfadiazine-trimethoprim combinations

Additive combinations are those that neither antagonize nor synergize each other.

1. Lincomycin (50 S ribosomal subunit) and aminoglycosides (30 S ribosomal subunit)
2. Penicillin and erythromycin

Antagonistic combinations are those that result in an antimicrobial effect less than either of the individual drugs alone. Avoid concomitant use of:

1. Static protein synthesis and cidal cell wall synthesis inhibitors
   a. Chloramphenicol and ampicillin
   b. Tetracycline and penicillin
2. Protein synthesis inhibitors in same class or acting at same site
   a. Chloramphenicol and lincomycin or erythromycin—50 S ribosomal subunit
   b. Tetracycline and aminoglycosides—30 S ribosomal subunit

RATIONAL EMPIRIC ANTIMICROBIAL THERAPY

The following discussion outlines the approach to empiric therapy for infections of the various organ systems. Greater detail on the specifics of the infective organisms may be found in the appropriate chapter on that organ system. These guidelines for "first-guess" empiric therapy are provided simply as a starting point for therapeutic choices when culture and sensitivity results are not available. A Gram stain of appropriate material should be examined to narrow the therapeutic choices whenever possible.

Circulatory Infections: Bacteremia, Septicemia, Endotoxemia

As the chances of positive blood cultures are small, the first goal in the presence of bacteremia should be to identify the original site of infection. For example, if a soft tissue wound is present, a culture and sensitivity test of material from this site should be performed. If intestinal trauma is evident, it should be assumed that a mixed infection with gram-positive, gram-negative, and anaerobic organisms is present. If no infected site is obvious, the blood should be cultured for aerobic and anaerobic organisms several times, particularly just before a fever spike.

Common aerobic organisms involved in bacteremias include *Staphylococcus*, *Streptococcus*, *Escherichia coli*, *Klebsiella*, *Enterobacter*, and *Pseudomonas* spp. Life-threatening endotoxemia is most commonly associated with the gram-negative organisms. Empiric therapy for these organisms should include an aminoglycoside alone or the synergistic broad spectrum combination of an aminoglycoside with a penicillin or cephalosporin given separately by the intravenous route. One study of bacteremia indicated that more than 90% of all bacteria were sensitive to gentamicin. Aminoglycosides and penicillins or cephalosporins may inactivate each other if co-administered in the same syringe. For resistant *Pseudomonas*, ticarcillin or carbenicillin and amikacin may be indicated.

Common anaerobic organisms involved in circulatory infections include *Clostridium* and *Bacteroides*. In virtually all cases, therapy against anaerobes is chosen empirically. Five classes of antimicrobials are effective against anaerobes. High doses of penicillin may be effective, although resistance appears to be increasing. Chloramphenicol, clindamycin, metronidazole, cefoxitin, and moxalactam are others. Chloramphenicol is the most active against all strains of anaerobic bacteria; therefore it is considered by some to be the drug of choice for empiric treatment of anaerobic infections. However, the in vivo activity of chloramphenicol occasionally is less than that in vitro.

Regardless of the drugs chosen, the therapy should proceed with aggressive intravenous administration. Calculation of the appropriate loading dose is possible using the following formula.

$$\text{Loading dose (mg/kg)}$$
$$= \text{Vd (liters/kg)} \times \text{target concentration (mg/ml)} \times 1000$$
$$\text{where Vd} = \text{Volume of distribution at steady state}$$

Alternatively, a loading dose of two times the maintenance dose can be administered. The administration of a loading dose is safest with penicillins and cephalosporins and is more dangerous with aminoglycosides because of their nephrotoxicity.

Cardiac Infections

Bacterial endocarditis is most commonly caused by *Staphylococcus aureus*, *Escherichia coli*, and β-hemolytic streptococci. A definitive diagnosis should be sought with multiple cultures or culture of extracardiac sites of original infection. If no culture results are available, treatment with ampicillin and gentamicin or cephalosporin is generally recommended. The *S. aureus* organism is generally sensitive to gentamicin and cephalosporin, but β-hemolytic streptococcus are frequently resistant to gentamicin but sensitive to ampicillin or cephalosporins. *E. coli* are most sensitive to gentamicin, and many are resistant to the cephalosporins and ampicillin. Anaerobes are often sensitive to ampicillin.

The use of aminoglycosides should be accompanied by careful monitoring of renal function using serial creatinine measurements and examination of urinary sediment for casts. Therapeutic drug monitoring of the serum gentamicin concentrations can help prevent nephrotoxicity. When starting therapy, the ampicillin or cephalothin should be administered intravenously at a dose of 20–40 mg/kg q6–8h. Gentamicin is administered intramuscularly at 2 mg/kg q8h. Following improvement, oral therapy with ampicillin or cephalexin may be continued at a dose of 20 mg/kg q8h for 6–8 weeks. The blood should be cultured again 7 days and 1 month after therapy is discontinued to confirm control of the infection.

See also Chapter 6.

Traumatic or Soft Tissue Infections

In dogs, surgical wounds not involving the alimentary canal often involve penicillinase-producing *Staphylococcus aureus,* and those in cats commonly involve the *Pasteurella* species. At the present time, the recommended agents for prophylaxis or control of staphylococcal infections are parenteral cefazolin (Ancef, Eli Lilly) or oral cefadroxil (Cefa-Tabs, Fort Dodge). About one-fourth of all infections, particularly those involving oropharyngeal, pleuropulmonary, and intraabdominal sites, are anaerobes. *Bacteroides fragilis* is the most common anaerobe, and clavulanic acid-amoxicillin (Clavamox, Beecham) and clindamycin (Antirobe, Upjohn) are the agents of choice for this anaerobe. For surgical procedures near the alimentary canal, gentamicin and cefazolin, or cefoxitin and cefotetan, are recommended.

See also Chapter 12.

Bite Wounds, Traumatic and Contaminated Wounds. Currently Clavamox is the preferred antimicrobial combination for bite wounds, which involve a mixture of obligate and facultative bacteria of oral origin *(Streptococcus, Pasteurella,* penicillinase-producing *Staphylococcus).* Other drugs used empirically for initial therapy include oxacillin, dicloxacillin, cephalosporins, tetracyclines, and trimethoprim-sulfadiazine. For outpatient management of traumatic wounds or abscesses, Clavamox and enrofloxacin (Baytril, Haver, Mobay Animal Health) are rational empiric choices. For serious polymicrobial aerobic and anaerobic infections, combinations of enrofloxacin and metronidazole given intravenously have been advocated.

Burns. The most common organisms involved in burn wounds are *Pseudomonas, Staphylococcus, Proteus, Klebsiella,* and *Candida* spp. Topical drugs recommended for initial therapy include silver sulfadiazine, polymyxin-neomycin-bacitracin (triple antibiotic), and gentamicin creams. Systemic drugs used for burns include aminoglycosides, oxacillin, dicloxacillin, and Clavamox.

Respiratory Infections

See also Chapter 7 and Table 7-1 (doses).

Upper Respiratory Tract. Pharyngeal, tonsillar, and nasal infections frequently involve multiple organisms. Bacterial culture of these areas is often difficult to interpret because of the abundant normal flora present. It is a common mistake to assume that a purulent nasal discharge is diagnostic of a primary bacterial infection. However, even with viral infections such as feline viral rhinotracheitis or calicivirus, suppression of the normal flora may be clinically beneficial. Therefore, the use of broad spectrum antimicrobials such as ampicillin, amoxicillin, cephalosporin, or chloramphenicol, for several days is often indicated. Following nasal surgery, administration of an antimicrobial agent is often beneficial. Tonsillitis and pharyngitis frequently respond to 5–7 days of oral ampicillin therapy. Chlamydial infections in the cat should be treated with a tetracycline.

Lower Respiratory Tract. Bacterial pneumonia in the dog is commonly caused by *Escherichia coli, Klebsiella* spp., *Pasteurella* spp., *Pseudomonas* spp., *Bordetella bronchiseptica,* or *Streptococcus zooepidemicus.* In the cat, *Bordetella* and *Pasteurella* are commonly observed. About two-thirds of the infecting organisms are gram-negative *(Pseudomonas, E. coli, Klebsiella)* and are resistant to commonly used antimicrobials. In most cases, a culture and sensitivity test of a transtracheal wash sample is recommended. While waiting for the results, trimethoprim-sulfa (Tribrissen) or chloramphenicol is a rational choice. Severe infections may merit the use of parenteral aminoglycosides to which the offending organisms are frequently sensitive. With bronchial infections, the more lipid-soluble drugs (e.g., chloramphenicol) and larger drugs such as macrolides, penetrate the tissue better. When bronchial secretions are severe, gentamicin might be less effective because it penetrates secretions poorly.

Common gram-positive organisms causing pneumonia are the α- and β-hemolytic streptococci and *Staphylococcus* spp. For these organisms, the empiric choices are cephalexin, trimethoprim-sulfa, clavulanic acid-amoxicillin, amoxicillin, or ampicillin, in approximate decreasing preference.

For anaerobes, clindamycin and metronidazole are the most frequent choices. When mycoplasmal infection is suspected, erythromycin, clindamycin, or a tetracycline is indicated.

The routes of therapy for lower respiratory tract infections depend on the severity of the disease. Aerosolization of antimicrobials is debatably efficacious for *Bordetella* infection in kennel cough, where the organism is attached to tracheobronchial epithelium. Standard treatment for *Bordetella* includes tetracyclines, trimethoprim-sulfa, cephalosporins, or chloramphenicol.

For pyothorax, intravenous ampicillin or cephalothin (20 mg/kg q6–8h), chloramphenicol, or trimethoprim-sulfa are rational choices. Clindamycin and metronidazole should be considered if an anaerobic infection is suspected.

Urinary Tract Infections

See also Chapter 11 and Tables 11-2 and 11-3.

When one region of the urinary tract is infected, consider that the entire tract is at risk. Therefore a cytologic examination of the urine and Gram stain are always recommended prior to choosing antimicrobial therapy. Particularly in cats, it is important to distinguish inflammation from bacterial infection. Routine prophylactic antimicrobial therapy is discouraged when urinary catheterization is performed. In cats, *Escherichia coli* predominates in animals following urinary catheterization. *Staphylococcus* and *Streptococcus* are common following urethrostomy surgery.

In the urinary tract of dogs and cats, about three-fourths of infections are caused by gram-negative organisms including *E. coli, Proteus, Klebsiella, Pseudomonas,* and *Enterobacter,* in decreasing frequency. The remaining one-fourth of urinary tract infections is due to either α-hemolytic *Streptococcus* or *Staphylococcus.* Two or more organisms may be found in about one-fifth of the cases.

If culture and gram stain are not possible or are pending, administer a broad spectrum agent reaching high concentrations in the urine for lower urinary tract infection (UTI) and reaching high concentrations in serum and, if possible, in urine, for upper UTI. The aminopenicillins (ampicillin, amoxicillin) and the cephalosporins are secreted into the urine and reach high concentrations. Fortunately, the in vitro sensitivity of microorganisms correlate highly with clinical success. In one study, *Staphylococcus, E. coli, Streptococcus, Proteus,* and *Klebsiella* spp. responded to agents to which they showed in vitro sensitivity in more than 80% of cases. A quantitative determination of the bacterial numbers in a cystocentesis or catheterized urine sample from a patient with UTI should generally exceed 10^5 bacteria. When bacterial counts are intermediate (10^3–10^{5}/ml), contamination during collection should be suspected. Determination of the minimum inhibitory concentration (MIC) of antimicrobial agents should be factored into the therapeutic decision when possible.

The first episode of a UTI should be treated for at least 10–14 days. The duration of therapy in UTIs should always be monitored by the use of urine cultures rather than reliance on clinical signs or even examination of the urine sediment. If possible, the urine should be cultured 4–7 days after discontinuing therapy and again 7–10 days after therapy. Recurrence of the same organism is generally rapid.

With recurrent UTIs the possibility of predisposing factors such as urinary calculi or a prostatic infection should be considered. In these cases, therapy, generally with ampicillin for gram-positive infections and trimethoprim-sulfa, nitrofurantoin, or cephalexin for gram-negative infections, must be administered for at least 4–6 weeks and may be necessary for an indefinite period until sterilization of the urine is achieved. The fluoroquinolones, e.g., norfloxacin and enrofloxacin, are recommended for recurrent gram-negative infections with *Pseudomonas, Proteus,* or *Klebsiella* spp. After sterilization of the urine, preventive single evening doses of one-half to two-thirds the daily dose of the urinary antiseptics nitrofurantoin, methenamine, or the antimicrobial combination trimethoprim-sulfa may be required.

When UTI is documented in male dogs, it should be assumed that prostatic infection occurs concurrently. Antibiotics that penetrate the blood-prostate barrier should be used to treat all male dogs with UTI (see the following section and Chapter 11).

Pyelonephritis. Chronic pyelonephritis should be treated for at least 6 weeks with an antimicrobial that has good tissue penetrance, e.g., chloramphenicol, trimethoprim, or the fluoroquinolones (enrofloxacin, norfloxacin, ciprofloxacin). Of course, if concomitant renal insufficiency exists, the tetracyclines (except doxycycline) and aminoglycosides should be avoided.

Reproductive Tract Infections

With infections of the reproductive tract, the penetration characteristics of an antimicrobial drug are important.

Prostatitis. Initially for acute prostatitis, the blood-prostate barrier is damaged and allows penetration of most drugs into the prostatic acinus. However, after reestablishment of the blood-prostate barrier in chronic prostatitis, the acidic infected prostatic fluid allows the basic antibiotics (pKa < 7), e.g., erythromycin, clindamycin, oleandomycin, norfloxacin, and trimethoprim, to penetrate more readily. Chloramphenicol, because of its high lipid solubility, also penetrates prostatic tissue well. As a result, if the infective organism is gram-positive, erythromycin, clindamycin, chloramphenicol, and trimethoprim-sulfa are the preferred drugs. If the organism is gram-negative, chloramphenicol or trimethoprim-sulfa is preferred. Second line drugs for gram-negative infections include carbenicillin and the quinolones. Antimicrobial therapy should be continued for at least 6 weeks. Urine and prostatic fluid should be recultured several days and 1 month following discontinuation of therapy.

Canine Brucellosis. Brucellosis may cause endometritis, epididymitis, and prostatitis in the dog. The recommended treatment is minocycline (12.5 mg/kg PO q12h) and dihydrostreptomycin (5 mg/kg IM or SC q12h for 7 days) or trimethoprim-sulfa (15 mg/kg PO q12h) given for two 2-week courses separated by 2 weeks.

Vaginitis. In puppies, vaginitis is generally a self-limiting condition and responds to douching with vinegar (diluted 1:4 with water) or povidone-iodine (diluted 1:40 with water) (Betadine). Persistent cases in adults generally involve *Escherichia coli, Proteus, Staphylococcus,* or *Streptococcus* spp. Effective drugs for this condition are chloramphenicol, amoxicillin, and lincomycin.

Pyometra and Metritis. Prompt implementation of antimicrobial and supportive therapy is indicated in all cases. Ovariohysterectomy is the preferred treatment, with culture and sensitivity tests performed on the uterine contents. *E. coli* infection is observed in most cases, with *Proteus* and *Streptococcus* also being found occasionally. The empiric drugs of choice are chloramphenicol and trimethoprim-sulfa. When nonsurgical treatment has been chosen, the intrauterine infusion of antiseptic or antibiotic solutions is of little value.

Gastrointestinal and Hepatic Infections

The gastrointestinal tract carries its normal flora which is susceptible to disruption by antimicrobial agents. Although they are difficult to culture, anaerobes predominate distally to the ileum. Bacterial overgrowth may be the result of oral administration of broad spectrum antimicrobial agents. This condition may be managed with the use of tylosin and tetracyclines.

Antimicrobial therapy is, contrary to popular practice, not indicated for routine treatment of nonspecific acute or chronic gastrointestinal disease. The only specific indications for antibacterial treatment are invasive bacterial infection and potentially, *Clostridium perfringens* enterotoxin producers. Following the mucosal damage caused by parvovirus and hemorrhagic gastroenteritis, intraabdominal sepsis or endotoxemia (or both) may result. *Escherichia coli* is the most common microorganism involved.

The incidence of bacterial pathogens causing diarrheal conditions is rare in the dog and cat. *Salmonella, Shigella,* and some strains of *E. coli* are the invasive primary pathogens of the gut. *Yersinia, Campylobacter,* and *Salmonella* species produce an enterotoxin leading to a secretory diarrhea. *Salmonella* and *Campylobacter* are public health hazards. The use of antibiotics to treat *Salmonella* is controversial because frequent and indiscriminate use of antimicrobials has led to a considerable number of resistant strains. For the individual animal, treatment may prolong the carrier state. Antimicrobial treatment is therefore recommended only when systemic illness is present or the animal is immunosuppressed. The antimicrobials effective against *Salmonella* include chloramphenicol, trimethoprim-sulfa, and amoxicillin. For *Campylobacter,* erythromycin is the drug of choice followed by gentamicin, chloramphenicol, and tetracyclines. *Yersinia* may be managed with chloramphenicol, gentamicin, tetracyclines, cephalosporins, or trimethoprim-sulfa. For *Clostridium,* ampicillum, cephalosporins, chloramphenicol, clindarmycin, linocomycin, and metronidazole should be effective.

When the intestine has been damaged, local and systemic anaerobic infections, particularly with *Bacteroides* spp., should be suspected. Antimicrobial choices for control of anaerobes includes ampicillin, cephalosporins, chloramphenicol, clindamycin, lincomycin, and metronidazole.

Hepatobiliary infections often involve *E. coli, Staphylococcus, Pasteurella,* and the anaerobic *Clostridium.* For the aerobes, kanamycin, gentamicin, chloramphenicol, streptomycin, cephalosporins, and ampi(amoxi)cillin. Given the microbes likely involved, hepatobiliary infections may be managed with ampicillin (11–22 mg/kg PO or IV q8h) and metronidazole (Flagyl, Searle) at 15 mg/kg IV or PO q8–12h.

Because of their extensive hepatic metabolism, hetacillin, tetracyclines, erythromycin, doxycycline, rifampin, clindamycin, and nafcillin are poor choices in the presence of liver disease. See also Chapters 8 and 9.

Nervous System Infections

For activity within most parts of the nervous system and particularly for entrance into the cerebrospinal fluid (CSF), an antimicrobial must have high lipid solubility. Although the penicillins may enter an inflamed site during acute infection, once the infection requires chronic therapy and the inflammation subsides, the drug is excluded and even actively transported out of the CSF. Drugs with the highest ability to penetrate the CNS include chloramphenicol, the sulfas, trimethoprim, and metronidazole. The tetracyclines, minocycline and doxycycline, and erythromycin may cross into the CSF more readily when inflammation exists. For the specific indication of CNS toxoplasmosis, clindamycin is the drug of choice. However, the synergistic combination of sulfonamides and pyrimethamine may also be recommended.

See also Chapter 13.

Ocular Infections

Many of the same antimicrobial agents used to treat CNS infections can be used for intraocular infections. Chloramphenicol (22–55 mg/kg PO q8h) is a good choice systemically or topically as an ointment due to its penetrability and its action against *Chlamydia* and *Mycoplasma.*

The choice of a topical antimicrobial for superficial ocular infections depends on the predominant organism involved. For gram-positive infections, sulfacetamide or neomycin-polymyxin-bacitracin (triple antibiotic) may be used. For gram-negative infections, gentamicin or polymyxin is appropriate.

Staphylococcus and *Streptococcus* are commonly involved in bacterial conjunctivitis. Therefore bacitracin, chloramphenicol, neomycin, and gentamicin are appropriate. A good initial choice would be the combination of bacitracin, neomycin, and polymyxin B (Neomycin, Burroughs Wellcome) applied four times or more daily. If effective, improvement should be observed in 2–5 days;

treatment should be continued 1 week beyond resolution. Systemic antimicrobials are indicated when a conjunctival infection is chronic and deep-seated.

For superficial corneal ulcers, neomycin is appropriate. However, for deep ulcers, the topical use of gentamicin ointment or solution (Schering) given every 1–4 hours is recommended. For superficial epithelial ulcers, chloramphenicol could also be used. Again, gentamicin is appropriate for deeper infections.

For deep ulcers that may involve *Pseudomonas*, gentamicin and tobramycin (Alcon Laboratories) are appropriate; and topical carbenicillin (Geopen, Roerig) is used for gentamicin-resistant strains. Gentamicin and carbenicillin synergize when used concomitantly. However, as the physical combination of high concentrations of these drugs can result in inactivation of the drugs, gentamicin and carbenicillin should not be administered in the same syringe. The reader is referred to Tables 14-7 and 14-8 for first choice drugs to treat external ocular infections.

See also Chapter 14.

Dermatologic Infections

The most common microbes involved in superficial pyodermas are the coagulase-positive penicillinase-producing *Staphylococcus* spp. Deep pyodermas often also feature gram-negative organisms, fungi, and *Mycoplasma*. Most infections can be characterized as microabscesses. The primary infection, usually due to the *Staphylococcus* organism, may be managed successfully by using high doses of such antimicrobials; however, resistance is relatively frequent.

The preferred antimicrobials for empiric use in dermatologic infections include dicloxacillin, oxacillin, high doses of amoxicillin and clavulanic acid (Clavamox, Beecham; 14–22 mg/kg three times daily), cephalosporins, erythromycin, and lincomycin. Erythromycin and lincomycin should be used only as primary choices and not for recurrences because cross-resistance between these drugs is observed and resistance develops quickly. Trimethoprim-sulfadiazine may be suitable but is not as efficacious with deep pyodermas. Chloramphenicol is an inexpensive choice; but because it is bacteriostatic it may not be as effective. Gentamicin and other aminoglycosides should be reserved for life-threatening deep infections. The fluoroquinolone enrofloxacin also may be appropriate for pyodermas. Mycobacterial pyodermas respond to high doses of penicillin (80,000–100,000 units/kg/day) or erythromycin, cephalosporins, and minocycline. Nocardiosis is most appropriately treated with trimethoprim-sulfa.

Bacterial otitis externa may be managed with chloramphenicol, neomycin, or the combination of polymyxin and neomycin. The moist otic infections should be managed with a topical solution, and the dry otitides should be managed with an ointment formulation. As *Pseudomonas* may be resistant to chloramphenicol, aminoglycosides may be added to Domeboro's solution or Tris-EDTA when these infections are encountered. However, because of their ototoxicity, the aminoglycosides should be avoided when the tympanic membrane is ruptured.

The successful treatment of otitis media requires a protracted (4–6 week) course of one of the following drugs or combinations: chloramphenicol, trimethoprim-sulfa, cephalosporins, and clavulanic acid-amoxicillin.

See also Chapter 3.

Orthopedic Infections

Sterile orthopedic surgery is considered by some to be an adequate risk to merit prophylactic antimicrobial therapy, particularly if the procedure is long in duration. When a known infection is encountered, the potential risk indicates that a culture of the wound or joint fluid is mandatory. With all treatment regimens, treatment should be continued for no less than 4–6 weeks.

Osteomyelitis most commonly involves *Staphylococcus, Streptococcus, Escherichia coli, Proteus,* or *Pseudomonas* spp. For the gram-negative organisms, gentamicin and amikacin are commonly effective. Cephalosporins (cephalothin, cephradine, cephalexin, cefazolin) are commonly effective against the gram-positive organisms. However, when penicillinase-producing *Staphylococcus* is involved, oxacillin and cloxacillin may be effective. Acute bacteremic osteomyelitis justifies the combination of oxacillin and gentamicin. For suspected anaerobes, in addition to the penicillins and third generation cephalosporins (e.g., moxalactam), clindamycin (Cleocin and Antirobe, Upjohn; 11 mg/kg q8h IV or q12h PO) may be used. With septic polyarthritis *Mycoplasma* or *Streptococcus* may also be present, and diskospondylitis may be caused by *Staphylococcus, Brucella, E. coli, Pasteurella* or *Proteus.* Nonetheless, similar choices of antimicrobials would be indicated.

See also Chapter 12.

SPECIAL TOPICS IN ANTIMICROBIAL THERAPY

Prophylactic Therapy

The use of antimicrobials in anticipation or prevention of an infection is a common misuse of these agents. Improper use of antimicrobials can lead to the development of resistant strains, which may adversely affect that patient or a future patient exposed to nosocomial infections of the practice environment. However, there are rational and acceptable applications of antimicrobials when an infection is not present. Such applications include primarily the use of antimicrobials in patients at high risk for infection, e.g., diabetics, patients immunosuppressed by disease, susceptible patient age (young or old), or use of drugs. The empiric use of antimicrobials upon placement of intravenous or urinary catheters results in the high number of nosocomial infections in intensive care units that are resistant to multiple drugs. For example, ampicillin has been a commonly chosen agent for "prophylactic" use in small animal practice, and studies have shown that this drug is only 37% effective against *Staphylococcus* spp. and only 55% effective for *Escherichia coli.* The preferable approach is to use absolute asepsis when placing and maintaining catheters. Intravenous catheters should be changed every 2–3 days and low trauma catheters employed where possible. Duration of urinary catheterization should be minimized as the incidence of infection parallels the duration of catheter maintenance.

Nosocomial infections may be predisposed by the following factors: age (young or old), severity of disease, duration of hospitalization, use of invasive support systems, and, importantly, previous use of antimicrobials. The longer a patient is in the hospital and the more extensive the use of catheters and indwelling feeding and oxygen tubes, the more likely is that patient to contract a nosocomial infection. Previous antimicrobial use results in the development of resistant strains and the potential suppression of endogenous flora that normally keep pathogenic enteric bacterial strains in check. The antimicrobials with the greatest potential to suppress this mechanism of *colonization resistance* include ampicillin, cloxacillin, amoxicillin, chloramphenicol, furazolidone, and the tetracyclines. Note that these agents tend to be broad spectrum agents. Antimicrobials that generally do not have this detrimental effect include the cephalosporins, aminoglycosides, natural penicillins given parenterally, trimethoprim-sulfa, and the sulfonamides. Those antimicrobial agents that may be useful for reducing the pathogenic flora of the gastrointestinal tract include oral neomycin and polymyxin. Unfortunately, these drugs may also destroy a significant portion of the normal enteric microflora.

Common Nosocomial Infections in Small Animal Practice

The following bacteria have been associated most frequently with nosocomial infections: *Klebsiella* spp., resistant *E. coli,* and *Serratia, Proteus, Pseudomonas* spp. Each of these organisms may develop plasmid resistance whereby the organism, without being directly exposed to selection by a given antimicrobial, may obtain genetic material from another microbe that was exposed and developed resistance.

Surgical Prophylaxis

It is useful to classify wounds prior to deciding whether antimicrobial use is indicated. For **clean** *wounds,* antimicrobials are not indicated. For **clean contaminated** *wounds,* such as surgical wounds in the alimentary, respiratory, and urogenital tracts, antimicrobial therapy should be considered as an option. Cystotomy, ovariohysterectomy with metritis, nephrotomy, pulmonary lobectomy, tracheal surgery, gastrostomy, esophagostomy, and bowel resection are included in this category. **Contaminated** *wounds,* those where there is inflammation but no pus, also might be appropriately treated with antimicrobials. Extensive burns, operations near infected tissue, placement of prostheses, and long surgical procedures fit into this category. **Dirty or infected** *wounds,* where there is purulent material or perforation of an infected viscus, are clear indications for antimicrobial therapy. Any wound caused by trauma that is 4 hours or more old (beyond the "golden period" for a wound) should be considered to be infected.

The approach to initial therapy for a wound infection should take into consideration the pharmacokinetics of the drug administered. The goal is to achieve early, high concentrations of the drug in tissue no later than the time of a surgical incision. Drugs that are rapidly distributed, such as the synthetic penicillins and cephalosporins, are commonly used to achieve intraoperative antimicrobial tissue levels. These drugs reach peak levels within 1 hour, are bactericidal, and are only weakly protein-bound so they are more likely to penetrate fibrin clots.

General Guidelines for Intraoperative Antimicrobial Administration

1. Intermittent intravenous boluses of ampicillin produce two to four times higher tissue concentrations than does a continuous infusion.
2. Concentrations should be maintained through surgery (repeat every 4 hours).
3. It is commonly recommended to administer a dose at the end of surgery, because the animal is immunosuppressed briefly by anesthesia and stress, and the drug is not allowed to diffuse away from the surgical site as rapidly.
4. Drug administration should be no longer than 24–72 hours postsurgically, as the risk of superinfection and emergence of resistant organisms is greater beyond this period.

Concurrent Use of Antimicrobials and Glucocorticoids

The decision to use a combination of antimicrobials and glucocorticoids often has its roots in the desire to treat an undiagnosed inflammatory or febrile condition. Caution should be used when employing these combination preparations. Generally, the drugs are included in the combination at inappropriate dosages. More importantly, glucocorticoids have adverse effects on the host's defense mechanisms by suppressing inflammation and cell-mediated immunity, decreasing interferon synthesis, slowing wound healing (decreased collagen synthesis), impairing phagocytosis and killing of microbes, and impairing the manifestation of one of the hallmarks of infection, fever.

The immunosuppressive potential of glucocorticoid usage is, to a great extent, determined by the duration of administration. For *short-term* use (< 7 days), glucocorticoids may have beneficial effects if they suppress the results of severe acute inflammation. For any application of glucocorticoids with an antimicrobial, a bactericidal agent should be chosen, as bacteriostatic agents require full participation of cell-mediated immunity to contain an infection. In most cases projected for *long-term* glucocorticoid use, the combination with antimicrobials is not rational unless there is evidence for infection together with the need to treat with immunosuppressive drugs (including the glucocorticoids). Although patients on chronic glucocorticoid therapy are at greater risk of infection, prophylaxis is *not indicated.* As an alternative to antimicrobial prophylaxis, the

TABLE 15-2. Protozoal Infections in the Dog and Cat

Enteric	Species Affected	Extraintestinal	Species Affected
Giardia	D, C	Toxoplasma gondii	D,C
Pentatrichomonas hominis	D, C	Babesia spp.	D,C
Entamoeba histolytica	D, C	Cytauxzoon felis	C
Balantidium coli	D	Trypanosoma spp.	D,C
Cystoisospora spp.	D, C	Leishmania spp.	D,C
Sarcocystis spp.	D, C	Encephalitozoon cuniculi	D,C
Hammondia spp.	D, C	Hepatozoon canis	D,C
Besnoitia spp.	C	Pneumocystis carinii	D
Cryptosporidium	D, C		
Toxoplasma gondii	C		

D = dog; C = cat.

clinician should monitor the animal frequently (physical, complete blood count, urinalysis), recognizing that glucocorticoids may suppress fever. In one study, two-thirds of the dogs receiving long-term glucocorticoids for skin disease were observed with nonclinical infections. Nonetheless, prophylactic antimicrobial therapy carries with it a risk of resistant strains of bacteria developing. Therefore, vigilance and appropriate treatment according to culture and sensitivity results is the most rational approach.

ANTIPROTOZOAL DRUGS

Protozoans cause a wide variety of clinical syndromes in the dog and cat. Both enteric and extraintestinal infections occur (Table 15-2). The reader is referred to individual chapters for full discussion of each antiprotozoal agent and therapeutic protocols. The following is a brief discussion of the drugs with antiprotozoal activity currently used in small animal medicine.

Antibiotics

Several antibiotics have antiprotozoal activity. Please refer to the previous sections and Table 15-1 of this chapter for more complete discussion of the pharmacokinetics of the following drugs. Sulfonamides induce their antibacterial effect by inhibiting nucleic acid synthesis. Several drugs in this class have been shown to be effective for the treatment of enteric coccidiosis. Sulfadimethoxine (Albon, Roche Animal Health and Nutrition) is the drug used most frequently. Sulfonamides combined with trimethoprim (Tribrissen,

Coopers Animal Health; Di-Trim, Syntex Animal Health), a related diami-nopyrimidine antibiotic, have been used for the treatment of *Pneumocystis carinii* infections in humans as well as successfully for the treatment of clinical feline toxoplasmosis. Long-term utilization of these drugs can lead to bone marrow suppression resulting from folic acid antagonism. The cat is more susceptible to these effects. Keratoconjunctivitis sicca and polyarthritis have developed in some dogs treated with trimethoprim-sulfa combination therapy. Hepatotoxicity resulting from sulfonamide hypersensitivity occurs occasionally. Pyrimethamine (Daraprim, Burroughs Wellcome) is a diaminopyrimidine that has been used in combination with sulfonamides for the treatment of toxoplasmosis. The combination of pyrimethamine with sulfonamides administered by intramuscular injection has prevented oocyst excretion in experimentally infected cats. This drug combination has also controlled clinical symptoms of toxoplasmosis in dogs and cats. Pyrimethamine is a potent folic acid antagonist and readily induces bone marrow suppression within days to weeks of administration, especially in the cat. If used, folic acid or folinic acid supplementation is recommended (see Chapter 16).

Furazolidone (Furoxone, Norwich Eaton Pharmaceuticals) is a nitrofuran that exerts its effect by interfering with intermediary metabolism. This drug is not well absorbed following oral administration. It has been effective in the treatment of both enteric coccidiosis and giardiasis in the dog and cat. Anorexia is the primary side effect.

Clindamycin hydrochloride (Antirobe, Upjohn) is a lincosamide antibiotic whose mechanism of action is inhibition of protein synthesis. This drug has been used successfully for the treatment of clinical toxoplasmosis and can reduce the numbers of *Toxoplasma gondii* oocysts shed by infected cats (see Chapter 16). This drug has been used for the treatment of cryptosporidiosis in humans with variable results. Toxicity studies have failed to identify serious side effects in the dog and cat other than gastrointestinal irritation.

The mechanism of action of the tetracycline derivatives is inhibition of protein synthesis. These drugs have been used to successfully treat human balantidiasis. Clinical hepatozoonosis in a cat has responded to oxytetracycline combined with primaquine.

Fumagillin (Fugillin, Upjohn) is an antibiotic that may be valuable as a therapeutic agent for the treatment of encephalitozoonosis in the dog and cat. This drug is not currently commercially available.

Monensin (Elancoban, Elanco, UK) is an antibiotic with anticoccidial effects. This drug has been used to successfully suppress *T. gondii* oocyst shedding (see Chapter 16). There are no significant toxicities when used in the cat.

Aromatic Diamidines

The major drugs among the aromatic diamidines are pentamidine isethionate (Pentam 300, LyphoMed), diminazene aceturate (Berenil, Hoechst, UK), and imidocarb dipropionate (Imidocarb, Burroughs Wellcome). Berenil and Imidocarb are currently unavailable in the United States. The mechanism of antiprotozoal activity of these drugs is inhibition of nucleic acid metabolism. The primary use is the treatment of babesiosis in the dog and cat. The drugs are static but rapidly decrease the number of circulating *Babesia,* lessening clinical signs of disease. Each agent has variable effects on different species of *Babesia.* Pentamidine also has effect against some *Leishmania* spp. and *Pneumocystis carinii.* Imidocarb also has been used to decrease numbers of circulating *Hepatozoon* organisms in the dog, but its effect on clinical illness is undetermined. Diamidine administration frequently induces hypotension, pain and swelling at the injection site, anaphylaxis, vomiting, diarrhea, nausea, and central nervous system disturbances.

Acridine Dyes

Quinacrine hydrochloride (Atabrine, Winthrop-Breon) is a drug commonly used for the treatment of giardiasis in the dog. This drug has controlled clinical signs of giardiasis in cats but does not always totally eliminate organism shedding. The mechanism of action against *Giardia* has not been ascertained, but the drug probably interferes with nucleic acid synthesis. Multiple side effects, including fever, pruritus, vomiting, anorexia, red urine, hepatotoxicity, and neurologic signs have been reported.

Primaquine phosphate (Winthrop-Breon) is a synthetic 8-aminoquinolone derivative structurally similar to quinacrine. This drug has been used successfully for the treatment of hepatozoonosis in the dog and the cat.

Azonaphthalene Dyes

Intravenous injection of trypan blue has been used to treat babesiosis in the dog. It is not as effective as the aromatic diamidines, and its use is no longer recommended.

Nitroimidazoles

Metronidazole (Flagyl, Searle) is the drug of choice for treatment of giardiasis in the dog and cat. It is also the primary therapy for *Entamoeba histolytica, Balantidium coli,* and *Pentatrichomonas hominis* infections. The likely mechanism against protozoans is related to the development of reduction products, which lead to disruption of DNA and inhibition of nucleic acid synthesis. The primary side effect is gastrointestinal irritation; however, neurologic signs, glossitis, stomatitis, and gastrointestinal *Candida* overgrowth have been reported. Ipronidazole (Ipropan, Hoffman-LaRoche) is a nitroimidazole that has been used in the water to treat giardiasis in kennel situations.

Quinoline Derivatives

Nifurtimox (Lampit, Bayer A-G, Leverkusen-Bayerwerk, West Germany) has been used successfully to treat *Trypanosoma cruzi* infection in the dog. The mechanism of action is currently unknown. The drug is active only against the circulating phases of the organism, and so recurrence of clinical disease is common. Adverse effects include gastrointestinal irritation, muscle pain, and weight loss.

Oral administration of diiodohydroxyquin (Yodoxin, Glenwood) is effective against *Balantidium coli* and *Entamoeba histolytica* infections. The mechanism of action is not known. Side effects include diarrhea, abdominal pain, and neurologic signs.

Miscellaneous Agents

The pentavalent antimonials sodium antimony gluconate (Pentostam, Wellcome Foundation, UK) and meglumine antimoniate (Glucantime, Rhodia) reportedly have activity against *Leishmania* in the dog. Long-term intramuscular or intravenous administration is required, and many dogs are not cured. Renal and cardiac toxicity is possible.

Ketoconazole (Nizoral, Janssen) is an imidazole used primarily for the treatment of systemic mycoses (see Chapter 16). This drug reportedly has been used to cure leishmaniasis in dogs. Amprolium (Corid, MSD AgVet) is a coccidiostatic drug used to treat or prevent intestinal coccidial infections in the dog. Thiamine deficiency can result from overdosage, leading to reversible central nervous system signs. Anorexia, diarrhea, and depression are other common side effects.

SUGGESTED READINGS

Antibacterials

Antimicrobial therapy. J Am Vet Med Assoc 1984;185(10):entire issue.

Barr FS, Jackson JW, Cantrell KB: Is anyone immune to the problems of susceptibility testing? Vet Med 1986;81:429.

Brown SA: Treatment of gram-negative infections. Vet Clin North Am 1988;18:1141.

Calvert CA, Greene CE, Hardie EM: Cardiovascular infections in dogs: epizootiology, clinical manifestations, and prognosis. J Am Vet Med Assoc 1985;187:612.

Center SA: Hepatobiliary infections. In: Green CE, ed. Clinical Microbiology and Infectious Diseases of the Dog and Cat. Philadelphia: WB Saunders, 1990;146.

Codner EC: Choosing a treatment course for dogs with pyoderma. Vet Med 1988;83:995.

Dow SW: Bacteremia in dogs and cats. In: Kirk RW, ed. Current Veterinary Therapy X. Philadelphia: WB Saunders, 1989;1077.

Dow SW: Management of anaerobic infections. Vet Clin North Am 1988;18:1167.

Ford RB, Aronson AL: Antimicrobial drugs and infectious diseases. In: Davis LE, ed. Handbook of Small Animal Therapeutics. New York: Churchill Livingstone, 1985;45.

Greene CE, Ferguson DC: Antibacterial chemotherapy. In: Greene CE, ed. Clinical Microbiology and Infectious Diseases of the Dog and Cat. Philadelphia: WB Saunders, 1990;461.

Hardie EM: Endotoxemia. In: Greene CE, ed. Clinical Microbiology and Infectious Diseases of the Dog and Cat. Philadelphia: WB Saunders, 1990;494.

Johnston DE, ed: The Bristol Veterinary Handbook of Antimicrobial Therapy, 2nd ed. Evansville: Bristol Meyers U.S. Pharmaceutical and Nutritional Group 1987;1.

Kalant H, Roschlau WHE, eds. Principles of Medical Pharmacology, 5th ed. New York: BC Decker, 1989;530.

Papich MG: Therapy of gram-positive bacterial infections. Vet Clin North Am 1988; 18:1267.

Penwick RC: Perioperative antimicobial chemoprophylaxis in gastrointestinal surgery. J Am Anim Hosp Assoc 1988;24(2):133–145.

Rosin E: Empirical selection of antibiotics in small animal surgery. Compend Contin Ed (Small Animal) 1990;12(2):231–232

Antiprotozoals

Abbitt B, Huey RL, Eugster AK, Syler J: Treatment of giardiasis in adult greyhounds using ipronidazole-medicated water. J Am Vet Med Assoc 1986;188:67.

Breitschwerdt E: Babesiosis. In: Green CE, ed. Clinical Microbiology and Infectious Diseases of the Dog and Cat, 1st ed. Philadelphia: WB Saunders, 1984;796.

Brightman AH, Slonka GF: A review of five clinical cases of giardiasis in cats. J Am Anim Hosp Assoc 1976;12:492.

Dubey JP, Yeary RA: Anticoccidial activity of 2-sulfamoyl-4-diaminodiphenylsulfone sulfadiazine, pyrimethamine, and clindamycin in cats infected with *Toxoplasma gondii.* Can Vet J 1977;18:51.

Frenkel JK, Smith DD: Inhibitory effects of monensin on shedding of *Toxoplasma* oocysts by cats. J Parasitol 1982;68:851.

Garett A: Visceral leishmaniasis. Southwest Vet 1978;31:125.

Giger U, Werner LL, Millichamp NJ, Gorman NT: Sulfadiazine-induced allergy in six Doberman pinschers. J Am Vet Med Assoc 1985;186:479.

Greene CE, Cook JR, Mahaffey EA: Clindamycin for treatment of *Toxoplasma* polymyositis in a dog. J Am Vet Med Assoc 1985;187:631.

Hughes WT: *Pneumocystis carinii.* In: Mandell GL, Douglas RG, Bennett JE, eds. Principles and Practice of Infectious Diseases. New York: John Wiley & Sons, 1979;2137.

Lappin MR, Greene CE, Winston S, et al: Clinical feline toxoplasmosis: serologic diagnosis and therapeutic management of 15 cases. J Vet Intern Med 1989; 3:139.

Ogunkoya AB, Adejanju JB, Aliu Yo: Experiences with the use of Imizol in treating parasites in Nigeria. J Small Anim Pract 1981;22:775.

Szabo JR, Pang V, Shadduck JA: Encephalitozoonosis. In: Green CE, ed. Clinical Microbiology and Infectious Diseases of the Dog and Cat, 1st ed. Philadelphia: WB Saunders, 1984:781.

Tippit TS: Canine trypanosomiasis (Chagas' disease). Southwest Vet 1978;31:97.

Van Amstel S. Hepatozoonoses in 'n kat. J S Afr Vet Assoc 1979;50:215.

CHAPTER SIXTEEN

Infectious Diseases

Michael R. Lappin

This chapter details the therapy for a select group of viral, bacterial, fungal, rickettsial, and protozoal agents that infect the dog and the cat. The reader is referred to individual chapters for further discussion of other infectious diseases and for further coverage of drugs and potential drug reactions.

VIRAL DISEASES

Feline leukemia virus, feline infectious peritonitis virus, and feline immunodeficiency virus are three of the most common viruses that infect domestic cats. Each of these viruses can induce a multitude of clinical syndromes. Unfortunately, there is no primary therapeutic agent universally effective for the treatment of infection. Usually, supportive therapy for the control of clinical signs of disease is all that can be offered. The following is a brief discussion of each infectious agent and the clinical management of common syndromes.

FeLV Infection

Feline leukemia virus (FeLV) is in the virus family Retroviridae, subfamily Oncovirinae. Infection by this subfamily of viruses can result in the development of neoplasia. More commonly, FeLV infection leads to immunosuppression and predisposition to other infectious diseases including toxoplasmosis, cryptococcosis, hemobartonellosis, feline infectious peritonitis, pyothorax, and bacterial rhinitis and stomatitis. The virus also can induce multiple hematologic abnormalities, fever, cachexia, abortion, infertility, glomerulonephritis, polyarthritis, osteochondromatosis, fading kitten syndrome, and distinctive lymphadenopathy.

Confirmation of FeLV infection in practice is primarily based on the demonstration of FeLV antigens using immunofluorescent antibody (peripheral blood leukocytes, platelets, or bone marrow smears) or ELISA (serum, saliva, or tears). A positive immunofluorescent antibody test generally indicates persistent viremia. Positive ELISA results from healthy cats should be rechecked to rule out transient viremia. Once the presence of viremia is documented, multiple therapeutic options exist, depending on the primary clinical syndrome.

Standard Therapy. Most cats with FeLV infection have secondary infections due to immunosuppression induced by the virus or its products. Chronic rhinitis and stomatitis often respond to oral administration of broad spectrum antibiotics. Many cases have overgrowth of anaerobic organisms and so often respond to antibiotics such as the penicillin derivatives, metronidazole, and clindamycin hydrochloride. Metronidazole (Flagyl, Searle) administered at a dosage of 10–15 mg/kg PO three times daily, amoxicillin (Amoxitabs, Smith-Kline Beecham) at a dosage of 11 mg/kg PO twice daily, or clindamycin hydrochloride (Antirobe, Upjohn) at a dosage of 5.5–11.0 mg/kg PO one or two times daily are often effective at decreasing local inflammation due to the bacterial component of the disease, but they rarely lead to a cure. Often these drugs can be used on a once daily or every other day administration schedule to minimize oral discomfort or congestion due to rhinitis. Metronidazole is generally safe but has been associated with anorexia, hepatotoxicity, diarrhea, and central nervous system (CNS) disease. Clindamycin is not currently approved for use in the cat, but toxicity studies have identified no significant side effects other than occasional gastrointestinal irritation (see section on toxoplasmosis). Gentamicin sulfate combined with betamethasone (Gentacin Durafilm, Schering) instilled into the nares twice daily also has been used successfully by the author.

Cases of lymphocytic-plasmacytic gingivitis have been documented in some cats with FeLV infection. Therapy with glucocorticoids, azathioprine, and gold salts combined with maintenance of good oral hygiene have been attempted with variable success (see section on disorders of the oral cavity). Topical therapy using 1% chloramphenicol solution (Chloromycetin, Parke-Davis) in fluocinolone acetonide-dimethylsulfoxide solution (Synotic, Syntex) (80 mg Chloromycetin added to 8 ml Synotic) applied to the gums twice daily reduces inflammation and discomfort in some cats. This solution also may be instilled into the nares twice daily to relieve congestion in cats with rhinitis. The management of systemic mycotic infections is discussed later in this chapter. The management of pyothorax is covered later in this chapter and in Chapter 7.

Fever associated with FeLV infection may be due to the virus or to secondary invaders. The indication for antipyretic therapy is unknown. Weight loss and anorexia also can be induced by the virus or by secondary invaders. Secondary infections should be managed primarily. Diazepam (Valium, Roche) administered at 0.2 mg/kg IV up to three times daily often stimulates immediate ingestion of food but rarely results in the consumption of total caloric needs. Oxazepam (Serax, Wyeth) administered at 1.25–2.5 mg PO up to three times daily may stimulate appetite within 20 minutes after administration. Unfortunately, the appetite-stimulating effects of the benzodiazepine derivatives are usually transient. Enteral nutrition can be supplied via force feeding or nasogastric, pharyngostomy, gastrostomy, or jejunostomy tube.

Hematologic abnormalities associated with FeLV infection include nonregenerative anemia, regenerative anemia associated with hemolysis (approximately

10% of the cats with anemia), neutropenia, thrombocytopenia, and pancytopenia, which often are FeLV strain-specific abnormalities. Nonregenerative anemia, neutropenia, thrombocytopenia, and pancytopenia may be due to myeloproliferative disease, direct viral destruction of precursor cells, or possibly immune reactions induced by the virus and directed at precursor or circulating cells. Coombs'-positive hemolytic anemias that develop in some cases may result from viral induction of red blood cell membrane changes or from secondary infection with *Haemobartonella felis*. When concurrent *H. felis* infection exists, tetracycline administered at a dosage of 22 mg/kg PO three times daily for 14–21 days is indicated. See the section on rickettsial diseases in this chapter for further discussion.

Administration of supportive therapies such as hematinic agents, vitamin B_{12}, folic acid, and anabolic steroids generally has been unsuccessful in the management of the nonregenerative anemia. Immunosuppressive therapy may be required for the management of hemolytic anemia. Prednisone (Deltasone, Upjohn) administered at a dosage of 2.2 mg/kg PO daily is often successful. For severe or refractory disease, azathioprine (Imuran, Burroughs Wellcome) can be administered at a dosage of 0.5–1.0 mg/kg PO every other day. Blood transfusions are required in some cases but should be administered only if the packed cell volume (PCV) is less than 10 or severe clinical signs exist. Information concerning immunosuppressive therapy for the treatment of other hematologic abnormalities is limited, and this form of therapy may be contraindicated. Prophylactic antibiotic therapy may be indicated in cats with severe neutropenia. A bactericidal, broad spectrum drug with few side effects should be chosen, e.g., amoxicillin (Amoxitabs, SmithKline Beecham) administered at a dosage of 11 mg/kg PO twice daily during neutropenic episodes.

There is no known specific therapy for abortion, infertility, osteochondromatosis, CNS disease, or the fading kitten syndrome. Abortion and infertility should be managed in a breeding operation by testing and removing viremic cats. Glomerulonephritis is thought to be due to persistent FeLV antigenemia and subsequent immune complex deposition. Polyarthritis also may be due to immune-complex deposition. Immunosuppressive therapy for the treatment of glomerulonephritis and polyarthritis may decrease inflammation but is controversial, as many of the affected animals are already immunosuppressed by the virus. Extracorporeal immunoabsorption can be used to remove immune complexes but is not routinely available. See Chapter 11 for a further discussion of the management of glomerulonephritis. Distinctive lymphadenopathy often resolves spontaneously but may progress to lymphosarcoma. See the Suggested Readings list for reviews of the treatment of lymphosarcoma.

The prognosis for persistently viremic cats is guarded. It has been estimated that 83% of persistently viremic cats die of FeLV-related diseases within 3.5 years. The prognosis varies based on the clinical syndrome and initial response to therapy.

Antiviral and Investigational Therapies. Optimal therapy for all FeLV-related syndromes would involve clearing the body of the virus. Several antiviral drugs have been evaluated for treatment of FeLV infection. No therapeutic agent has been shown to clear the body of the organism following persistent viremia. Zidovudine (Retrovir, Burroughs Wellcome) inhibits reverse transcriptase. When administered to cats at a dosage 10–20 mg/kg PO divided twice daily for 6 weeks and initiated within the first 14–21 days after infection, this drug can block the development of persistent viremia. When given to viremic cats, zidovudine only decreases the viral antigen load. Passive immunotherapy, the transfer of serum from immune cats to viremic cats, has aided in the treatment of some cases of lymphosarcoma but has not changed the level of viremia. Immune system stimulation using drugs such as interferon or levamisole has been attempted with little clinical benefit noted. Oral administration of alpha interferon has reportedly led to cessation of viremia and improvement in clinical signs of some cats. Blood constituents such as fibronectin also may be valuable adjunct therapeutic agents for the treatment of lymphosarcoma. Bone marrow transplantation from immune cats to FeLV-infected cats following whole body irradiation shows promise for the clearance of viremia. Human recombinant erythropoietin (Epogen, Amgen, Inc.) has improved the non-regenerative anemia in some cats.

FIPV Infection

Feline infectious peritonitis virus (FIPV) is a coronavirus that is likely transmitted via the feces or in utero. It is possible that some cats become infected by contact with oronasal secretions or urine from infected cats. Most cats with FIPV infection are purebred. The peak incidence of infection is between 6 and 12 months of age, with an increased incidence also seen in cats 14–15 years of age.

After exposure to the organism a combination of humoral and cell-mediated immune responses develop. If the cell-mediated response is adequate, the viremia is terminated and the cat should not develop clinical signs of disease. If cell-mediated immune responses are suboptimal, two forms of disease are recognized, both of which result from the development of vasculitis. Vasculitis is caused by the formation and deposition of small immune complexes during the strong humoral antibody response to infection. The effusive form is fulminating and develops in cats that have a poor cell-mediated immune response. This form is characterized by the presence of fibrinous serositis leading to the development of pleural or peritoneal effusions. Noneffusive FIPV infection is characterized by the development of pyogranulomatous lesions in the parenchymal organs, CNS, and eyes. This form of disease develops in cats with partial cell-mediated immune responses.

Clinical signs can be diverse, as the vasculitis can occur in most body tissues. Fever, anorexia, weight loss, lethargy, and malaise can occur with either form of disease. Progressive abdominal distention and respiratory distress due to the development of effusion are common in the effusive form. Renal, CNS and ocular abnormalities are common with the noneffusive form. Both anterior uveitis and choroiditis are common in cats with the noneffusive form. CNS manifestations are variable. Hematologic and biochemical abnormalities associated with clinical illness are not pathognomonic. Mild normocytic, normochromic anemia, neutrophilic leukocytosis, lymphopenia, azotemia, hyperbilirubinemia, increased liver enzymes, and hyperproteinemia characterized by hyperglobulinemia are common findings. The effusion is classified as a non-septic exudate. A presumptive diagnosis of FIPV infection is made based on clinical and laboratory findings, FIPV serology, and the exclusion of other diseases causing similar syndromes. Definitive diagnosis can be based only on the histopathologic presence of the virus or characteristic lesions. Concurrent FeLV infection is common.

Standard Therapy. Supportive care and administration of glucocorticoids or cytotoxic agents to control inflammation induced by immune-complex deposition are the most commonly prescribed treatment regimens. Prednisone (Deltasone, Upjohn) at a dosage of 2.2–4.4 mg/kg PO daily alone or in combination with cytotoxic agents such as cyclophosphamide (Cytoxan, Bristol-Myers Oncology) at a dosage of 2–4 mg/kg PO daily for 4 days each week have reportedly induced clinical remission in some cats. Cyclophosphamide is particularly valuable because it purportedly exerts its effects primarily on B lymphocytes and thus may decrease immune complex formation. When combination therapy is used, ampicillin (Ampicillin trihydrate capsules, Lederle) at a dosage of 22 mg/kg PO three times daily has also been administered. It has been difficult to assess the response to therapy, as spontaneous remission occurs in some cats. Dyspnea associated with the effusive form can be lessened by pleural or peritoneal centesis. Ocular manifestations of disease are generally treated topically with anti-inflammatory agents, e.g., 1% prednisone acetate (EconoPred, Alcon) one drop applied to the affected eye(s) three or four times daily; however, posterior segment disease may also require systemic anti-inflammatory therapy (see Chapter 14).

The primary side effect from the use of immunosuppressive drugs is that the drugs may induce dissemination of the virus. They also predispose the animal to secondary infections. The use of prednisolone or prednisone in cats with renal involvement may increase the degree of azotemia. Cyclophosphamide has been associated with hemorrhagic cystitis and may predispose to the development of transitional cell carcinoma of the lower urinary tract. The prognosis with either form of FIPV infection is grave. The more common effusive form often has more rapid progression. Response to therapy is nonspecific, varies with the form of FIPV infection, and is generally monitored by improved attitude and appetite. Concurrent FeLV infection generally results in poorer prognosis.

Investigational Therapy. Antiviral agents such as ribavirin (Virazole, ICN Pharmaceuticals) and immunomodulating agents such as recombinant DNA human α-interferon (Hoffman-LaRoche) have shown promise for the treatment of FIPV infection. Optimally, drug therapy should be aimed at strengthening the cell-mediated immune system responses against FIPV while suppressing the humoral immune responses against the virus and concurrently killing the virus itself. Although work with interferon has shown promise, no drug is currently available that definitively increases survival time or cures infection.

Feline Immunodeficiency Viral Infection

The feline immunodeficiency virus (FIV) is a member of the virus family Retroviridae, subfamily Lentivirinae. This virus leads to persistent, lifelong infection commonly leading to an immunodeficiency syndrome that predisposes the host to the development of chronic infections. Aggressive biting behavior is thought to be the primary route of transmission. The virus replicates in T lymphocytes. After exposure, the virus disseminates throughout the body, initially leading to low-grade fever and generalized lymphadenopathy. Anemia and lowered leukocyte counts are common sequelae. After a latent period of variable length, immunodeficiency develops as the terminal stage of infection.

Clinical signs are diverse owing to the wide range of secondary infectious agents associated with immunodeficiency. Elevated body temperature; chronic weight loss; chronic small bowel diarrhea; gingivitis; recurrent skin infection (bacterial and demodicosis), respiratory, ear, and urinary tract infections; abortion; uveitis; and neurologic disease are common sequelae to the infection.

Currently, diagnosis is made by detecting antibodies formed against the virus in the serum. Because persistent infection occurs, a positive titer is considered evidence of lifelong infection. Tests for the detection of virus antigen are being developed. Once infection is confirmed, there are multiple therapeutic options depending on the clinical signs of the disease. Many of these cats are clinically healthy, and therapeutic intervention is not required.

Standard Therapy. The primary management of FIV-infected, clinically ill cats includes supportive care and administration of antibiotics to control secondary infections. Rhinitis and stomatitis are commonly improved by the administration of drugs effective for the treatment of anaerobic infections. Metronidazole (Flagyl, Searle) administered at a dosage of 10–15 mg/kg PO three times daily, amoxicillin (Amoxitabs, SmithKline Beecham) at a dosage of 11 mg/kg PO twice daily, or clindamycin hydrochloride (Antirobe, Upjohn) at a dosage of 5.5–11.0 mg/kg PO one or two times daily are commonly used. Chronic infections of other organ systems such as the skin, ears, urinary tract, and gastrointestinal tract are managed as discussed in previous sections and chapters. The major difference in the management of these cases is that immunosuppression results in most cats, requiring long-term therapy or multiple treatment periods for the management of recurrent disease. Clinical feline toxoplasmosis occurs frequently as a sequela of immunodeficiency

induced by FIV infection. Treatment with clindamycin hydrochloride as discussed in the section on toxoplasmosis has been successful in some cases, but
clinical signs are more difficult to control than in cats that are not immunosuppressed. Resolution of demodicosis was reported in one cat following the
application of a 2% lime sulfur solution (Lym Dyp, DVM) to the skin every fifth
day for 7 months. Lymphoma has been diagnosed in a cat co-infected with
FeLV; it is not known what role FIV played in the pathogenesis of the
neoplasia. The prognosis is variable with FIV-infected cats. Supportive care and
control of secondary infections has extended the life-span of some infected
cats considerably.

Investigational Therapy. Drugs that inhibit reverse transcriptase and directly inhibit the virus are needed. Zidovudine (Retrovir, see FeLV), an antiviral
drug that has been successful in some cases of the acquired immunodeficiency
syndrome (AIDS) in humans, may be helpful in some cases of FIV, but its side
effects are severe in cats. Immunostimulators such as interleukin-2 and γ-
interferon may ultimately be prescribed, but information is still lacking.

BACTERIAL DISEASES

There are multiple bacterial agents that infect dogs and cats as primary or
secondary invaders. Many of these agents are discussed in individual chapters
on systems. This chapter discusses a number of the bacterial diseases that have
been shown to infect the dog and cat, or about which new information is
available. They include anaerobic infections, *Mycoplasma* infections, *Actinomyces* spp., nocardiosis, and *Borrelia burgdorferi* (Lyme disease).

Anaerobic Infections

Anaerobic infections occur frequently in dogs and cats. Improvements in
culture techniques have increased the recognition of clinical diseases caused by
anaerobes. The most important obligate anaerobic bacteria include *Bacteroides,
Fusobacterium, Peptostreptococcus, Actinomyces*, and *Clostridium*. Anaerobes are
common normal flora of the oropharynx, gastrointestinal tract, and female
reproductive tract. Anaerobic infections are also initiated commonly by bite
wounds and tend to develop in areas of devitalized tissue. The most common
clinical infections with anaerobic bacterial involvement include bite wounds,
bacterial endocarditis, gingivitis, retrobulbar abscesses, pyothorax, peritonitis,
osteomyelitis, rhinitis/sinusitis, and CNS infections.

Diagnosis is based on historical findings (e.g., bite wound induction of
infection, the presence of chronic infection, previous poor response to antibiotics); physical findings (e.g., infections with gas production, foul-smelling
exudates, wounds with large amounts of necrotic tissue, or infection of closed

TABLE 16-1. Antibiotics Commonly Used for the Treatment
of Anaerobic Infections

Drug/Manufacturer	Dosage	Route of Administration
Penicillin G (Pfizerpen, Pfizer)	D & C: 22,000 U/kg 4–6× daily	IM, IV
Ampicillin sodium (Omnipen N, Wyeth)	D & C: 22 mg/kg 3× daily	IM, IV
Ampicillin (Ampicillin, Lederle)	D & C: 22 mg/kg 3× daily	PO
Amoxicillin (Amoxitabs, SmithKline Beecham)	D: 11–22 mg/kg 2–3× daily C: 11 mg/kg 2–3× daily	PO PO
Clindamycin (Antirobe, Upjohn)	D: 5.5–11.0 mg/kg C: 11.0 mg/kg 1–2 × daily	PO
Metronidazole (Flagyl, Searle)	D & C: 10–50 mg/kg 2–3× daily	PO
Chloramphenicol (Chloramphenicol capsules, Rugby)	D: 15–25 mg/kg 3× daily C: 22 mg/kg 2× daily	PO PO
Chloramphenicol (Chloromycetin, Parke-Davis)	D: 15–25 mg/kg 3× daily C: 22 mg/kg, 2× daily	IV IV

D = dog; C = cat; IM = intramuscular; IV = intravenous; PO = oral.

body spaces such as pyothorax, peritonitis, or pyometra); cytologic evaluation of tissue discharges (anaerobic infections often have multiple morphologic forms present); and results of culture techniques.

Standard Therapy. Aggressive surgical débridement and drainage comprise an important part of the management of anaerobic infections. Surgical débridement improves tissue blood flow and tissue oxygenation and removes necrotic tissue that had provided an optimal environment for the organism. Establishment of drainage often leads to the resolution of localized abscesses even without concurrent administration of antibiotic therapy.

Table 16-1 lists the drugs most frequently used in the treatment of anaerobic infections. In general, higher dosages of drugs and longer treatment duration (weeks to months) are indicated for anaerobic infections. Aminoglycosides and polymyxins have no activity against anaerobic bacteria. Sulfonamides have questionable effect against anaerobes in vivo. Intravenous therapy is often indicated for the first several days in animals with severe clinical signs and, in particular, cases of bacterial endocarditis. Side effects associated with each of these drugs are covered in Chapter 15.

The prognosis with anaerobic infections varies with the organ system affected. Bacterial endocarditis, CNS infection, pyothorax, and diffuse peritonitis often have a grave prognosis. However, if high dose, appropriate antibiotic therapy is initiated early in the course of the disease and surgical drainage is achieved in appropriate cases, many animals can be saved. Pyometra can be managed with ovariohysterectomy. Alternatively, in the expensive breeding animal, the combination of chloramphenicol (Chloramphenicol capsules, Rugby) administered at a dosage of 15–25 mg/kg PO three times daily for 14 days with induction of uterine emptying by the administration of prostaglandin $F_2\alpha$ (Lutalyse, Upjohn) at a dosage of 25–50 μg/kg IM or SC twice daily to effect may possibly maintain the reproductive tract for future breeding.

Alternative Therapy. Erythromycin and tetracycline derivatives are also effective for the treatment of some anaerobic infections. Unfortunately, these drugs have a narrow spectrum against aerobic bacteria. Second generation cephalosporins such as cefoxitin (Mefoxin, Merck) at a dosage of 22 mg/kg IV three times daily is effective against most obligate anaerobes as well as coliforms. This drug is often indicated for the treatment of critically ill animals with unknown bacterial etiologies. The primary problem with its use is its considerable expense. Third generation cephalosporins such as ceftriaxone (Rocephin Injectable, Roche) also are active against obligate anaerobes but are expensive.

Mycoplasma *Infections*

Mycoplasma and *Ureaplasma* are facultative anaerobes intermediate in size between viruses and other bacteria. They differ from other bacteria in that they lack a cell wall. This characteristic makes them susceptible to environmental factors but resistant to antibiotics that inhibit cell wall synthesis such as the penicillins. This class of bacteria is often found as commensals of the conjunctival, genital, and oronasal mucous membranes.

Several species of *Mycoplasma* and *Ureaplasma* infect the dog or cat, occasionally leading to clinical disease. The organisms are usually species-specific. The most common clinical presentations include cystitis, pneumonitis, conjunctivitis, pleuritis, and arthritis. Infertility associated with these organisms can be due to orchitis and epididymitis, endometritis, early embryonic death, embryonal or fetal resorption, abortion, stillborn pups, or neonatal death. Diagnosis is primarily based on organism demonstration by culture. Reports of clinical disease in the dog and cat are relatively rare, which may be a reflection of the failure of clinicians to properly handle specimens for *Mycoplasma* culture or a failure to request *Mycoplasma* isolation by the laboratory.

Standard Therapy. Either chloramphenicol (Chloramphenicol capsules, Rugby) at a dosage of 15–25 mg/kg PO three times daily in the dog or 22 mg/kg PO twice daily in the cat or tetracycline (Panmycin, Upjohn) at a dosage of 22 mg/kg PO three times daily for at least 14 days are the drugs of choice for the treatment of *Mycoplasma* or *Ureaplasma* infections. If lower respiratory infection is present, concurrent therapy for pneumonitis as discussed in Chapter 7 may be indicated. Topical therapy with chloramphenicol (Chlorofair, Pharmafair) or tetracycline (Terramycin, Pfizer) ophthalmic ointments may speed resolution of conjunctivitis (see Chapter 14). In cats with conjunctivitis alone, polysystemic therapies are not required. Instillation of a 1% povidone-iodine solution (Betadine, Purdue Frederick) into the genital tract two or three times daily may be beneficial in cases with infertility. The prognosis is good with most cases of infection. Therapy is monitored by response. In cases of infertility, records concerning conception rates, litter size, and number of weaned puppies should be kept and compared.

Alternative Therapy. Alternative therapeutic agents include erythromycin, spectinomycin, clindamycin, lincomycin, tylosin, and the fluoroquinolones. Erythromycin (Erythromycin tablets, Abbott) at a dosage of 22 mg/kg PO q8h for 14 days, although potentially less effective than chloramphenicol or tetracyclines, is safe for use during early pregnancy. Clindamycin (Antirobe, Upjohn) at a dosage of 11–22 mg/kg PO divided twice daily can be effective, but its safety when used in pregnant animals is undetermined.

Actinomycosis and Nocardiosis

Actinomyces are anaerobic or microaerophilic organisms that commonly live as commensals on the oral mucous membranes of animals. Infection is generally initiated by foreign bodies or trauma penetrating the mucous membranes with resultant infection of the underlying tissues. Active adult hunting dogs are most commonly infected. Most commonly, actinomycosis leads to localized abscesses, usually involving the head and neck. Pyothorax, peritonitis, osteomyelitis, and disseminated infections also occur. Nocardiosis is caused by a saprophytic, aerobic organism that infects animals most commonly by inhalation or wound contamination. Nocardiosis is much less commonly diagnosed than actinomycosis. Nocardiosis can cause localized abscesses, pyothorax, osteomyelitis, and disseminated infections. Disseminated infections occur more commonly than with actinomycosis, and the symptoms that result often are confused with canine distemper virus infection.

The exudate from animals infected by *Actinomyces* is generally yellow to gray but can have the classic "tomato soup" appearance. *Nocardia* infections frequently lead to a serosanguineous discharge. Sulfur granules are soft, mucoid clumps of organisms; they are found most frequently with actinomycosis. The presence of gram-positive, branching filamentous rods in exudates are suggestive of actinomycosis or nocardiosis. *Nocardia* organisms are acid-fast, whereas *Actinomyces* are not. Definitive diagnosis is based on culture techniques.

Standard Therapy. As discussed for anaerobic infections in a previous section of this chapter, primary management of actinomycosis and nocardiosis involves surgical drainage or débridement and long-term appropriate antibiotic therapy. Excision of local subcutaneous abscesses is also possible occasionally. Treatment of body cavity effusions should include drainage and lavage. For pyothorax, large-bore tubes should be placed bilaterally and lavage performed with lactated Ringer's solution or 0.9% sodium chloride using 10–20 ml of solution per kilogram per side each lavage. After instillation of the lavage solution, the animal should be moved to distribute the fluid, followed by removal of the fluid after 20–30 minutes. Lavage should be repeated three times daily, and it should be continued until no organisms are seen cytologically; it requires 10–14 days in most animals. Lavage by repeated thoracocentesis has generally been unsuccessful, and the placement of chest tubes is recommended. Occasionally, severe intrathoracic scarring and loculation of pus or the presence of foreign material necessitates surgical exploration and débridement of the chest cavity using median sternotomy. Surgery is not indicated for disseminated disease.

Antibiotic therapy is indicated in all cases of actinomycosis or nocardiosis. Many drugs have been shown to have in vitro and in vivo activity against these organisms. Penicillin V (Veetids, Squibb) at a dosage of 8–50 mg/kg PO q8h has been used successfully for the treatment of actinomycosis. Alternatively, ampicillin (Lederle) at a dosage of 20–40 mg/kg PO, SC, IM, or IV q6–8h can be used. Side effects associated with the use of these drugs are rare. There is more variability in response to antibiotics for nocardiosis than for actinomycosis. Sulfadiazine (Lilly) given at dosages up to 80 mg/kg PO q8h have most frequently been recommended in the human literature. Combinations of sulfonamides and trimethoprim (Ditrim, Syntex) at a dosage of 15 mg/kg PO twice daily for 3–6 months may be successful for the management of some cases. Sulfonamide hypersensitivity has led to a variety of side effects including hepatopathies, keratoconjunctivitis sicca, macrocytic anemia, and nonerosive polyarthritis in Doberman pinschers. I generally institute combination therapy with penicillin V and trimethoprim-sulfadiazine at the dosage schedules listed above in all cases of suspected actinomycosis or nocardiosis.

Antibiotic therapy should be continued for weeks to months after diagnosis. Human patients commonly are treated for months to years. Continuous antibiotic therapy has been required in some human and dog cases. Prompt initiation and long-term administration of the appropriate therapy combined with drainage if indicated should lead to the recovery of many animals infected by *Actinomyces*. The overall mortality rate for nocardiosis in dogs has been estimated to be 56% (Hardie, 1984). Disseminated disease carries the worst prognosis. Therapeutic response monitoring varies with the type of infection. Improvement of clinical signs of malaise, fever, and depression can indicate a positive response to antibiotics. Pyothorax is monitored initially by cytologically examining lavage fluid and then by thoracic radiography after tube removal. Recheck radiographs should be made monthly until pleural disease has resolved and then monthly for several months after discontinuing antibiotic therapy. Recurrence of pyothorax is not uncommon. If trimethoprim-sulfadiazine is used, periodic rechecks of complete blood cell counts and monitoring for the development of keratoconjunctivitis sicca is recommended (see Chapter 14). The use of this drug in Doberman pinschers should be avoided owing to the potential for development of nonerosive polyarthritis.

Alternative Therapy. Poor therapeutic response generally is associated with inadequate drainage of subcutaneous masses, inadequate lavage of cases of pyothorax, or antibiotic resistance. Alternative drugs for the treatment of actinomycosis include cephalosporins, macrolide antibiotics including erythromycin, lincomycin, and clindamycin, tetracyclines, and tetracycline derivatives such as doxycycline. Alternative drugs for the treatment of nocardiosis include ampicillin combined with erythromycin (synergistic), doxycycline, minocycline, and amikacin. See Chapter 15 for toxicities associated with each of these drugs. Monitoring of therapy is as discussed above. Information is not available concerning the prognosis associated with resistant infections.

Borrelia burgdorferi *Infection (Lyme Disease)*

Serologic evidence of infection of dogs with *Borrelia burgdorferi* has been documented. This organism is a tick-borne spirochete with wide distribution in the United States. The nymphal stage of the tick genus *Ixodes* is most important in the transmission of the organism to humans. Adult ticks often feed on dogs. Clinical signs of disease develop in only a small percentage of the dogs that are infected. The pathogenesis of clinical signs probably requires persistence of the organism in the host tissues.

Acute clinical signs of disease include lameness, fever, anorexia, lymphadenopathy, and general malaise. Chronic clinical signs are more common in dogs and are manifested primarily as an intermittent, recurrent, nonerosive arthritis that generally involves more than one joint. There is limited information available concerning renal, neurologic, and cardiologic manifestations of the disease in the dog. Atrioventricular block and glomerulonephritis have been documented in dogs seropositive for Lyme borreliosis, but it is not known if these disease manifestations were induced by the organism.

Cytology of joint taps from infected dogs generally reveals a purulent exudate with most of the cells being polymorphonuclear leukocytes. In acute infections, the volume of fluid obtained is often minimal. Definitive diagnosis is made by culturing the organism from affected joints, the blood, or the cerebrospinal fluid (CSF), which requires special techniques and specimen handling. Unfortunately, the organism is rarely recovered. The organism also can be detected in tissues evaluated by histopathology. Serology can be used to confirm exposure to the organism. Immunoglobulin G class antibody titers may be positive for months after the infection and are present in dogs with both clinical and subclinical infection. Immunoglobulin M class antibody titers generally are positive only for weeks after the infection and so may be more consistent with recent infection. However, the presence of antibodies to *Borrelia burgdorferi* confirms only exposure, not necessarily active, clinical disease.

Standard Therapy. If a clinical infection is strongly suspected, several antibiotics can be used. Ampicillin (Ampicillin trihydrate capsules, Lederle) at a dosage of 22 mg/kg PO three times daily for 10–14 days, tetracycline (Panamycin, Upjohn) at a dosage of 22 mg/kg PO three times daily for 10–14 days, or erythromycin (Erythromycin tablets, Abbott) at a dosage of 22 mg/kg PO three times daily for 10–14 days can be used. Ampicillin should be used in pregnant animals. Erythromycin and tetracycline are commonly associated with gastrointestinal irritation. Aspirin can be administered for pain relief (see Chapter 12). Exercise restriction is recommended during the initial treatment period. The prognosis is good with acute phase disease. Treatment of dogs during the acute phase of the disease may lessen the likelihood of developing chronic disease. Cases with chronic disease may have a more variable response to therapy. Therapeutic effectiveness is monitored by resolution of clinical signs. Alternatively, recheck cytology of joint taps can be performed to document resolution of inflammatory changes. Degenerative joint disease can develop as a sequela to infection. See Chapter 12 for a discussion of the management of degenerative joint disease.

Alternative Therapy. Alternative therapeutic regimens used in humans include penicillin G (Pfizerpen, Pfizer) administered intravenously every 6 hours for 14–21 days, ceftriaxone (Rocephin injectable, Roche) administered intravenously for 14 days, or doxycycline (Vibramycin, Pfizer) administered orally for 30 days. Dosages and dosage schedules for the use of these drugs for the treatment of canine Lyme borreliosis have not been determined. Ceftriaxone is usually cost-prohibitive. Appropriate therapy for the management of cardiac, neurologic, or renal abnormalities has not been determined.

FUNGAL DISEASES

A summary of the fungal diseases (see Chapter 3 for a discussion of dermatophytes) infecting the dog or the cat and the primary organ systems involved with each agent are listed in Table 16-2. These agents are often distributed geographically. Blastomycosis and histoplasmosis are diagnosed most frequently in the Mississippi, Missouri, and Ohio River valleys and the mid-Atlantic states. Coccidioidomycosis is most commonly diagnosed in the southwestern United States and California. The other fungal diseases are less well defined geographically.

Fungal disease is diagnosed using a combination of cytologic, histopathologic, culture, and serologic techniques. Therapeutic options vary based on the

TABLE 16-2. Common Canine and Feline Fungal Diseases

Agent or Disease	Species Infected	Organ Involvement
Blastomycosis	D & C	D: P,S,L,O,MS,G,CNS C: P,S,O,CNS
Cryptococcosis	D & C	D: CNS,O,S,MS,UR C: UR,CNS,O,S
Histoplasmosis	D & C	D: P,GI,H,O,CNS,MS,S C: P,GI,MS,S,H,O
Coccidioidomycosis	D & C	D: P,MS,S,O,CNS,CA C: P,S,O
Sporotrichosis	D & C	D & C: S,DI-rare
Aspergillosis	D: common C: rare	D: UR,DI-rare,MS,DS,CNS C: UR-rare,P,GI
Penicilliosis	D & C: rare	D: UR C: P,UR,O
Candida	D & C	Localized: D & C Systemic: D only—PM,MS,L

D = dog; C = cat; P = pulmonary; S = skin; L = lymphatic; O = ocular; MS = osteomyelitis; G = male genitalia; CNS = central nervous system; UR = upper respiratory; GI = gastrointestinal; H = hepatic; CA = cardiac; DI = disseminated; DS = discospondylitis; PM = polymyositis.

organism that is identified and the organ system involved. Table 16-3 lists the commonly used antifungal drugs and their dosages. The following is a brief discussion of the use of these drugs for the treatment of various fungal diseases. See Chapter 15 for additional information on side effects and drug interactions.

Standard Therapy. If amphotericin B (Fungizone, Squibb) is used alone, it is generally administered at the dosages listed in Table 16-3 with a total cumulative dosage of 10 mg/kg in the dog and 4–5 mg/kg in the cat. One-half the calculated dose is given during the initial treatment as a trial. Amphotericin B can be administered using either rapid or slow intravenous infusion techniques. If the rapid infusion technique is utilized, the reconstituted drug is added to 30 ml of 5% dextrose solution which is administered over 5 minutes through a butterfly catheter. Ten milliliters of 5% dextrose solution flush is administered both before and after the amphotericin B. When the slow infusion technique is chosen, the reconstituted amphotericin B is added to 250–500 ml of 5% dextrose solution which is administered over 4–6 hours. The rapid intravenous infusion technique should be used in reasonably healthy animals with normal renal function. The slow infusion technique is used in severely ill animals or animals with renal insufficiency. The rapid infusion technique is generally recommended in cats.

TABLE 16-3. Antifungal Drugs

Drug/Manufacturer	Dosage	Organism
Amphotericin B (Fungizone, Squibb)	D: 0.5 mg/kg IV 3 times weekly C: 0.25 mg/kg IV 3 times weekly	B,H,Cr,Ca,Co,S,A
Ketoconazole (Nizoral, Janssen)	D: 10–30 mg/kg PO daily C: 10–20 mg/kg PO daily	Ca,B,H,Co,Cr,S,A
Flucytosine (Ancobin, Roche)	D & C: 30–50 mg/kg PO 4 times daily	Cr
K iodide (SSKI, Upsher-Smith)	D: 20–40 mg/kg PO 3 times daily C: 20 mg/kg PO twice daily	S
Enilconazole (Imaverol, Pitman-Moore)	D: 20 mg/kg nasal flush divided twice daily	A,P

B = *Blastomyces*; Ca = *Candida*; H = *Histoplasma*; Cr = *Cryptococcus*; Co = *Coccidioides*; S = *Sporothrix*; A = *Aspergillus*; P = *Penicillium*. D = dog; C = cat; IV = intravenous; PO = oral.

Amphotericin B commonly induces anorexia, vomiting, phlebitis, elevated body temperature, and renal dysfunction. The blood urea nitrogen (BUN) should be monitored during therapy. If the BUN exceeds 30 mg/dl, therapy should be discontinued until renal function normalizes. Pretreatment intravenous administration of 0.9% sodium chloride solution at a fluid administration rate of 2 ml/kg/hr for several hours prior to administration of amphotericin B may decrease the adverse renal effects. Intravenous infusion of 12.5 g of mannitol concurrently with amphotericin B may decrease renal toxicity but also may decrease the overall cure rate.

Ketoconazole (Nizoral, Janssen) administered alone at the dosages listed in Table 16-3 has been used successfully to treat many of the fungal diseases. The total daily dosage should be administered divided two or three times daily. Primary side effects include anorexia, alopecia, hepatotoxicity, and vomiting. If side effects occur in the cat, alternate-day therapy may be indicated. This drug should not be used alone if the animal is critically ill or suffers from gastrointestinal malabsorption. Higher dosages (approximately 40 mg/kg/day) are required in animals with CNS disease, disseminated disease, or bone involvement.

Flucytosine (Ancobin, Roche) is used primarily for the treatment of cryptococcosis (Table 16-3). This drug crosses the blood-brain barrier well and so may be indicated in cases of CNS cryptococcosis. Primary side effects include vomiting, diarrhea, hepatotoxicity, cutaneous reactions, and bone marrow suppression.

Administration of potassium iodide (SSKI, Upsher-Smith) has been effective for the management of sporotrichosis (Table 16-3). Reversible side effects include anorexia, vomiting, and cutaneous reactions.

There have been a number of therapeutic agents used for the treatment of nasal aspergillosis or penicilliosis. Rhinotomy with and without the administration of thiabendazole (Equizole, MSD AgVet) at a dosage of 20 mg/kg PO one or two times daily and ketoconazole at the dosages listed in Table 16-3 have generally led to an improvement rate of less than 50%. The treatment of choice for this disease appears to be the nasal instillation of enilconazole (Imaverol, Pitman-Moore). The primary drawback of this therapeutic option is that it requires placement of tubes into the nasal cavity and potentially the sinuses. However, a much greater cure rate has been seen compared to previously evaluated techniques.

Combination therapy is commonly indicated in animals poorly responsive to a therapeutic agent when used alone or in animals showing toxicity or potential toxicity from individual drugs. Drug combinations can also be synergistic in some instances and often are recommended as the initial therapeutic protocol. The combination of amphotericin B and ketoconazole is commonly used and has been effective for the management of blastomycosis, histoplasmosis, coccidioidomycosis, and cryptococcosis. In this protocol, amphotericin B is given as described above to a total cumulative dosage of 4–6 mg/kg. Ketoconazole is administered from the beginning of amphotericin B administration at a dosage of 10 mg/kg PO daily and continued for at least 2–3 months. The combination of amphotericin B and flucytosine is superior for the treatment of cryptococcosis, particularly if CNS disease is present. The cumulative dosage of amphotericin B should be decreased to 4–6 mg/kg. The flucytosine is administered using standard protocols (Table 16-3).

Therapy is monitored primarily by clinical response, resolution of radiographic abnormalities, and resolution of organism isolation. Serologic monitoring probably is valuable only for cryptococcosis. Cryptococcal antigen titers diminish during successful therapy. Treatment should be continued for several weeks after resolution of disease with the exception of amphotericin B. The prognosis for the various fungal diseases varies but is generally guarded if polysystemic manifestations exist. CNS disease carries a grave prognosis. Recurrence of systemic fungal diseases is common. See Chapter 14 for a discussion of the manifestations and treatment of ocular fungal diseases.

Alternative or Investigational Therapies. Itraconazole (Janssen) and fluconazole (Pfizer) are imidazole derivatives that are closely related to ketoconazole. These drugs are currently under investigation. Promising results have been seen with itraconazole for the treatment of nasal aspergillosis, blastomycosis, and cryptococcosis. Itraconazole maintains higher plasma levels than does ketoconazole and has been used successfully for the treatment of CNS cryptococcosis in rabbits. In vitro activity against *Sporothrix* has been demonstrated. Fluconazole reaches high levels in the CNS and may prove to be effective for the management of several mycotic infections. Ketoconazole administered at the dosages listed in Table 16-3 is the second drug of choice for

TABLE 16-4. Common Canine and Feline Rickettsial Diseases

Agent	Species Infected	Organ Involvement or Clinical Sign
Rickettsia rickettsii (Rocky Mountain spotted fever)	D	F,AN,V,D,ON,DE,WL,C, L,PM,AP,PE,EP,M,RH,CNS,DY
Ehrlichia canis (ehrlichiosis)	D	Acute: F,ON,AN,DY,L,CNS Chronic: DE,WL,PMM, AP,EP,PE,AU,RH,CNS,L,SP
Ehrlichia equi	D	Similar to *E. canis* except milder signs
Ehrlichia platys (Infectious cyclic thrombocytopenia)	D	PE (rare), AU
Neorickettsia helminthoeca (salmon poisoning)	D	F,AN,D,M,DE,V,ON,L
Neorickettsia elokominica	D	As for *N. helminthoeca*
Haemobartonella canis	D	DE,PMM (rare)
Haemobartonella felis	C	DE,WK,AN,WL,PMM,SP,IC,F

D = dog; C = cat; F = fever; AN = anorexia; V = vomiting; D = diarrhea; DE = depression; WL = weight loss; ON = oculonasal discharge; C = cough; L = lymphadenopathy; PM = muscle pain; AP = abdominal pain; PE = petechia; EP = epistaxis, M = melena; AU = anterior uveitis; RH = retinal hemorrhage; CNS = central nervous system; DY = dyspnea; PMM = pale mucous membranes; SP = splenomegaly; WK = weakness; IC = icterus.

the treatment of dogs and cats with sporotrichosis if potassium iodide fails or is not tolerated by the patient.

RICKETTSIAL DISEASES

A summary of the common rickettsial diseases affecting dogs and cats in the United States is presented in Table 16-4. Rocky Mountain spotted fever (RMSF) and the *Ehrlichia* species are transmitted primarily by ticks and occur most commonly in the southern and southeastern states. The agents causing salmon poisoning and Elokomin fluke fever (salmon disease complex) are transmitted by flukes *(Nanophyetus salmincola)* that parasitize fish, particularly salmon, and so are limited geographically to the Pacific Northwest. Dogs are infected after ingestion of parasitized fish. The intermediate host of *Haemobartonella felis* is unknown but is thought to be fleas. *Haemobartonella canis* is transmitted by ticks. These rickettsia occur nationwide.

The clinical syndromes vary with the organism. RMSF and *Ehrlichia canis* (canine ehrlichiosis) are the most commonly diagnosed rickettsial diseases. Canine ehrlichiosis has acute, subclinical, and chronic phases. The acute phase is essentially indistinguishable from clinical RMSF. Affected dogs often develop fever, malaise, lymphadenopathy, hepatosplenomegaly, vomiting, diarrhea, petechiation, epistaxis, and CNS disease. Polyarthritis can occur as well. Cases with chronic phase ehrlichiosis commonly develop bone marrow suppression leading to pancytopenia. Nonregenerative anemia and thrombocytopenia are common. Clinical signs are similar to those of acute phase ehrlichiosis but are often more vague. *Ehrlichia equi* causes clinical syndromes similar to those induced by *E. canis* and is discussed under canine ehrlichiosis.

Ehrlichia platys parasitizes platelets, leading to cyclic thrombocytopenia and occasionally anterior uveitis. Both species of *Haemobartonella* can cause anemia. *Haemobartonella canis* infections are usually subclinical unless the animal is immunocompromised, usually by splenectomy. Elokomin fluke fever and salmon poisoning have clinical signs similar to those of RMSF and acute phase ehrlichiosis, but gastrointestinal signs predominate. These signs often include vomiting and diarrhea with melena or hematochezia.

Serologic tests are available to aid in the diagnosis of RMSF and *E. canis* and *E. platys* infections. Because *E. canis* causes persistent infection and ultimately chronic clinical syndromes, any positive antibody titer is significant and indicates that therapy should be administered. Many dogs infected with *Rickettsia rickettsii* (the etiologic agent of RMSF) develop subclinical infection and clear the organism without therapy. Thus a positive antibody titer for *R. rickettsii* indicates only exposure and not necessarily clinical disease. Infection by *Haemobartonella* spp. is usually detected by demonstrating the organism in parasitized red blood cells. Elokomin fluke fever and salmon poisoning are generally diagnosed by a combination of clinical signs of disease, history, and demonstration of the intermediate host fluke eggs in feces.

Standard Therapy. Intravenous fluid therapy is usually indicated in anorectic animals or those with vomiting or diarrhea. The primary therapeutic agent used for the treatment of rickettsial infections is tetracycline and its derivatives. Tetracycline (Panmycin, Upjohn) should be administered at a dosage of 22 mg/kg PO three times daily for 14–21 days. Oxytetracycline (Liquimycin Injectable, Pfizer) is available for intravenous administration to anorectic patients. The most common significant side effects of the tetracyclines include gastrointestinal irritation and induction of fever, especially in cats. Tetracyclines may lead to dental discoloration if used in young animals. Variable gastrointestinal absorption occurs with this product. For a complete discussion of potential toxicities, see Chapter 15. Doxycycline (Vibramycin, Pfizer), a synthetic tetracycline derivative, is more fat-soluble than tetracycline and leads to less gastrointestinal irritation. The greater fat solubility results in improved absorption from the gastrointestinal tract and greater penetration across the blood-brain barrier. Hence this drug may be superior to tetracycline for the treatment of rickettsial infections causing CNS signs. Doxycycline is given at a dosage of 5 mg/kg PO daily for 7–10 days for the treatment of *Haemobartonella felis* and acute phase canine ehrlichiosis. For severe cases, a dosage of 5 mg/kg PO twice daily for 14–21 days is indicated.

The prognosis for most rickettsial diseases is good if therapeutic intervention is begun promptly. Fever, petechiation, vomiting, diarrhea, epistaxis, and thrombocytopenia often resolve within days after initiation of therapy. Occasionally, severe cases of RMSF, Elokomin fluke fever, and salmon poisoning progress rapidly and are poorly responsive to therapy. The bone marrow suppression that often occurs secondary to chronic phase ehrlichiosis may not respond for weeks to months following therapy. Infrequently, the bone marrow suppression associated with chronic phase ehrlichiosis results in a nonregenerative anemia severe enough to require blood transfusion. The anemia associated with *Haemobartonella* spp. also may become severe enough to require blood transfusion. Anabolic steroids such as stanozolol (Winstrol V, Winthrop) at a dosage of 0.5–2.0 mg PO twice daily in the cat and 1–4 mg PO twice daily in the dog or nandrolone decanoate (Deca-Durabolin, Organon) at a dosage of 100 mg IM weekly (dog) can be used in an attempt to support or stimulate erythropoiesis. However, the results from the use of anabolic steroids have been disappointing.

The pathogenesis of acute phase ehrlichiosis, RMSF, and *Haemobartonella* spp. infections may include immune-mediated events leading to the destruction of red blood cells and thrombocytes. Thus, some authors have advocated the administration of immunosuppressive doses of corticosteroids to acutely affected animals. Prednisone (Deltasone, Upjohn) at a dosage of 2.2 mg/kg PO divided twice daily during the first 3–4 days after diagnosis is beneficial in some cases. Generally, this therapy should be reserved for those cases showing initially poor response to tetracycline therapy alone or those in which phagocytosis of red blood cells or platelets has been demonstrated on cytologic evaluation of bone marrow aspiration. Vincristine (Oncovin, Lilly) at a dosage of 0.01 mg/kg IV weekly has been used to stimulate bone marrow release of platelets in severely thrombocytopenic animals.

Nanophyetus salmincola infection in dogs with the salmon disease complex can be treated with fenbendazole (Panacur, Hoechst) at a dosage of 50 mg/kg PO daily for 10–14 days or until trematode eggs are no longer present in feces.

Dogs with ehrlichiosis are subject to reinfection. The organism is not passed transovarially in the tick and so can be eliminated in the environment by tick control or by treating all dogs through a generation of ticks. If tick control is not feasible, tetracycline should be administered at a dosage of 6.6 mg/kg PO daily for at least 200 days. Long-term tetracycline therapy is not helpful in the control of RMSF, as the tick vector passes the organism transovarially and maintains a sylvan cycle in small rodents in the environment.

Alternative and Investigational Therapy. Chloramphenicol (Chloramphenicol capsules, Rugby) administered at a dosage of 22 mg/kg PO three times daily in dogs or twice daily in cats has been used successfully to control the clinical signs of most rickettsial infections. The duration of therapy should be 14–21 days. The primary side effect is bone marrow suppression, which is more likely to develop in cats. Weekly complete blood counts should be monitored when this drug is used. Enrofloxacin has been successful in the treatment of experimentally-induced RMSF in dogs.

Imidocarb dipropionate has been administered at a dosage of 5–7 mg/kg IM given twice over a 14-day period for the successful treatment of canine ehrlichiosis. Alternatively, success has been seen using this drug and dosage after a single intramuscular injection. Some patients develop pain at the injection site, salivation, oculonasal discharge, diarrhea, tremors, and dyspnea following administration of this drug. Imidocarb is not currently licensed for use in the United States.

FELINE TOXOPLASMOSIS

The most common protozoan parasite leading to polysystemic clinical illness in the dog and cat is *Toxoplasma gondii*. This ubiquitous organism has been found in all areas of the world that have cats. The cat is the definitive host of this parasite and is the only known species that completes the sexual phase of the organism, which leads to the passage of oocysts in feces (enteroepithelial cycle). An extraintestinal cycle occurs in both dogs and cats and occasionally leads to the development of clinical signs of disease.

Clinical signs are generally not associated with the enteroepithelial cycle in cats. The most common clinical syndromes resulting from the extraintestinal cycle in cats include fever, malaise, anorexia, weight loss, pneumonitis, icterus, CNS disease, stillbirth or neonatal death, and ocular diseases including anterior uveitis and retinochoroiditis. In the dog, clinical signs are divided into those involving the neuromuscular, respiratory, and gastrointestinal systems. Ocular disease appears to be less common in the dog than in the cat.

The antemortem diagnosis of clinical toxoplasmosis is made by combining clinical signs and serologic evidence of active infection with response to anti-*Toxoplasma* drugs or organism demonstration. Often in neonatal or immunosuppressed animals the course of the disease is rapid, and the diagnosis is often made postmortem. When an antemortem diagnosis is made, several drugs have been used with some success for shortening the oocyst shedding period and controlling the clinical signs of the disease.

Standard Therapy. Clindamycin hydrochloride (Antirobe, Upjohn) at a dosage of 25 mg/kg PO divided two or three times daily for 21 days has been used successfully to manage clinical signs of the disease associated with the extraintestinal cycle in cats. This drug has also been used successfully in the treatment of *T. gondii*-induced polymyositis in a dog (see Chapter 12). The drug is available in an injectable formulation (Cleocin, Upjohn) for use intramuscularly in anorectic or vomiting animals. Side effects other than mild gastrointestinal irritation have not been identified in cats. When side effects occur, they have most commonly been characterized by occasional vomiting during the early phases of treatment and short-term (1–2 days) diarrhea following drug withdrawal. Specific treatment of toxicity other than resting of the gastrointestinal tract has not been required. Pseudomembranous colitis and coagulopathies associated with the use of this drug in humans have not been documented in cats or dogs.

Clinical signs not involving the eyes generally resolve within days after initiating therapy. Treatment protocols of fewer than 14 days' duration often have been associated with exacerbations of clinical signs, which has been attributed to the fact that anti-*T. gondii* drugs only inhibit replication and cannot totally clear the body of the organism. Some information suggests that clindamycin can penetrate the blood-brain barrier and may be effective in the management of CNS toxoplasmosis. The administration of clindamycin leads to resolution of retinochoroiditis in most affected cats. Anterior uveitis has been difficult to manage with anti-*Toxoplasma* drugs. It is likely that anterior uveitis associated with toxoplasmosis is not due to organism replication but to immune-mediated events, explaining the poor response to anti-*Toxoplasma* drugs. Anti-inflammatory agents are usually indicated for the management of anterior uveitis induced by toxoplasmosis. Topical administration of 1% prednisone acetate (EconoPred, Alcon) using a dosage schedule of 1–2 drops applied to the affected eye(s) three or four times daily is sufficient for the control of inflammation in some cases. *T. gondii* seropositive cats with uveitis are more likely to have decreased intraocular inflammation if they are treated with clindamycin combined with glucocorticoids than if treated with glucocorticoids alone. See Chapter 14 for a full discussion of the management of anterior uveitis.

Drugs that inhibit folic acid metabolism are effective anti-*Toxoplasma* drugs. Classically, pyrimethamine (Daraprim, Burroughs Wellcome) at a dosage of 0.5–1.0 mg/kg PO divided two or three times daily combined with rapidly acting sulfonamides such as sulfadiazine (Sulfadiazine, Lilly) at a dosage of 60–120 mg/kg PO divided two or three times daily have been used frequently in humans and cats. A primary problem associated with this drug combination is bone marrow suppression induced by folic acid inhibition. Also, cats often become anorectic and depressed following initiation of therapy. If this drug combination is used, folic acid (folic acid tablets, Lilly) at a dosage of 50 mg PO daily, baker's yeast at a dosage of 100 mg/kg/day PO, or folinic acid at a dosage of 1 mg/kg PO daily should be administered to avert side effects. Trimethoprim-sulfadiazine (Ditrim, Syntex) at a dosage of 15 mg/kg PO twice daily for 14–21 days has anti-*Toxoplasma* effects but has been used in only a limited number of cases. This drug and dosage schedule have been used by the author for the successful management of ocular and CNS toxoplasmosis. The side effects are less severe than those that occur with pyrimethamine, but complete blood cell counts should be monitored if therapy is continued for more than 2 weeks.

The effectiveness of therapy is monitored by resolution of signs. Serology is an ineffective tool for monitoring because serum antibody titers remain elevated for months to years following treatment. The prognosis for resolution of clinical signs not involving the eyes has been good. Ocular signs commonly recur. Cats co-infected by the feline immunodeficiency virus have a poorer prognosis.

The oocyst shedding period in cats is short and generally not recognized in clinical practice, as clinical signs of disease rarely occur. Several nonpathogenic coccidian parasites infecting cats have oocysts indistinguishable from those of *T. gondii*. Because *T. gondii* also infects humans, when oocysts measuring 10 × 12 μm in diameter are found in a fecal sample from a cat they should be assumed to be *T. gondii* and therapy administered to attempt to decrease oocyst numbers. Pyrimethamine at a dosage of 2.0 mg/kg PO daily, sulfonamides at a dosage of 100 mg/kg PO daily, clindamycin at a dosage of 25–50 mg/kg PO daily, or monensin (Rumensin, Elanco) 0.02% concentration by weight in dry food can shorten the oocyst shedding period.

Investigational Therapy. Many drugs have been shown to have anti-*Toxoplasma* effect in vitro. Most of the drugs evaluated to date have been either macrolide antibiotics or folate antagonists. None of these compounds has been evaluated for use in dogs or cats.

SUGGESTED READINGS

Viral Diseases

August JR: Coronavirus infections in cats: an internist's perspective. In: Proceedings of the Eastern States Veterinary Conference, 1989;4.

Barr MC, Barlough JE: Feline immunodeficiency virus. Cornell Feline Health Center Information Bulletin 1989;10:1.

Beck ER, Harris CK, Macy DW: Feline leukemia virus: infection and treatment. Comp Contin Educ Pract Vet 1986;8:567.

Cotter SM: Treatment of lymphoma and leukemia with cyclophosphamide, vincristine, and prednisone. II. Treatment of cats. J Am Anim Hosp Assoc 1983;19:166.

Gasper PW, Fulton R, Thrall MA: Bone marrow transplant in cats. In: Proceedings of the 51st Annual Conference for Veterinarians, Colorado Veterinary Medical Association 1990;374.

Kiehl AR, Macy DW: Feline leukemia virus: testing and prophylaxis. Comp Contin Educ Pract Vet 1985;7:1038.

Lutz H, Hansen B, Horzinck MC: Feline infectious peritonitis (FIP)—the present state of knowledge. J Small Anim Pract 1986;27:108.

Macy DW: Management of the FeLV-positive patient. In: Kirk RW, ed. Current Veterinary Therapy X. Philadelphia: WB Saunders, 1989:1069.

Mooney SC, Hayes AA, MacEwen EG, et al: Treatment and prognostic factors in lymphoma in cats: 103 cases (1977–1981). J Am Vet Med Assoc 1989;194:696.

Rojko JL, Hardy WB: Feline leukemia virus and other retroviruses. In: Sherding RG, ed. The Cat: Diseases and Clinical Management. New York: Churchill Livingstone, 1989;229.

Sparger EE: Feline T-lymphotrophic lentivirus infection. In: Proceedings of the 4th Kal Kan Seminar and Eastern States Veterinary Conference, 1988;9.

Weiss RC: A virologist's approach to treatment of feline infectious peritonitis. In: Proceedings of the Eastern States Veterinary Conference, 1989;14.

Bacterial Diseases

Abramowicz M, ed: Treatment of lyme disease. Med Lett 1988;30:65.

Ackerman N, Grain E, Castleman W: Canine nocardiosis. J Am Anim Hosp Assoc 1982;18:147.

Dow SW: Anaerobic infections in dogs and cats. In: Kirk RW, ed. Current Veterinary Therapy X. Philadelphia: WB Saunders 1989;1082.

Dow SW, Jones RL, Adney WF: Anaerobic bacterial infections and responses to treatment in dogs and cats: review of 36 cases (1983–1985). J Am Vet Med Assoc 1986;189:930.

Dow SW, Jones RL, Rosychuk RAW: Bacteriologic specimens: selection, collection, and transport for optimum results. Comp Contin Educ Pract Vet 1989;11:686.

Grauer GF, Burgess EC, Cooley AJ, Hagee JH: Renal lesions associated with *Borrelia burgdorferi* infection in a dog. J Am Vet Med Assoc 1988;193:237.

Greene RT: Canine Lyme borreliosis. In: Kirk RW, ed. Current Veterinary Therapy X. Philadelphia: WB Saunders 1989;1086.

Harari J, Lincoln J: Pharmacologic features of clindamycin in dogs and cats. J Am Vet Med Assoc 1989;195:124.

Hardie EM: Actinomycosis and nocardiosis. In: Greene CE, ed. Clinical Microbiology and Infectious Diseases of the Dog and Cat. Philadelphia: WB Saunders, 1984;663.

Hardie EM, Barsanti JA: Treatment of canine actinomycosis. J Am Vet Med Assoc 1982;180:537.

Hirsh DC, Indiveri ML, Jang SS, Biberstein EL: Changes in prevalence and susceptibility of obligate anaerobes in clinical veterinary practice. J Am Vet Med Assoc 1985;186:1086.

Jang SS, Ling GV, Yamamoto R, Wolf AM: *Mycoplasma* as a cause of canine urinary tract infection. J Am Vet Med Assoc 1984;185:45.

Lein DH: Canine mycoplasma, ureaplasma, and bacterial infertility. In: Kirk RW, ed. Current Veterinary Therapy IX. Philadelphia: WB Saunders, 1986;1240.

Levy SA, Duray PH: Complete heart block in a dog seropositive for *Borrelia burgdorferi*, similarity to human Lyme carditis. J Vet Intern Med 1988;2:138.

Neer TM: Clinical pharmacologic features of fluoroquinolone antimicrobial drugs. J Am Vet Med Assoc 1988;193:577.

Pedersen NC: Mycoplasmosis. In: Pedersen NC, ed. Feline Infectious Diseases. Goleta, CA: American Veterinary Publications, 1988;215.

Rosendal S: Canine mycoplasmas: their ecologic niche and role in disease. J Am Vet Med Assoc 1982;180:1212.

Fungal Diseases

Harvey CE: Nasal aspergillosis and penicillinosis in dogs: results of treatment with thiabendazole. J Am Vet Med Assoc 1984;184:48.

Legendre AM, Selcer BA, Edwards DF, Stevens R: Treatment of canine blastomycosis with amphotericin B and ketoconazole. J Am Vet Med Assoc 1984;184:1249.

Moriello KA: Ketaconazole: clinical pharmacology and therapeutic recommendations. J Am Vet Med Assoc 1986;188:303.

Noxon JO: Systemic antifungal chemotherapy. In: Kirk RW, ed. Current Veterinary Therapy X. Philadelphia: WB Saunders, 1989;1101.

Sharp N: Nasal aspergillosis. In: Kirk RW, ed. Current Veterinary Therapy X. Philadelphia: WB Saunders, 1989;1106.

Rickettsial Diseases

Cowell RL, Tyler RD, Clinkenbeard KD, Meinkoth JH: Ehrlichiosis and polyarthritis in three dogs. J Am Vet Med Assoc 1988;192:1093.

Glaze MB, Gaunt SD: Uveitis associated with *Ehrlichia platys* infection in a dog. J Am Vet Med Assoc 1986;188:916.

Greene CE, Burgdofer W, Cavagnolo R, et al: Rocky Mountain spotted fever in dogs and its differentiation from canine ehrlichiosis. J Am Vet Med Assoc 1985;186:465.

Hibler SC, Hoskins JD, Greene CE: Rickettsial infections in dogs. Part I. Rocky Mountain spotted fever and *Coxiella* infections. Comp Contin Educ Pract Vet 1985;7:856.

Hibler SC, Hoskins JD, Greene CE: Rickettsial infections in dogs. Part II. Ehrlichiosis and infectious thrombocytopenia. Comp Contin Educ Pract Vet 1986;8:106.

Hibler SC, Hoskins JD, Greene CE: Rickettsial infections in dogs. Part III. Salmon disease complex and hemobartonellosis. Comp Contin Educ Pract Vet 1986;8:251.

Toxoplasmosis

Dubey JP: Toxoplasmosis in dogs. Canine Pract 1985;12:7.

Dubey JP: Toxoplasmosis in cats. Feline Pract 1986;16:12.

Greene CE, Cook JR, Mahaffey EA: Clindamycin for treatment of *Toxoplasma* polymyositis in a dog. J Am Vet Med Assoc 1985;187:631.

Lappin MR: Feline toxoplasmosis. In: Kirk RW, ed. Current Veterinary Therapy X. Philadelphia: WB Saunders, 1989;1112.

Lappin MR, Greene CE, Winston S, et al: Clinical feline toxoplasmosis: serologic diagnosis and therapeutic management of 15 cases. J Vet Intern Med 1989;3:139.

CHAPTER SEVENTEEN

Medical Emergencies

Cynthia M. Otto

Emergencies can occur at any time of the day or night and even within the relatively controlled environment of a veterinary hospital. The most critical matter in successful management of an emergency involves the ability to recognize and treat life-threatening problems.

It is also important to realize that the emergency patient's condition is changing constantly, and therefore completion of a thorough initial physical examination and laboratory database is crucial. Monitoring procedures should be used to look for changes in status, response to therapy, and complications of both the original insult and any therapeutic interventions (see the section at the end of this chapter for a description of monitoring procedures).

RESPIRATORY EMERGENCIES

Respiratory failure is the most life-threatening emergency seen. The underlying problems that result in animals presenting in respiratory distress are varied and may not always reflect a primary respiratory problem. Successful management of these situations requires a complete and thorough physical examination to identify the source of the problem. The ability to identify the source guides therapeutic and diagnostic decisions and minimizes risk of inappropriate or unnecessary intervention. Respiratory emergencies can be divided into four main categories according to the location of the primary problem: 1) upper airway; 2) lower airway; 3) pleural/extrapulmonary; and 4) metabolic.

Upper Airway Emergencies

Common upper airway emergencies include obstruction, elongated soft palate, stenotic nares, laryngeal edema, laryngeal paralysis, and collapsing trachea. Acute upper airway emergencies are most often associated with partial or complete airway obstruction. They may present with forced inspiration, stridor, hyperthermia, or acute cyanosis and collapse. Intrathoracic obstruction of the trachea may present with expiratory dyspnea. Rupture or laceration of the upper airway results in subcutaneous emphysema or pneumomediastinum. Cats and dogs with pharyngeal or tracheal foreign bodies and dogs with collapsing trachea often present with a severe cough. Successful treatment depends on prompt removal of the obstruction. Specific therapy depends on the cause of the obstruction. Obstructions can be classified as functional or physical. Functional obstructions include collapsing trachea, stenotic nares, elongated soft palate, and partial laryngeal paralysis, whereas physical obstructions include foreign body, trauma, tumor, laryngeal or soft palate edema, and complete laryngeal paralysis.

Standard Therapy. *Upper Airway Obstruction.* Complete airway obstruction, regardless of etiology, requires urgent care; immediate removal of the obstruction must be accomplished. Some upper airway foreign bodies may be dislodged by suspending the animal from its hind limbs and applying a sudden sharp compression to the abdomen (similar to the Heimlich maneuver).

For partial obstructions oxygen therapy may be of benefit, but oxygen alone is rarely adequate. Initially placing the animal in an oxygen cage may allow the patient enough relief that it calms down, and it is then safer to complete an evaluation and institute primary care. If an oxygen cage is not available, administration of oxygen by mask or nasal oxygen catheter may be of benefit; however, if this measure further stresses the animal, it may induce respiratory arrest. See Table 17-1 for recommendations for oxygen therapy.

Once the patient is stable, radiographs may help identify a foreign body, tracheal collapse, or area of regional atelectasis suggestive of obstruction of a bronchus. A complete airway examination under light anesthesia is necessary to evaluate laryngeal function and look for obstruction. The external and internal pharyngeal areas should be carefully examined both digitally and visually. Visual evaluation of the pharynx is greatly facilitated by the use of a laryngoscope. A bronchoscope may be required to identify and remove a foreign body lodged beyond the pharynx.

If the animal is in respiratory distress and the obstruction cannot be reached or removed, an emergency tracheostomy must be performed to provide a patent airway. If the obstruction is not complete or is located distal to the thoracic inlet, a transtracheal oxygen catheter can be placed, and oxygen therapy can be used to stabilize the animal until appropriate surgical intervention can be accomplished. Animals with airway obstruction from any cause often have complicating components of laryngeal inflammation and edema and anxiety. Administration of anti-inflammatory dosages of glucocorticoids such as prednisolone sodium succinate (Solu-Delta-Cortef, Upjohn) administered at a dosage of 0.5 mg/kg IV once or twice daily or dexamethasone sodium phosphate (Azium SP, Schering) at a dosage of 0.1 mg/kg IV once (may be repeated in 12–24 hours if necessary) may minimize laryngeal edema.

Anxiety increases respiratory rate, exacerbates laryngeal edema, and raises body temperature often to dangerous levels. Although minimal handling and

TABLE 17-1. Methods of Oxygen Administration to Emergency Patients

Method	Recommended Flow and % O_2	Comments
Mask	3–5 L/min	Poor animal compliance
Cage	40% O_2	Minimizes stress but difficult to handle and monitor patient; high cost; difficult to regulate temperature and humidity
Intranasal catheter[a]	100–200 ml/kg/min, 40% O_2	Decreased volume of O_2 required; allows animal to be handled; low cost
Transtracheal catheter[b]	50–100 ml/kg/min, 40% O_2	Same as nasal catheter but also can be used for partial obstructions; can be used for high frequency jet ventilation (HFJV); may induce cough, tracheal irritation, or necrosis (if used long term with HFJV)
Endotracheal	100% O_2 (short-term) 30–40% O_2 (long-term)	Requires chemical restraint; can deliver 100% oxygen; can ventilate
Tracheostomy tube	30–40% O_2	For long-term use (> 12 hr) must use O_2 mix to achieve 30–40% inspired O_2

[a]Sovereign feeding tube (5–8 Fr), Monoject.
[b]I Cath (18 g), Delmed Inc.

oxygen are beneficial, the use of sedatives is often necessary. Acepromazine maleate (Techamerica) at a dosage of 0.05–0.20 mg/kg IV, IM, or SC once or twice daily (maximum dosage per animal is not to exceed 3 mg) or 0.4–1.0 mg/kg PO once daily can be used in animals with a stable cardiovascular system. Alternatively, in depressed or critical patients diazepam (Valium, Roche) can be used at a dosage of 0.1–0.4 mg/kg IV q1–2h as necessary. Narcotics are usually not recommended as they increase the tendency to pant and often induce nausea and vomiting, which can lead to increased vagal tone and cardiac or respiratory arrest. However, caution must be used with any sedative. Acepromazine has potential hypotensive effects, and it should also be avoided in patients with decreased liver function. Sedation may decrease respiratory drive and result in respiratory arrest. An endotracheal tube and method of positive pressure ventilation must be readily available. Placement of an intravenous catheter for drug or fluid administration is recommended prior to sedation.

Pulmonary edema often accompanies or follows upper airway obstruction. It should be anticipated, and if it occurs, it should be treated with oxygen and diuretics. Glucocorticoids and bronchodilators may be useful. See the section on pulmonary edema in this chapter for details.

Elongated Soft Palate, Stenotic Nares. These congenital abnormalities, if severe enough, can cause respiratory distress and require surgical correction. Stabilization prior to surgery involves administration of oxygen, anti-inflammatory dosages of prednisolone or dexamethasone (see Table 17-2 for dosages), and cage rest.

TABLE 17-2.   Selected Emergency Drugs for Dogs and Cats

All dosages are the same for dogs and cats unless specifically indicated.

Antibiotics

Aminoglycosides

Gentamicin (Gentocin, Schering): 2.2 mg/kg SC q8h
  The initial dose may be given IV, but SC administration has been shown to be less toxic and should be considered. Side effects include nephrotoxicity and ototoxicity.

Cephalosporins

Cephalexin (Keflex, Dista): 22 mg/kg PO q8h

Cephalothin Sodium (Keflin, Lilly): 22–44 mg/kg IV, IM, q6h to q8h

Cefotaxime Sodium (Claforan, Hoechst-Roussel): dogs 22 mg/kg IV, IM, or SC q8h

Penicillins

Ampicillin (Ampicillin, Elkins-Sinn Inc.): 22–44 mg/kg IV, IM, SC, or PO q6h to q8h

Dicloxacillin (Dicloxacillin Sodium Capsules, Lederle): 5–25 mg/kg PO q8h

Other antibiotics

Tetracycline (Tetracycline HCl Capsules, Danbury): dogs 22–44 mg/kg PO q8h; cats 20 mg/kg PO q8h
  Side effects include discoloration of teeth in immature animals and renal toxicity.

Trimethoprim sulfadiazine (Tribrissen, Coopers): 15–22 mg/kg (combined) PO, SC q12h
  Tribrissen has been associated with sterile abscesses when given SC, particularly when using 48% suspension. Other side effects include keratoconjunctivitis sicca, drug eruptions, and joint swelling.

Anticoagulants/Antithrombotics

Aspirin: dogs 5 mg/kg q24h; cats 25 mg/kg every third day to decrease platelet aggregation in thromboembolism and heartworm disease

Heparin (Heparin Sodium Injection, Elkins-Sinn): 50–200 U/kg SC q8h for DIC; for anticoagulation, 220 U/kg SC initial dose (although some recommend IV) followed in 3 hours by maintenance of 66–200 units/kg SC q6h to q8h.

Streptokinase (Kabikinase, Smith Kline & French): 90,000 IU IV for 30 minutes followed by 45,000 IU/hr for 2.5 hours for cats with aortic thromboemboli (investigational)

Tissue plasminogen activator (Alteplase, Genentech): 0.25–1.00 mg/kg/hr IV infusion for a total dosage of 1–10 mg/kg (investigational).
  Current cost is about $3000 per 50 mg. Half of the cats in one study died during its infusion.

TABLE 17-2. Selected Emergency Drugs for Dogs and Cats *(continued)*

All dosages are the same for dogs and cats unless specifically indicated.

Antidotes/Reversal Agents

Activated charcoal: 1–5 g/kg administered in a slurry 1 g/5–10 ml of water; may repeat this dose 3–4 times daily for up to 2–3 days to decrease absorption of ingested toxins.

Ascorbic acid (vitamin C): 30 mg/kg PO q6h for a total of 7 treatments.
 To be used with *N*-acetylcysteine for treatment of methemoglobinemias.

1% Methylene blue solution (Methylene Blue Injection, Eklins-Sinn): 8.8 mg/kg (0.9 ml/kg) slowly IV
 In cats it may produce Heinz body anemia.

N-Acetylcysteine 5% solution (Mucomyst, Mead Johnson Pharmaceuticals): 140 mg/kg PO loading dose followed by 3–5 treatments administered q6h at 70 mg/kg PO, as an antidote for acetaminophen or other methemoglobinemias

Naloxone hydrochloride (Naloxone HCl, Quad): 0.01–0.20 mg/kg IM, IV or SC for reversal of narcotics

Protamine sulfate (Protamine Sulfate, Lilly): 1 mg/100 units of heparin slowly IV, for heparin overdose resulting in overt hemorrhage (maximum of 50 mg/10 minutes)
 The dosage is decreased by 50% for every elapsed hour since heparin administration. Protamine may result in hemorrhage for which there is no antidote!

Vitamin K_1 (Aquamephyton, Mephyton, Merck Sharp & Dohme): 1.0–2.5 mg/kg SC; then in 12 hours start 1.0–2.5 mg/kg PO daily (can be divided in 2–3 doses) for 5–7 days for use in hepatic failure and first generation coumarin (Warfarin) toxicity; administer 2.5–5 mg/kg SC followed in 12 hours by 2.5–5 mg/kg PO daily divided in 2–3 doses for 6 weeks for second generation coumarin toxicity
 Always recheck coagulation status 2 days after last vitamin K dose; if it remains prolonged, vitamin K therapy should be continued. IV administration is associated with a risk of anaphylaxis and is not recommended. IM injections are not recommended in patients with coagulation abnormalities. Use of vitamin K_3 is ineffective for treatment of rodenticide toxicity and is associated with Heinz body anemia, hemoglobinuria, urobilinogenuria, methemoglobinemia, cyanosis, and hepatic damage.

Yohimbine (Yobine, Lloyd Laboratories): 0.1–0.4 mg/kg IV for reversal of Xylazine

Antihistamines

Cimetidine (see GI drugs)

Diphenhydramine (Benedryl, Parke Davis):
 2–4 mg/kg *slowly* IV (IV administration is not recommended in cats), IM, or SC for allergic reactions (to be effective must be given soon after the reaction begins)
 0.5–2.0 mg/kg SC 30 minutes prior to administration of blood decreases the incidence and severity of acute plasma reactions

Antioxidants

Desferoxamine (Desferal, Ciba-Geigy): 25–50 mg/kg IM (or *slowly* IV) as soon as resuscitation is initiated

(continued)

TABLE 17-2. Selected Emergency Drugs for Dogs and Cats *(continued)*

All dosages are the same for dogs and cats unless specifically indicated.

DMSO (Domoso, Syntex): Dilute 1:4 in 0.9% NaCl and inject 1.1 g/kg for dogs and
550 mg/kg for cats, slowly IV q12h

Cardiac Drugs

Antiarrhythmics

Atropine (Atropine Sulfate Injection, Elkins-Sinn): 0.02–0.05 mg/kg IV for
bradyarrhythmias

Lidocaine (Lidocaine, Elkins-Sinn):
   Dog: 1–2 mg/kg IV bolus, followed by IV infusion of 0.1% solution at 30–50
   μg/kg/min for ventricular tachyarrhythmias
   Cat: *if necessary*, 0.25–0.50 mg/kg IV slowly. The cat is very sensitive to neurotoxic
   side effects. The drug of choice for ventricular arrhythmias in the cat is
   propranolol (Inderal Injectable, Ayerst), 0.1 mg boluses IV repeated to effect

CPR drugs

Calcium gluconate (10% solution) (Calcium Gluconate Injection, Elkins-Sinn): 10
mg/kg IV
   If used, calcium gluconate solution should be administered early following
   electrical mechanical dissociation (EMD). Routine use of calcium in CPR has
   fallen into disfavor and is not recommended unless hyperkalemia or the use of
   calcium channel blockers precedes the arrest.

Epinephrine (Adrenalin Chloride, Parke Davis):
   Standard CPR dose 0.01–0.02 mg/kg (0.1–0.2 ml of 1:10,000 epinephrine/kg) IV
   q5min
   High dose epinephrine (for better brain perfusion and neurologic outcome)
   0.1–0.2 mg/kg (0.1–0.2 ml of 1:1,000 epinephrine/kg) IV q5min.

Inotropes

Dobutamine (Dobutrex, Lilly): 2.5–10 μg/kg/min constant IV infusion
   Higher doses of dobutamine (>20 μg/kg/min) may result in tachycardia.
   Dobutamine should not be used in patients with atrial fibrillation because it
   enhances A-V conduction.

Dopamine (Dopamine, Elkins-Sinn): 2–8 μg/kg/min constant IV infusion
   Lower doses (2–5 μg/kg/min) of dopamine are used to improve renal perfusion;
   higher doses (5–10 μg/kg/min) may result in vasoconstriction and poor organ
   perfusion. Dopamine is light sensitive and should be protected from light at all
   times.

Vasodilators

Acepromazine maleate (Acepromazine Maleate, Techamerica): 0.2–0.4 mg/kg SC
q8h for vasodilation
   See sedatives for comments.

Hydralazine (Hydralazine, Lederle): 0.5–1.0 mg/kg PO q8h–q12h as a vasodilator

Central Nervous System Drugs

Analgesics
Aspirin:
   Dog: 10 mg/kg PO q8h to q12h
   Cat: 10 mg/kg PO every third day

TABLE 17-2. Selected Emergency Drugs for Dogs and Cats *(continued)*

All dosages are the same for dogs and cats unless specifically indicated.

Side effects include increased bleeding time (decreased platelet aggregation) and gastric irritation/ulceration.

Butorphanol (Torbugesic, Fort Dodge):
 Dog: 0.2–0.4 mg/kg IM, SC, IV
 Cat: 0.2 mg/kg IM, SC as necessary
   Side effects include nausea and vomiting (occur half as frequently as with morphine).

Meperidine (Demerol, Winthrop):
 Dog: 2–6 mg/kg IM or SC
 Cat: 2–4 mg/kg IM or SC given q4–6h as necessary for sedation and pain relief

Morphine (Morphine, Astra):
 Dog: 1–2 mg/kg IM or SC
 Cat: 0.1 mg/kg IM or SC as necessary, may provide sedation and pain relief
   Use with caution in cats! Side effects include initial excitement, panting, salivation, nausea, vomiting, urination, defecation, bradycardia and hypotension (due to histamine release). Contraindicated for both dogs and cats in acute uremia, toxemia, seizure disorders, and hypovolemic shock.

Oxymorphone (Numorphan, Dupont): 0.06–0.14 mg/kg IV, IM, SC as necessary for sedation and pain relief
   May produce excitement in cats and should be combined with a tranquilizer such as acepromazine or diazepam.

Pentazocine (Talwin-V, Winthrop): dog, 0.5–1.0 mg/kg IM for pain relief
   Side effects include mydriasis and apprehension, occasionally ataxia and disorientation.

Anesthetics

Ketamine hydrochloride (Ketaset, Bristol): 4.4–11.0 mg/kg IV used in combination with Valium (0.11–0.22 mg/kg IV), for short-term anesthesia or as an induction agent

Ketaset (0.5–1.0 mg/kg IV) and Valium (0.05 mg/kg IV)
This combination is moderately safe and usually provides about 15 minutes of sedation in a sick cat.

Thiopental (Pentothal, Abbott) and lidocaine (Lidocaine, Elkins-Sinn): 4.4 mg/kg IV of each as an initial dose, with a maximum dosage of 8.8 mg/kg (use separate syringes, start with thiopental) for short-term anesthesia or as an induction agent

Sedatives

Acepromazine maleate (Techamerica): 0.05–0.20 mg/kg IV, IM, SC, q12h to q24h (maximum parenteral dose per animal is not to exceed 3 mg; for sedation, control of anxiety
   Not to be used in animals with hepatic dysfunction or seizures. Acepromazine may produce severe hypotension, particularly when given IV.

Demerol: See analgesics.

Diazepam (Valium, Roche): 0.1–0.4 mg/kg IV q1–2h as necessary; 0.5–2.0 mg/kg PO as necessary for sedation or control of anxiety in depressed or critical patients; 2.5–5.0 mg/animal IV repeated up to 3 times within 20 minutes for control of seizures

(continued)

TABLE 17-2.   Selected Emergency Drugs for Dogs and Cats *(continued)*

All dosages are the same for dogs and cats unless specifically indicated.

Midazolam (Versed, Roche): 0.2 mg/kg IV, IM as necessary for sedation
    Versed may cause initial excitement.

Morphine: See analgesics.

Oxymorphone: See analgesics.

Pentobarbital (Nembutal Sodium, Abbott; Pentobarbital Sodium, Elkins-Sinn): 2.2
mg/kg IV as necessary for diazepam-resistant seizures; 2–4 mg/kg IV or deep IM as
necessary for sedation; 1–6 mg/kg IV as necessary for anesthesia followed by 1–4
mg/kg/hr infusion
    Schedule II controlled substance.

Phenobarbital (Phenobarbital Sodium, Elkins-Sinn): 2–6 mg/kg IV, IM as necessary,
for sedation
    Schedule IV controlled substance
    Side effects for both pentobarbital and phenobarbital include induction of liver
    enzymes (which results in many drug interactions), depression of respiration,
    laryngospasm, and decreased intestinal motility.

Corticosteroids

Prednisolone sodium succinate (Solu-Delta-Cortef, Upjohn): 0.5 mg/kg IV q12h to
q24h, for laryngeal edema, inflammation of airways, and as an antipyretic; 1–2
mg/kg IV as a single dose, for acute asthma; 22–44 mg/kg IV once, for shock and
EMD.

Prednisone tablets: 1–2 mg/kg PO q12h gradually tapering the dosage and frequency
over several weeks for immunosuppressive therapy

Dexamethasone sodium phosphate (Azium SP, Schering): 0.1 mg/kg IV, usually a
one-time dose, but may be repeated in 12–24 hours if necessary for laryngeal
edema, inflammation of airways, or as an antipyretic; 0.2–0.5 mg/kg IV or deep IM
once for acute asthma; 2–4 mg/kg IV once for shock or EMD; 0.2–0.4 mg/kg PO
daily gradually tapering the dose and frequency over several weeks for
immunosuppressive therapy (prednisone is recommended for long-term
immunosuppressive therapy)
    Side effects of prolonged glucocorticoid therapy include polyuria, polydypsia,
    polyphagia, immunosuppression, adrenal suppression, thromboembolism, hair
    loss, gastric ulcers, and weakening of collagen structures.

Gastrointestinal Drugs

Anthelmintics

Pyrantel pamoate (Nemex, Pfizer): 10 mg/kg PO for hookworms and roundworms,
repeat in 21 days
    Safe for administration to puppies and kittens.

Antiemetics/Protectants

Barium sulfate 30% w/v: 5–10 ml/kg PO acts as a coating agent and appears to slow
or stop active GI hemorrhage.
    Pneumonitis can be associated with aspiration of barium; perforated ulcers will
    result in barium peritonitis.

TABLE 17-2. Selected Emergency Drugs for Dogs and Cats *(continued)*

All dosages are the same for dogs and cats unless specifically indicated.

Cimetidine (Tagamet, SmithKline & French): 5–10 mg/kg q6h to q12h PO, IM, IV to decrease gastric acid secretion
   Side effects in humans include gynecomastia, mental confusion, vomiting, seizures, bacterial overgrowth in the GI tract, multiple drug interactions through decreased gastric acid, and inhibition of liver P450 enzymes.

Sucralfate (Carafate, Marion): 500 mg PO q6h if <20 kg, 1 g PO q6h if >20 kg on an empty stomach; acts to coat gastric ulcers
   The drug is not absorbed systemically; no reported adverse side effects.

Cathartics

Mineral oil: 0.5–2.0 ml/kg given by stomach tube followed by a saline cathartic in 30–40 minutes.
   Do not use vegetable oil because it is absorbed and may facilitate absorption of lipid-soluble toxins. Side effects include aspiration pneumonitis and diarrhea.

Sodium sulfate (GoLytley, Braintree), magnesium sulfate: 1 g/kg PO q12h to q24h
   Sodium sulfate is a safer cathartic than magnesium sulfate. Side effects from sodium sulfate include sodium overload or water deprivation syndrome. Magnesium sulfate may cause CNS depression.

Emetics

Apomorphine (Apomorphine, Lilly): ¼–½ tablet in the conjunctival sac (flush tablet out of conjunctival sac once emesis begins); 0.04 mg/kg IV; 0.08 mg/kg IM, SC.
   Reversal agent is Naloxone (see antidotes and reversal agents).

Syrup of ipecac (Ipecac Syrup, Roxane): 1–2 mg/kg, with a maximum dose of 15 ml
   It is only 50% effective and can have cardiotoxic effects.

Xylazine (Rompun, Haver): 0.66 mg/kg IM once
   The most effective emetic in cats. This dose is lower than the dose for sedation. Reversal agent is yohimbine (see antidotes and reversal agents).

Miscellaneous Drugs

Alkalinizing Agents

Sodium bicarbonate: 1 mEq/kg by slow IV infusion as needed for acidosis, or 50 mg/kg (1 tsp powder equals 2 g) PO q8h to q12h
   It is important to monitor urine pH: if pH <7, increase dose or frequency; if pH >9 reduce dose or frequency.

Drugs that Promote Diuresis

10% Dextrose for diuresis: See Chapter 11

Furosemide (Lasix, American Hoescht): 2–4 mg/kg IV SC q6–8h; cats 2.5 mg/kg IV, IM, SC once or twice daily at 6- to 8-hour intervals (some clinicians recommend a maximum single dose of 5 mg in cats)

Mannitol (Mannitol Injection, Abbott): 1–2 g/kg IV q6–8h as necessary, for osmotic diuresis or treatment of cerebral edema
   It should not be used in hyperosmolar or anuric states.

(continued)

TABLE 17-2. Selected Emergency Drugs for Dogs and Cats *(continued)*

All dosages are the same for dogs and cats unless specifically indicated.

Miscellaneous Agents

Calcium gluconate (10% solution): 1.0–1.5 ml/kg slowly (over 20 minutes) IV to effect for hypocalcemic seizures
  Monitor for bradycardia during infusion.

Desmopressin acetate (DDAVP, Rorer Pharmaceuticals): 1 µg/kg SC
  DDAVP increases von Willebrand factor within 30 minutes in normal dogs and in some dogs with von Willebrand's disease. No clinically significant side effects are recognized in dogs. It has been associated with platelet aggregation in some people with von Willebrand's disease.

50% Dextrose: 0.5 ml/kg diluted 1:3 in 0.9% saline or lactated Ringer's IV for hypoglycemia

Dipyrone monohydrate (Dipyrone, Vedco): 25 mg/kg IV, IM, SC; may repeat q8h
  May falsely suppress body temperature for 48–72 hours.

Specialty Fluids

Hetastarch (Hespan, Dupont Pharmaceuticals): maximum rate of 22 ml/kg/hr

7% NaCl: 3–5 ml/kg slow IV infusion over 3–5 minutes

Urinary Acidifiers

Ammonium chloride: Dogs 100 mg/kg PO q12h; Cats 20 mg/kg PO q12h.

Ascorbic acid (vitamin C): Dogs 100–500 mg or cats 100 mg PO q8h
  The use of acidifiers is contraindicated in animals with metabolic acidosis.

Respiratory Drugs

Bronchodilators

Epinephrine (Adrenalin Chloride, Parke Davis; Epinephrine Injection, Astra): 0.5–1.0 ml 1:10,000 (0.05–0.10 mg) IM or SC once as alternative therapy in nonresponsive asthmatic crisis in cats

Theophylline ethylenediamine (Aminophylline, Elkins-Sinn):
  Dogs: 8–10 mg/kg PO, IM, or slowly IV q8h
  Cats: 6.6 mg/kg PO q12h or 4 mg/kg IM or *slowly* IV q8h to q12h
  For collapsing trachea, bronchitis, adjunct therapy in pneumonia (stimulates diaphragm), and asthma

Terbutaline (Brethine, Geigy): dogs 0.11 mg/kg q8h to q12h, cats 0.625 mg per cat, PO q8h to q12h for collapsing trachea, bronchitis, adjunct therapy in pneumonia, and asthma

Cough Suppressants

Butorphanol tartrate (Torbutrol, Fort Dodge): dogs 0.5–1.0 mg/kg PO q8h or 0.05–0.10 mg/kg SC, IV q6h to q12h as an antitussive

Hydrocodone (Hycodan, Dupont Pharmaceuticals): dog 0.25–0.50 mg/kg PO q12h as an antitussive

Laryngeal Edema. Laryngeal edema is characterized by swelling of structures in the laryngeal and pharyngeal areas that interferes with breathing. It may be induced by excess panting, anxiety, or allergic reactions to insect bites.

Therapy includes the administration of anti-inflammatory dosages of glucocorticoids to decrease the edema and minimize continued inflammation. In animals with acute or life-threatening laryngeal edema, intravenous administration of anti-inflammatory dosages of prednisolone or dexamethasone is recommended because of the rapid onset of action (see Table 17-2 for dosages). Antihistamines may be of some use, particularly for allergic laryngeal edema. To be effective, antihistamines must be given prior to histamine release. They are also useful as calming agents. Diphenhydramine (Benadryl, Parke Davis) can be administered at the dosage of 2–4 mg/kg *slowly* IV (IV administration not recommended in cats), IM, or SC at the time of presentation.

Sedatives may be beneficial to limit progression of edema associated with panting or anxiety. Hyperventilation increases body temperature and exacerbates laryngeal edema. If the animal is hemodynamically stable, acepromazine can be used as a sedative (see Table 17-2 for dosages). Alternatively, meperidine (Demerol, Winthrop) at a dosage of 2–5 mg/kg IM or SC in dogs or 2–4 mg/kg IM or SC in cats given every 4–6 hours as necessary, or morphine (Astra) when given at a dosage of 1–2 mg/kg IM or SC in dogs or 0.1 mg/kg IM or SC in cats (some authors recommend never using morphine in cats because of the potential excitatory effects) may provide adequate sedation. Narcotics may induce nausea, vomiting, or panting, which may cause further distress to the patient. Whenever narcotics are used in cats, they must be given in combination with a tranquilizer such as acepromazine or diazepam to minimize the excitatory effects (see Table 17-2 for dosages).

Diuretics are not indicated unless there is concomitant pulmonary edema.

Laryngeal Paralysis. Laryngeal paralysis causes respiratory distress, which is often worse after exercise or in hot weather. Clinical signs include stridor and often a change in voice. The acquired form is most common in older giant or large breed dogs. It may be associated with trauma or peripheral neuropathies (e.g., hypothyroidism), or it may be idiopathic. Congenital forms are more common in Siberian huskies, Bouviers, and sled dogs.

Emergency therapy of laryngeal paralysis is directed at preventing life-threatening airway obstruction. Forced respirations across the narrowed airway lead to secondary laryngeal edema and further compromise of the airway. Initial therapy is directed at treatment of laryngeal edema. Therapy includes sedatives and anti-inflammatory dosages of glucocorticoids. Refer to the previous section on treatment of laryngeal edema for details of therapy.

Definitive treatment for laryngeal paralysis involves surgical removal of the obstruction (the vocal folds or arytenoid cartilages) from the laryngeal lumen. Various surgical procedures have been described elsewhere.

Collapsing Trachea. Collapsing trachea is characterized by a honking type of cough (if extrathoracic) or expiratory dyspnea and cough (if intrathoracic).

It is most commonly seen in middle-aged toy and small breed dogs. Obesity and concurrent cardiopulmonary problems are common.

Sedation is often required, and the recommendations for sedatives can be found in the previous section on laryngeal edema.

Cough suppressants can be used to break the cycle of irritation and edema formation, but they should not be used in the presence of pneumonia. Commonly used antitussives include hydrocodone (Hycodan, Dupont Pharmaceuticals) at a dosage of 0.25–0.50 mg/kg PO twice daily (in the dog) and butorphanol tartrate (Torbutrol, Fort Dodge) at a dosage of 0.5–1.0 mg/kg PO three times daily or 0.05–0.10 mg/kg SC or IV two to four times daily (in the dog).

Bronchodilators have been recommended for acute and chronic management of tracheal collapse. Theophylline ethylenediamine (Aminophylline, Elkins Sinn) can be administered at a dosage of 8–10 mg/kg PO, IM, or slowly IV three times daily in dogs. The dosage for cats is 6.6 mg/kg PO twice daily or 4 mg/kg IM or *slowly* IV two or three times daily. Terbutaline (Brethine, Geigy) may be administered at a dosage of 0.11 mg/kg two or three times daily PO in the dog and 0.625 mg PO twice daily in the cat.

Glucocorticoids must be used cautiously but may help control edema and inflammation in the event of tracheal collapse. Weakened cartilage appears to be a contributing factor to the development of tracheal collapse, and the collapse can be exacerbated by glucocorticoid therapy. When glucocorticoids are used, they should be administered at anti-inflammatory dosages. Prednisolone is the corticosteroid of choice for rapid onset of anti-inflammatory effects; alternatively, dexamethasone, can be given (see Table 17-2 for dosages).

Monitoring. The patient with an upper airway emergency should be monitored closely during the first 24 hours. Respirations, temperature, pulse, mucous membrane color, and capillary refill time provide an indication of response to therapy or development of complications. Arterial blood gases are essential if the animal requires ventilation. See the monitoring guidelines in the last section of this chapter.

Alternative Therapy. *Tracheostomy.* An emergency tracheostomy must be performed in patients for which an airway cannot be obtained. The surgical technique is described in detail in many surgical texts. The most critical factor is rapid establishment of a patent airway. If the animal has been hypoxic for an extended period, positive pressure ventilation with 100% oxygen or even complete cardiopulmonary resuscitation may be required.

If the animal is conscious, sedation with intravenous ketamine hydrochloride (Ketaset, Bristol) and diazepam can be used. A combination of thiopental (Pentothal, Abbott) and lidocaine (Lidocaine, Elkins-Sinn) is an alternative that also has minimal cardiopulmonary depressant effects (see Table 17-2 for dosages). In very depressed patients, local anesthesia may be adequate. Once an airway is established, isoflurane (Forane, Anaquest) or halothane (Halocarbon Laboratories) general anesthesia can be used to maintain a surgical plane.

Depending on the cause of obstruction, a permanent or temporary tracheostomy can be established. Indications for permanent tracheostomies include patients requiring long-term tracheostomy maintenance, laryngeal reconstruction or resection, radiation therapy of the upper airway, or severe laryngeal paralysis or collapse. Complications associated with permanent tracheostomies include an increased risk of aspiration pneumonia, risk of mucous plugs or inhaled foreign bodies, water obstructing the airway, and loss of voice.

Proper management of a tracheostomy tube includes hydration, systemically and by nebulization. The inspired air should be humidified and ideally should be warmed. Because of excess respiratory loss when the nasal cavity is bypassed, animals with tracheostomy tubes may require two to three times maintenance oral or intravenous fluids (lactated Ringer's solution, about 4–6 ml/kg/hr) (see Chapter 1).

In animals with severe tracheal irritation, the accumulation of mucus requires that the tube be cleaned or suctioned as frequently as every 15 minutes. In animals with minimal mucous buildup, the tube should be cleaned or suctioned using sterile technique at least every 6 hours. Prior to suctioning, 5–15 ml of sterile saline should be instilled to hydrate the respiratory tree, loosen the mucus, and facilitate suctioning. Prior to removing the tracheostomy tube for cleaning, the patient should be hyperventilated with 100% oxygen. Regular coupage or clapping on the chest to facilitate removal of deep secretions should be performed every 4–6 hours. The wound dressing should be changed and the wound cleaned at least daily. When the tube is no longer needed, it should be removed and the wound allowed to granulate closed.

Complications of tracheostomy tube placement include infection, loss of tube, aspiration pneumonia, tracheal stenosis, dysphagia, tracheoesophageal fistulas, and tracheal necrosis.

Ventilatory Support. When an emergency patient is unable to provide adequate oxygenation and ventilation, the use of mechanical ventilation is indicated. There are several alternatives for providing artificial ventilation (Table 17-3). Intermittent positive pressure (IPP) is one of the most frequently used forms of ventilation for short term support. It is accomplished by hand or by using a mechanical ventilator. Guidelines for controlled ventilation are outlined in Table 17-4. IPP expands the lungs and delivers oxygen at designated intervals. Between respirations there is no additional pressure applied to the airway. Positive end-expiratory pressure (PEEP) and continuous positive airway pressure (CPAP) maintain pressure within the airway at the end of expiration and throughout the entire respiratory cycle, respectively. The increased airway pressures help to prevent alveolar collapse. Either CPAP or PEEP should be tried if IPP does not result in arterial $PO_2 > 60$ mm Hg on 100% O_2. Elevations in airway pressure should be adjusted in 5 cm H_2O

TABLE 17-3.   Use of Ventilators in Dogs and Cats

Indications

1. Acute brain swelling (use hyperventilation to reduce intracranial pressure)
2. Respiratory insufficiency
   a. Inadequate ventilation
   b. Inadequate gas exchange
   c. Inadequate delivery of oxygen and removal of CO_2 from tissues (cyanosis, gasping for breath)
3. Laboratory indications
   a. Arterial PO_2 < 60 mm Hg (oxygen therapy alone should be tried first unless the arterial PCO_2 is also elevated)
   b. Arterial PCO_2 > 55 mm Hg

Contraindications

1. Closed pneumothorax, if air cannot be drained from the chest
2. Pulmonary contusions (may increase pulmonary hemorrhage)
3. Tracheal avulsion (do not ventilate until the distal portion of the trachea is secured)

Equipment

1. Endotracheal/tracheostomy tube with a low pressure, high volume cuff (Portex)
2. Transtracheal catheter for high frequency jet ventilation
3. Suction catheters and suction pump
4. Oxygen source with controlled method of adjusting the fractional inspired oxygen (FIO_2) (Precision Medical)
5. Ventilator
   a. Short term ventilation by hand: Ambu bag (Lederle)/anesthetic machine with a rebreathing bag
   b. Mechanical ventilators suitable for long or short term
      (i) Volume-limited ventilator (Metomatic, Ohio Medical Products)
      (ii) Pressure-limited ventilator (Mark 8 Respirator, Bird Corp.)
      (iii) High pressure jet ventilator (Ohmeda)
6. Humidification system for inspired gases to supply 30 g H_2O per liter of air inspired

Adapted from Pascoe PJ: Short-term ventilatory support. In: Kirk RW, ed. *Current Veterinary Therapy IX*. Philadelphia, WB Saunders, 1986; 269.

increments and evaluated by arterial blood gases. Mechanical ventilation is usually not tolerated by conscious cats or dogs. Therefore some form of chemical restraint is frequently required (Table 17-5) as well as intensive monitoring. High frequency jet ventilation (HFJV) ventilates the patient with small volumes at a rate of 60–1800 cycles per minute. It is well tolerated by conscious animals when used with a transtracheal catheter. HFJV can also be used in conjunction with an endotracheal or tracheostomy tube. Although HFJV has been used successfully for management in both human and veterinary patients, it is still investigational and requires further evaluation to eliminate complications such as tracheal necrosis caused by the transtracheal catheter.

TABLE 17-4. Guidelines for Controlled Ventilation in Dogs and Cats

Respiratory rate	8–12 breaths/minute
Tidal volume	15–20 ml/kg ideal body wt.
Peak airway pressure	15–20 cm H_2O
Inspiratory time	1.5–2.0 seconds
Expiratory time	2–3 seconds
Inspiratory/expiratory (I/E) ratio	1:2–1:3
Desired arterial PCO_2	40 mm Hg 20–30 mm Hg to decrease intracranial pressure

TABLE 17-5. Chemical Restraint for Mechanical Ventilation in the Dog

Drug	Dosage
Oxymorphone[a]	0.2 mg/kg IV initially then repeat with 0.05–0.10 mg/kg IV q1–2h or less frequently as needed
Oxymorphone plus	Dosage as above
diazepam[b]	0.2–0.5 mg/kg IV initially and repeat with 0.2 mg/kg IV q1–2h alternately with oxymorphone
Fentanyl[c]	10 μg/kg IV loading dose then either 0.3–0.6 μg/kg/min IV infusion or 5–10 μg/kg IV q30 minutes or less frequently as needed
Fentanyl plus	Dosage as above
diazepam	Dosage as above then 0.25–0.5 mg/kg/hr IV or initial bolus then repeat 0.2 mg/kg IV q1h alternately with fentanyl
Fentanyl plus	Dosage as above
midazolam[d]	0.2 mg/kg IV loading dose then 0.1–0.3 mg/kg/hr IV infusion
Pentobarbital	1–5 mg/kg IV loading dose then 1–4 mg/kg/hr infusion
Atracurium[e] plus adequate sedation using one of the above combinations	0.20 mg/kg IV initial dose then 0.15 mg/kg IV as needed (approximately q30 minutes) or initial dose then 3–8 μg/kg/min IV infusion

[a]Numorphan, Dupont. [b]Valium, Roche. [c]Sublimaze, Janssen. [d]Versed, Hoffman-LaRoche. [e]Tracrium, Burroughs Wellcome.
From Moon PF, Concannon, KT: Mechanical ventilation. In: Kirk RW, ed. Current Veterinary Therapy XI. Philadelphia: WB Saunders. (In press.)

One of the frequent complications of mechanical ventilation is the development of pneumonia. It can result from decreased mucociliary clearance due to the presence of the endotracheal tube and suppression of cough reflex by sedatives. Tracheal necrosis, stenosis, and development of tracheoesophageal fistulas due to the endotracheal/tracheostomy tube or HFVJ catheter have been reported following ventilator use. If the mix of gases is not properly controlled, oxygen toxicity results after delivery of 100% O_2 for more than 12 hours. Atelectasis and pulmonary congestion can result from the long-term anesthesia or heavy sedation necessary to maintain an animal on a ventilator. Decreased cardiac output results from prolonged increased intrathoracic pressure during the inspiratory phase of ventilation. This decrease is further exacerbated by hypovolemia. Dehydration contributes to hypovolemia and promotes the formation of thick pulmonary mucous plugs. Adequate hydration and humidification of inspired gases can prevent this complication. Pneumothorax can result from excessive positive pressure; there is an increased risk in lungs with underlying pathology.

Prognosis of upper airway emergencies depends on the underlying etiology and the ability to correct it. If a foreign body can be removed, the prognosis is guarded to good, depending on the severity of complications seen. The complications of upper airway obstruction can be as mild as edema or as severe as tracheal pressure necrosis. Complications following surgery for thoracotomy and airway resection due to trauma or a foreign body include infection, dehiscence, pneumothorax, or death. Tracheal collapse that cannot be managed medically has a guarded prognosis. Elongated soft palates, stenotic nares, and laryngeal paralysis can all be treated surgically. The prognosis is variable but usually fair to good. Congenital laryngeal paralysis is more difficult to treat than the acquired form because of the associated tracheal abnormalities. Correction of underlying metabolic or neurologic problems usually does not resolve the laryngeal paralysis but is important for the well-being of the animal and the prevention of further complications. Resection of airway tumors carries a guarded prognosis depending on the histopathology and biologic behavior of the tumor type.

Lower Airway Emergencies

Patients with respiratory emergencies of the lower airway (from the carina to the alveolus, including lung parenchyma) often present with rapid, labored breathing and hypoxia. Therapy for lower airway emergencies depends on the underlying etiology. Empiric therapy may worsen certain conditions. For example, identification of respiratory distress and pulmonary crackles could be caused by pulmonary edema or pneumonia. The administration of diuretics to patients with pneumonia increases viscosity of secretions, causes dehydration, and makes management more difficult. Physical examination is an important tool for differentiating causes of lower airway disease. Extensive diagnostics can be dangerous to the patient and should be obtained only after the patient is stabilized.

Asthma (Allergic Bronchitis). Asthmatic patients often present with coughing, wheezing, and cyanosis. Respirations are typically characterized by a normal inspiration with a prolonged forced expiration followed by an extra expiratory effort. Cats presenting with acute episodes of asthma are usually unstable patients. Diagnostic procedures may further compromise these patients, precipitating respiratory arrest. Minimal stress and restraint are necessary. Oxygen therapy alone cannot eliminate the respiratory distress. To treat these patients, a high index of suspicion is necessary, and a good visual examination from a distance coupled with auscultation, palpation, and percussion of the thorax is required.

Standard Therapy. Treatment of an asthmatic crisis (most commonly seen in cats) consists of administration of rapid-acting glucocorticoids. Prednisolone sodium succinate (Solu-Delta-Cortef) is recommended at a dosage of 1–2 mg/kg IV as a single dose. Another rapid-acting glucocorticoid that is available in a parenteral form is dexamethasone (Azium SP). It can be given at a dosage of 0.2–0.5 mg/kg IV or deep IM once. Glucocorticoids should decrease inflammation and potentially prevent ongoing damage through cell membrane stabilization during the acute crisis. Anti-inflammatory dosages may be adequate to control signs in less critical cases (Table 17-2). Asthma is an ongoing problem and often requires chronic therapy (see Chapter 7).

Oxygen therapy may be beneficial; however decreasing inflammation by glucocorticoid administration is essential. The least stressful method of oxygen delivery is usually use of an oxygen cage. These patients are often unstable, and the stress of an oxygen mask may cause respiratory collapse. See Table 17-1 for further recommendations regarding oxygen therapy.

Bronchodilators may be useful for the treatment of asthma. Aminophylline or terbutaline, a β-adrenergic agonist, may improve respiratory function (see Table 17-2 for dosages).

One of the cornerstones of therapy for the patient with asthma in severe respiratory distress is to minimize stress and unnecessary handling.

Alternative Therapy. For patients that do not respond to glucocorticoid administration, epinephrine (Adrenalin Chloride, Parke Davis; Epinephrine Injection, Astra) is the second line of therapy. The recommended dosage is 0.5–1.0 ml of a 1:10,000 dilution IM or SC once. If the animal has not responded in 15–30 minutes, an alternative diagnosis should be pursued. If the animal is stable, radiographs should be performed to substantiate the diagnosis. Feline heartworm disease and lung parasites should be ruled out.

Prognosis for controlling asthma is fair to good. Long-term management may require alternate day prednisone therapy for life or intermittently (see Chapter 7).

Pneumonia. Patients often present with fever, pulmonary crackles, and dyspnea. Depending on the duration and extent of the disease, they may be debilitated or cyanotic. The history may help identify an underlying cause such as a viral infection, megaesophagus, laryngeal dysfunction, immunosuppression, immunoglobulin A (IgA) deficiency, feline immunodeficiency virus (FIV) or feline leukemia virus (FeLV) infection, glucocorticoid administration, or cancer chemotherapy. The extent of pulmonary involvement, the physical condition of the animal, and the underlying etiology influence the prognosis and likely response to therapy (see Chapter 7).

Standard Therapy. Initial therapy consists of providing oxygen. Administration by nasal catheter is contraindicated if the animal has increased upper airway secretions. The flow of oxygen may form bubbles in the secretions and obstruct the airway.

Fluid therapy is used to rehydrate the patient and replace ongoing pulmonary losses. Dehydration makes pulmonary mucus thick and difficult to clear. Overhydration may cause pulmonary edema and further compromise respiratory function. Fluid therapy is also important to maintain good renal perfusion when using aminoglycosides. A balanced electrolyte solution such as lactated or acetated Ringer's is recommended. Initially the patient may require rapid rehydration over 2–4 hours (% dehydration × body weight in kilograms = the number of *liters* of fluid for deficit replacement). At that time hydration status should be reevaluated [packed cell volume (PCV), total solids (TS), body weight, clinical appearance] and the fluid administration adjusted accordingly. Approximately twice maintenance may be required each day, but individuals vary dramatically and require close monitoring (see Chapter 1).

Antibiotics are necessary for bacterial pneumonia. In critically ill patients, a *safe*, bactericidal, intravenous antibiotic should be used to initiate therapy. See Chapter 7 for details of antibiotic and long-term therapy of pneumonia.

Coupage consists of clapping on the chest for 10 minutes four to six times a day followed by exercise. It is useful to stimulate the removal of mucus from the lungs.

Nebulization is a method for microaerosolizing fluids or drugs. In humans, nebulization helps keep airways moist and delivers drugs to the lungs. Disposable nebulizers can be obtained from hospital supply companies. Dosages and efficacy of nebulized drugs are not established for veterinary patients. Nebulization of 0.9% saline in conjunction with physical therapy and systemic antibiotics and bronchodilators (Table 17-2) may make the patient more comfortable and facilitate resolution of pneumonia (see Chapter 7 for further information).

Bronchodilators are useful for keeping bronchioles patent. Aminophylline may further increase respiratory function by stimulating the diaphragm. Another available bronchodilator is the β-adrenergic agonist, terbutaline. See Table 17-2 for dosage recommendations and Chapter 7 for further information.

Monitoring. Animals presenting in respiratory distress due to pneumonia require intensive nursing care and monitoring. Respiratory rate, temperature, heart rate and rhythm, mucous membrane color, and capillary refill time should be evaluated as frequently as every 1–2 hours during initial stabilization. Arterial blood gases are essential if ventilators are to be used and are useful for monitoring response to therapy.

Because hydration is particularly important in these patients, PCV/TS and central venous pressure (CVP) should be evaluated every 4–6 hours and fluid therapy adjusted accordingly. Another indicator of hydration is body weight, which should be recorded at least once or twice daily.

In addition to changes in heart rate and respiratory rate, sepsis often causes hypoglycemia. Blood glucose can be checked along with the PCV and TS.

Urine specific gravity and sediment must be examined daily if aminoglycosides are being used. The presence of casts or loss of concentrating ability (in the face of dehydration) are indications to discontinue aminoglycosides.

Alternative Therapy. If medical therapy is not adequate to maintain oxygenation, artificial ventilation should be instituted. See Tables 17-3, 17-4, and 17-5 for recommendations on the use of ventilators.

The prognosis is guarded, if the underlying cause cannot be eliminated. Mild cases in otherwise healthy animals usually respond well.

Noncardiogenic Pulmonary Edema. Pulmonary edema can often complicate syndromes of electrical shock, smoke inhalation (see Carbon Monoxide Poisoning), toxins, drowning, uremia, shock, heat stroke (see Hyperthermia), pulmonary hypertension, and airway obstruction. The accumulation of fluid within the lung parenchyma creates a diffusion barrier for oxygen.

Standard Therapy. Administration of 100% oxygen helps increase arterial PO_2 and lowers pulmonary arterial pressure. See Table 17-1 for methods of administration.

Positive pressure ventilation helps to fully inflate the lungs. Accumulation of fluid within the lungs increases the tendency for alveolar collapse and further compromises oxygenation. See Tables 17-3, 17-4, and 17-5 for details on ventilation.

Furosemide (Lasix, American Hoescht) at a dosage of 2-4 mg/kg IV or SC q8-12h in dogs or 2.5 mg/kg IV, IM, or SC once to twice daily at 6 to 8 hour intervals in cats (some clinicians recommend a maximum dosage of 5 mg in cats) helps eliminate the fluid accumulation in the lungs. Any diuretic may induce dehydration and azotemia if supplemental fluids are not given. Furosemide may increase the nephrotoxicity of some drugs, e.g., gentamicin (Gentocin, Schering).

The use of glucocorticoids may be associated with an increased risk of secondary pneumonia; however, in some cases of acute pulmonary edema the antiinflammatory effects are beneficial. If used, prednisolone or dexamethasone can be administered at antiinflammatory dosages (see Table 17-2 for dosages).

Bronchodilators may be helpful in reducing bronchospasm. Aminophylline is available in both oral and parenteral forms. Terbutaline is also useful for the management of bronchospasm; however, it is available only in an oral preparation. See Table 17-2 for dosage recommendations and Chapter 7 for further information.

The most critical period is the first 12 hours following the onset of pulmonary edema. Fulminant pulmonary edema is life-threatening, and aggressive treatment must be initiated immediately. Resolution or treatment of the inciting cause is obviously necessary for successful management of patients with pulmonary edema.

Monitoring. Respiratory and pulse rate and character, temperature, mucous membrane color, and capillary refill time will help guide further therapeutics and identify complications. Monitoring should be frequent for the first 12–24 hours.

Cardiogenic Pulmonary Edema. Refer to Chapter 6 for discussion of management of left heart failure.

Arterial blood gases and blood pressure monitoring are ideal for these patients. Refer to the last section in this chapter for discussion of monitoring techniques.

Pulmonary Contusions. Pulmonary contusions are a frequent consequence of thoracic trauma. Contusions result in focal areas of increased vascular permeability and accumulation of fluid and blood within the lung. The best treatment for contusions is supportive care and includes cage rest and oxygen therapy (Table 17-1). The goal is to minimize respiratory distress. In animals who present in shock with pulmonary contusions, fluids should be administered cautiously (see section below). Bruising of the lung predisposes to "leaky" capillaries, and pulmonary edema is more likely to occur even with mild overhydration. If an animal with pulmonary contusions requires emergency surgery, caution should be maintained to avoid overzealous positive pressure ventilation. The damaged lung may not be able to withstand high airway pressures, predisposing it to rupture and development of pneumothorax.

Standard Therapy. The use of an oxygen mask, intranasal oxygen, or an oxygen cage helps provide 40% inspired oxygen (see Table 17-1 for details). Fluid therapy should be appropriate for treatment of shock but closely monitored to prevent fluid overload and pulmonary edema. If the patient is in shock, fluids are given at the standard shock dose, 90 ml/kg/hr. The lungs should be auscultated every 5–10 minutes during fluid administration. If evidence of pulmonary edema occurs, the fluids should be stopped or decreased to maintenance rate (about 1–2 ml/kg/hr) depending on the cardiovascular stability of the patient. Alternatively, if the patient is not in hypodynamic shock but requires some fluid support, fluids should be started at the rate of about 4–6 ml/kg/hr with frequent auscultation of the lungs and evaluation of the heart rate and pulse for signs of developing hypodynamic shock. Colloids such as Hetastarch (Hespan, Dupont Pharmaceuticals) or hypertonic saline 7% (see discussion of therapy for circulatory shock in this chapter) might provide an alternative to standard crystalloid fluid therapy in these patients.

If anesthesia or controlled ventilation is used, caution should be exercised with positive pressure ventilation. Excessive force may result in the development of pulmonary hemorrhage or pneumothorax. In many cases of thoracic trauma, clinical signs of pneumothorax or traumatic myocarditis do not occur immediately. Because of these risks, the respiratory rate and effort, pulse character and rhythm, and electrocardiogram (ECG) should be monitored regularly (every 4–6 hours) for the first 24–48 hours.

Prognosis for recovery from mild to moderate pulmonary contusions alone is good. Animals with severe pulmonary contusions usually die rapidly of intrapulmonary hemorrhage. Other traumatic injuries may complicate therapy and recovery.

Pulmonary Thromboembolism. Thromboembolism is a difficult premortem diagnosis. Although thromboembolism can affect any organ, thrombi to the lungs have a relatively high incidence and dramatic effects. The signs associated with thromboembolism are variable depending on the organ(s) that experiences sudden loss of blood supply. Aortic thromboemboli are associated with feline cardiomyopathy. For discussion of this condition, refer to the section on cardiovascular emergencies.

The presenting signs with pulmonary thromboembolism can be as severe as sudden death or as mild as increased respiratory rate and effort. Other signs that may be seen include fever, tachycardia, pale mucous membranes, weakness, cough and possibly hemoptysis. Radiographs may show signs of regional consolidation, but this does not occur immediately. There are many pathologic states that predispose to the development of thromboembolism, particularly pulmonary thromboembolism. These include hyperadrenocorticism (Cushing's syndrome), disseminated intravascular coagulation (DIC), intravenous catheterization, bacterial endocarditis, nephrotic syndrome, and heartworm disease.

Standard Therapy. Pulmonary thromboembolism is difficult to diagnose, and there is no specific therapy. Supportive care with cage rest and oxygen may help. The goal is to prevent the occurrence in high risk patients.

Aspirin may be used in dogs at a dosage of 5 mg/kg PO daily to decrease platelet aggregation when the clinician anticipates an increased risk of pulmonary thromboembolism. Administration of aspirin should be continued for as long as the animal is thought to be at risk for thromboembolism, unless adverse side effects such as nausea, gastrointestinal hemorrhage, and ulcers are noted. Experimental work using feline platelets suggests that aspirin is less effective at decreasing in vitro platelet aggregation. Aspirin is still frequently recommended prophylactically in feline patients at increased risk of thromboembolism. See Table 17-2 for dosage recommendations. Aspirin is not recommended in patients with platelet counts of less than 50,000/mm^3 because of increased risk of hemorrhage. Aspirin is used in some patients with severe pulmonary changes who are undergoing treatment for heartworm disease (see Chapter 6).

If DIC is present, heparin may help control the hypercoagulability and reduce the risk of thromboembolism. See the section on hyperthermia in this chapter for further information on heparin therapy and treatment recommendations for DIC.

Prognosis is guarded, depending on the success of the treatment of the underlying disease.

Investigational Therapy. Most of the investigational work on thromboembolism in veterinary medicine has been done in cats with aortic thromboembolism. Tissue plasminogen activator (Alteplase, Genentech) has been infused intravenously at a dosage of 0.25–1.00 mg/kg/hr for a total dose of 1–10 mg/kg. Current cost is about $3000 per 50 mg. Half of the cats in one study died during its infusion. Streptokinase (Kabikinase, Smith Kline & French) has also been investigated. In one study, it was given at an intravenous dosage of 90,000 IU for 30 minutes followed by 45,000 IU/hr for 2.5 hours to cats with aortic thromboemboli. These cats showed no statistically significant improvement when compared to untreated cats. There were no adverse side effects of therapy.

PLEURAL AND EXTRAPULMONARY EMERGENCIES

Although the histories may vary widely, patients with diseases or conditions that cause a space-occupying lesion within the thoracic cavity present with similar clinical findings. The most common presenting complaint is dyspnea characterized by rapid, shallow respirations and often postural changes such as orthopnea. Initial management depends on findings from a complete physical examination. Thoracic palpation, auscultation, and percussion combined with observations of the respiratory pattern suggest a problem originating in the pleural space. These animals often have severely compromised ventilation because of collapsed lung fields. Stress (which increases the metabolic rate and oxygen demand), sedation (which may decrease the respiratory drive), or changing the patient's position (i.e., turning it on its back for thoracic radiographs, which further limits the available lung space), may result in respiratory arrest.

Standard Therapy. The preferred initial management is to remove the cause of poor ventilation ability: remove the fluid or air. It can often be accomplished by thoracocentesis. The animal should be allowed to remain in the most comfortable position possible to maximize ventilation. Oxygen should be administered by mask (if tolerated) or nasal oxygen catheter. An area between the seventh and ninth intercostal spaces should be clipped and prepared with a sterile scrub. A 19 to 22 gauge butterfly needle with a stopcock (turned off to the outside air) and a 20 to 60 cc syringe attached should be used to penetrate the skin, intercostal muscles, and pleura on the cranial aspect of the rib. These tissues are highly innervated, and the patient often jumps when the needle passes through them. The needle should be directed straight in; and once within the pleural space, it should not be redirected because it would increase the risk of lacerating the lung (especially on a negative tap). In animals with hyperresonant thoracic percussion suggesting pneumothorax the needle should be placed more dorsally, whereas in those with dull percussion or decreased thoracic compliance the needle should be placed more ventrally. Fluids aspirated should always be saved for cytologic evaluation and possible culture or chemistries in order to determine the definitive therapy required. Both sides of the thorax should be aspirated and the volume removed recorded.

Alternative Therapy. If thoracocentesis must be repeated more than two or three times within 24 hours, placement of a chest tube should be considered. The diameter of the tube should be as large as the mainstem bronchi. The method for chest tube placement is described in detail in many surgery texts.

Pleural Effusions

Pleural effusions can be categorized as transudates, modified transudates, and exudates. Initial management involves relief of respiratory distress and evaluation of the fluid in order to provide definitive care. Transudates are low protein fluids often associated with hypoproteinemia. The cause of a modified transudate is often more difficult to identify. It is an expected finding with right heart failure but can also occur with neoplasia, diaphragmatic hernias, and lung lobe torsions. Exudates may be infected (e.g., bacterial, viral, or fungal) or noninfected (e.g., pyogranulomatous inflammation). Those that are infected often require both systemic and local antibiotic therapy as well as drainage of the exudate, or removal of the nidus if possible. The choice of antibiotics should be based on initial cytology and Gram stain and should be changed if necessary according to culture results.

Other forms of pleural effusion that do not fit into a specific category of the above classification system are hemothorax, chylothorax, and neoplastic effusions. Hemothorax is an uncommon finding and is usually associated with severe trauma, rupture of a tumor, or a bleeding diathesis. Chylothorax can be divided into true chylous effusions characterized by the presence of lymph and chylomicrons, and pseudochylous effusions that do not contain chylomicrons and are usually associated with feline cardiomyopathy. Neoplastic effusions can appear as modified transudates or exudates. They are often difficult to diagnose based on cytology and may require pleural biopsy.

Standard Therapy. Pleural effusions are usually slow to accumulate. The most critical therapy is to immediately improve ventilation by thoracocentesis. Once the animal is stable, further treatment should be directed at the underlying cause. If pleural effusion is secondary to right heart failure, proper cardiac support should be initiated (see Chapter 6 for discussion of treatment strategies).

The use of diuretics does not resolve most effusions, although these drugs may help prevent recurrence if the effusion is due to heart failure. Furosemide is usually the diuretic of choice (see Table 17-2 for dosage recommendations). Administration of diuretics may induce dehydration and prerenal azotemia if supplemental fluids (oral or parenteral) are not provided. Furosemide may increase the nephrotoxicity of some drugs, e.g., gentamicin.

Diaphragmatic hernias can also produce pleural effusion. They are often emergencies, and definitive care is described in a later section of this chapter.

Long-term management of pleural effusion depends on the etiology and is discussed in Chapter 7.

Prognosis depends on the underlying etiology and the response to thoracocentesis.

Monitoring. Respiratory rate and effort, heart rate and rhythm, temperature, mucous membrane color, and CRT are important tools for evaluating therapy and identifying complications or recurrence of pleural effusion.

Arterial blood gases may be beneficial if the animal does not respond to withdrawal of the fluid. They also help evaluate the need for, and effectiveness of, oxygen therapy. Repeated percussion and auscultation can be used as indications of recurrence of fluid if a chest tube is not in place. Refer to the last section of this chapter for further discussion of monitoring techniques.

Alternative Therapy. If repeated thoracocentesis is necessary, placement of a chest tube may be required while medical management is being pursued. The procedure for chest tube placement is described in standard texts of veterinary surgery. If a chest tube has been placed, the amount of fluid withdrawn should be recorded every 4 hours. If an etiology cannot be identified and pleural effusion persists, surgical management with a pleural-peritoneal shunt or chemical pleurodesis may be required.

Chemical pleurodesis can be performed in dogs by instilling tetracycline at a dosage of 35 mg/kg diluted in 75 ml of sterile water into the pleural space, preferably through a chest tube, followed by 200 ml of air. The water and air should be drained after 2 hours. The process is painful, and success is variable. Other drugs have been used for chemical pleurodesis but are either less effective or have more side effects and therefore are not recommended. They include quinacrine HCl (Atabrine, Winthrop-Breon), bleomycin (Blenoxane, Bristol-Myers), and talc.

Prognosis is guarded. In many animals, repeated thoracocentesis or chemical pleurodesis provides only a palliative treatment; however, some animals with idiopathic pleural effusion respond favorably and survive for years.

Monitoring. In addition to the monitoring described above for pleural effusions, it is necessary to monitor the amount of fluid produced. The chest drains may be removed when the fluid aspirated is less than 50–100 ml in 24 hours.

Pneumothorax

Pneumothorax is the accumulation of air within the pleural space. It can be categorized according to etiology into spontaneous or traumatic.

Spontaneous pneumothorax is also called a closed pneumothorax because there are no wounds communicating with the outside. Spontaneous pneumothorax in dogs is usually secondary to bullous emphysema, neoplasia, parasites (e.g., *Dirofilaria immitis, Paragonimus kellicoti, Ecchinococcus granulosus*), and pneumonia (bacterial and viral). Initial management is the same as for a simple, traumatic, closed pneumothorax (see description of treatment that follows). Long-term management and prognosis depend on the etiology and amount of lung involvement.

Simple pneumothorax is an incidental finding in many trauma cases. Small amounts of free air in the pleural space not associated with respiratory difficulty do not require definitive treatment. Simple pneumothorax can be severe and require immediate thoracocentesis. Open simple pneumothorax is associated with a sucking chest wound. The wound should be sealed immediately with a sterile Vaseline-covered gauze sponge to prevent more air from entering the chest. Closed, simple pneumothorax is usually the result of a leak in an airway due to trauma, overzealous positive pressure ventilation, or fine needle aspiration of the lung. Many of the leaks seal over in 24–48 hours, but some require surgery.

Tension pneumothorax occurs when air continuously enters the pleural space from either a leak in the lung (closed) or the atmosphere (open) and cannot escape. This type of pneumothorax is rapidly fatal. It increases the intrathoracic pressure and results in collapse of the lungs and impairment of venous return. The net effect is cardiopulmonary collapse. It requires immediate release of the pressure within the pleural space. Chest tube placement is the most effective method for rapid removal of large volumes of air.

Standard Therapy. Mild cases of pneumothorax that are not producing clinical signs may require only cage rest. It is important that all trauma patients have 24–48 hours of cage rest following trauma because pneumothorax can occur during that time. Cage rest minimizes the risk of pneumothorax and, if it does occur, may minimize the severity of signs. Thoracocentesis (see above for technique) is essential to allow reexpansion of the lungs and resolve the crisis.

If thoracocentesis is required more than twice in 24 hours or a tension pneumothorax is present, a chest tube should be placed. For chest tube placement, most dogs require only a local anesthetic, such as 2% lidocaine (Lidocaine, Elkins-Sinn) in a line block. It is beneficial to anesthetize the pleura, as it is highly innervated. Cats usually require sedation. The combination of ketamine (Ketaset, Bristol) 0.5–1.0 mg/kg IV and diazepam (Valium, Roche) 0.05 mg/kg IV, is usually adequate for 15 minutes of sedation in a sick cat. Be sure to be prepared to intubate and ventilate. Sedation removes the respiratory drive and may result in severe hypoxia and pulmonary collapse. Refer to a recent veterinary surgical textbook for a technique for chest tube placement.

Simple pneumothorax frequently resolves spontaneously if it is mild. More severe cases often recover if they are recognized and treated appropriately. Spontaneous pneumothorax has a guarded prognosis due to underlying lung pathology and recurrence. Tension pneumothorax has a poor prognosis unless it is recognized and treated immediately. If it can be converted to a simple pneumothorax, the prognosis improves.

Monitoring. Respiratory rate and effort, heart rate and rhythm, temperature, mucous membrane color, and capillary refill time are important tools for evaluating therapy and identifying complications or recurrence of pleural effusion. Percussion and auscultation help identify recurrence of pneumothorax prior to respiratory compromise. If chest tubes are in place, the amount of air withdrawn should be recorded every 4 hours. Arterial blood gases can be important, particularly in trauma patients with pulmonary contusions or spontaneous pneumothorax with diffuse pulmonary involvement. Traumatized patients may also have complications of internal hemorrhage that can be evaluated by checking heart rate and PCV and TS. A further complication of thoracic trauma is traumatic myocarditis, and an ECG should be checked at 24, 48, and 72 hours (or sooner if pulse irregularities are noted). Refer to the last section of this chapter for discussion of monitoring techniques.

Alternative Therapy. If chest tubes are not able to eliminate the accumulation of air, or the volume of air does not decrease within 2–3 days, surgery may be required to identify the leak. Once a leak is identified, the surgeon may be able to seal it, or removal of the affected lobe may be necessary.

Another alternative is chemical pleurodesis with tetracycline to increase fibrin deposition (see Pleural Effusion, Alternative Therapy). Thoracotomy and pleurodesis are painful procedures.

If the source of the leak is removed, the rest of the lung is normal, and the animal survives surgery, the prognosis is fair to good.

Monitoring. Immediate monitoring is the same as with conventional therapy, with the addition of observing the surgery site. Long-term monitoring for recurrence by the owners is necessary, particularly in animals with spontaneous pneumothorax. They can be taught to monitor the respiratory rate and character as well as thoracic percussion.

Investigational Therapy. Fibrin glue (Histocryl, B. Braun Melsungen AG) to seal bronchopleural fistulas has been used in humans, but there is limited experience with this procedure in veterinary medicine.

Diaphragmatic Hernia

Diaphragmatic hernias are most commonly caused by trauma in the small animal population. A hernia may not be identified for weeks following trauma. Congenital hernias are most commonly peritoneopericardial, and they may be incidental findings or responsible for respiratory distress. Respiratory function in patients with traumatic diaphragmatic hernias may be complicated by pulmonary contusions, pneumothorax, pleural effusion or pulmonary edema in addition to pulmonary atelectasis. Although no patient with a diaphragmatic hernia should be considered stable, herniation of the stomach is an indication for emergency surgery. Entrapment of the stomach within the thorax can lead to gastric dilation, which further compromises respiratory function and decreases venous return, thereby limiting cardiac output.

Clinical signs are variable according to the extent of herniation and presence of other lung pathology. Signs may be intermittent as organs move freely from one cavity to the other. Physical examination may reveal muffled heart sounds and dull percussion (unless a gas-distended stomach is trapped within the thorax). Intestinal sounds auscultated in the thorax are neither reliable nor consistent in diagnosing a diaphragmatic hernia. Abdominal palpation in small patients with large hernias may reveal a decrease in palpable structures. Radiography or ultrasonography is necessary to confirm the diagnosis, but the patient should be stabilized as much as possible prior to diagnostic procedures.

Standard Therapy. Definitive treatment of a diaphragmatic hernia requires surgery. Prior to surgery, the animal should be stabilized. Oxygen may improve the animal's condition temporarily but does not improve the ability to ventilate, which is the limiting factor. See Table 17-1 for oxygen therapy guidelines.

Particularly in trauma cases, hypovolemic shock may be present. Signs to look for include tachypnea, tachycardia, pale mucous membranes, weak, thready pulses, and cold extremities. These signs suggest later stages of shock, and vigorous therapy is necessary to prevent irreversible shock. See a later section in this chapter for recommendations on treatment of shock.

Diaphragmatic hernias may be further complicated by the accumulation of pleural fluid. Thoracocentesis (see above for technique) may be required to improve lung expansion.

Prognosis is guarded. The most critical time is during stabilization prior to surgery and at anesthesia induction. The most common causes of death are limited tidal volume, multiple organ failure, and shock. Any of these problems can be exacerbated by attempting diagnostic procedures prior to stabilization. If the patient survives the first 24 hours following surgery, the prognosis improves considerably.

Monitoring. Careful monitoring of respiratory rate and character is important. Depending on the nature of the hernia, abdominal viscera may move in and out of the thoracic cavity, which may cause intermittent respiratory distress. Sudden entrapment of a bowel loop may induce rapid shallow respirations associated with pain. Because patients may have sudden changes in the character of their respirations, frequent monitoring is necessary while waiting for surgery. Even if the animal has been stable for several weeks, displacement of the stomach or strangulation of the bowel within the hernia could lead to acute respiratory collapse. Early increases in respiratory rate and the development of shallow breathing suggest the need to reassess the patient and consider emergency surgery.

Temperature should be monitored at frequent intervals in patients with diaphragmatic hernias. A decrease in rectal temperature (< 99°F, or 37°C) is a sign of poor perfusion and often accompanies shock. Increased temperature may be associated with bowel strangulation and endotoxemia or sepsis. Antibiotic therapy (cephalosporins or aminoglycosides—see Table 17-2 for dosage information) is indicated if bowel compromise is suspected. If the temperature is greater than 105°F (40.5°C) despite appropriate fluid and antibiotic therapy, another cause for the elevation should be evaluated. Antipyretics such as aspirin, glucocorticoids, or dipyrone monohydrate (Vedco) (see Table 17-2 for dosage information) should be used only as a last resort to decrease temperature, as response to antibiotics is best monitored by resolution of the fever.

Heart rate and rhythm, mucous membrane color, and capillary refill time should be monitored routinely. Trauma patients should be watched closely for complications of the trauma. Routine monitoring of PCV, TS, and ECG are useful. Arterial blood gases may be useful for evaluating respiratory function and may be used to guide the decision to perform immediate surgery.

Once the animal has been stabilized, or if it does not improve despite medical therapy, surgery should be performed. The surgical technique for diaphragmatic hernia repair is described in detail in surgical texts.

Alternative Therapy. If the animal is not able to ventilate adequately, positive pressure ventilation should be started while preparing the animal for surgery (Tables 17-3, 17-4, and 17-5). If there are concurrent pulmonary contusions, ventilation increases the risk of further pulmonary hemorrhage or rupture of an airway and must be done carefully.

If the animal requires ventilation, the prognosis for surviving surgery is poor. If the patient survives surgery and the first 24 hours afterward, prognosis improves.

Monitoring. Monitoring is the same as for standard therapy, with the addition of monitoring ventilation.

Flail Chest

Unlike the previous extrapulmonary syndromes causing respiratory distress, a flail chest results not in a space-occupying mass within the pleural cavity but a disruption in the chest wall. It can be induced by animal bites to the thorax ("big dog/little dog") or blunt trauma.

A flail segment is characterized by dorsal and ventral fractures of three or more adjacent ribs. During breathing, the segment is influenced by intrathoracic pressure. It is sucked in during inspiration and moves out on expiration. This injury decreases the ability of the thorax to create adequate pressure changes. In addition, the amount of force required to break the ribs and create a flail segment is significant and usually results in pulmonary contusions. Pulmonary tissue can be further damaged by the sharp edges of fractured ribs. Respiratory effort is also limited owing to pain. Puncture wounds can produce a pneumothorax, which leads to further respiratory compromise.

Diagnosis can be made by observation of paradoxical movement of the segment during respirations (as the chest expands during inspiration the negative pressure built up in the thorax sucks the flail segment inward). In large or hairy animals, palpation may be the only way to identify a flail segment.

Standard Therapy. Stabilize the patient. The animal should be placed in lateral recumbency with the injured side down (to maximize inflation of the uninjured lung), and then oxygen is administered (see Table 17-1 for techniques). Animals with trauma severe enough to produce a flail chest usually present in shock. It is important to start treatment for shock immediately (see a later section in this chapter for specific therapy of shock). Fluids should be given, but the animal should be closely monitored for development of pulmonary edema (see the section on pulmonary contusions).

Once the patient is hemodynamically stable, the flail segment must be stabilized. It may be done under local anesthesia with external fixation devices, depending on the extent of damage. The technique has been described in veterinary surgical texts. Dog bites require extensive surgical débridement and repair. Extensive fractures may require internal fixation or chest wall reconstruction. Bandaging the thorax is not appropriate because it compromises ventilation and promotes further injury to the lung.

If the flail chest is associated with animal bites, the most important steps in treatment are débridement and copious lavage of wounds. Use of prophylactic antibiotics is controversial. One retrospective study reported no difference between survival in animals receiving antibiotics following bite wounds and those that did not. There are currently no prospective studies in the veterinary literature to substantiate the usefulness of antibiotics. If they are used, a broad spectrum antibiotic is recommended. Trimethoprim-sulfadiazine (Tribrissen, Coopers) has good tissue penetration, has a broad spectrum of activity, and is relatively inexpensive (see Table 17-2 for dosage recommendations). One report in the literature on humans recommended the use of dicloxacillin (Dicloxacillin Sodium Capsules, Lederle) or cephalexin (Keflex, Dista).

Pain compromises respirations. Control of pain can be accomplished with a combination of stabilizing the segment, administering local anesthetics, and using systemic analgesics. For local anesthesia, 0.5–1.0 ml of 0.5% bupivacaine (Maracaine, Winthrop Laboratories) is administered in the area of the intercostal nerves on the caudal aspect of each rib in the involved area and extending three ribs cranial and caudal. Prior to injection the syringe plunger should be aspirated to confirm that the intercostal vessels have not been penetrated. Although any local anesthetic can be used at the above dosage, bupivacaine is preferred because it has the longest duration (4–6 hours) of action of the local anesthetics. It also has the lowest toxic threshold of the local anesthetics.

Opioids are the most commonly used systemic pain relievers. They are available in parenteral forms. Traditionally, morphine, oxymorphone (Numorphan, Dupont), and meperidine (Demerol, Winthrop) have been used for pain management. These drugs are controlled substances; and in addition to their analgesic properties, they produce central nervous system (CNS) depression. Some of the newer opioid drugs, such as pentazocine (Talwin-V, Winthrop) and butorphanol (Torbugesic, Fort Dodge), lack sedative effects and are not as closely regulated. All narcotics cause some respiratory depression, but the pain relief may result in better gas exchange. See Table 17-2 for dosing information.

Although sedatives do not provide pain relief, combined with an analgesic agent they may relax the patient and therefore improve ventilation. Phenothiazines (e.g., acepromazine) have significant cardiovascular effects and should be avoided or used with extreme caution and only in stable patients.

Phenobarbital (Phenobarbital Sodium Injection, Elkins-Sinn) and pentobarbital (Nembutal Sodium, Abbott; Pentobarbital Sodium Injection, Elkins-Sinn) provide a longer duration of sedation. Diazepam and the water-soluble midazolam (Versed, Roche) must be given more frequently and in combination with an analgesic. See Table 17-2 for dosing information.

Prognosis is guarded. In animals with significant associated pulmonary damage or infection the prognosis is poorer, and the amount of nursing care required increases.

Monitoring. Contusions result in areas of dull percussion and decreased lung sounds. Respiratory rate and character and thoracic percussion should be monitored frequently during the first 24–48 hours.

Shock may be associated with the trauma causing flail chest. This problem should be anticipated by closely monitoring the heart rate and rhythm, temperature, mucous membrane color, and capillary refill time. Trauma may also result in hemorrhage. By monitoring heart rate, respiratory rate, PCV, and TS, shock can be recognized before either hypovolemic shock or hypoxia develops.

Septic shock is a potential sequela to bite wound-induced flail chest. Blood glucose may drop rapidly during sepsis and should be monitored regularly. Arterial blood gases help determine lung function in these patients. ECG evaluation should be performed in all animals with traumatic chest injuries to evaluate for traumatic myocarditis.

Alternative Therapy. If conservative management with external fixation devices fails to stabilize the flail segment, reconstructive thoracic surgery is indicated. Various methods have been described. Extensive débridement of bite wounds might also result in the need for reconstructive surgery.

Success of this technique depends on the experience of the surgeon, extent of the defect, underlying pulmonary damage, and nursing care. Prognosis is guarded.

METABOLIC CAUSES
OF RESPIRATORY EMERGENCIES

Patients with certain diseases that originate as metabolic abnormalities present in respiratory distress. Application of common therapy for respiratory disorders rarely resolves the problem. It is important to perform a complete physical examination to identify underlying metabolic abnormalities. In addition, an emergency laboratory database—PCV, TS, blood urea nitrogen (Azostick, Ames), blood glucose (Chemstrip BG, Boehringer Mannheim), urinalysis, and blood smear—helps differentiate the source of the problem.

Anemia

Many disease processes can result in anemia. Therefore anemia is not a diagnosis but a sign. In an emergency situation it is important to identify the presence of anemia and prevent tissue hypoxia that can lead to further organ failure, shock, or death. The severity of clinical signs associated with anemia is related to both the severity of the anemia and rate at which the anemia developed. An animal may manifest severe respiratory distress due to hypoxia when its PCV is 20% if the hematocrit decrease occurred acutely, e.g., from hemorrhage or hemolysis. An animal with a PCV of 10% may show minimal signs if the anemia has occurred over weeks to months. Once the presence of anemia is identified, characterization of the anemia helps in long-term management and prognosis.

Animals with signs of hypoxia secondary to anemia are usually identified by rapid respiratory and heart rates. They are often lethargic, exercise intolerant, and anorexic. Mucous membranes are pale to white, or if icterus is present they are yellow. Presence of bilirubin or hemoglobin in plasma and urine can occur with hemolysis. Splenomegaly may also be present.

Standard Therapy. (See Chapter 5 for additional information.) For animals with clinical signs of hypoxia due to anemia, the only effective therapy is to provide a source of hemoglobin to carry oxygen. The decision to administer blood should not be based on an absolute packed cell volume but on the animal's clinical condition. Administration of oxygen alone does not significantly help the patient. The animal should be kept in a stress-free environment and quiet to minimize tissue oxygen demand.

Whole Blood Transfusions. *All blood products alter biochemical, hematologic, and some serologic tests. Obtain diagnostic samples prior to transfusions.*

Various blood components can be administered depending on the needs of the patient and the availability of the components. Fresh whole blood has the advantage that it contains clotting factors and platelets. It is indicated in animals bleeding from coagulation factor deficiencies, DIC, and thrombocytopenia; however, fresh whole blood administration does not produce a noticeable increase in platelet numbers. Blood transfusion does result in alterations of coagulation profiles; therefore any coagulation study should be performed *prior to* blood administration.

Stored whole blood provides red blood cells and protein. It is useful for replacement of chronic or acute blood loss unassociated with a coagulopathy. The shelf life of stored blood depends on the anticoagulant used (Table 17-6).

Packed red blood cells (RBCs) can be given either fresh or stored. They are most useful in animals with normal plasma protein concentrations. They should be reconstituted with *0.9% saline*. The volume of saline used to resuspend the packed RBCs should be adequate to allow the cells to flow freely. Typically, one volume of saline and three or four volumes of packed RBCs are used. If the patient requires fluid volume also, larger volumes of saline can be used. If the patient is hypothermic, the packed cells may be mixed with warm, usually 103°F (39°C), saline. One study demonstrated no adverse effects on RBC viability when using 158°F (70°C) normal (0.9%) saline to reconstitute the cells for immediate administration. Incubation of RBCs at 113°F (45°C) for an hour, however, causes increased

TABLE 17-6. Anticoagulants Used for Dogs and Cats

Anticoagulant	FDA Shelf Life [a] (days)	Dosage
Heparin[b]	Not for storage (use within 24 hr)	5–10 units/ml blood
ACD[c]	21 days (feline 30 days)[d]	1 ml/5 ml blood
CPD[c]	21 days (28 days)[d]	1 ml/5 ml blood
CPD-A1[c]	35 days	1 ml/5 ml blood

[a]As licensed by the FDA. The shelf-life, or maximum allowed storage time, is defined as the expectation that at least 70% of the transfused cells remain in the recipient's circulation 24 hours after transfusion. [b]Elkins-Sinn. [c]Fenwal. [d]Reported red blood cell viability if different from FDA guidelines.

fragility and hemolysis. Therefore, caution should be used to avoid overheating the RBCs. Administration of antihistamines, e.g., diphenhydramine (Benadryl, Parke Davis) at a dosage of 0.5–2.0 mg/kg SC, 30 minutes prior to administration of blood decreases the incidence and severity of acute plasma reactions. See Table 17-7 for general recommendations regarding administration of blood products.

Transfusion reactions can be classified as immune or nonimmune mediated. Non-immune-mediated reactions tend to be less severe and include signs of volume overload (vomiting, coughing, pulmonary edema) and fever. Volume overload can be associated with an excess total volume or too rapid rate of administration.

Immunologic reactions can occur immediately or as a delayed reaction. Signs that have been associated with immune hemolysis are restlessness, urticaria and pruritus, tremors, vomiting, fever, change in respiratory rate, tachycardia, renal failure, and convulsions. Anaphylactic reactions can also occur during blood transfusions. Prevention by proper crossmatching is ideal (see Chapter 5).

Monitoring. Baseline values should be obtained *prior* to transfusion. Rectal temperature should be recorded every 30 minutes during a transfusion. Elevations in body temperature could be associated with either immune or nonimmune transfusion reactions. If body temperature begins to rise and is not a result of improved perfusion, the rate of infusion should be decreased. If other clinical signs accompany the increase in temperature, the transfusion should be stopped. Temperature should be followed at regular intervals for at least 48 hours following the transfusion.

Mucous membrane color should improve with transfusion. It should be evaluated during transfusion and continue to be checked at regular intervals for 48 hours following administration of blood products. Pallor following transfusion might be associated with a delayed transfusion reaction. The capillary refill time (CRT) is a rough guide to the state of perfusion and is influenced by both local and central perfusion. Transfusion reactions may result in hypotension and increased CRT.

Pulse should be monitored every 30 minutes during the transfusion. The pulse rate should decrease as the PCV increases. Irregular rhythms are associated with

TABLE 17-7. Blood Administration Recommendations for Dogs and Cats

Blood products should be warmed to 37°C and administered through a commercial blood filter (Travenol).

Volume

1. Milliliters of donor blood = [(2.2 × kg body wt) × 40 (dog) or 30 (cat)] × [(desired hematocrit − recipient hematocrit)/donor hematocrit].

2. 2.2 ml of blood/kg of body weight raises the packed cell volume (PCV) about 1%, assuming a donor PCV of 40%.

3. Maximum recommended volume is 22 ml/kg/day.

Rate

1. Start at a rate of 0.25 ml/kg over 30 minutes; if no adverse effects are seen, the rate can be increased.

2. The absolute rate of administration depends on the needs of the animal and the ability to tolerate the transfusion. In normovolemic patients with normal cardiac function, 5–10 ml/kg/hr can be used. Administration of the blood over a maximum time period of 6 hours has been recommended.

3. The rate in cardiac patients should not exceed 4 ml/kg/hr.

4. Hypovolemic patients may be given up to 22 ml/kg/hr.

administration of cold blood or transfusion reactions. Transfusion reactions also can result in hypotension and shock, which are associated with rapid, weak pulses.

Sudden changes in respiratory rate or character are often associated with transfusion reactions. Rapid infusion rates commonly cause dyspnea, which usually resolves as the rate is decreased. Either tachypnea associated with other clinical signs or apnea is suggestive of a more serious transfusion reaction, and the infusion should be stopped immediately. If the animal stops breathing, it should be intubated and ventilated. Respirations should become more relaxed, deeper, and slower as the PCV increases.

PCV and TS should be measured *prior to* transfusion. In order to evaluate progress during the transfusion, the PCV and TS can be measured on blood from a peripheral vein. If the measured PCV exceeds the desired PCV or the plasma TS are greater than 8 (with adequate hydration), the transfusion should be stopped. If the PCV has not significantly increased, sources of ongoing blood loss should be evaluated and a larger volume of blood considered. The PCV and TS should be measured following completion of transfusion and should be monitored daily for 3–4 days following transfusion. A slight drop in PCV can be expected over the first 48 hours. Plasma color should be noted, looking for evidence of hemolysis.

Specific Therapy for Common Causes of Anemia. See Chapters 5, 8, and 11 for information on specific treatment of common causes of anemia.

Anemia as an Acute Emergency. Acute anemia is often associated with blood loss or red blood cell lysis. Hemorrhage can result from numerous causes. Signs of regeneration may not be apparent for the first 4–5 days following acute hemorrhage or if chronic hemorrhage has led to iron deficiency. The most common causes of hemolytic anemias are immune-mediated reactions, parasitic infestations, and toxins. Clinical signs of hypoxia due to anemia include rapid and often weak pulses. If present, these signs are an indication for transfusion. Thoracic auscultation may reveal a functional murmur. Animals with acute anemia also are at risk for hypovolemic or hypoxia-induced shock. Elevations in temperature can be associated with hemolysis, drug therapy, or infectious agents.

Standard Therapy. Therapy of blood loss requires the use of whole blood (or in some cases of chronic loss, packed RBCs) plus additional therapy depending on the cause of the hemorrhage. In cases with a bleeding diathesis, to determine the most effective therapy a coagulation profile or activated clotting time, platelet count, and mucosal bleeding time should be performed *prior* to therapy. Blood given for treatment of bleeding diatheses should always be fresh so as to provide clotting factors and platelets.

Some common causes of abnormal coagulation seen in veterinary medicine include hepatic failure and vitamin K antagonists (e.g., coumarin-like rodenticides). Treatment includes supportive care and treatment with vitamin K_1 (see Table 17-2 for dosage information). Von Willebrand's disease (VWD) is a deficiency in von Willebrand factor and results in platelet defects and often concurrent factor VIII deficiency. VWD can be treated with desmopressin acetate (DDAVP, Rorer Pharmaceuticals). The recommended dosage of DDAVP is 1 μg/kg SC. The effect is to increase von Willebrand factor within 30 minutes in normal dogs and some dogs with VWD. It has been used to treat animals with VWD prior to surgery and to pretreat blood donors in order to increase von Willebrand factor in the collected blood. No clinically significant side effects are known. Treatment of thrombocytopenias requires determination and treatment of the inciting cause. Treatment of disseminated intravascular coagulation (DIC) is discussed in the section below on hyperthermia.

Another source of hemorrhage is gastrointestinal ulceration, which is treated with sucralfate, cimetidine, or barium sulfate (see Chapter 8). Additionally, the cause of ulceration must be treated. If the animal is receiving nonsteroidal anti-inflammatory drugs (NSAIDs) or glucocorticoids, they should be discontinued. Parasites can also contribute to blood loss. Appropriate use of pyrethrin-based flea shampoo for removal of fleas and ticks and anthelmintics for elimination of intestinal parasites help resolve ongoing blood loss contributing to anemia. In patients with traumatic blood loss, the goal of therapy is to stop active hemorrhage.

Treatment of anemia associated with RBC lysis requires the use of whole blood or packed cells for transfusions. In immune-mediated hemolytic anemia, transfusions should be given only if absolutely necessary. Treatment usually consists of immunosuppressive dosages of glucocorticoids (see Table 17-2 for dosage information) and elimination of any predisposing factors such as drugs (see Chapter 5 for details). Parasitic causes of hemolysis include *Haemobartonella*, which is treatable with tetracycline (see Table 17-2 for dosage information), and cytauxzoonosis, which is fatal and has no specific therapy. Hemolysis associated with zinc ingestion (pennies minted after 1982 and zinc-plated bolts) has been described. Treatment is to eliminate the source (surgery) and provide supportive care.

Prognosis is based on the underlying disease and the initial response to therapy.

Monitoring. (See previous section in this chapter on monitoring during transfusions.) Hypoxia due to anemia results in rapid, gasping respirations. This important clinical sign indicates the immediate need for blood administration. Respirations rapidly return to normal following administration of blood. Animals with a PCV of 15% or less should be watched closely for signs of hypoxia. Mucous membrane color may be misleading, as poor perfusion, as well as anemia, can produce pallor.

Temperature should be monitored regularly to evaluate the response to therapy. If temperature decreases, hypoperfusion or shock should be considered.

The PCV and TS are two of the most important long-term monitoring procedures for the anemic patient. In order for PCV and TS to be of value, the clinician *must* have baseline values. Acute changes in PCV are more likely to be associated with alterations in heart rate and respiratory rate. Decreases in PCV suggest ongoing disease or hemodilution. However, repeated blood sampling, particularly in small animals, can create blood loss anemia. Do not remove more than 5% of a sick animal's blood volume (e.g., do not remove more than about 4.5 ml/kg). Increases in PCV can be due to response to therapy or dehydration. Plasma color can be useful for diagnosis and monitoring the progression of the hemolytic disease.

Alternative Therapy. In some animals the use of blood transfusions can be reserved for alternative therapy. If the animal fails to respond to medical therapy or transfusions, there is currently no alternative therapy.

Investigational Therapy. Many companies are currently producing purified hemoglobin products for intravenous infusion in humans. Clinical trials in animals have been started. Current purified hemoglobin products are stable polymers of bovine hemoglobin. One example is Oxyglobin (Biopure). Oxyglobin can be infused without crossmatching and has oxygen carrying capacity similar to that of whole blood. The preparation is isotonic and because of the size of the polymer helps maintain intravascular oncotic pressure. Following infusion, the polymerized hemoglobin persists for several days in the dog. Side effects reported to date are minimal and appear to be reversible (elevations in blood urea nitrogen and creatinine). It has potential for use in the treatment of hemorrhagic shock, hemolytic anemia, and any other condition for which packed RBCs would be indicated.

Recombinant human erythropoietin (Epogen, Amgen) has been used successfully to increase the hematocrit of humans with chronic renal insufficiency. Early experimental results in both dogs and cats with anemia of chronic renal failure showed promising therapeutic results; however, pro-longed administration may result in the formation of antibodies against the erythropoietin. It may provide a therapeutic alternative in the future.

Methemoglobinemia. Acquired methemoglobinemia (usually recognized by the brown color of the blood) results from compounds that oxidize the iron in hemoglobin, making it incapable of carrying oxygen. There are several compounds capable of inducing methemoglobinemia in dogs and cats. Most commonly recognized is acetaminophen in cats. Toxic signs can occur after ingestion of doses as low as 163 mg. Dogs are also susceptible to the toxic effects; however, the toxic dose is much higher (200 mg/kg). Other compounds such as nitrates, chlorates, benzocaine, and methionine (in cats) are also capable of producing methemoglobinemia.

Standard Therapy. Initial therapy, as with any toxin, is to limit exposure or absorption and facilitate elimination (see the section in this chapter on intoxications). Administration of oxygen is advised. N-Acetylcysteine is given orally as a 5% solution at 140 mg/kg loading dose, followed by three to five treatments administered every 6 hours at a dosage of 70 mg/kg PO. Ascorbic acid should also be administered at a dosage of 30 mg/kg PO q6h for a total of seven treatments.

Alternative Therapy. An alternative treatment is the administration of 1% methylene blue solution *slowly* intravenously at a dosage of 8.8 mg/kg (0.9 ml/kg). This dosage may be repeated if necessary. Methylene blue is *not recommended in cats* as it may produce Heinz body anemia.

If the animal fails to respond, exchange transfusion (replacing the patient's blood with transfused blood) may provide adequate oxygen-carrying capacity provided the source of the toxin is removed.

Monitoring. Patients being treated for methemoglobinemia need to be monitored for changes in their respiratory rate and character, heart rate, and mucous membrane color. Blood smears should be checked for the presence of Heinz body anemia prior to therapy and after the administration of methylene blue.

Prognosis is guarded. If the animal is treated early and survives the first 24 hours, the prognosis improves.

Carbon Monoxide/Smoke Inhalation. Carbon monoxide (CO) poisoning is the primary cause of fire-related deaths. Carbon monoxide is a colorless, odorless gas that has a much higher affinity for hemoglobin than does oxygen. The effect of exposure to CO is that oxygen is displaced from hemoglobin, resulting in tissue hypoxia. Clinical signs include bright red mucous membranes and skin (unless masked by poor peripheral perfusion due to shock), shortness of breath, dyspnea, and confusion. These signs may progress to irritability, nausea, vomiting, incoordination, convulsions, and finally respiratory failure and death. If the animal survives the exposure to CO, pulmonary edema and pneumonia are often complicating sequelae. Pneumonia is a result of inhaled toxins, smoke-altered pulmonary macrophage function, and rarely direct thermal injury. The severity of pulmonary damage may not be evident for 24–72 hours.

Standard Therapy. The first step in therapy for CO poisoning is the administration of 100% oxygen. It may require placement of an endotracheal tube if laryngeal spasm is present.

If signs of shock are present, treatment requires intravenous fluids (90 ml/kg in an hour) or a vasopressor such as dopamine at a dosage of 2–8 μg/kg/min by IV infusion. Higher dosages may cause severe vasoconstriction and should be used only if cardiac output is adequate. Caution must be used during fluid administration, as pulmonary edema is often present. Hypertonic saline may be useful; however, the efficacy and safety of hypertonic saline administration have not been evaluated in patients with CO poisoning.

Bronchospasm is usually associated with frequent coughing in these patients. Bronchodilators, e.g., aminophylline and terbutaline, may be used to decrease bronchospasm. (See Table 17-2 for dosage information.)

Glucocorticoids have been associated with increased mortality and are *not* recommended. Antibiotics administered prophylactically are not recommended either because they predispose to the development of resistant bacterial infection. If pneumonia occurs, antibiotic therapy should be initiated based on transtracheal wash cytology and culture results. The development of bacterial pneumonia is associated with a poor prognosis.

Monitoring. Intensive monitoring of patients with CO poisoning or smoke inhalation is necessary during the initial 24 hours. Temperature, pulse, and respiratory rate should be watched for signs of increases that may be associated with hypoxia, shock, or pneumonia. Regular auscultation of the lungs helps identify crackles that may be associated with overhydration or pneumonia. Monitoring trends in mucous membrane color and capillary refill time will also guide therapy. Arterial blood gases are useful for determining oxygen delivery and are essential if a ventilator is to be used. Radiographs are useful for monitoring the patient's progress and should be obtained at regular intervals. It is important to realize that radiographic signs may not occur for 24 hours.

Carboxyhemoglobin concentrations can be determined at human hospitals. Contact the laboratory at your local hospital for sampling requirements.

Alternative Therapy. If the animal is in advanced stages of CO-induced hypoxia (disorientation, collapse, convulsions), sedation and positive pressure ventilation are necessary. Extreme caution must be used when managing the endotracheal tube in order to minimize the risk of introducing infection to an already damaged lung. (Refer to the section in this chapter on the use of ventilators.)

Metabolic Acidosis. Metabolic acidosis results from the accumulation of endogenous or exogenous acids within the bloodstream. Examples of endogenous acids include lactic acid, ketoacids, and uremic acids. Exogenous acids are most commonly associated with toxins such as ethylene glycol or acetylsalicyclic acid (aspirin). The body responds to the accumulation of acid by increasing its removal of carbon dioxide (part of the body's buffering system).

The clinical manifestations include an increased rate and depth of respirations (Kussmaul respirations). Physical examination, history, and a minimum laboratory database help direct attention to metabolic acidosis. Toxins causing metabolic acidosis often result in an increased anion gap owing to the presence of unmeasured anions of acids.

Standard Therapy. See Chapter 1 for discussion of treatment.

Pain. Pain compromises respirations. It may limit thoracic excursion and decrease ventilation, resulting in poor oxygenation and respiratory acidosis. Pain can also produce respiratory alkalosis due to hyperventilation. Control of pain can be accomplished by a combination of resolution of the underlying pathology, administration of local anesthetics, and use of systemic analgesics.

Standard Therapy. See Chapter 12 for a discussion on the use of analgesics.

CARDIOVASCULAR EMERGENCIES

Shock

Shock is defined as decreased effective circulating blood volume. The three most common categories of shock seen in veterinary medicine are hypovolemic, septic, and cardiogenic. The goals of therapy for shock are to improve tissue perfusion and minimize the sequelae to hypoperfusion. Cardiogenic shock is a result of acute failure of the heart to pump an effective volume. This type of shock must be differentiated from septic or hypovolemic shock because fluid loading a patient in cardiogenic shock increases the cardiac work load and further compromises circulation. Treatment of cardiogenic shock must be based on the treatment of acute heart failure (e.g., ruptured chordae tendineae, acute pericardial effusion, acute aortic insufficiency associated with bacterial endocarditis). Treatment recommendations for heart failure are discussed in Chapter 6.

Hypovolemic shock is most commonly seen in traumatized patients. Hypovolemia does not necessarily mean blood loss. Many patients develop vasodilation, and blood pools in the veins, decreasing return to the heart. Septic shock is associated with volume redistribution; however, it is often complicated by fluid loss into the gastrointestinal tract and interstitium. In either case the best therapy is to reestablish tissue perfusion through volume expansion. Protracted periods of marginal perfusion lead to organ dysfunction or failure.

Standard Therapy. Fluid therapy is the most important part of therapy for shock. Initial therapy involves the administration of a warm (100°–103°F), balanced, crystalloid or colloid solution. In hypovolemic animals with normal cardiac function, lactated Ringer's or acetated Ringer's solution should be administered rapidly. The recommended shock dose is 90 ml/kg IV in an hour. Colloids such as hetastarch (Hespan, Dupont Pharmaceuticals) or plasma at a dosage of 22 ml/kg/hr are even better than crystalloids for maintaining perfusion in patients in shock. The cost of such products often prohibits their routine use. If poor perfusion is a result of massive blood loss, ideally whole blood should be administered at a rate not to exceed 22 ml/kg/hr IV. If sufficient volumes of whole blood are unavailable, the supplemental volume of crystalloids given should equal (22 ml/kg − volume of blood administered) × 3. Control of hemorrhage is essential as well.

Oxygen therapy is important for shock because as tissues are reperfused their oxygen demand increases. Administration of 100% oxygen may be useful initially and may require endotracheal tube placement and ventilation.

The use of glucocorticoids for treatment of shock is controversial; however, whenever they are used they should be administered early in the treatment regimen and not repeated. Prednisolone (Solu-Delta-Cortef) is recommended at a dosage of 22–44 mg/kg IV once. Another rapid-acting glucocorticoid that is available in a parenteral form is dexamethasone sodium phosphate (Azium SP), with a recommended dosage of 2–4 mg/kg IV once.

Signs of septic shock are frequently associated with gram-negative bacteria, and appropriate intravenous broad spectrum antibiotics, such as a cephalosporin or aminoglycoside and penicillin, should be used (see Table 17-2 for dosage information). When using an aminoglycoside, be sure that the animal is well hydrated, as these drugs may produce nephrotoxicity.

Monitoring. Animals being treated for shock require continuous monitoring. Blood pressure and volume are the two most critical factors. Use of blood pressure monitors, central venous pressure (CVP), heart rate, respiratory rate, and urine output can guide therapy. (Refer to the last section of this chapter on common monitoring techniques for further discussion.) The use of positive inotropes such as dopamine (see Table 17-2 for dosage information) is indicated if blood pressure cannot be maintained above 60 mm Hg. PCV and TS are important measures of hemorrhagic shock and for evaluating fluid therapy. Blood gases are essential for determination and monitoring of acid-base balance. Once stabilized, these patients require diligent monitoring to identify early signs of recurrence of shock. Predisposing factors must also be corrected and appropriate parameters used to monitor response to therapy.

Investigational Therapy. Although still considered investigational, the success of clinical trials suggests that hypertonic saline (HS) will be used routinely in the near future. An advantage of using HS is the ability to administer a small volume over a short duration. Studies report improvement in cardiac output, arterial blood pressure, and acid-base status when using HS to resuscitate animals suffering from experimentally induced hypovolemic shock. The recommended dosage of 7% NaCl given as a slow intravenous infusion (3–5 minutes) is 3–5 ml/kg. It has been used at this same dosage in solution as 7% NaCl in 6% dextran 70 (a colloid) with promising results. HS can be used effectively to initially stabilize an animal; *however*, definitive care (e.g., control of hemorrhage, cardiac inotropic support) must be pursued. Side effects of HS are limited; however, there is significant controversy regarding the use of HS in patients who are actively hemorrhaging. Some investigational studies have reported an increase in hemorrhage, possibly associated with improved circulation. HS should be avoided in hypernatremic and hyperosmolar (e.g., suspect ethylene glycol intoxication) patients. The beneficial effects of HS do not persist if the underlying cause of shock is not treated.

Many companies are currently producing purified hemoglobin products for intravenous infusion in humans. They have potential for use in treatment of hemorrhagic shock, hemolytic anemia, and any other situation in which packed RBCs would be indicated. Refer to the section in this chapter on anemia for further discussion of polymerized hemoglobin.

Free radical scavengers, e.g., superoxide dismutase, catalase (not available for clinical use), and DMSO (Domoso, Syntex), have been advocated for treatment of shock as well as in the postresuscitative patient. See the section on investigational therapy for cardiopulmonary resuscitation for details on the use of free radical scavengers.

Cardiopulmonary Resuscitation

Standard Therapy. Closed-chest cardiopulmonary resuscitation (CPR) can be effective in small to medium-sized dogs and cats. Cardiac output resulting from closed-chest CPR may not be adequate in large or deep-chested dogs. Animals with thoracic disease, pleural effusions, pneumothorax, or rib fractures should receive open-chest CPR.

The recommended cardiac massage rate is 80–120 compressions per minute. In some deep-chested dogs, external compressions appear to be more effective if the animal is in dorsal recumbency. In small animals, compressions completely encircling the thorax may improve cardiac output.

Ventilation should be performed simultaneous with thoracic compressions. Ventilation rates for cats are 12–15 breaths per minute (bpm), small dogs 20–25 bpm, and large dogs 20 bpm. Too rapid ventilation causes persistently increased intrathoracic pressure, which interferes with venous return to the heart and results in worse cardiac output.

Several techniques are available that dramatically increase venous return and prevent pooling of blood in the periphery. The easiest one is the use of abdominal counterpressure, which is done by alternating compressions between the thorax and abdomen. Although effective, abdominal counterpressure does increase the risk of abdominal organ injury. Alternatively, a veterinary modification (marketed for investigational use only: pneumatic device, Jobst) of the inflatable human antishock trousers (also referred to as MAST— military antishock trousers) can be used to compress the hind limbs and abdomen forcing blood back to the heart. A practical alternative to MAST trousers is to use elastic tape to wrap the hind limbs and caudal abdomen. After CPR this wrap must be removed slowly and the cranial binding loosened prior to caudal or distal binding.

TABLE 17-8. Recommended Settings for Defibrillation for Dogs and Cats

Cats

External 0.5–10 (W-s)*/kg
Internal 0.2–0.4 (W-s)/kg

Start low and do not increase until the third attempt. The maximum setting should not exceed 100 W-s.

Dogs:

<7 kg	External 2 W-s/kg
8–40 kg	External 5 W-s/kg
>40 kg	External 5–10 W-s/kg
All sizes	Internal 0.2–0.4 W-s/kg

*W-s = Watt-seconds.

Open cardiac massage is indicated when closed chest CPR is inadequate. Reasons to anticipate the need for open cardiac massage include large body size, thoracic disease, low systemic blood pressure despite shock doses (90 ml/kg IV in 1 hour) of fluids, and failure to respond to conventional therapy. Studies show that in some animals that fail to respond to closed-chest CPR, if open cardiac massage is started within 3–5 minutes the prognosis improves. The recommended cardiac massage rate is 80–120 compressions per minute. When performing internal cardiac massage, in order to optimize flow out of the heart, it is important to begin pressure at the apex of the heart and gradually squeeze up toward the base.

Ventricular fibrillation can be converted to normal sinus rhythm by applying a current to the heart. It can be administered externally or internally (directly on the heart). An ECG monitor is essential to identify the rhythm and evaluate the success of defibrillation. Cats are less susceptible to ventricular fibrillation than dogs. See Table 17-8 for recommended settings for defibrillation.

Epinephrine is the most valuable drug for CPR. The standard dosage is 0.01–0.02 mg/kg (or 1:10,000 epinephrine 0.1–0.2 ml/kg) IV every 5 minutes. Many investigational and clinical studies are now recommending the use of high dose epinephrine (0.1–0.2 mg/kg or 1:1000 epinephrine 0.1–0.2 ml/kg IV given every 5 minutes) for better brain perfusion and neurologic outcome.

Oxygen should be delivered at a fractional inspired oxygen (FIO_2) of 100% by endotracheal tube or tracheostomy.

Although volume resuscitation is important in animals in shock, fluids should be administered with caution to patients that are well hydrated or overhydrated at the time of arrest. Shock doses (90 ml/kg IV in 1 hour) may be started initially, but close monitoring (checking pulse, respirations, lung sounds, and CVP every 5–10 minutes) of the patient should be done to individualize treatment and prevent complications (refer to the last section of this chapter on monitoring for further discussion). Volume loading an animal with adequate prearrest blood volume may lead to decreased coronary and cerebral blood flow.

For bradyarrhythmias, atropine should be administered. The recommended dosage is 0.02–0.04 mg/kg IV given initially. If there is a response, atropine may be repeated as necessary to maintain the heart rate above 60 beats/minute in the dog and 100–120 beats/minute in the cat. Atropine may cause tachycardia, which results in increased myocardial oxygen demand and decreased ventricular filling. Lidocaine is used for treatment of ventricular arrhythmias (see Chapter 6). Ventricular fibrillation as the presenting arrhythmia is recognized much less commonly in domestic animals than in the human population; therefore lidocaine should be administered only if the rhythm is known. The drug of choice for ventricular arrhythmias in the cat is propranolol given in intravenous boluses of 0.1 mg repeated to effect. In the cat, lidocaine can be used at a dosage of 0.25–0.50 mg/kg IV slowly if necessary.

Alternative Therapy. If fluid support and epinephrine do not improve cardiac output, alternative therapy would be use of an agent to improve cardiac contractility. Dopamine (Elkins-Sinn) or dobutamine (Dobutrex, Lilly) can be administered intravenously for inotropic support. Both must be administered in a constant infusion drip. The recommended administration rate for both drugs is 2–10 μg/kg/min. Lower dosages of dopamine (2–5 μg/kg/min) are used to improve renal perfusion. Higher dosages (5–10 μg/kg/min) may result in vasoconstriction and poor organ perfusion. Dopamine is light sensitive and should be protected from light at all times. Higher dosages of dobutamine (> 20 μg/kg/min) may result in tachycardia. Dobutamine should not be used in patients with atrial fibrillation because it enhances atrioventricular conduction. *Do not use isoproterenol* (Isuprel, Winthrop Breon), as it causes peripheral vasodilation, which negates any beneficial effects of increased contractility.

Animals undergoing CPR that demonstrate electrical activity of the heart but fail to produce cardiac contractions are experiencing electrical mechanical dissociation (EMD). In this situation the one-time administration of rapid-acting glucocorticoids, such as prednisolone (Solu-Delta-Cortef) at a dosage of 22–44 mg/kg IV or dexamethasone sodium phosphate (Azium SP) at a dosage of 2–4 mg/kg IV, may be beneficial. Some clinicians recommend the administration of calcium gluconate (10% solution) at a dosage of 10 mg/kg IV. If used, calcium gluconate solution should be administered early following EMD. Routine use of calcium for CPR has fallen into disfavor and is not recommended unless hyperkalemia or the use of calcium channel blockers precedes the arrest.

Another drug that has been part of the standard treatment for CPR is sodium bicarbonate. Current research suggests that unless the animal is in a confirmed state of acidosis based on blood gases or TCO_2, sodium bicarbonate may be harmful. Sodium bicarbonate may be given at a dosage of 1 mEq/kg IV based on confirmed acidosis. The administration of sodium bicarbonate inappropriately increases the load of CO_2 in an animal that is already having compromised respiration and may also promote paradoxical cellular acidosis. Routine use of sodium bicarbonate is not recommended.

The route of drug administration has significant influence on the response to therapy. The ideal route of administration is through a central venous catheter. Use of this route is frequently impossible, and alternative routes may be necessary. The intratracheal route is effective for several drugs such as lidocaine, epinephrine, and atropine. When given intratracheally, the recommended intravenous dose should be doubled and the drug diluted 1:3 in sterile water for intratracheal injection. For fluids and other drugs not recommended for intratracheal administration, use of a peripheral vein is advised. If venous access is impossible or too time-consuming, placement of an intraosseous catheter is recommended. Studies show that administration of many drugs by the intraosseous route provides more rapid peak action than administration in a peripheral vein. Intraosseous catheters can be placed rapidly and are indicated in animals with hypovolemia and peripheral vein collapse. The use of intracardiac injections is not advised unless the heart can be visualized (open chest resuscitation). There is no indication for intraperitoneal, intramuscular, or subcutaneous administration of drugs used for CPR. Poor perfusion prevents absorption of the drugs or fluids and may lead to further complications.

Monitoring. Although ECG monitors only electrical activity, not mechanical activity, it is essential to determine the rhythm present and dictate the best pharmacologic intervention. Most common presenting arrhythmias in dogs and cats are EMD and asystole. The most common presenting arrhythmia in humans is ventricular fibrillation. It is worth noting that myocardial infarction is the most common cause of cardiac arrest in the human population. It is not a commonly recognized problem in the pet population, and therefore caution must be used when trying to extrapolate CPR recommendations and information based on human studies.

Although direct blood pressure monitoring is the most informative, it is impractical in most situations. The Doppler blood pressure monitor can be used to indirectly measure peripheral blood pressure. It can also be used during CPR to qualitatively evaluate blood flow to the brain. It is done by placing the probe in the conjunctival sac. The flow to the ocular arteries may correlate with flow to the brain. The pupillary reflex is not a good monitor of response to CPR or prognosis. Short term hypoxia often results in temporary loss of the pupils' response to light.

Patients that survive cardiac arrest often have abnormal neurologic function including blindness, disorientation, and paresis or paralysis. Depending on the duration of brain hypoxia, these abnormalities may persist, or they may resolve over days to weeks.

The prognosis for animals with cardiopulmonary arrest is poor. Most of the animals that survive are young, healthy animals that had an arrest while undergoing an anesthetic episode. Some studies show an improved survival with more aggressive treatment such as using internal cardiac massage early during the resuscitative effort. The survival rate drops dramatically with duration of the arrest. After 20 minutes of CPR the survival rate is negligible.

Terminally ill patients are not good candidates for CPR. The clinician should have prior owner consent in high risk patients for permission either not to resuscitate (DNR) or to perform open chest massage.

Investigational Therapy. Many investigations have identified oxygen-derived free radicals as mediators of neurologic and other tissue damage after arrest. There are several free radical scavengers that have been used with some success. Superoxide dismutase, catalase (not available for clinical use), and dimethylsulfoxide (DMSO) (Domoso, Syntex—dilute 1:4 in 0.9% NaCl and inject 1.1g/kg for dogs and 550 mg/kg for cats slowly IV twice daily) are examples. (Note: DMSO is not approved for parenteral use.) DMSO is an organic solvent and can be readily absorbed across the skin. Always wear gloves when handling DMSO. Another drug that is directed at free radical-mediated damage is the iron chelator desferoxamine mesylate (Desferal, Ciba-Geigy). The recommended dosage of desferoxamine is 25–50 mg/kg IM (or *slowly* IV) as soon as resuscitation is initiated. Rapid IV infusion can cause hypotension.

Although high dose epinephrine (0.1–0.2 mg/kg IV given every 5 minutes) is still considered investigational, there is much work under way to convince the American Heart Association to adopt it as the recommended dosage for CPR.

Calcium entry blockers have been used to improve neurologic outcome following CPR. Nimodipine (not available for clinical use) has been demonstrated to improve neurologic outcome when administered at a dosage of 10 μg/kg IV, or 1 μg/kg/min for 10 hours. Because of their tendency to produce hypotension, calcium entry blockers may actually make the postarrest patient worse. Until further investigation is completed these drugs are not recommended.

Feline Aortic Thromboembolism

Cats typically present with an acute onset of pain and cold, pulseless limb(s). Lower motor neuron (LMN) paresis or paralysis often involves one or both rear limbs but may also affect the forelimbs. Nail beds are cyanotic and do not bleed when cut to the vascular ungual process.

Standard Therapy. Standard therapy is directed at treatment of heart failure, as this syndrome is most frequently associated with cardiomyopathy, and specific therapy for thromboembolism. See Chapter 6 for more information on treatment of heart failure.

Heparin is used for anticoagulation at an initial dosage of 220 units/kg SC followed by 66–200 units/kg SC three or four times daily. Some authors recommend 220 units/kg IV followed in 3 hours by a maintenance dosage of 66 units/kg SC four times daily. The activated partial thromboplastin time (aPTT) should be slightly prolonged (1.5 times the preheparin aPTT is the guideline for humans) at 3-4 hours after the subcutaneous heparin dose. In the event of heparin overdose and overt hemorrhage, protamine sulfate (Lilly) should be administered slowly intravenously at a dosage of 1 mg/100 units of heparin; the dosage is decreased by 50% for every elapsed hour since heparin administration. Protamine should be used cautiously because it may result in hemorrhage for which there is no antidote.

Acepromazine can be used at a dosage of 0.2–0.4 mg/kg SC three times daily for vasodilation. Alternatively, hydralazine (Lederle) can be used as a vasodilator at a dosage of 0.5–1.0 mg/kg PO two or three times daily. Hydralazine may cause reflex tachycardia and complicate the heart failure.

Aspirin has been recommended for antiplatelet therapy at a dosage of 25 mg/kg every third day.

Investigational Therapy. Tissue plasminogen activator (Alteplase) at a dosage of 0.25–1.00 mg/kg/hr for a total dosage of 1–10 mg/kg has been investigated. The cost is $3000 per 50 mg. Half of the cats in one study died during its infusion.

Streptokinase (Kabikinase, Smith Kline & French) given at a dosage of 90,000 IU IV over a period of 30 minutes, followed by 45,000 IU/hour for 2.5 hours in cats with aortic thromboemboli, produced no statistically significant improvement when compared to untreated cats. There were no adverse side effects of therapy.

THERMODYNAMIC EMERGENCIES

Hyperthermia

Hyperthermia can be associated with multiple causes. The most frequent causes of an elevated rectal temperature in veterinary medicine are an increased environmental temperature, failure to dissipate heat (e.g., respiratory disease), increased heat production (e.g., seizures), and fever.

Regardless of the cause of hyperthermia, an acute elevation in rectal temperature of more than 109.4°F (43°C) or a persistently elevated body temperature of more than 106°F (41°C) leads to the same physiologic response. The effects of hyperthermia are twofold. First is the direct effect of heat on body proteins, which results in inactivation of enzymes and destruction of cell membranes and subsequent organ failure. The second effect is a consequence of severe dehydration and hemoconcentration, which leads to sludging of blood in the microvasculature, tissue hypoxia, and DIC.

Anticipation of the organ systems affected is critical to management of a hyperthermic patient. The critical organs and the potential effects of hyperthermia are listed in Table 17-9.

TABLE 17-9.   Effects of Hyperthermia in Dogs and Cats

Organ	Effect
Brain	Irreversible brain damage, blindness, seizures
Kidneys	Acute renal failure
GI tract	Bacteria/toxin absorption, slough of GI mucosa/GI hemorrhage
Liver	Coagulation necrosis, failure to clear bacteria and toxins, elevated enzymes
Heart	Ischemia, arrhythmias, arrest
Lungs	Pulmonary edema, hemorrhage
Blood vessels	DIC

Standard Therapy. If the patient is seizuring or having muscle tremors that are generating heat, one of the first steps is to control the seizures or tremors. Diazepam (Valium) is usually effective for control of seizures when given intravenously at a dosage of 2.5–5.0 mg/animal. Diazepam has a duration of 20 minutes to 1 hour and may need to be repeated. If it must be repeated more than three or four times, pentobarbital sodium at a dosage of 2.2 mg/kg IV is recommended. Pentobarbital sodium usually has a longer duration of action but needs to be dosed according to the patient's needs. Hypoglycemia may also induce seizures. If the animal has a blood glucose of less than 60 mg/dl and is seizuring, glucose at a dosage of 0.5 ml 50% dextrose/kg diluted 1:3 in 0.9% saline or lactated Ringer's solution should be given intravenously. The animal may need continuous glucose infusion, either as 5% dextrose or 5% dextrose in lactated Ringer's administered at a dosage of 1–6 ml/kg/hr IV. Another cause of seizures or tremors is hypocalcemia. If hypocalcemia has been documented, seizures can be controlled with 10% calcium gluconate 1.0–1.5 ml/kg IV slowly (over 20 minutes), while monitoring for bradycardia.

In animals with upper airway obstruction and hyperthermia, anxiety increases the respiratory drive, promoting laryngeal swelling and thereby making respirations and cooling less effective. In order to control anxiety, diazepam or acepromazine can be used (see Table 17-2 for dosage information). Acepromazine should be used only if hyperthermia is due to hyperventilation and the animal is hemodynamically stable.

Hypovolemic and septic shock can occur as a result of hyperthermia. Aggressive therapy of shock is important. Shock doses of crystalloid fluids are 90 ml/kg IV. If an intravenous catheter cannot be established, the intraosseous route should be used. Additional fluids must be given to correct dehydration and replace ongoing losses. Hyperthermic patients typically have fluid and electrolyte losses due to third spacing in the gastrointestinal tract and vasculitis. Hemorrhage can occur from direct organ and vessel damage, or it can be

TABLE 17-10. Methods of Cooling in Dogs and Cats

When cooling an animal, cool only to 103°F (39.4°C).

Chilled IV fluids
Alcohol: poured on foot pads, or whole body
Ice/ice water: on head or whole body
Gastric lavage: effective but requires anesthesia and placement of an endotracheal tube to prevent aspiration
Ice water enemas: effective but lose ability to monitor rectal temperature
Peritoneal lavage with cool lactated Ringer's solution at 10–20 ml/kg (see section in this chapter on intoxications for further description)

due to DIC. Fluid administration is important for maintaining renal perfusion. Acute renal failure is a frequent consequence of hyperthermia and must be anticipated. Vasculitis predisposes to pulmonary edema, so fluid therapy must be appropriately monitored and adjusted. Both plasma and colloids (22 ml/kg/hr IV maximum) are effective for therapy of shock in hyperthermia; however, blood should be avoided, as these patients are usually hemoconcentrated and developing DIC.

Glucocorticoids are usually administered in pharmacologic dosages (prednisolone 22–44 mg/kg or dexamethasone 2–4 mg/kg IV one time). Although controversial, it appears that there are benefits when glucocorticoids are administered early in the treatment of shock.

Antibiotics are recommended for hyperthermic patients. Those chosen should have a broad spectrum of bactericidal activity and be available in intravenous preparations (e.g., cephalosporins or broad spectrum penicillins; see Table 17-2 for dosage information). The most likely bacteria to consider are enterics, gram negatives, and anaerobes that are absorbed across the damaged gastrointestinal tract. Avoid aminoglycosides as renal failure is common in hyperthermia. Cephalosporins are effective, although they have minimal activity against anaerobes (except third generation cephalosporins, e.g., cefotaxime sodium, Claforan, Hoechst-Roussel).

Whenever cooling the hyperthermic animal, cool only to 103°F (39.4°C), or there may be a loss of normal thermoregulatory control, and hypothermia will become a problem. In animals with heat stroke, immersion into ice water causes peripheral vasoconstriction. These peripheral vessels are already engorged with thick, viscous blood secondary to severe hemoconcentration. Constriction of these vessels results in rupture of many small vessels and increased exposure of damaged vascular endothelium leading to activation of the clotting cascade and DIC. Refer to Table 17-10 for common methods of cooling the hyperthermic patient.

Monitoring. Routine and frequent monitoring of temperature, pulse, respirations, ECG, blood glucose, blood pressure, and CVP are useful for evaluating response to treatment. Sudden changes in these parameters guide the clinician to early recognition of problems and improve the chances of correcting them. See the last section in this chapter for details.

With severe hyperthermia both PCV and total solids are dramatically elevated, reflecting severe dehydration and hemoconcentration. With fluid therapy, PCV and TS should return to normal; however, ongoing disease processes such as DIC and sepsis may change this prediction. DIC leads to vasculitis and hemorrhage, decreasing both the PCV and TS. Hyperthermia predisposes to sepsis, which causes vasculitis and a decrease in plasma proteins. Hypoproteinemia and anemia are common sequelae and may require replacement therapy.

Patients with acute renal failure secondary to hyperthermia often present with anuric renal failure. Urine output should be 1–2 ml/kg/hr in the dog and 0.5–1.0 ml/kg/hr in the cat. *However*, it can be evaluated only following rehydration. If urine output is greater than the fluid volume administered, fluids administered must be increased to prevent dehydration.

The prognosis for hyperthermia is guarded. If there are signs of sepsis and DIC, the chance of recovery is minimal. If animals survive the initial insult, renal failure is frequently the limiting factor in long term survival.

Disseminated Intravascular Coagulation. If DIC is present, heparin therapy may be initiated. The recommended dosage is 50–200 units/kg SC q8h. Once initiated, therapy must be continued until all signs of DIC are eliminated or for at least 3 days. To discontinue heparin therapy, the dosage is halved daily over 3–4 days. Premature discontinuation of heparin or failure to taper the dosage may result in rebound hypercoagulability. Dosage adjustments are based on the results of activated clotting times and platelet counts. If the activated clotting time (ACT) measured *prior* to administration of heparin (8 hours after the last dose) is longer than the initial ACT baseline, or the platelet count is decreasing, the dosage is increased by 25–50%. If the ACT has returned to control values and platelet counts are normal, heparin dosage is decreased by 50%. Another method of monitoring heparin therapy is to look for prolongation of the aPTT of 1.5–2.0 times the control value. The aPTT is performed *following* the administration of heparin. Initiation of heparin therapy early in the course of DIC appears to be associated with increased survival.

Plasma and cryoprecipitate provide fresh clotting factors. Whole blood may be necessary if DIC is leading to blood loss; however, whole blood may fuel the progression of DIC. Platelet counts are not markedly increased by transfusion therapy. All blood products should be fresh or fresh-frozen. Incubation of the blood products with heparin (5–75 units/kg body weight) for 30 minutes helps activate the antithrombin III present and is useful for treatment of DIC.

Antithrombin III replacement therapy is investigational and not currently available for routine use.

Monitoring. DIC produces a prolonged ACT, prolonged aPTT (most sensitive), prothrombin time, and thrombin time (most specific), and decreased platelets. Animals with late DIC have fibrin degradation products in their blood and frequently low plasma fibrinogen. With treatment of DIC, removal of the inciting cause, and appropriate therapy (e.g., heparin, plasma), the ACT should return to normal when measured immediately prior to administration of heparin.

Thrombocytopenia is often an early sign of DIC and frequently precedes prolonged clotting times. Thrombocytopenia, however, is not pathognomonic for DIC, so it must be interpreted with caution. Platelet counts of less than $50,000/\mu l$ may be associated with spontaneous hemorrhage. Increasing platelet counts following therapy are an indication of improvement and, when coupled with return of clotting times to normal, are an indication of resolution of DIC.

Hypothermia

Hypothermia is associated with exposure to cold temperatures and poor peripheral perfusion. In veterinary medicine, most cases of hypothermia in adult animals, unless associated with an anesthetic episode, are secondary to poor peripheral perfusion. Monitoring the rectal temperature may be misleading. In low perfusion states the body selectively shunts blood to vital organs, causing a decrease in perfusion of secondary organs such as the skin or gastrointestinal tract. A low rectal temperature therefore may not reflect the animal's core body temperature. Application of external heat to the skin causes vasodilation and results in redistribution of blood, causing further compromise to the vital organs. With hypothermia induced by poor perfusion, the first goal of therapy is to improve perfusion. The cause of poor perfusion should be identified. The most common causes are decreased effective circulating blood volume (shock) or poor cardiac output (heart failure).

Therapy is aimed at the underlying pathology and consists of increasing the blood volume by administering fluids or improving cardiac output by treating heart failure.

Exposure hypothermia is most common in neonates or animals that are debilitated. Central rewarming and minimizing ongoing losses constitute the primary treatment (see below). Neonates are often hypoglycemic in addition to hypothermic. At low body temperatures the intestinal tract does not function normally. Feeding is not recommended until the body temperature is returned to normal. Corn syrup or 50% dextrose is absorbed directly across the oral mucosa to increase the blood glucose concentration. Alternatively, glucose may be administered parenterally (intravenously or intraosseously). Refer to Table 17-2 for dosage recommendations.

Standard Therapy. (See the section on treatment of shock in this chapter and the section on heart failure in Chapter 6 for additional details.)

The metabolism of drugs is altered at low body temperatures. Avoid any unnecessary drugs until the temperature has returned to normal. Myocardial response to defibrillation is also diminished during hypothermia.

With hypothermia secondary to poor perfusion, the cardiovascular system should be stabilized using volume resuscitation (see Chapter 1 and the section in this chapter on treatment of shock) or inotropes such as dopamine or dobutamine (see Chapter 6) prior to rewarming. The safest and most effective method of rewarming is to warm the core of the body. Many methods are used to increase body heat. Administration of intravenous fluids warmed to 100°–103°F (37.7°–39.4°C) can help centrally warm the animal while increasing circulating blood volume. If packed RBCs need to be given, they can be reconstituted with saline that has been warmed to 100°–103°F (37.7°–39.4°C). Providing a warm environment for the patient is useful while avoiding direct application of heat. It can be provided by warming the air the animal is breathing in an incubator or with an infrared heat lamp (*do not* aim the lamp directly on the patient) If heating pads are to be used, those that heat by circulating warm water (Aquamatic K Pad, American Hospital Supply) are safer than electrical heating pads and should be wrapped around the torso leaving the extremities free. *Remember* that direct cutaneous heating by either infrared lamp or heating pad can lead to peripheral vasodilation, cardiovascular collapse, and severe burns.

Another important part of the care of a hypothermic patient is to prevent additional heat loss. This can be achieved by wrapping the animal in blankets or plastic (garbage bags or plastic film).

Alternative Treatment. Gastric lavage must be done under anesthesia or in an unconscious patient, with an inflated endotracheal tube in place. Warm water (5–10 ml/kg) should be administered by stomach tube and then aspirated off. This process should be performed several times.

Peritoneal lavage can be performed using a balanced electrolyte solution at a dosage of 20 ml/kg warmed to 109°F–113°F (43°C to 45°C). The fluid instilled should be allowed to remain for 5–10 minutes and then be drained. (*Note:* You may recover only 10% of the volume infused.) This process can be repeated, being cautious not to overdistend the abdominal cavity and compromise the thorax.

Investigational Therapy. Thoracic lavage is sometimes used to treat hypothermia. The procedure is similar to that for peritoneal lavage. Warmed, sterile, balanced electrolyte solution is instilled into the thorax through one chest tube and drained through a second tube. This step allows warming of blood at the level of the heart. In one investigational study, thoracic lavage was found to be superior to other methods of rewarming severely hypothermic dogs.

Complications following hypothermia are various. Hypothermia is irreversible if body temperature drops below 75°F (24°C). Cardiac arrhythmias can occur that are usually ventricular in origin. Antiarrhythmic drugs should be avoided until the animal is rewarmed and then given only if arrhythmias persist and result in decreased perfusion. Pulmonary edema, bronchopneumonia, and acute pancreatitis have been reported following hypothermia.

Exposure-related hypothermia with a temperature of more than 92°F (33°C) carries a fair to good prognosis depending on the length of the exposure and presence of concurrent or predisposing problems (e.g., coma). Hypothermia due to poor peripheral perfusion from shock carries a guarded prognosis; however, early aggressive therapy can improve the outcome. The underlying condition is also important for determining outcome. Poor cardiac output resulting in hypothermia carries a guarded to grave prognosis and is frequently seen with dilated cardiomyopathy and severe left heart failure.

Monitoring. Body temperature should be monitored continuously initially to evaluate efficacy of therapy. The body temperature should increase by at least 1°F (0.55°C) per hour. It should continue to be monitored every 4–6 hours for the next 24–48 hours. Failure to maintain body temperature is a poor prognostic indicator.

Hypothermic animals have slower metabolism and often have a depressed heart rate and respiratory rate initially. These parameters should return to normal with therapy. Auscultation of the lungs is important for evaluating pulmonary edema associated with rewarming. Rapid respirations may be associated with poor perfusion; and if present, the cause of hypothermia should be evaluated carefully and addressed.

On presentation, most hypothermic animals have pale mucous membranes and a prolonged capillary refill time. If the mucous membrane color and capillary refill time do not return to normal with rewarming, other causes, such as anemia and poor cardiac output, must be evaluated.

A baseline ECG may help identify an underlying cardiac abnormality and should be performed in all patients with rectal temperatures less than 92°F (33°C). If arrhythmias are present, ECGs should be performed at regular intervals. In patients with a body temperature of less than 92°F (33°C), constant monitoring of the ECG during rewarming is useful for identifying arrhythmias. If there are no initial ECG abnormalities or clinical signs suggestive of heart disease, repeated ECGs can be reserved for use if palpable irregularities in the pulse develop.

Fluid therapy should be evaluated repeatedly. The use of PCV, TS, blood pressure, CVP, and body weight can guide changes in fluid therapy. Both severe hypothermia and poor perfusion can result in decreased renal function. Urine output should be monitored closely.

See the section on monitoring later in this chapter for more details.

INTOXICATIONS

Standard Therapy. The goals of therapy in any form of intoxication are to eliminate exposure to the toxin, decrease absorption, and increase elimination. To eliminate exposure, the source of the intoxicant must be identified and removed. Client education is the single most important tool when treating intoxications because prevention is much more effective than treatment.

If an animal has been exposed to a toxin, the first step of treatment is to decrease absorption. With topical toxins, the animal should be bathed in a non-toxic detergent soap with good degreasing power (e.g., Dawn detergent, Procter & Gamble). Particularly in cats, topical toxins are also ingested during grooming, and treatment to decrease gastrointestinal absorption should be employed.

Treatment of enteral toxins requires more aggressive therapy. If the ingestion occurred within 4 hours of presentation, induction of emesis should be attempted *unless* the animal has an altered mental status, decreased gag reflex, or is known to have ingested a strong acid or base, a petroleum distillate, tranquilizers, or antiemetics. Hydrogen peroxide given orally, although recommended by some texts, has variable effects. Syrup of ipecac can be administered at 1–2 mg/kg PO with a maximum dosage of 15 ml. It is effective in only about half of all cases and can have cardiotoxic effects if it is not vomited. It also reduces the efficacy of activated charcoal.

The recommended dosage of apomorphine (Lilly) is one-fourth to one-half a tablet in the conjunctival sac. The tablet should be flushed out of the conjunctival sac once emesis begins. Alternatively, apomorphine can be given at a dosage of 0.04 mg/kg IV or 0.08 mg/kg IM or SC. It has been used at this dose in cats as well. Apomorphine may cause respiratory depression or pro-tracted emesis. These signs can be controlled with a narcotic antagonist such as naloxone hydrochloride (Quad) at a dosage of 0.01–0.20 mg/kg IM, IV, or SC. Xylazine (Rompun, Haver) at a dosage of 0.66 mg/kg IM is the most effective emetic in cats. This dosage is lower than that used for sedation. Side effects include sedation, bradycardia, and decreased cardiac output. Yohimbine (Yobine, Lloyd Laboratories) is an antagonist of xylazine and may reverse the effects when administered at a dosage of 0.1–0.4 mg/kg IV.

Gastric lavage is an effective mechanism for eliminating toxins from the stomach within 2 hours of ingestion. In an unconscious patient it must be performed under anesthesia or with an inflated endotracheal tube in place. The endotracheal tube should extend 2 inches rostral to the teeth, and the head should be tilted down to minimize the risk of aspiration. Warm water (5–10 ml/kg) should be administered by a large-bore stomach tube and then imme-diately aspirated off. This process should be performed 10–15 times. Activated charcoal can be instilled following completion of lavage. Caution should be taken to use minimum force when infusing the lavage fluid to minimize forcing the toxin into the duodenum and to minimize pressure on a stomach that may be weakened. The stomach tube should be premeasured to extend from the tip of the nose to the xiphoid cartilage and never placed forcefully.

Use of activated charcoal is one of the most effective ways to limit intestinal absorption of toxins. The type of activated charcoal used greatly influences its ability to absorb the toxin. The best forms are of petroleum or vegetable origin. A product is available that is two to three times more absorptive than standard formulations and has been shown to be more effective in preventing the absorption of toxins (SuperChar-Vet, Gulf Biosystems). The standard dosage is

1–5 g/kg administered in a slurry 1 g/5–10 ml of water. Many currently available products are premixed. Activated charcoal slurries should be administered by stomach tube. It is recommended that the above dosage be repeated three or four times daily for up to 2–3 days. Side effects are limited to the presence of black feces that stain carpet and clothing.

The use of cathartics in addition to activated charcoal is debatable. Many activated charcoal solutions contain cathartics. The administration of a cathartic is meant to speed transit of the toxin through the gastrointestinal tract, but it may decrease the contact time for the activated charcoal. Some research studies show support for use of cathartics, whereas others show that activated charcoal alone is more effective. Sodium sulfate (GoLytley, Braintree) is a safer cathartic than magnesium sulfate. The dosage of either sodium sulfate or magnesium sulfate is 1 g/kg PO. Side effects from sodium sulfate include sodium overload or water deprivation syndrome. Magnesium sulfate may cause CNS depression. Mineral oil is given by stomach tube. The recommended dosage is 5–10 ml/kg followed by a saline cathartic in 30–40 minutes. Do not use vegetable oil because it is absorbed and may facilitate absorption of lipid-soluble toxins. Side effects include aspiration pneumonitis, if mineral oil is given per os or vomited, and diarrhea. Warm soapy enemas may also speed the elimination of toxins and minimize colonic absorption. *Do not* use hypertonic sodium phosphate enemas (Fleet enema, Fleet) in cats or small dogs.

Parenteral intoxications can occur by either cutaneous absorption or parenteral administration. The goal of therapy is to increase elimination. Many toxins are eliminated by the kidneys. Therefore diuresis hastens elimination and decreases the concentrations in the body. Fluid diuresis using a balanced electrolyte solution is recommended at a rate of 6.6 ml/kg/hr IV (three times the maintenance dose). Once the animal is hydrated, the addition of an osmotic (e.g., mannitol; Mannitol Injection, Abbott; or 10% dextrose) or loop diuretic such as furosemide (see Table 17-2 for dosage information) may facilitate elimination. Furosemide may induce dehydration if supplemental fluids are not administered. It increases the nephrotoxicity of some drugs, e.g., gentamicin. Certain compounds are excreted more rapidly, depending on the pH of the urine. Urinary acidifiers are useful for increasing the elimination of some alkaline toxins. Ammonium chloride at a dosage of 100 mg/kg (dogs) or 20 mg/kg (cats) PO twice daily, and ascorbic acid (vitamin C) at a dosage of 100–500 mg (dogs) or 100 mg (cats) PO three times daily can be used as acidifiers. The use of acidifiers is contraindicated in animals with metabolic acidosis. Alkalinizing agents can increase the removal of acid compounds. Sodium bicarbonate at a dosage of 1 mEq/kg IV or 50 mg/kg (1 tsp baking soda equals 2 g) PO two or three times daily is often used. It is important to monitor urine pH. If the urine pH is less than 7, increase the dosage of sodium bicarbonate or frequency of administration. If the urine pH is more than 9, reduce the dosage or frequency.

Peritoneal dialysis is a labor-intensive procedure that can be effective in eliminating toxins, particularly in anuric or oliguric patients. It is effective for removing some toxins, e.g., ethylene glycol and aspirin, even if renal function is maintained. Peritoneal dialysis requires sterile placement of a peritoneal catheter (Peritoneal Dialysis Catheter, Travenol). A large-bore cephalic catheter may be adequate for short-term dialysis. Dialysate fluid is infused into the peritoneal cavity at a dosage of 10–20 ml/kg and left for 1–4 hours before draining. Rapid exchanges increase the elimination of substances that diffuse quickly across the peritoneum.

Monitoring. Specific monitoring depends on the type of toxin involved. If an intoxication is suspected but confirmation is not possible, monitoring procedures should include regular assessment of temperature, pulse (ECG if indicated by irregularities of pulse), respirations, mucous membrane color, capillary refill time, neurologic status, and urine output. Laboratory evaluation of the patient, particularly electrolytes and acid-base status (TCO_2 or arterial blood gases) and complete urinalysis, is often useful for directing and monitoring therapy. If fluid therapy is used, routine monitoring of PCV, TS, CVP, body weight, and urine output is helpful.

Prognosis depends on the type of intoxication and the time elapsed between exposure and treatment. Early aggressive treatment often provides favorable results.

The following are phone numbers of veterinary toxicology hotlines:

Illinois   1-800-548-2423 Clients or veterinarians, charge is $25/case
Georgia   (404) 542-6751

> For veterinarians in Georgia, Alabama, South Carolina, North Carolina, Tennessee, and Florida only.

> Requires a membership fee.

MONITORING EMERGENCY PATIENTS

Common Noninvasive Monitoring Techniques

Body Weight. An accurate initial body weight is important. Serial body weights every 12–24 hours are excellent guides for monitoring hydration and nutritional status.

Capillary Refill Time. Capillary refill time is a rough guide to the state of tissue perfusion and is influenced by both local and central perfusion. The most valuable information obtained from capillary refill time is the trend seen. Normal capillary refill time is between 1 and 2 seconds. Times exceeding 2 seconds usually are indications of poor perfusion (either local or systemic). Times much less than 1 second suggest hyperdynamic states, e.g., early shock or sepsis.

Mucous Membranes. Mucous membrane color can be a guide to perfusion and oxygenation. Changes in color from pink to white (suggesting hypoperfusion or anemia), red (suggesting the development of hyperdynamic shock or sepsis), blue (suggesting cyanosis), or brown (suggesting methemoglobinemia) can serve as an indication of response to therapy or the development of new problems.

Percussion/Auscultation. Repeated percussion and auscultation can be used to identify the presence of pleural effusion or pneumothorax. Dull-sounding areas are suggestive of fluid or soft tissue structures (collapsed lung or abdominal organs that are abnormal), but percussion over the heart also sounds dull. Hollow resonance suggests air. Thoracocentesis, or if the animal is stable, radiographs can be used to confirm presence of fluid or air.

Pulse Rate and Character. The heart rate increases in hypoxic animals, and rates of more than 180 beats/minute in the dog and 240 beats/minute in the cat may not allow adequate ventricular filling time. Declining heart rates are often associated with increased vagal tone, which may occur just prior to arrest. General parameters for monitoring for bradycardia are heart rates of less than 60 beats/minute in awake dogs (some sleeping or athletic dogs may have normal resting heart rates as low as 40 beats/minute) and less than 120 beats/minute in the cat. Animals with severe hypothermia may have bradycardia that resolves with rewarming. Pulse character is especially important in animals presenting in heart failure. Decreasing pulse quality is associated with poor cardiac output and suggests the need for inotropic or volume support. The development of rapid, thready pulses suggests shock due to sepsis or hypovolemia secondary to dehydration. An irregular rhythm may result from chronic hypoxia and may require specific antiarrhythmic therapy if arrhythmias result in decreased perfusion and persist despite supplemental oxygen and fluid support.

Respiratory Rate and Character. Respiratory rate and character are the most important monitoring tools for animals in acute respiratory distress. Subtle changes in rate or character often precede a respiratory crisis. The character of respirations includes the inspiratory and expiratory effort and duration and the presence of respiratory sounds, either normal or abnormal. Decreased respiratory effort is an indication of successful therapy. It is important to monitor these animals continuously because they may relapse or develop respiratory complications that can result in rapid decompensation and death. Auscultation can be used to monitor for the presence of crackles. Crackles may be associated with overhydration, pulmonary edema, or developing pneumonia. Rapid, shallow respirations are associated with pleural effusions, pneumothorax, or other space-occupying pleural abnormalities. The sudden development of rapid respirations may be associated with hypoxia due to poor ventilation or poor perfusion. Pain, anxiety, or the need to urinate may also stimulate an increased respiratory rate.

Common Invasive Monitoring Techniques

Blood Glucose. With sepsis the blood glucose concentration often drops to a value less than 60 mg/dl. Blood glucose values can be monitored quickly and economically using a blood glucose strip (Chemstrip bG, Boehringer Mannheim) and glucose meter (Accuchek II, Boehringer Mannheim). Hypoglycemia can also occur in pediatric patients and toy breeds that are anorexic (see Chapter 4). Blood glucose does not help in the evaluation of nutritional status of most other patients unless it is used to monitor for hyperglycemia during hyperalimentation or total parenteral nutrition.

Packed Cell Volume and Total Solids. Baseline packed cell volume (PCV) and total solids (TS) are useful parameters in all trauma patients. They help assess the efficacy of fluid therapy in all patients (see Chapter 1). PCV and TS should be rechecked following administration of shock doses of fluids. Ongoing hemorrhage is usually associated with an inappropriate decrease in PCV and TS for the amount of fluids given or despite cessation of fluid therapy. In a patient that presents in a dehydrated state, a decrease in PCV and TS is expected following rehydration. If the PCV and TS increase despite fluid therapy, the volume of fluids given should be increased. PCV and TS can also be used to evaluate for overhydration and development of anemia. Plasma color can identify hemolysis and icterus. The presence of icterus can often be seen in septic animals or those with hepatic damage or trauma.

Temperature. Rectal temperature is an important guide to patient status. Changes in rectal temperature can reflect changes in perfusion (decreased temperature occurs in shock), development of infection (increased temperature may be associated with the development of infection or lack of response to antibiotics), or failure to cool. Empiric administration of antipyretics is contraindicated. Temperature should not be artificially lowered because it eliminates an important therapeutic monitoring device and one of the body's natural defense mechanisms. If the temperature is higher than 105°F (40.5°C) despite appropriate fluid and antibiotic therapy, fever may be a result of tissue injury, then judicious use of antipyretics may be indicated.

Because the lungs are the primary route for cooling in the dog and cat, and interference with the normal pulmonary defense mechanisms may allow the development of pneumonia, rectal temperature should be closely monitored in patients with respiratory disorders. In addition, diseases producing pulmonary edema may also damage the normal pulmonary protective mechanisms. In animals with respiratory distress, depending on the presenting temperature and the ability of the clinician to resolve the respiratory distress, rectal temperature should be evaluated every 2–4 hours. If the animal is in an oxygen cage without a system for cooling, the temperature should be checked even more frequently. Trends of increasing rectal temperature or temperatures of more than 105°F (40.5°C) mandate reevaluation of the patient to look for a cause of decreased heat dissipation or fever. Neoplastic conditions may be associated with fevers.

Urine Specific Gravity and Sediment. Measurement of urine specific gravity is essential *prior to starting fluid therapy*, especially for patients that will be receiving aminoglycosides. Daily urine specific gravity and urine sediment should be evaluated in animals on nephrotoxic drugs. If the animal is not on fluids (i.e., it is maintaining its own hydration well) urine specific gravity decreases during the initial stages of nephrotoxicity. If the animal is on fluids, the specific gravity is not useful. Evaluation of the urine sediment for casts is helpful for determining when to stop aminoglycoside therapy (see Chapters 11 and 15). Toxicity usually occurs in 5–7 days. High fevers can also cause cast formation.

Advanced Monitoring Techniques

Arterial Blood Gases. (See Chapter 1 for additional information.)

Arterial blood gases help evaluate acid-base status and the need for, and effectiveness of, oxygen therapy. Normal blood pH is 7.35–7.45. Blood pH less than 7.35 signifies acidemia; pH more than 7.45 represents alkalemia. This information is essential in animals that are receiving ventilatory support. Elevation of PCO_2 with normal or decreased PO_2 is an indication that ventilatory support is needed. In diseases involving the pleural space, abnormal blood gases are also an indication of the need for more aggressive therapy. If thoracocentesis alone does not improve respiratory function, as indicated by persistent PO_2 of less than 60 mm Hg, ventilatory support, placement of chest drains, or thoracotomy may be required. High PCO_2 is not expected in cases of pleural effusion or pneumothorax unless there is concurrent pulmonary disease or airway obstruction. Low PCO_2 with low PO_2 suggests the need for oxygen therapy. Respiratory acidosis (increased PCO_2) is associated with decreased ventilation or decreased removal of CO_2. Respiratory alkalosis (decreased PCO_2) is associated with hyperventilation (e.g., hypoxia, anxiety, or pain). Metabolic acidosis stimulates an increased respiratory rate to eliminate excess acid. Correction may require bicarbonate therapy, improved perfusion, or correction of the underlying metabolic derangement. Metabolic alkalosis is not as common. Definitive treatment requires correction of the underlying disease; however, acidifying fluids (e.g., 0.9% saline, Ringer's solution) may be helpful for returning the acid-base balance toward normal.

Blood Pressure. Blood pressure can be monitored using direct or indirect methods. Direct monitoring requires placing an arterial line, which is not practical in most situations. An alternative method for monitoring blood pressure is the use of a Doppler Blood Pressure Monitor (Parks Medical Electronics). This device allows indirect measurement of blood pressure. If this equipment is unavailable, trends in blood pressure can be followed by palpation of pulses. As a general rule, the dorsal metatarsal pulse can be palpated when the blood pressure is more than 80 mm Hg, and the femoral pulse can be palpated when the blood pressure is more than 60 mm Hg. Mean blood pressure of less than 60 mm Hg is associated with poor renal perfusion and decreased urine production. Decreasing blood pressure can be associated with poor cardiac output or vasodilation.

Central Venous Pressure. The CVP is measured using a manometer connected to a central venous catheter, and it measures the pressure in the right heart. Normal CVP is 3–8 cm H_2O. The CVP measurements should always be taken with the animal in the same position and the manometer at the level of the right heart. Elevations in CVP are associated with increased right heart pressure, which can be a result of right heart failure or fluid overload. Small increases in CVP are expected with aggressive fluid therapy and represent an expansion of circulating blood volume. Trends in CVP measurements are more important than single values. Increases of more than 3 cm H_2O or a CVP of more than 10 cm H_2O warrant reevaluation of the patient's fluid therapy and cardiovascular status.

Electrocardiogram. A baseline ECG is valuable in trauma patients. Any animal with chest trauma has a high risk of traumatic myocarditis. The presence of an irregular heart rate or pulses of abnormal character suggests the need for an ECG. Traumatic myocarditis usually is not evident for 24–48 hours after injury. Many cases of traumatic myocarditis do not require treatment unless there is decreased perfusion associated with the arrhythmias. Hypoxia can also lead to disturbances of the ECG, but often oxygen therapy alone reverses these abnormalities.

Fluid or Air Withdrawn from the Pleural Space. The character of the fluid and volume of fluid and air removed from the thorax by thoracocentesis or chest tube should be evaluated. Changes in fluid character from clear to cloudy suggest infection and prompt repeated cytologic evaluation and culture. Decreasing volumes (< 1 ml/kg/day) of fluid and absence of air can be used to guide the decision to remove the chest tubes. When chest tubes are present, they should be continuously suctioned or aspirated every 4 hours.

Urine Output. Adequate urine output is defined as 2.2–4.4 ml/kg/hr in the dog or 1.1–2.2 ml/kg/hr in the cat—in a *hydrated* patient. Hypotension (mean blood pressure < 60 mm Hg) results in poor renal perfusion and decreased urine output. Toxins such as ethylene glycol also produce anuric renal failure (see Chapter 11). Urine output should be monitored with aseptic intermittent catheterization or an indwelling urinary catheter and collection unit. If this setup is not practical, an indwelling catheter can be placed but must be maintained as a closed system to minimize the risk of urinary tract infection.

SUGGESTED READINGS

General Information

Crowe DT: Performing life-saving cardiovascular surgery. Vet Med 1989;84 Jan:77.
Haskins SC: Monitoring the critically ill patient. Vet Clin North Am [Small Anim Pract] 1989;19:1059.
Kirk RW, Bistner SI: Handbook of Veterinary Procedures & Emergency Treatment, 4th ed. Philadelphia: WB Saunders, 1985.

Slatter DH, ed: Textbook of Small Animal Surgery, Vols. 1 and 2. Philadelphia: WB Saunders, 1985.

Respiratory Emergencies

Aron DN: Laryngeal paralysis. In: Kirk RW, ed. Current Veterinary Therapy X. Philadelphia: WB Saunders, 1989;343.

Birchard SJ, Fossum TW: Chylothorax in the dog and cat. Vet Clin North Am [Small Anim Pract] 1987;17:271.

Bjorling DE: High-frequency ventilation: a review. Vet Surg 1986;15:399.

Christopher MM: Pleural effusions. Vet Clin North Am [Small Anim Pract] 1987;17:255.

Crowe DT: Managing respiration in the critical patient. Vet Med 1989;84 Jan.55.

Fingland RB: Tracheal collapse. In: Kirk RW, ed. Current Veterinary Therapy X. Philadelphia: WB Saunders, 1989;353.

Harpster N: Pulmonary edema. In: Kirk RW, ed. Current Veterinary Therapy X. Philadelphia: WB Saunders, 1989;385.

Harvey CE: Tracheotomy and tracheostomy. In: Kirk RW, ed. Current Veterinary Therapy IX. Philadelphia: WB Saunders, 1986;262.

Hedlund CS: Surgical diseases of the trachea. Vet Clin North Am [Small Anim Pract] 1987;17:301.

Kramek BA, Caywood DD: Pneumothorax. Vet Clin North Am [Small Anim Pract] 1987;17:285.

Levine SH: Diaphragmatic hernia. Vet Clin North Am [Small Anim Pract] 1987;17:411.

Murtaugh RJ, Spaulding GL: Initial management of respiratory emergencies. In: Kirk RW, ed. Current Veterinary Therapy X. Philadelphia: WB Saunders, 1989;195.

Pascoe PJ: Oxygen and ventilatory support for the critical patient. Semin Vet Med Surg (Small Anim) 1989;3:202.

Pascoe PJ: Short-term ventilatory support. In: Kirk RW, ed. Current Veterinary Therapy IX. Philadelphia: WB Saunders, 1986;269.

Potthoff A, Carithers RW: Pain and analgesia in dogs and cats. Comp Contin Educ Pract Vet 1989;11:887.

Raffe MR: Management of pain in the traumatized animal. Semin Vet Med Surg (Small Anim) 1988;3:210.

Shaer M: The diagnosis and treatment of metabolic and respiratory acidosis. In: Kirk RW, ed. Current Veterinary Therapy IX. Philadelphia: WB Saunders, 1986;59.

Spackman CJA, Caywood DD: Management of thoracic trauma and chest wall reconstruction. Vet Clin North Am [Small Anim Pract] 1987;17:431.

Tams TR: Pneumonia. In: Kirk RW, ed. Current Veterinary Therapy X. Philadelphia: WB Saunders, 1989;376.

Venker-van Haagen AJ: Laryngeal diseases of dogs and cats. In: Kirk RW, ed. Current Veterinary Therapy IX. Philadelphia: WB Saunders, 1986;265.

Cardiovascular Emergencies

Auer LK, Bell K: Feline blood transfusion reactions. In: Kirk RW, ed. Current Veterinary Therapy IX. Philadelphia: WB Saunders, 1986;515.

Authement JM, Wolfsheimer KJ, Catchings S: Canine blood component therapy: product preparation, storage, and administration. J Am Anim Hosp Assoc 1987;23:483.

Crowe DT: Cardiopulmonary resuscitation in the dog: a review and proposed new guidelines (part I). Seminars Vet Med Surg (Small Anim) 1988;3:321.

Crowe DT: Cardiopulmonary resuscitation in the dog: a review and proposed new guidelines (part II). Seminars Vet Med Surg (Small Anim) 1988;3:328.

Feldman BF: Thrombosis—diagnosis and treatment. In: Kirk RW, ed. Current Veterinary Therapy IX. Philadelphia: WB Saunders, 1986;505.

Goodwin JK, Schaer M: Septic shock. Vet Clin North Am [Small Anim Pract] 1989;19:1239.

Haskins SC: Cardiopulmonary resuscitation. In: Kirk RW, ed. Current Veterinary Therapy IX. Philadelphia: WB Saunders, 1989;330.

Henik RA, Wingfield WE: Cardiopulmonary resuscitation in cats. Semin Vet Med Surg (Small Anim) 1988;3:185.

Muir WW: Brain hypoperfusion post-resuscitation. Vet Clin North Am [Small Anim Pract] 1989;19:1151.

Otto CM, Kaufman GM, Crowe DT: Intraosseous infusions of therapeutics. Compend Contin Educ Vet 1989;11:421.

Pichler ME, Turnwald GH: Blood transfusion in the dog and cat. Part I. Physiology, collection, storage, and indications for whole blood therapy. Comp Contin Educ Pract Vet 1985;7:64.

Pion PD, Kittleson MD: Therapy for feline aortic thromboembolism. In: Kirk RW, ed. Current Veterinary Therapy X. Philadelphia: WB Saunders, 1989;295.

Schertel ER, Muir WW: Shock: pathophysiology, monitoring, and therapy. In: Kirk RW, ed. Current Veterinary Therapy X. Philadelphia: WB Saunders, 1989;316.

Slappendel RJ: Disseminated intravascular coagulation. In: Kirk RW, ed. Current Veterinary Therapy IX. Philadelphia: WB Saunders, 1989;451.

Turnwald GH, Pichler ME: Blood transfusion in the dog and cat. Part II. Administration, adverse effects and component therapy. Comp Contin Educ Pract Vet 1985;7:115.

Thermodynamic Emergencies

Johnson KE: Pathophysiology of heatstroke. Comp Contin Educ Pract Vet 1982;4:141.

Krum SH, Osborne CA: Heatstroke in the dog: a polysystemic disorder. J Am Vet Med Assoc 1977;170:531.

Smith M: Hypothermia. Comp Contin Educ Pract Vet 1985;7:321.

Intoxications

Bailey EM: Emergency and general treatment of poisonings. In: Kirk RW, ed. Current Veterinary Therapy IX. Philadelphia: WB Saunders, 1986;135.

Oehme FW: Aspirin and acetaminophen. In: Kirk RW, ed. Current Veterinary Therapy IX. Philadelphia: WB Saunders, 1986;188.

Approximate Drug Dosages

Generic Name and Brand Name—Manufacturer	Dosage (mg/kg)*	Chapter	Suggested Use
Acepromazine maleate Acepromazine Maleate—Techamerica	D: 0.05–0.20, IV,IM,SC q12–24h C: 0.05–0.20 IV,IM,SC q12–24h	17	Sedation
Acetaminophen Tylenol—McNeil	D: 10 PO q8h	2	Pyrexia
Acetazolamide Diamox—Lederle	D: 5–15 PO q8–12h C: 5–15 PO q8–12h	14	Glaucoma
Acetylcysteine (10%) Mucomyst—Bristol	D: 1 drop into eye q1h C: 1 drop into eye q1h D: 140 PO then 70 q6h PO C: 140 PO then 70 q6h PO	14 17	Ocular ulcers Acetaminophen toxicity
Activated charcoal	1 g/5–10 ml water D: 1–5 g/kg PO q6–8h C: 1–5 g/kg PO q6–8h	17	Adsorption of intestinal toxins
Albendazole	C: 25 PO q12h	7	*Paragonimus* (lung fluke) infection
Allopurinol Zyloprim—Burroughs-Wellcome	D: 10–20 PO q24h C: 10–20 PO q24h	11	Urate urolithiasis
Aluminum acetate solution Domeboro's Solution—Miles	D: Apply topically q8–12h C: Apply topically q8–12h	3	Contact dermatitis
Aluminum hydroxide and magnesium hydroxide suspension Amphogel 500 liquid—Wyeth Gelusil II liquid—Parke-Davis	D: 5–10 ml PO q3–4h C: 5–10 ml PO q3–4h	8	Gastric ulcers

*Doses per administration at specified intervals, expressed as milligrams per kilogram unless otherwise stated.

Drug	Dosage (mg/kg)	References	Indication
Amikacin Amiglyde-V—Fort Dodge	D: 5 IV, SC, IM q8h C: 5 IV, SC, IM q8h	8, 15	Enteric bacterial infections
	D: 5.5 SQ q8h C: 5.5 SQ q8h	11	Urinary tract infections
Amitraz Mitaban, liquid conc.—Upjohn	D: Dilute 1:9 in mineral oil, apply periocularly q3days C: Dilute 1:9 in mineral oil, apply periocularly q7days	14	Demodectic blepharitis
Ammonium chloride	D: Apply topically q2weeks	3	Demodicosis
	D: 100–200 PO q12h C: 20 PO q12h	11, 17	Urinary acidifying agent
Amoxicillin Amoxitabs—Smith Kline & French	D: 11–22 PO q8–12h C: 11–22 PO q8–12h	7, 8, 11, 16	Bacterial infections
Amoxicillin (aqueous)	D: 40–50 mg total subconjunctivally q24h C: 40–50 mg total subconjunctivally q24h	14	Ocular bacterial infections
Amoxicillin and clavulanic acid Clavamox—Beecham	D: 13.75–22.0 PO q8h C: 13.75–22.0 PO q8h	3, 7, 12, 15	Pyoderma, bacterial rhinitis and sinusitis, orthopedic infections, bacterial blepharitis
Amphotericin B Fungizone—Squibb	D: 0.50 IV 3 times weekly C: 0.25 IV 3 times weekly	16	Mycotic infections
Ampicillin Ampicillin—Lederle	D: 10–50 IV, SC, IM q6–8h C: 10–50 IV, SC, IM q6–8h	6, 7, 8, 15, 16	Bacterial infections
Ampicillin trihydrate capsules—Lederle	D: 10–50 PO q8–12h C: 10–40 PO q8–12h	6, 7, 8, 9, 11, 15, 16	Bacterial infections

(continued)

Generic Name and Brand Name—Manufacturer	Dosage (mg/kg)*	Chapter	Suggested Use
Ampicillin (aqueous)	D: 40–100 mg total subconjunctivally q24h C: 40–100 mg total subconjunctivally q24h	14	Ocular infections
Ampicillin (A) and gentamicin (G) Ampicillin—Lederle Gentocin—Schering	D: A, 20 IV q8h; G, 2.2 IV q6–8h C: A, 20 IV q8h; G, 2.2 IV q6–8h	9	Septicemia with acute hepatic failure
Amprolium Corid—Merck Sharp & Dohme	D: 100–200 mg total PO q24h for 7–10 days	8	Coccidiosis
Apomorphine Apomorphine—Lilly	D: 0.25–0.50 tablet in conjunctival sac; 0.04 IV or 0.08 IM, SC C: 0.25–0.50 tablet in conjunctival sac; 0.04 IV or 0.08 IM, SC	17	Emetic
Ascorbic acid (vitamin C)	D: 30 PO q6h C: 30 PO q6h	17	Methemoglobinemia
	D: 100–500 mg total PO q8h C: 100 mg total PO q8h	17	Urinary acidifying agent
	D: 25 PO q24h C: 25 PO q24h	9	Copper-toxicity hepatitis, chronic hepatic insufficiency

Drug	Dosage	Ref.	Indication
Aspirin	D: 10 PO q8–12h C: 10 PO q48–72h	2	Pyrexia
	D: 5 PO q24h C: 25 PO q72h	6, 17	Pulmonary arterial disease, pulmonary thromboembolism
	D: 15–25 PO q8–12h C: 10–15 PO q48h (max. 25 PO q24h)	12	Musculoskeletal diseases, degenerative joint disease
Atropine Atropine sulfate injection—Elkins-Sinn 1%	D: 0.02–0.05 IV C: 0.02–0.05 IV	6, 17	Bradyarrhythmias
	D: Instill into eye q6–24h	14	Ocular pain
Auranofil Ridaura—Smith Kline & French	D: 0.05–0.20 PO q12h	3	Autoimmune skin disease
Aurothioglucose Solganol—Schering	D: See Ch. 3 for protocol C: See Ch. 3 for protocol	3	Autoimmune skin disease
Azathioprine Imuran—Burroughs Wellcome	D: 2.0 PO q24h C: 2.0 PO q24h	8, 12	Lymphocytic-plasmacytic enteritis, canine rheumatoid arthritis
	D: 0.5–1.0 PO q48h	16	Autoimmune hemolytic anemia
	D: 3 PO q24h, taper to 1 q24h C: 3 PO q24h, taper to 1 q24h	5	Systemic lupus erythematosus
	D: 3 PO q24h, taper to 1 q48h C: 3 PO q24h, taper to 1 q48h	5	Thrombocytopenia
	D: See Ch. 3 for protocol C: See Ch. 3 for protocol	3	Autoimmune skin disease
Azathioprine (A) and prednisolone (P)	D: A, 1.0 PO q24h; P, 0.5 PO q24h	9	Chronic hepatitis

(continued)

Generic Name and Brand Name—Manufacturer	Dosage (mg/kg)*	Chapter	Suggested Use
Bacitracin/neomycin/polymyxin B Neosporin—Burroughs Wellcome	D: 1–2 drops into eye q4–6h C: 1–2 drops into eye q4–6h	14	Ocular infections
Bacitracin/polymyxin B/neomycin/hydrocortisone Cortisporin—Burroughs Wellcome	D: Thin film into eye q6–8h C: Thin film into eye q6–8h	14	Bacterial blepharitis
Baclofen Lioresal—Geigy	D: 1–2 PO q8h	11	Urethral hyperreflexia, reflex dyssynergia
Baker's yeast	D: 100 PO q24h C: 100 PO q24h	16	Prevent folic acid deficiency when using pyrimethamine and sulfadiazine
Benzoyl peroxide (2.5–5.0%) OxyDex Gel—DVM, Inc.	D: Apply topically as directed C: Apply topically as directed	3	Dermatitis
Benzyl benzoate solution	D: Apply periocularly	14	Demodectic blepharitis
Betaxolol Hydrochloride Betoptic—Alcon	D: 1 drop into eye q12h C: 1 drop into eye q12h	14	Glaucoma
Bethanechol Urecholine—Merck Sharp & Dohme	D: 5–15 mg total PO q8h C: 1.25–5.00 mg total PO q8h	11	Bladder atony
Bisacodyl Dulcolax—Boehringer	D: 5–20 mg total PO q24h C: 5 mg total PO q24h	8	Constipation
Bismuth subsalicylate Corrective Mixture—SmithKline Beecham Pepto-Bismol—Norwich-Eaton	D: 2.5 ml/kg PO q4–6h C: 1–2 ml/kg PO q8h	8	Diarrhea
Bovine thyrotropin Dermathycin—Coopers Thytropar—Armour	D: 0.1 U/kg IV C: 1 U/kg IV	4	Testing for hypothyroidism

Drug	Dose	Ref.	Indication
Bunamide Scolaban—Burroughs Wellcome	D: 25–50 mg total C: 25–50 mg total	8	*Taenia* infection
Bupivacaine (0.5%) Maracaine—Winthrop	D: 0.5–1.0 ml SC C: 0.5–1.0 ml SC	17	Local anesthesia
Butamisol Styquin—American Cyanamid	D: 2.4 SC repeat at 21 and 70 days	8	Ancylostomiasis and trichuriasis
Butorphanol Torbugesic—Fort Dodge	D: 0.4 IM q6h	10	Pancreatitis
	D: 0.2–0.4 IM, SC, IV C: 0.2 IM, SC	10, 17	Pain relief
Torbutrol—Fort Dodge	D: 0.5–1.0 PO q6–12h; 0.05–0.10 SC, IV q6–12h C: 0.5 PO q6–12h	7, 17	Cough suppressant
Calcium gluconate Calcium gluconate tablets—Elkins-Sinn	D: 1–4 g PO divided q8–12h C: 0.5–1.0 g PO q24h	4	Hypocalcemia
Calcium gluconate injection 10%—Elkins-Sinn	D: 10 IV C: 10 IV	17	Electrical mechanical dissociation
	D: 1.0–1.5 ml/kg slowly (over 20 min.) IV to effect C: 1.0–1.5 ml/kg slowly (over 20 min.) IV to effect	17	Hypocalcemic seizures
	D: 0.5 IV slowly over 10–20 minutes C: 0.5 IV slowly over 10–20 minutes	6	Hyperkalemic myocardial toxicity

(continued)

Generic Name and Brand Name—Manufacturer	Dosage (mg/kg)*	Chapter	Suggested Use
Captan 50% powder Orthocide Garden Fungicide—Ortho	D: Dilute 1.5 tsp/L water, apply topically q12h C: Dilute 1.5 tsp/L water, apply topically q12h	3	Dermatophytosis
Captopril Capoten—Squibb	D: 0.5–1.5 PO q8h C: 0.5–1.5 PO q8h	6	Congestive heart failure
	D: 0.5–2.0 PO q8–12h C: 0.5–2.0 PO q8–12h	11	Vasodilation
Carbaryl Sevin—Union Carbide	D: Apply topically as directed C: Apply topically as directed	3	Fleas
Mitox—Norden	D: Instill a few drops into ear C: Instill a few drops into ear	3	Ear mites
Carbenicillin Geopen—Roerig	D: Instill 100–250 mg total into eye q1–2h C: Instill 100–250 mg total into eye q1–2h	14	Ocular ulcers
	D: 15–60 IM, IV, PO q8h	15	Bacterial infections
Cefaclor Ceclor—Lilly	D: 20 PO q8h C: 20 PO q8h	6	Infective endocarditis
Cefadroxil Cefa-Tabs—Fort Dodge	D: 15.4–30.0 PO q8–12h C: 15.4–30.0 PO q8–12h	3, 12, 15	Pyoderma, soft tissue and orthopedic infections
Cefamandole Mandol—Lilly	D: 15 IV, IM q4–6h C: 15 IV, IM q4–6h	15	Bacterial infections

Cefazolin Kefzol—Lilly Ancef—Smith Kline & French	D: 15–25 IV, IM, SC q6–8h C: 15–25 IV q6–8h	12, 15	Diskospondylitis, bacterial inflammatory arthritis, soft tissue infections
Cefazolin (C) and gentamicin (G) Ancef—Smith Kline & French Kefzol—Lilly Gentocin—Schering	D: C–22 IV; G–2.2 IV q8h C: C–22 IV; G–2.2 IV q8h	12	Bacterial osteomyelitis
Cefotaxime Claforan–Hoechst Roussel	D: 20–80 IV, IM, SC q6–8h C: 20–80 IV, IM, SC q6–8h	15, 17	Bacterial infections
Cefoxitin Mefoxin—Merck Sharp & Dohme	D: 22 IV q8h, 6–40 q4–6h C: 22 IV q8h, 6–40 q4–6h	15, 16	Anaerobic infections
Ceftazidime Fortaz–Glaxo	D: 35 IM, SC q8–12h C: 35 IM, SC q8–12h	15	Bacterial infections
Cephalexin Keflex–Dista	D: 8–22.0 PO q8h C: 8–22.0 PO q8h	3, 7, 11, 12, 13, 15, 17	Bacterial infections
	D: 22–30 PO q8h	12	Diskospondylitis
Cephalothin Keflin—Lilly	D: 15–40 IV, IM, SC q6–8h C: 15–40 IV, IM, SC q6–8h	6, 7, 15	Bacterial endocarditis
Cephalothin (aqueous)	D: 22–30 IV, IM, SC 6–8h	12	Diskospondylitis
	D: 25–100 mg total subconjunctivally q24h C: 25–100 mg total subconjunctivally q24h	14	Ocular infections
Cephapirin sodium Cefadyl—Bristol-Myers	D: 20–40 IV q6–8h C: 20–40 IV q6–8h	7, 9, 12, 15	Bacterial infections

(continued)

Generic Name and Brand Name—Manufacturer	Dosage (mg/kg)*	Chapter	Suggested Use
Cephradine Velosef—Squibb	D: 20–40 PO q8h C: 20–40 PO q8h	3, 7, 9, 12, 13	Bacterial infections
	D: 12–25 IV, IM, SC, q8h C: 12–25 IV, IM, SC, q8h	3, 7, 9, 12, 13	Bacterial infections
Chlorambucil Leukeran—Burroughs Wellcome	D: 2 mg/m²/day PO C: 2 mg/m²/day PO	5	Systemic lupus erythematosus
Chloramphenicol Chloramphenicol capsules—Rugby	D: 15–55 PO q6–8h C: 15–50 PO q8–12h	3, 7, 11, 15, 16	Bacterial, rickettsial, and mycoplasma infections
Chloramphenicol	D: 20 SC q8h C: 20 SC q8h	10	Pancreatitis
Chloramphenicol Chloroptic—Allergan Chlorofair—Pharmafair	D: 40–100 mg total instill into eye q4–6h C: 40–100 mg total instill into eye q4–6h	14	Ocular infections
Chloramphenicol (sodium succinate suspension) Chloromycetin sodium succinate—Parke-Davis	D: 40–100 mg total subconjunctivally q24h C: 40–100 mg total subconjunctivally q24h	14	Ocular infections
	D: 15–25 PO, IV q8h C: 22 PO, IV q12h	16	Anaerobic infections
Chloramphenicol/polymyxin B/hydrocortisone Ophthocort—Parke-Davis	D: Instill into eye q4–6h C: Instill into eye q4–6h	14	External hordeolums
Chloramphenicol and fluocinolone acetonide-DMSO Chloromycetin—Parke-Davis Synotic—Syntex	D: Apply to gingiva q12h C: Apply to gingiva q12h	16	Gingivitis

Drug / Manufacturer	Dose		Indication
Chlorhexidine Nolvasan Solution—Fort Dodge	D: 25 cc/L water; apply topically q12–24h C: 25 cc/L water; apply topically q12–24h	3	Dermatitis
Chlorpheniramine Chlor-Trimeton—Schering	D: 2–12 mg total PO q8–12h C: 2–4 mg total PO q12h	3	Atopy
Chlorpromazine Thorazine—SmithKline Beecham	D: 0.5 IM or IV q6–8h C: 0.5 IM or IV q6–8h	8	Vomiting
Chlortetracycline	D: 20 PO q8h C: 20 PO q8h	8	Intestinal bacterial overgrowth
Chlorothiazide Diuril—Merck Sharp & Dohme	D: 20–40 PO q12–24h C: 20–40 PO q12–24h	11	Diuresis
	D: 12–25 PO q12h C: 12–25 PO q12h	6	Congestive heart failure
Cimetidine Tagamet—SmithKline Beecham	D: 5–10 PO, IV, SC q6–12h C: 5–10 PO, IV, SC q6–12h	8, 9, 10, 17	Decrease gastric acid secretion
Ciprofloxacin Cipro—Miles	D: 5–22 PO q12h C: 5–22 PO q12h	12, 15	Bacterial osteomyelitis
Clindamycin Antirobe—Upjohn	D: 5–22 IV, IM, PO q8–12h C: 5.5–11.0 PO q12–24h	7, 11, 12, 15, 16	Anaerobic bacterial infections
	C: 25 IV, IM, PO divided q8h C: 25–50 PO q24h	12 16	Toxoplasmosis *Toxoplasma* oocyst shedding
Cleocin—Upjohn	D: 11–20 IV, IM, PO q8h	12	Diskospondylitis
	D: 20 IV q8h C: 20 IV q8h	10	Pancreatitis

(continued,

Generic Name and Brand Name—Manufacturer	Dosage (mg/kg)*	Chapter	Suggested Use
Clonazepam Klonopin—Roche	D: 0.02–0.50 PO q12h C: 0.02–0.50 PO q12h	13	Seizures
Clotrimazole Mycelex—Miles Lotrimin—Schering	D: Apply topically q12h C: Apply topically q12h	3	Dermatophytosis, pyoderma
Cloxacillin Cloxapen—Beecham	D: 10–22 IV, IM, PO q6–8h C: 22.0 q8h	3, 12, 15	Diskospondylitis, pyoderma
Colchicine Colchicine tablets—West-ward	D: 0.03 PO q24h	9	Fibrotic liver disease
Cyclophosphamide Cytoxan—Mead Johnson	D: See Chs. 3 & 5 for protocol C: See Chs. 3 & 5 for protocol C: 2–4 PO q24h	3, 5 12 16	Autoimmune hemolytic anemia, thrombocytopenia Canine rheumatoid arthritis Feline infectious peritonitis
Cyclosporine	D: 10–30 PO divided q12h C: 10–30 PO divided q12h	3	Autoimmune skin disease
2% in corn oil Sandimmune—Sandoz	D: 1 drop into eye q6–8h C: 1 drop into eye q6–8h D: See Chapter 14 for protocol	14 14	Pannus Keratoconjunctivitis sicca
Cyproheptadine Periactin—Merck Sharp & Dohme	D: 0.3–2.0 PO q12h C: 2–4 PO q24h	3 2	Atopy Anorexia
Cythioate Proban—Haver-Mobay	D: 3 PO twice weekly	3	Fleas

Drug	Dose		Indication
D,L-Methionine	D: 100 PO q12h C: 100 PO q12h	11	Urinary acidifying agent
D-penicillamine Cuprimine—Merck Sharp & Dohme	D: 14 PO q12h C: 14 PO q12h	11	Cystine urolith prevention
DMSO Domoso—Syntex	D: 10-15 PO q12h	9	Copper-toxicity hepatitis
	D: Dilute 1:4 in 0.9% saline, 1.1g/kg slow IV q12h C: Dilute 1:4 in 0.9% saline, 550 slow IV q12h	17	Shock
Dapsone Avlosulfon—Ayerst	D: 1 PO q8-12h C: 1 PO q8-12h	3	Pemphigus foliaceus
Dehydrocholic acid Decholin—Miles	D: 10-15 PO q8h C: 10-15 PO q8h	9	Cholangiohepatitis
Demecarium bromide Humorsol—Merck Sharp & Dohme	D: 1 drop into eye q12-24h C: 1 drop into eye q12-24h	14	Glaucoma
Desmopressin acetate DDAVP—USV DDAVP—Rorer	D: 5-20 µg IN or conjunctival sac q12-24h C: 5-20 µg IN or conjunctival sac q12-24h	4	Diabetes insipidus
	D: 1 µ/kg SC once	17	von Willebrand's disease
Desoxycorticosterone acetate Percorten acetate—Ciba	D: 0.5-5.0 mg total IM q24h C: 0.5-1.0 mg total IM q24h	4	Hypoadrenocorticism
Desoxycorticosterone pivilate Percorten pivilate—Ciba	D: 25-100 mg total IM every 3-4 weeks C: 12.5 mg total IM monthly	4	Hypoadrenocorticism

(continued)

Generic Name and Brand Name—Manufacturer	Dosage (mg/kg)*	Chapter	Suggested Use
Dexamethasone Azium—Schering	D: 0.5–1.0 IV once then prednisone PO C: 0.5–1.0 IV once then prednisone PO	5	Autoimmune hemolytic anemia
	D: 0.15 IV or IM q8h for 1 day C: 0.15 IV or IM q8h for 1 day	7	Laryngeal edema
	D: 0.03–0.10 PO q48h C: 0.5 PO q1week	3	Autoimmune skin disease
Maxidex—Alcon Decadron—Merck Sharp & Dohme Dexacidin—CooperVision	D: Instill 1–2 mg total into eye q4–6h C: Instill 1–2 mg total into eye q4–6h	14	External hordeolums
Dexamethasone sodium phosphate Azium SP—Schering	D: 2–4 IV once C: 2–4 IV once	17	Shock
	D: 0.1 IV C: 0.1 IV	17	Antipyretic, laryngeal edema, anti-inflammatory
	D: 0.2–0.5 IV or deep IM C: 0.2–0.5 IV or deep IM	17	Asthma
Dexamethasone/polymyxin B/neomycin Maxitrol—Alcon Dexasporin—Pharmafair	D: Instill into eye q4–6h C: Instill into eye q4–6h	14	Bacterial blepharitis

Drug	Dosage		Indication
Diazepam Valium—Roche	D: 0.1–0.50 IV C: 0.1–0.50 IV	6, 12, 17	Sedation
	D: 0.05–0.20 IV q12h or 1 mg total PO q12–24h C: 0.2 IV q12h	2, 9, 17	Anorexia
	D: 3–5 mg total IV C: 3–5 mg total IV	9, 13, 17	Seizures
	D: 0.2 PO q8h C: 2.5 mg total PO q8h	11	Urethral hyperreflexia, reflex dyssynergia
	D: 10 mg total PO q12h	12	Hereditary myopathy of Labrador retrievers
Diazoxide Proglycem—Schering	D: 10–60 PO divided q12h	4	Hypoglycemia (chronic) caused by insulinoma
Dichlorphenamide Daranide—Merck Sharp & Dohme	D: 2.2 PO q8–12h C: 2.2 PO q8–12h	14	Glaucoma
Dicloxacillin Dicloxacillin sodium capsules—Lederle	D: 5–25 PO q8h C: 5–25 PO q8h	3, 15, 17	Bacterial infections
Diethylcarbamazine Caracide—American Cyanamid	D: 2.5–3.0 PO q24h	6	Heartworm preventative
	D: 6.6 PO q24h C: 6.6 PO q24h	8	Ascariasis preventative
Diethylstilbestrol	D: 0.1 mg total PO q24h; taper to q1week C: 0.05–0.1 mg total PO q24h; taper to q1week	11	Urinary incontinence
	D: 0.2 mg C: 0.2 mg	11	Benign prostatic hyperplasia

(continued)

Generic Name and Brand Name—Manufacturer	Dosage (mg/kg) *	Chapter	Suggested Use
Digitoxin Crystodigin—Eli Lilly	D: 0.03 PO q8–12h	6	Congestive heart failure
Digoxin Cardoxin—Evsco Lanoxin—Burroughs Wellcome	D: 0.004–0.008 PO q12h C: 0.002–0.008 PO q24h	6	Congestive heart failure
Dihydrotachysterol Dihydrotachysterol—Philips Roxane	D: 0.3 PO q24h for 3–4 days then 0.01–0.02 PO q24h C: 0.3 PO q24h for 3–4 days then 0.01–0.02 PO q24h	4	Hypocalcemia with hypoparathyroidism, hyperthyroidism
Diltiazem Cardizem—Marion Laboratory	D: 1 PO q8h C: 7.5–15.0 mg total PO q8h	6	Arrhythmias
Dimenhydrinate Dramamine—Searle	D: 25–50 mg total PO q8h C: 12.5 mg total PO q8h	8	Vomiting
Dioctyl sodium sulfosuccinate (enema solution) Colace—Mead Johnson	D: 5–10 mg total in warm water; administer 5–10 ml/kg per rectum C: 5–10 mg total in warm water; administer 5–10 ml/kg per rectum	8	Constipation
Diphenhydramine Benadryl—Parke-Davis	D: 2–4 IM, SC, slow IV C: 2–4 IM, SC	3, 17	Atopy, larngyeal edema
	D: 2 IV C: 2 IV	5	Anaphylaxis
	D: 0.5–2.0 SC 30 min prior to blood or plasma transfusion	17	Prevent blood or plasma transfusion reaction

Drug — Manufacturer	Dose	Ref.	Indication
Diphenoxylate Lomotil—Searle	D: 0.1 PO q6-8h C: 0.25 mg total PO q12h	8	Diarrhea, acute colitis
Dipivefrin hydrochloride Propine—Allergan	D: 1 drop into eye q12h C: 1 drop into eye q12h	14	Glaucoma
Dipyrone Novin—Haver	D: 25 SC, IM, IV C: 25 SC, IM, IV	2	Pyrexia
Disophenol DNP—American Cyanamid	D: 10 SC; repeat in 2-3 weeks C: 10 SC; repeat in 2-3 weeks	8	Ancyclostomiasis
Dobutamine Dobutrex—Eli Lilly	D: 5-15 µg/kg/min IV C: 5-15 µg/kg/min IV	6, 17	Congestive heart failure
Dopamine Intropin—American Critical Care Dopastat—Parke-Davis Dopamine—Elkins-Sinn	D: 5-15 µg/kg/min IV C: 5-15 µg/kg/min IV D: 2-5 µg/kg/min IV C: 2-5 µg/kg/min IV	6 6, 17	Complete atrioventricular block Congestive heart failure
Doxycycline Vibramycin—Pfizer	D: 0.5 µg/kg/min IV infusion C: 0.5 µg/kg/min IV infusion	1	Hypokalemia
	D: 3-20 PO or IV q12h C: 3-20 PO or IV q12h	8, 15, 16	Bacterial and rickettsial infections
Echothiophate iodide Phospholine Iodide—Ayerst	D: 1 drop into eye q12-24h C: 1 drop into eye q12-24h	14	Glaucoma
Econazole cream Spectrazole—Ortho	D: Apply topically q12h C: Apply topically q12h	3	Dermatophytosis
Edrophonium Tensilon—ICN Pharmaceuticals	D: 0.1 IV C: 0.1 IV	6	Supraventricular tachycardia
Enalapril Vasotec—Merck Sharp & Dohme	D: 0.25-0.50 PO q12-24h	6	Congestive heart failure

(*continued*)

Generic Name and Brand Name—Manufacturer	Dosage (mg/kg)*	Chapter	Suggested Use
Enilconazole Imaverol—Pitman-Moore	D: 20 IN flush, divided q12h	16	Aspergillosis, penicilliosis
Enrofloxacin Baytril—Mobay Animal Health	D: 2.5–15 PO q12h C: 2.5–5.0 PO q12h	3, 11, 12, 15	Bacterial infections
Epinephrine Epinephrine injection—Astra Adrenalin Chloride—Parke-Davis	D: 0.5–1.0 ml 1:10,000 dilution IM, SC C: 0.5–1.0 ml 1:10,000 dilution IM	17	Asthma
	D: 0.01–0.02 (0.1–0.2 ml 1:10,000) IV q5min C: 0.01–0.02 (0.1–0.2 ml 1:10,000) IV q5min	17	Cardiovascular emergencies
Epifrin—Allergan Glaucon—Alcon	D: 1 drop into eye q8–12h C: 1 drop into eye q8–12h	14	Glaucoma
Ergonovine	D: 0.2 IM once C: 0.2 IM once	11	Metritis
Erythromycin Erythromycin Tablets—Abbott	D: 10–22 q8h C: 10–22 q8h	3, 8, 15, 16	Bacterial infections, *Mycoplasma* infections
Erythromycin—Pharmafair	D: Thin film into eye q4–6h C: Thin film into eye q4–6h	14	Bacterial blepharitis
Ethoxzolamide Cardrase—Upjohn	D: 5 PO q12h C: 5 PO q12h	14	Glaucoma
Fenbendazole Panacur—Hoechst-Roussel	D: 25–50 PO for 3–5 consecutive days C: 25–50 PO for 3–5 consecutive days	7, 8, 16	Endoparasites, lungworms

580

Fentanyl Sublimaze—Janssen	D: 10 mg/kg IV initially, then either 0.3–0.6 µg/kg/min IV infusion or 5–10 µg/kg IV q30min	17	Restraint for mechanical ventilation
Fentanyl (F) and diazepam (D) Sublimaze—Janssen Valium—Roche	D: F, 10 µg/kg IV initially, then either 0.3–0.6 µg/kg/min IV infusion or 5–10 µg/kg IV q30min; D, 0.2–0.5 IV, then 0.2 IV q1h alternating with F	17	Restraint for mechanical ventilation
Fentanyl (F) and midazolam (M) Sublimaze—Janssen Versed—Hoffman LaRoche	D: F, 10 µg/kg IV initially, then either 0.3–0.6 µg/kg/min IV infusion or 5–10 µg/kg/min IV q30min; M, 0.2 IV initially, then 0.1–0.3 q1h IV infusion	17	Restraint for mechanical ventilation
Fenthion ProSpot—Haver-Mobay Spotton (20% w/v)—Bayvet	D: 4–8 topically q2weeks D: 20 topically q3weeks	3	Fleas
Flucytosine Ancobin—Roche	D: 30–50 PO q6h C: 30–50 PO q6h	16	Cryptococcosis
Fludrocortisone acetate Florinef—Squibb	D: 0.5 mg/5 kg PO q24h C: 0.1 mg once PO q24h	4	Hypoadrenocorticism
Flunixin meglumine Banamine—Schering	D: 1.1 IV (give only twice)	8	Gastric dilatation, volvulus
Fluocinolone and DMSO Synotic—Syntex	D: Apply topically q12h C: Apply topically q12h	3	Acral lick granuloma
Flurometholone FML—Allergan	D: Instill into eye q4–6h C: Instill into eye q4–6h	14	Bacterial blepharitis

(continued)

Generic Name and Brand Name—Manufacturer	Dosage (mg/kg) *	Chapter	Suggested Use
Folate (folic acid)	D: 1 mg total PO q24h C: 1 mg total PO q24h	5	Anemia
	D: 50 mg total PO q24h C: 50 mg total PO q24h	16	Prevent folic acid deficiency when using pyrimethamine and sulfadiazine
Folinic acid	D: 1 PO q24h C: 1 PO q24h	15	Prevent folic acid deficiency when using pyrimethamine and sulfadiazine
Furosemide Lasix—Hoechst-Roussel Disal—Techamerica	D: 1–4 PO q12h C: 1 PO q12–24h	6	Congestive heart failure
	D: 2–4 IV, IM, SC q6–8h C: Not to exceed 2 IV or IM q6–8h	6, 17	Pulmonary edema
	D: 2.0–4.0 PO q8h	11	Calcium homeostasis disorders
	D: 2–8 IV C: 2–8 IV	11, 17	Loop diuresis
Furosemide and dopamine Lasix—Hoechst-Roussel (L) Inotropin—Anar-Stone (I)	D: L, 2–8 IV, I-1–5 µg/kg/min IV C: L, 2–8 IV, I-1–5 µg/kg/min IV	11	Loop diuresis and vasodilator
Gentamicin Gentocin—Schering	D: 2–4 IM, SC, IV q6–12h C: 2–4 IM, SC, IV q6–12h	6, 7, 8, 11, 15	Bacterial infections
	D: Instill into eye q4–6h C: Instill into eye q4–6h	14	External hordeolums

582

Drug	Indication	Ref	Dosage
Gentamicin (aqueous)	Ocular infections	14	D: 10–20 mg total subconjunctivally q24h C: 10–20 mg total subconjunctivally q24h
Gentamicin sulfate/betamethasone Gentocin Durafilm—Schering	Rhinitis	16	C: Instill into nares q12h
Gentamicin (G) and cephapirin (C) Gentocin—Schering Cefadyl—Bristol	Sepsis	9	D: G, 2.2 IV q6–8h, C, 20 IV q8h C: G, 2.2 IV q6–8h, C, 20 IV q8h
Glucagon Glucagon—Lilly	Hypoglycemia (acute)	4	D: 0.5–1.0 mg IV or IM once C: 0.5–1.0 mg IV or IM once
Glycerol/glycerine	Glaucoma	14	D: 1.4–1.6 g/kg PO q6–12h C: 1.4–1.6 g/kg PO q6–12h
Griseofulvin (microsize) Fulvicin-U/F—Schering	Dermatophytosis	3	D: 50 PO q24h or 25 PO q12h C: 50 PO q24h or 25 PO q12h
Griseofulvin (ultramicrosize) Gris-PEG—Herbert Laboratories	Dermatophytosis	3	D: 30 PO q24h C: 30 PO q24h
Haloprogin cream or solution Halotex—Westwood	Dermatophytosis	3	D: Apply topically q12h C: Apply topically q12h
Heparin Heparin sodium injection—Elkins-Sinn	DIC	5, 6, 10, 17	D: 50–200 units/kg SC q6–8h C: 30–200 units/kg SC q6h
	Anticoagulation	17	D: 220 U/kg SC then 66–200 U/kg SC q6–8h C: 220 U/kg SC then 66–200 U/kg SC q6–8h
	Pemphigus vulgaris	3	D: 100 IU/kg SC q12h

(continued)

Generic Name and Brand Name—Manufacturer	Dosage (mg/kg)*	Chapter	Suggested Use
Hetacillin Hetacin—K—Fort Dodge	D: 10–50 IM, IV, SC, PO q6–8h C: 10–20 PO q8–12h	15	Bacterial infections
Hydralazine Apresoline—Ciba Hydralazine—Lederle	D: 0.5–1.5 PO q8–12h C: 0.5–1.5 PO q8–12h	6, 17	Congestive heart failure, vasodilation
Hydrochlorothiazide Hydrodiuril—Merck Sharp & Dohme	D: 2–5 PO q12–24h C: 2–5 PO q12–24h	4, 11	Diuresis
Hydrocodone Hycodan—Dupont	D: 0.25–0.5 PO q8–12h C: 0.25–0.5 PO q8–12h	7, 17	Cough suppressant
Hydrocortisone Hydrocortisone acetate—Merck Sharp & Dohme Ophthocort—Parke-Davis	D: Instill into eye q4–6h C: Instill into eye q4–6h	14	Ocular inflammatory diseases
Cortef tablets—Upjohn	D: 0.1–0.5 PO q12h C: 0.1–0.5 PO q12h	4	Hypoadrenocorticism
	2.5 taper to 0.1–0.5 PO q12h	4	Adrenocortical tumors
Hydrocortisone/bacitracin/polymyxin/neomycin Vetropolycin-HC—Pitman-Moore	D: Instill into eye q4–6h C: Instill into eye q4–6h	14	Bacterial blepharitis
Hydroxyurea Hydrea—Squibb	D: 30 PO divided q24h; taper to 15 C: 30 PO divided q24h; taper to 15	5	Polycythemia
Hydroxyzine HCl Atarax—Roerig	D: 2 PO q8h	3	Atopy
Idoxuridine Stoxil—Smith Kline & French	C: Instill into eye q2h	14	Herpesvirus ulcerative keratitis

Drug	Dose		Indication
Imidocarb dipropionate	D: 5–7 IM	16	Canine ehrlichiosis
Imipramine	D: 5–15 mg total PO q12h	11	Urinary incontinence
Tofranil—Geigy	C: 2.5–5.0 mg total PO q12h		
Insulin	D: 0.5–1.0 units/kg SC	4	Diabetes mellitus
NHP	then adjust as needed		
Regular	D: See Chapter 4 for protocol	4	Diabetic ketoacidosis
	C: See Chapter 4 for protocol		
	D: 0.5 units/kg IV + 2–4 g	6	Sinoventricular conduction
	dextrose/unit insulin		due to severe hyperkalemia
	C: 0.5 units/kg IV + 2–4 g		
	dextrose/unit insulin		
PZI	C: 1–3.5 units/cat SC then adjust	4	Diabetes mellitus
Iron (ferrous sulfate & gluconate)	D: 100–200 μg/day PO	5	Anemia
Iron—American Pharmaceutical	C: 100–200 μg/day PO		
Iron dextran	D: 10–20 IM once	5	Anemia
Imferon—Merrell Dow	C: 10–20 IM once		
Irrigating solution (ophthalmic)	D: Flush eyes as needed	14	Ocular disease
Lactated Ringer's Inject. USP—Travenol	C: Flush eyes as needed		
Dacriose—IOLAB			
Sensitive Eyes—Bausch & Lomb			
Eye-Stream—Alcon			
Many others			
Isoflupredone/neomycin	D: Instill into eye q4–6h	14	Ocular disease
Neopredef—Upjohn	C: Instill into eye q4–6h		
Isoflurophate ophthalmic ointment	D: Apply periocularly as directed	14	Demodectic blepharitis
Floropryl—Merck Sharp & Dohme			

(continued)

585

Generic Name and Brand Name—Manufacturer	Dosage (mg/kg)*	Chapter	Suggested Use
Isopropamide Darbid—Smith Kline & French	D: 0.5–10 mg PO q8–12h	6	Bradycardia
Isotretinoin Accutane—Roche Dermatologics	D: 1 PO q24h	3	Granulomatous sebaceous adenitis
Itraconazole	D: 10 PO q24h	3	*Malassezia* skin infection
Ivermectin Heartgard—Merck Sharp & Dohme	D: 6 μg/kg PO monthly	6	Heartworm preventative
Kanamycin	D: 3.8 SC q8h; 5–15 IM, IV, SC q6–12h C: 3.8 SC q8h; 5–15 IM, IV, SC q6–12h	11, 15	Urinary tract infections
Ketamine hydrochloride (K) and diazepam (D) Ketaset—Bristol Valium—Roche	D: K, 4.4–11.0 IV, IM, D, 0.11–0.22 IV C: K, 0.5–1.0 IV; D, 0.05 IV	17	Sedation, anesthesia
Ketoconazole Nizoral—Janssen	D: 10 PO q24h C: 10 PO q24h	3	*Malassezia* infection
	D: 10–20 PO divided q24h C: 10–20 PO divided q24h	16	Mycotic infections
	D: See Ch. 4 for protocol	4	Adrenocortical tumors, hyperadrenocorticism

Drug	Dosage		Indications
L-thyroxine Synthroid—Flint Thyro-Tab—Vet-A-Mix Noroxine—Vortech Levoid—Nutrition Control Products Levothroid—Rorer Soloxine—Daniels	D: 0.02–0.40 PO q24h or divided q12h C: 0.1–0.2 mg PO q24h or divided q12h	4	Hypothyroidism
L-triiodothyronine Cytomel—Smith Kline & French Cytobin—Norden	D: 4–6 μg/kg PO q8h	4	Hypothyroidism
Lactulose Cephulac—Merrell Dow	D: 5 ml (3.3 g)/5–10 kg PO q6h C: 5 ml (3.3 g)/5–10 kg PO q6h	9	Chronic hepatic encephalopathy
Levamisole Levasole—Pitman-Moore	D: 8 PO	7	*Filaroides osleri* and *Capillaria aerophila* infection
Lidocaine Lidocaine—Elkins-Sinn	D: 1–4 IV bolus; see Table 6–9 C: 0.25–0.50 IV	6, 17	Ventricular tachyarrhythmias
Lime sulfur (2%) Lym Dyp—DVM	D: 25 ml/L water, apply topically q5days C: 25 ml/L water, apply topically q5days	3, 16	Dermatophytosis, demodicosis
Lincomycin	D: 15–25 PO q8h C: 15–25 PO q8h	3, 15	Pyoderma
Lincomycin (aqueous)	D: 50–150 mg total subconjunctivally q24h C: 50–150 mg total subconjunctivally q24h	14	Ocular infections
Loperamide Imodium—Ortho	D: 0.08 PO q8h	8	Diarrhea

(continued)

587

Generic Name and Brand Name—Manufacturer	Dosage (mg/kg)*	Chapter	Suggested Use
Mannitol	D: 0.25–1.00 g/kg IV C: 0.25–1.00 g/kg IV	13	Brain injury
	D: 1.0 IV over 30 minutes C: 1.0 IV over 30 minutes	11, 17	Osmotic diuresis
	D: 1.4–1.6 g/kg slow IV q6–12h C: 1.4–1.6 g/kg slow IV q6–12h	14	Glaucoma
Mebendazole Telmintic—Pitman Moore	D: 22 PO for 3–5 days	8	Intestinal parasitism
Medroxyprogesterone Depo-Provera—Upjohn	D: 10 IM, SC once, then q4–6 weeks as needed	3	Pruritus
Megestrol acetate Megace—Mead Johnson Ovaban—Schering	D: 2.5–5.0 mg/day total PO for 2 days then every 1–2 weeks	3	Pruritus
Meperidine Demerol—Winthrop	D: 2–6 IM, SC q4–6h C: 2–4 IM, SC q4–6h	17	Sedation
6-Mercaptopurine Purinethol—Burroughs Wellcome	D: 2.0 PO q24h	12	Canine rheumatoid arthritis
Metaisoproterenol Alupent—Boehringer Inhelheim	D: 2–3 PO q8h C: 2–3 PO q8h	6	Heart block
	D: 0.5 PO q6h	7	Chronic canine bronchitis
Methazolamide Neptazane—Lederle	D: 2.2 PO q8–12h C: 2.2 PO q8–12h	14	Glaucoma
Methenamine mandelate Mandelamine—Parke-Davis	D: 10 PO q6h C: 10 PO q6h	11	Urinary tract infections

Drug	Dosage		Indication
Methicillin (aqueous) Staphcillin injection—Bristol Myers	D: 20–100 mg total subconjunctivally q24h C: 20–100 mg total subconjunctivally q24h	14	Ocular infections
	D: 20–40 IM, IV q4–6h	15	Bacterial infections
Methimazole Tapazole—Lilly	C: 5 mg total PO q8–12h then adjust	4	Hyperthyroidism
Methylene blue (1% solution) Methylene Blue Injection—Elkins Sinn	D: 8.8 slow IV	17	Methemoglobinemia
Methylprednisolone Medrol—Upjohn	D: Start: 0.16–0.40 PO q12h Maint: 0.16–0.50 PO q48h	3	Allergic dermatitis
Methylprednisolone (soluble aqueous)	D: 10–20 mg total subconjunctivally C: 10–20 mg total subconjunctivally	14	Ocular inflammatory disease
Methylprednisolone acetate Depo-Medrol—Upjohn	C: 4 SC, IM	3	Allergic dermatitis
	C: 1.0–2.0 IM every 3–4 weeks	7	Feline allergic bronchitis
	C: 15–20 mg total IM every 3–4 weeks	8	Eosinophilic stomatitis
	C: 4 SC or 20 mg/cat SC	3	Eosinophilic granuloma
	C: 10 mg total IM monthly	4	Hypoadrenocorticism
Methylprednisolone sodium succinate Solu-Medrol—Upjohn	D: 30 IV then 5 mg/kg/hr for 24 hr C: 30 IV then 5 mg/kg/kg for 24 hr	13	Spinal cord injury

(continued)

Generic Name and Brand Name—Manufacturer	Dosage (mg/kg)*	Chapter	Suggested Use
Metoclopramide Reglan—Robins	D: 0.2–0.4 PO or SC q6–8h C: 0.2–0.4 PO or SC q6–8h	8, 9	Vomiting
Metronidazole Flagyl—Searle	D: 65 PO q24h or 20 PO q12h C: 65 PO q24h or 20 PO q12h	8	Giardiasis
Redi-Infusion—Elkins-Sinn Others	D: 7.5–50 PO q8–12h; 10 IV q8h C: 7.5–50 PO q8–12h; 10 IV q8h	7, 8, 9, 10, 15, 16	Bacterial rhinitis and sinusitis, septicemia, pancreatitis, suppurative cholangiohepatitis, stomatitis
Miconazole cream (solution) Conofite—Pitman-Moore Monostat—Ortho Micatin—Advanced Care	D: Apply topically q12–24h C: Apply topically q12–24h	3, 14	Dermatophytosis, mycotic blepharitis
Midazolam Versed—Roche	D: 0.2 IV, IM C: 0.2 IV, IM	17	Sedation
Milbemycin oxime Interceptor—Ciba-Geigy	D: 0.5 PO monthly	8	Ancylostomiasis and heartworm preventative
Mineral oil	D: 0.5–2.0 ml/kg PO then saline C: 0.5–2.0 ml/kg PO then saline	17	Cathartic
Mineral oil and petrolatum Laxatone—Evsco	C: 1–5 ml PO q24h	8	Hair balls
Minocycline	D: 5–15 PO q12h C: 5–15 PO q12h	15	Bacterial infections
Minocycline (M) and dihydrostreptomycin (D) Minocycline—Warner Chilcott Dihydrostreptomycin—Maurry	D: M, 12.5 PO q12h D: D, 5 IM, SC q12h for 7 days	15	Brucellosis

Drug—Manufacturer	Dose		Indication
Morphine Morphine—Astra	D: 1-2 IM, SC C: 0.1 IM, SC	17	Sedation
	D: 0.05-0.50 IV or IM once	6	Pulmonary edema
Nafcillin Unipen—Wyeth-Ayerst	D: 10 IV q6h C: 10 IV q6h	15	Bacterial infections
Naloxone hydrochloride Naloxone HCl—Quad	D: 0.01-0.20 IM, IV, SC C: 0.01-0.20 IM, IV, SC	17	Narcotic antagonist
Naltrexone Trexan—Dupont Pharmaceuticals	D: 2.2 PO q12-24h C: 2.2 PO q12-24h	3	Acral lick granuloma
Nandrolone decanoate Deca-Durabolin—Organon	D: 1-3 IM weekly C: 1-3 IM weekly	5	Anemia
Neomycin	D: 10-20 in water instill into colon C: 10-20 in water instill into colon	9	Hepatic encephalopathy
Neomycin/polymyxin B/dexamethasone Dexacidin—CooperVision	D: Instill into eye q4-6h C: Instill into eye q4-6h	14	External hordeolums
Neomycin/polymyxin/bacitracin Neosporin—Burroughs Wellcome	D: Instill into eye q6h C: Instill into eye 16h	14	Ocular ulcers
Neomycin/polymyxin B/bacitracin/hydrocortisone Cortisporin—Burroughs Wellcome	D: Instill into eye q4-6h C: Instill into eye q4-6h	14	External hordeolums, chalazion
Nitrofurantoin Macrodantin—Norwich-Eaton	D: 4.4-6 PO q8h C: 6 PO q8h	11	Urinary tract infections
Nitroglycerine ointment 2% Mitrol—Adria	D: 0.5-1.0 in. ribbon topically q8h C: 0.125-0.250 in. ribbon topically q8h	6	Pulmonary edema due to congestive heart failure

Generic Name and Brand Name—Manufacturer	Dosage (mg/kg)*	Chapter	Suggested Use
Norfloxacin Noroxin—Merck Sharp & Dohme	D: 5–20 PO q12h C: 5–20 PO q12h	11, 15	Urinary tract infections, bacterial prostatitis
o,p'-DDD Lysodren—Bristol	D: 25 PO q12h then 25 PO twice weekly C: 25–50 PO q24h	4	Pituitary-dependent hyperadrenocorticism
	D: 50–75 PO q24h taper to 100–200 PO weekly	4	Nonresectable adrenocortical tumor
Oxacillin Bactocil—Smith Kline Beecham	D: 7–22 IV, IM, SC, PO q6–8h C: 7–22 IV, IM, SC, PO q6–8h	3, 12, 15	Bacterial infections
Oxacillin (O) and gentamicin (G) Bactocil—Smith Kline Beecham Gentocin—Schering	D: O, 22 IV q8h; G, 2.2 IV q8h C: O, 22 IV q8h; G, 2.2 IV q8h	12	Osteomyelitis
Oxazepam Serax—Wyeth	D: 0.2–0.5 PO q12–24h C: 2.5 mg/cat PO C: 1.25–2.5 mg total PO 1–3 times daily	2, 9, 16	Anorexia Incontinence due to detrusor hyperreflexia
Oxybutynin Ditropan–MarionD: 0.2 PO q12h	D: 0.2 PO q12h	11	
OxyDex—DVM	D: Shampoo as directed C: Shampoo as directed	3	Dermatitis
Oxymethazoline (0.25%) Afrin Pediatric Nose Drops—Schering	D: Instill IN q24h C: Instill IN q24h	7	Bacterial rhinitis and sinusitis
Oxymorphone Numorphan—Dupont	D: 0.06–0.14 IV, IM, SC D: 0.2 IV initially then 0.05–0.10 q1–2h	17 17	Sedation Restraint for mechanical ventilation

Drug—Manufacturer	Dosage		Indication
Oxymorphone (O) and diazepam (D) Numorphan–Dupont Valium–Roche	D: 0, 0.2 IV initially then 0.05–0.10 q1–2h; D, 0.2–0.5 IV initially then 0.2 IV q1–2h	17	Restraint for mechanical ventilation
Oxytetracycline Terramycin—Pfizer	D: 10–20 PO q12h C: 10–20 PO q12h	5, 10, 15	Hemobartonellosis, intestinal bacterial overgrowth
Oxytocin	D: 0.25–0.50 U/kg IM C: 0.25–0.50 U/kg IM	11	Metritis
Oxymetholone Anadrol-5—Syntex	D: 2.5–5.0 PO q24h C: 2.5–5.0 PO q24h	5	Anemia
Pancreatic digestive enzymes Viokase-V—Robins Pancrezyme—Daniel's	D: 2.0 tsp/20 kg PO with food C: 2.0 tsp/20 kg PO with food	10	Exocrine pancreatic insufficiency
Penicillin	D: 80,000–100,000 U/kg/day C: 80,000–100,000 U/kg/day	3	Actinomycosis
Penicillin G	D: 22,000–88,000 U/kg PO q8–12h C: 22,000–88,000 U/kg PO q8–12h	11, 15	Urinary tract infections
Penicillin G (aqueous)	D: 300,000–1,000,000 U subconjunctivally q24h C: 300,000–1,000,000 U subconjunctivally q24h	14	Ocular infections
Penicillin V Veetids—Squibb	D: 8–50 PO q8h C: 8–50 PO q8h	11, 16	Urinary tract infections, actinomycosis, nocardiosis
Pentazocine Talwin-V—Winthrop	D: 0.5–1.0 IM q6h C: 0.5–1.0 IM q6h	10, 17	Analgesic

(continued)

Generic Name and Brand Name—Manufacturer	Dosage (mg/kg)*	Chapter	Suggested Use
Pentobarbital Pentobarbital Sodium Injection—Elkins-Sinn Nembutal Sodium—Abbott	D: 1-6 IV C: 1-6 IV D: 1-5 IV initially then 1-4 q1h IV infusion	9, 17 17	Control seizures, anesthesia Restraint for mechanical ventilation
Phenobarbital	D: 1.5–5.0 PO q12h C: 1.5–5.0 PO q12h	13	Control seizures
Phenobarbital Sodium Injection—Elkins-Sinn	D: 2–6 IV, IM C: 2–6 IV, IM	17	Sedation
Phenoxybenzamine Dibenzyline—SmithKline	D: 0.25 PO q12h C: 0.25 PO q12h	11	Urethral spasms
Phenylephrine (10%) AK-Dilate—Akorn	D: Instill into eye q4–6h C: Instill into eye q4–6h	14	Mydriatic
Phenylephrine HCl (0.25%) Neo-Synephrine—Winthrop	D: Instill IN q4–6h C: Instill IN q4–6h	7	Bacterial rhinitis and sinusitis
Phenylpropanolamine Ornade—SmithKline	D: 1.5 PO q12h C: 1.5 PO q12h	11	Urinary incontinence
Phosmet Paramite—Vet-Kem	D: Apply topically C: Apply topically	3	Ectoparasites
Phosphate binders Alternagel—Stuart Amphojel—Wyeth Basaljel—Wyeth	D: 10 PO q8h with food C: 10 PO q8h with food	11	Renal failure

594

Drug / Manufacturer	Dosage		Indication
Phytonadione Vet-A-K1—Professional Veterinary Labs Mephyton—Merck Sharp & Dohme AquaMephyton—Merck Sharp & Dohme Konakion—Roche	D: 2.5 SC once then 0.3–0.8 PO q8h C: 2.5 SC once then 0.3–0.8 PO q8h	5	Vitamin K deficiency
	D: 0.8–1.5 q12h C: 0.8–1.5 q12h	5	Indadione poisoning
Pilocarpine Pilocar—CooperVision	D: 1–2 drops into eye q8–12h C: 1–2 drops into eye q8–12h	14	Tear secretion
Pilocarpine/epinephrine E-Pilo-1—CooperVision	D: 1 drop into eye q8–12h C: 1 drop into eye q8–12h	14	Glaucoma
Piperacillin Pipracil—Lederle	D: 50–70 IM, IV q4–6h C: 50–70 IM, IV q4–6h	15	Bacterial infections
Pitressin tannate Pitressin Tannate—Parke-Davis	D: 2.5–5.0 units IM q36–48h C: 2.5 units IM q36–48h	4	Diabetes insipidus
Polyhydroxydine Xenodyne—Solvay	D: Apply topically as directed C: Apply topically as directed	3	Mycotic otitis
Potassium bromide	D: 20–60 PO q12h	13	Seizures
Potassium citrate Urocit-K—Mission Pharmacal	D: 35 PO 3 times daily C: 35 PO 3 times daily	11	Urinary alkalinizing agent
Potassium iodide SSKI—Upsher–Smith	C: 50–100 PO	4	Hyperthyroidism
	D: 20–40 PO q8h C: 20 PO q12h	16	Sporotrichosis

(continued)

Generic Name and Brand Name—Manufacturer	Dosage (mg/kg) *	Chapter	Suggested Use
Povidone-iodine ointment or solution Betadine—Perdue Frederick	D: Dilute 42 ml/L water, apply topically q12h C: Dilute 42 ml/L water, apply topically q12h	3	Dermatophytosis
	D: Dilute 1:300 with water; apply periocularly q12–24h C: Dilute 1:300 with water; apply periocularly q12–24h	14	Mycotic blepharitis
Praziquantel Droncit—Haver	D: 5 PO or IM C: 11–33 mg total; depends on weight	8	Tapeworm infection
Prazosin Minipress—Pfizer	D: 1 mg/15 kg PO q12h C: 0.25–1.00 mg total q12h	11	Hypertension
Prednisolone Prednisolone tablets—Roxane	D: 1.1–3.3 PO q12–24h C: 1.1–3.3 PO q12–24h	5	Thrombocytopenia, lupus erythematosus, anemia
		3	Granulomatous sebaceous adenitis, eosinophilic granuloma, autoimmune skin disease
		6	Thromboembolic lung disease
	D: Start: 1–2 PO q24h Maint: 0.5 PO q48h C: Start: 1–2 PO q24h Maint: 0.5 PO q48h	9	Chronic active hepatitis (dog) Lymphocytic cholangiohepatitis (cat)

Drug	No.	Dose	Indication
Prednisolone (continued)	11	D: 2.2–4.4 PO q24h	Calcium homeostasis disorders
	12	D: 0.02–0.10 PO q12h C: 0.02–0.10 PO q12h	Inflammatory polymyositis, masticatory muscle myositis, familial canine dermatomyositis; canine dermatomyositis, degenerative joint disease, hypertrophic osteodystrophy, arthritis
	3, 16	D: 0.25 PO q24h C: 0.25 PO q24h	Inflammation, anemia
	4	D: Start: 0.2–0.5 PO q12h Maint: 0.2–0.6 PO q48h C: Start: 1–2 PO q12h Maint: 1–2 PO q48h	Hypoadrenocorticism
	2		Anorexia
	3		Allergic dermatitis
Prednisolone acetate Pred Forte—Allergan Econopred—Alcon	14	D: Instill into eye q4–6h C: Instill into eye q4–6h	Ocular inflammatory diseases
Prednisolone sodium succinate Solu-Delta-Cortef—Upjohn	7, 8, 17	D: 0.5–1.0 IV q6–24h or IM q6h for 1 day C: 0.5–1.0 IV q6–24h or IM q6h for 1 day	Laryngeal edema, anti-inflammatory, antipyretic
	7	C: 10 IV	Allergic bronchitis

(continued)

Generic Name and Brand Name—Manufacturer	Dosage (mg/kg)*	Chapter	Suggested Use
Prednisolone sodium succinate (continued)	D: 10–20 IV; repeat in 6 hr C: 10–20 IV; repeat in 6 hr	10	Shock
	D: 1–2 IV then 0.1–0.5 IV q4–6h	4	Hypoadrenocorticism
	D: 22–44 IV C: 22–44 IV	17	Electrical mechanical dissociation, shock
	D: 1–2 IV C: 1–2 IV	17	Asthma
Prednisone Prednisone Tablets—Roxane Deltasone—Upjohn	D: 1.1–3.3 PO q12–24h C: 1.1–3.3 PO q12–24h	5	Thrombocytopenia, lupus erythematosus, anemia
		3	Granulomatous sebaceous adenitis, eosinophilic granuloma
		6	Thromboembolic lung disease
		11	Calcium homeostasis disorders
		12	Inflammatory polymyositis, masticatory muscle myositis, familial canine dermatomyositis, degenerative joint disease, hypertrophic osteodystrophy, arthritis
	D: 2.2–4.4 PO q24h C: 2.2–4.4 PO q24h	16	Inflammation, anemia

Drug	Dose		Indication
Prednisone (Continued)	D: 0.02–0.10 PO q12h	4	Hypoadrenocorticism
	C: 0.02–0.10 PO q12h		
	D: Start: 0.2–0.5 PO q12h	3	Allergic dermatitis
	Maint: 0.2–0.6 PO q48h		
	C: Start: 1–2 PO q12h		
	Maint: 1–2 PO q48h		
Primidone	D: 10–15 PO q8h	13	Seizures
Procainamide	D: 10–12 PO q6h; see also Table	6	Tachyarrhythmias
Pronestyl-ER—Squibb & Sons	6-9		
Procan-SR—Parke-Davis	D: 15–17 PO q8h		
Prochlorperazine	D: 0.5 IM or IV q6–8h	8	Vomiting
Compazine—SmithKline Beecham	C: 0.5 IM or IV q6–8h		
Propantheline	D: 3.75–15.00 mg total PO q8h;	6	Bradycardia
Pro-Banthine—Searle	0.5–1.0 PO q8h		
	D: 0.25 PO q8h	8	Diarrhea, acute colitis
	C: 0.25 PO q8h		
	D: 7.5–15.0 PO q8h	11	Urinary incontinence
	C: 5.0–7.5 PO q4–3h		
Proparacaine hydrochloride (0.5%)	D: Instill into eye as directed	14	Ocular anesthesia
Ophthetic—Allergan	C: Instill into eye as directed		
Propionibacterium acnes bacterin	D: See Chapter 3 for protocol	3	Pyoderma
Immunoregulin—Rhone Merieux			
Propranolol	D: 1 PO q8h or 20–40 mg total	6	Tachycardia
Inderal—Ayerst Laboratories	PO q8h		
	D: 10 mg total PO q8–12h for		
	large dogs		
	D: 2.5–5.0 mg total PO q6h for		
	small dogs		

(continued)

Generic Name and Brand Name—Manufacturer	Dosage (mg/kg)*	Chapter	*Suggested Use
Propranolol (Continued)	C: 2.5–5.0 mg PO q8–12h	4	Hyperthyroidism
	D: 0.2–1.0 mg PO q8–12h	11	Systemic hypertension
	C: 2.5–10.0 mg total PO q8–12h		
Propylthiouracil	C: 50 mg PO q8–12h then adjust	4	Hyperthyroidism
Prostaglandin F$_{2\alpha}$ Lutalyse—Upjohn	D: 25–50 µg/kg IM, SC q12h C: 25–50 µg/kg IM, SC q12h	16	Pyometra
	D: 0.25 SC repeat in 24 hours if needed	11	Metritis
	C: 0.10 SC repeat in 24 hours if needed		
Protamine sulfate Protamine Sulfate—Lilly	D: 1 mg/100 units heparin slow IV; maximum 50 mg/10 min C: 1 mg/100 units heparin slow IV; maximum 50 mg/10 min	17	Heparin overdose
Psyllium Metamucil—Searle	D: 1–5 tsp PO q24h C: 1–5 tsp PO q24h	8	Lymphocytic-plasmacytic colitis
Pyrantel pamoate Nemex, Strongid T—Pfizer	D: 15 PO; repeat in 21 days C: 15 PO; repeat in 21 days	8, 17	Ascarids, hookworms
Pyrethrins Oti-Care-M—ARC Laboratories Cerumite—Evasco	D: Instill into ear as directed C: Instill into ear as directed	3	Ear mites
Pyrimethamine	C: 2.0 PO q24h	16	Toxoplasma oocyst shedding

Drug	Dosage		Indication
Pyrimethamine (P) and sulfadiazine (S) Daraprim—Burroughs Wellcome Sulfadiazine—Lilly	D: P, 0.5–1.0 PO; S, 60–120 PO divided q8–12h C: P, 0.5–1.0 PO; S, 60–120 PO divided q8–12h	16	Toxoplasmosis
Quinacrine hydrochloride Atabrine—Winthrop	D: 9 PO q24h	8	Giardiasis
Quinidine Quinaglute—Berlex	D: Init: 8 PO q8h; increase by 50% until improvement	6	Supraventricular tachyarrhythmias Ventricular tachyarrhythmias
	D: 8–18 PO q8h	6	
Ranitidine Zantac—Glaxo	D: 2 PO or IV q8–12h C: 2 PO or IV q8–12h	8	Gastric ulcers, reflux esophagitis
Rifampin Rifadin—Marion Merrill Dow	D: 10–20 PO q12h	15	Bacterial infection
Rotenone Canex—Pitman-Moore	D: Dilute 1:3 in mineral oil, instill into ear q24h C: Dilute 1:3 in mineral oil, instill into ear q24h	3	Ear mites
Rotenone (1%) Goodwinol ointment—Goodwinol Products	D: Apply topically as directed C: Apply topically as directed	3	Demodicosis
Sebbafon—Winthrop Laboratories	D: Shampoo as directed	3	Dermatitis
Selenium disulfide shampoo (1%) Seleen—VetKem	D: Shampoo 1–2 times/week	3	*Malassezia* skin infection
Sodium bicarbonate	D: 1 mEq/kg IV over 15–30 minutes C: 1 mEq/kg IV over 15–30 minutes	6	Reduce serum potassium, correct severe metabolic acidosis

(continued)

Generic Name and Brand Name—Manufacturer	Dosage (mg/kg)*	Chapter	Suggested Use
Sodium bicarbonate (*Continued*)	D: 10–50 PO q8–12h C: 10–50 PO q8–12h	11, 17	Urinary alkalinizing agent
Sodium chloride	D: 50–100 PO q24h C: 50–100 PO q24h	11	Urolith control
Sodium EDTA Disodium versenate injection—Riker	D: 25–75 mg/kg/hr IV C: 25–75 mg/kg/hr IV	4	Hypercalcemia
Sodium hypochlorite (bleach)	D: Dilute 100 ml/L water, apply topically q12h C: Dilute 100 ml/L water, apply topically q12h	3	Dermatophytosis
Sodium levothyroxine Synthroid Injection—Boots-Flint	D: 100–200 µg IV	4	Myxedema coma
Sodium sulfate GoLytley—Braintree	D: 1 g/kg PO q12–24h C: 1 g/kg PO q12–24h	17	Cathartic
Spironolactone Aldactone—Searle	D: 1.0 PO q12h C: 1.0 PO q12h	9	Diuresis
Stanozolol Winstrol—Winthrop-Breon	D: 1–4 mg total PO q12h; 25–50 mg total IM once weekly C: 0.5–2 mg total PO q12h; 25–50 mg total IM once weekly	2, 16	Anorexia
Staphylococcal bacterin Staphage Lysate—Delmont	D: See protocol, Ch. 3 C: See protocol, Ch. 3	3	Recurrent pyoderma
	D: 0.2 ml SC 1–2 times weekly C: 0.2 ml SC 1–2 times weekly	14	Bacterial blepharitis

Drug	Dose		Indication
Streptomycin Streptomycin sulfate–Roerig	D: 11 IM, SC q6–12h C: 11 IM, SC q6–12h	15	Bacterial infections
Sucralfate Carafate—Marion	D: >20 kg, 1 g PO q8h; <20 kg, 0.5 g PO q8h C: 0.25–0.50 g PO q8–12h	6, 8, 9, 17	Gastric ulcers
	D: 1g/30kg PO q6h	8	Reflux esophagitis
Sulfacetamide sodium Blephamide—Allergan	D: Instill into eye as directed C: Instill into eye as directed	14	Bacterial blepharitis
Sulfadiazine Sulfadiazine—Lilly	D: 220 PO once then 110 q12h C: 220 PO once then 110 q12h	3, 15	Nocardiosis
Sulfadimethoxine Bactrovet—Pitman-Moore	D: 80 PO q8h C: 80 PO q8h	16	Nocardiosis and actinomycosis
	D: 25 q24h C: 25 q24h	3	Nocardiosis
	D: 50 PO once then 25 PO q24h C: 50 PO once then 25 PO q24h	8	Coccidiosis
Sulfasalazine Azulfidine—Pharmacia	D: 25–50 PO q8h C: 15 PO q8h	8	Lymphocytic-plasmacytic colitis
Sulfisoxazole	D: 22 PO q8h C: 22 PO q8h	11	Urinary tract infections
Sulfonamides	C: 100 PO q24h	16	*Toxoplasma* oocyst shedding
Syrup of ipecac Ipecac Syrup—Roxane	D: 1–2 PO C: 1–2 PO	17	Emetic

(continued)

603

Generic Name and Brand Name—Manufacturer	Dosage (mg/kg) *	Chapter	Suggested Use
Taurine	C: 250–500 mg total PO q12h	6	Congestive cardiomyopathy
Tear substitute (insert) Lacrisert—Merck Sharp & Dohme	D: Insert into conjunctival sac q8–24h C: Insert into conjunctival sac q8–24h	14	Keratoconjunctivitis sicca
Tear substitute (liquid) Adapt—Burton Parsons Adsorbotear—Alcon	D: Instill into eye q1–12h C: Instill into eye q1–12h	14	Keratoconjunctivitis sicca
Tear substitutes (ointment) Duolube—Muro Duratears—Alcon AKWA Tears—Akorn Lacri-Lube—Allergan	D: Instill into eye q1–12h C: Instill into eye q1–12h	14	Keratoconjunctivitis sicca
Terbutaline Brethine—Geigy	D: 0.1 PO q8–12h C: 0.1 PO q8h, 0.625 mg total PO q8–12h	7, 17	Bronchodilation, chronic canine bronchitis
	D: 2–3 PO q8h C: 2–3 PO q8h	6	Heart block
Terfenadine Seldane—Merrell Dow	D: 4–10 PO q12h	3	Atopy
Testosterone cypionate Depo-Testosterone—Upjohn	D: 2.2 IM in males C: 2.2 IM in males	11	Urinary incontinence
Testosterone propionate Androlane 50—Keene	D: 2.2 IM in males C: 2.2 IM in males	11	Urinary incontinence

Drug — Manufacturer	Dose	Ref.	Indication
Tetracycline Panmycin—Upjohn	D: 22 q8h C: 22 q8h	3	Subcutaneous infections
	D: 18–22 PO q8h C: 18–22 PO q8h	7, 11, 16	Bacterial rhinitis and sinusitis, urinary tract infections, rickettsial infections, Lyme disease, hemobartonellosis, *Mycoplasma* and *Ureaplasma* infections
	D: 25 PO q6–8h; 4.4–11.0 IV q8–12h C: 25 PO q6–8h; 4.4–11.0 IV q8–12h	15	Soft tissue infections
Tetracycline (T) and dihydrostreptomycin (D)	D: Instill 35 into pleural space, dilute in 75 ml water	17	Pleurodesis
	D: T, 22 PO q8h; D, 5 IM q12h	13	*Brucella canis* in CNS
Tetracycline (ophthalmic) Achromycin—Lederle	C: Instill into eye q4–6h	14	Complicated viral conjunctivitis
2,2,2 Tetramine Syprine—Merck Sharp & Dohme	D: 10–15 PO q12h	9	Copper toxicity hepatitis
Theophylline Theo-Dur—Key	D: 20 PO q12h	7	Chronic bronchitis
Slo-Bid Gyrocaps—Rorer	D: 10–15 PO q12h	6	Thromboembolic lung disease
	D: 20 PO q12–24h C: 10–20 PO q12–24h	7	Bronchodilation

(continued)

Generic Name and Brand Name—Manufacturer	Dosage (mg/kg)*	Chapter	Suggested Use
Theophylline ethylenediamine Aminophylline—Elkins-Sinn	D: 8–10 PO, IM or slow IV q8h C: 6.6 PO q12h; 4 IM or slow IV q8–12h	17	Bronchodilation
Thiabendazole Equizole—MSD Agvet	D: 20 PO q12–24h	16	Aspergillosis, penicillosis
Tresaderm—MSD Agvet	D: Apply topically q12h C: Apply topically q12h	3	Dermatophytosis
	D: Instill into ear as directed C: Instill into ear as directed	3	Ear mites, chiggers
Thiacetarsamide sodium Caparsolate—Abbott	D: 2.2 IV q12h for 2 days C: 2.2 IV q12h for 2 days; see Ch. 6	6	Heartworm adulticide
Ticarcillin	D: 40 PO q6h C: 40 PO q6h	11	Urinary tract infections
	D: 25–33 IV, SC q6–8h C: 25–33 IV, SC q6–8h	15	Bacterial infections
Timolol maleate Timoptic—Merck Sharp & Dohme	D: Instill 1 drop into eye q12h C: Instill 1 drop into eye q12h	14	Glaucoma
Tobramycin Tobrex—Alcon	D: Instill into eye q1–2h C: Instill into eye q1–2h	14	Ocular ulcers
Tobramycin (aqueous)	D: 10–20 mg subconjunctivally q24h C: 10–20 mg subconjunctivally q24h	14	Ocular infections
	D: 1.1 SC q8h C: 1.1 SC q8h	11, 15	Urinary tract infections

Tocainide Tonocard—Merck Sharp & Dohme	D: 20 PO q8h; 10 IV bolus	6	Ventricular tachyarrhythmias
Triamcinolone Vetalog—Solvay	D: Apply topically q6–12h C: Apply topically q6–12h	3	Acral lick granuloma
	D: 10–20 mg total subcorjunctivally C: 10–20 mg total subcorjunctivally	14	Ocular inflammatory diseases
Triamterene Dyrenium—Smith Kline Beecham	D: 1–2 PO q12–24h C: 1–2 PO q12–24h	6	Congestive heart failure
Trifluridine Viroptic—Burroughs Wellcome	C: Instill 1 drop into eye q2h	14	Herpesvirus ulcerative keratitis
Trimeprazine Temaril—Herbert	C: 1–2 PO q8h	3	Atopy
Trimethoprim sulfa Septra—Burroughs Wellcome Tribrissen 24%—Coopers Ditrim—Syntex	D: 13.2–22 IV, IM, SC, PO q12h C: 13.2–22 IV, IM, SC, PO q12h	3, 7, 8, 9, 10, 11, 15, 16	Sepsis with pancreatitis, pancreatitis, bacterial rhinitis and sinusitis, pyoderma, suppurative cholangiohepatitis, urinary tract infections, renal insufficiency, nocardiosis and actinomycosis, acute colitis, toxoplasmosis, soft tissue infections

(continued)

Generic Name and Brand Name—Manufacturer	Dosage (mg/kg)*	Chapter	Suggested Use
Trimethoprim sulfa (Continued)	D: 15–20 PO q12h; carrier state: 25–30 PO q12h C: 15–20 PO q12h; carrier state: 25–30 PO q12h	8	Enteric bacterial infections
Tropicamide (1%) Mydriacyl—Alcon	C: Instill into eye q6–24h	14	Ocular pain
Tylosin Tylan—Elanco	D: 1–2 tsp; mix with food C: 0.25 tsp q12h; mix with food	8	Lymphocytic-plasmacytic colitis
	D: 7–10 PO q8h; 6.6–11 IM q12–24h C: 7–10 PO q8h; 6.6–11 IM q12–24h	10, 15	Intestinal bacterial overgrowth
Valproic acid Depakene—Abbott	D: 60 PO q8h C: 60 PO q8h	13	Seizures
Vancomycin Vancocin—Lilly	D: 5–12 PO q8h C: 5–12 PO q8h	8	Pseudomembranous colitis
Vidarabine VIRA-A—Parke-Davis	C: Instill into eye q3h	14	Herpesvirus ulcerative keratitis
Vincristine Oncovin—Eli Lilly	D: 0.4 IV once	6	Thrombocytopenia associated with heartworm disease
	D: 0.02 IV once weekly C: 0.02 IV once weekly	5	Thrombocytopenia
Vitamin B12 Cyanocobalamin—Elkins-Sinn Others	D: 500–1000 μg weekly C: 500–1000 μg weekly	5	Anemia

Drug	Dose	Ref	Indication
Vitamin D Calciferol—Kremers-Urban Drisdol—Winthrop Deltalin—Lilly	D: 4000–6000 U/kg PO q24h, taper to 1000 U/kg/week C: 4000–6000 U/kg PO q24h, taper to 1000 U/kg/week	4	Hypocalcemia
Vitamin E Vitamin E capsule-Lederle	D: 400–500 IU PO q24h C: 400–500 IU PO q24h	10	Exocrine pancreatic insufficiency
Vitamin K_1 Aquamephyton—Merck Sharp & Dohme Mephyton—Merck Sharp & Dohme	D: 1–2 SC q12h C: 1–2 SC q12h	5, 9	Coagulopathy associated with suppurative cholangiohepatitis, vitamin K malabsorption
	D: 1.0–5.0 SC then 1.0–5.0 PO q8–12h C: 1.0–5.0 SC then 1.0–5.0 PO q8–12h	17	Coumarin toxicity, hepatic failure
Xylazine Rompun—Haver	D: 0.66 IM once	17	Emetic
Yohimbine Yobine—Lloyd	D: 0.1–0.4 IV C: 0.1–0.4 IV	17	Xylazine antagonist
Zinc sulfate, acetate, or gluconate	D: 5–10 PO q12h	9	Copper-toxicity hepatitis

INDEX

Page numbers followed by t or f indicate tables or figures respectively.

ISBN 0-397-50994-4